Clinical Obstetrics and Gynaecology

Fifth Edition

Clinical Obstetrics and Gynaecology

Elizabeth A. Layden, MBChB, DLM, MRCOG
Clinical Research Fellow in Medical Education
University of Edinburgh, Great Britain
Specialty Registrar in Obstetrics and Gynaecology
Simpson Centre for Reproductive Health
Royal Infirmary of Edinburgh
Edinburgh, Great Britain

Andrew Thomson, BSc, MBChB, MRCOG, MD
Consultant Obstetrician and Gynaecologist
Obstetrics & Gynaecology
Royal Alexandra Hospital
Paisley, Great Britain

Philip Owen, MBBCh, MD, FRCOG
Consultant Obstetrician and Gynaecologist
Princess Royal Maternity Hospital and Stobhill Hospital
Glasgow, Great Britain

Mayank Madhra, MBChB, MRCOG
Consultant Obstetrician and Gynaecologist
Simpson Centre for Reproductive Health
Royal Infirmary of Edinburgh
Edinburgh, Great Britain

Brian A. Magowan, FRCOG
Consultant Obstetrician and Gynaecologist
Borders General Hospital
Melrose, Scottish Borders, Great Britain

ELSEVIER

Notices

Practitioners and researchers must always rely on their own experience and knowledge in evaluating and using any information, methods, compounds or experiments described herein. Because of rapid advances in the medical sciences, in particular, independent verification of diagnoses and drug dosages should be made. To the fullest extent of the law, no responsibility is assumed by Elsevier, authors, editors or contributors for any injury and/or damage to persons or property as a matter of products liability, negligence or otherwise, or from any use or operation of any methods, products, instructions, or ideas contained in the material herein.

ISBN: 978-0-7020-8513-0

Content Strategist: Trinity Hutton
Content Project Manager: Shubham Dixit
Design: Patrick C. Ferguson
Illustration Coordinator: Narayanan Ramakrishnan
Marketing Manager: Deborah Watkins

Printed in Scotland.

Last digit is the print number: 9 8 7 6 5 4 3 2 1

This book is dedicated to the millions of women worldwide who will suffer disability, lose their babies, or lose their lives through the want of adequate reproductive healthcare.

Preface

Obstetrics and gynaecology is an evolving specialty, which is reflected in our fifth edition. We have fully updated and streamlined the textbook to reflect clinical advances such as non-invasive prenatal screening, added new chapters discussing some of the ethical and medicolegal challenges specific to obstetrics and gynaecology, and extended the section on practical guidance to make the most of your clinical time spent in this specialty. A new chapter of OSCE cases has also been added to allow you to practice this style of assessment, as well as 'single best answer' questions with which to test your learning.

The global COVID-19 pandemic has impacted all healthcare systems, and has had enormous direct and indirect effects on women's health. This fifth edition covers the impact of COVID-19 upon maternal, fetal and global healthcare, and includes updates on other epidemic diseases such as Zika virus.

There are many challenges that remain constant in obstetrics and gynaecology – a specialty which encompasses hugely varied topics, from assisted reproductive technology to gynaecological cancer care, fetal medicine to advanced laparoscopic gynaecological surgery and contraception to obstetric haemorrhage – with the associated complex clinical and ethical issues with which you will become familiar.

Although there have been many global advances, sadly, hundreds of thousands of women and babies are still dying each year from treatable complications of pregnancy, nearly all in low-resource settings. There are many remaining obstacles to improving their care. These are still ours – and, hopefully, now also yours – to overcome.

Wherever you study or practise obstetrics and gynaecology, a sound knowledge of the clinical aspects will underpin your understanding of this specialty and maximize your ability to learn about and contribute to the care of women. This book aims to provide you with that knowledge.

Elizabeth A. Layden

Andrew Thomson

Philip Owen

Mayank Madhra

Brian A. Magowan

Contributors

The editors would like to acknowledge and offer grateful thanks for the input of all previous editions' contributors, without whom this new edition would not have been possible.

Karema Al Rashid, MBBCh, MSc, PhD
Research Associate
University of Glasgow
Glasgow, Great Britain

Amrita Banerjee, MBBS, BSc (Hons), MRCOG
University College London Hospitals
London, Great Britain

Susan Brechin, MBBS, FFSRH, MD, MIPM, FHEA, ILM
Lead for Sexual Health and Blood Borne Viruses
NHS Fife
Kirkcaldy, Great Britain

Savita Brito-Mutunayagam, MBBS, MFSRH, DIPM
Specialist Registrar in Sexual and Reproductive Health
NHS Fife
Kirkcaldy, Great Britain

Audrey Brown, MBChB, MRCOG
Consultant in Sexual and Reproductive Healthcare
NHS Greater Glasgow and Clyde
Glasgow, Great Britain

Kevin Burton, MBChB, MD (Hons), MRCOG
Consultant Gynaecological Oncologist
NHS Greater Glasgow and Clyde
Glasgow, Great Britain

Sharon Cameron, MBChB, MD
Professor, Sexual and Reproductive Health
NHS Lothian
Edinburgh, Great Britain

Fraser Christie, MBChB, BSc (Hons), MRCPCH
Registrar, Neonatal Unit
Simpson Centre for Reproductive Health
Royal Infirmary of Edinburgh
Edinburgh, Great Britain

Dan Clutterbuck, FRCP, MRCGP, DFSRH
Consultant in Genitourinary and HIV Medicine
Clinical Lead for Sexual and Reproductive Health
NHS Lothian
Edinburgh, Great Britain
Honorary Clinical Senior Lecturer
University of Edinburgh
Edinburgh, Great Britain

Katie Cornthwaite, BA, MBBS, MRCOG
University of Bristol
Bristol, Great Britain
Doctor
North Bristol NHS Trust
Bristol, Great Britain

Kate Darlow, MBChB, MRCOG
Doctor
Obstetrics and Gynaecology
Borders General Hospital
Scottish Borders, Great Britain

Tim Draycott, MD, BSc, MBBS, FRCOG
Professor
University of Bristol
Bristol, Great Britain
Consultant Obstetrician
North Bristol NHS Trust
Bristol, Great Britain

Malcolm Farquharson, MBBS, MSc, PhD, MRCS, MRCOG
Consultant Gynaecological Oncologist
Glasgow Royal Infirmary
Glasgow, Great Britain

Amy Fitzgerald, MBBS
Registrar in Obstetrics and Gynaecology
O&G Clinical Care Unit
King Edward Memorial Hospital
Perth, Western Australia, Australia

Olivia Foster, MBChB
Obstetrics and Gynaecology
NHS Lothian
Edinburgh, Great Britain

David Gerber, MBChB, MRCPsych, MBA, FECSM
Consultant in Adult Psychiatry
Clinical Lead for Gender and Psychosexual Services
Sandyford Sexual Health
Glasgow, Great Britain

Janice Gibson, MBChB, MD, MRCOG
Maternal Fetal Medicine Consultant
Queen Elizabeth University Hospital
Glasgow, Great Britain

Karen Guerrero, FRCOG
Consultant Urogynaecologist
NHS Greater Glasgow and Clyde
Glasgow, Great Britain

Kirun Gunganah, MBBS, MRCP (UK), MRCP (Diabetes and Endocrinology), PGCME
Consultant in Diabetes and Endocrinology
Barts Health NHS Trust
London, Great Britain

Cameron Hinton, BSc (Hons), MBChB, MRCOG
Consultant Obstetrician
North Bristol NHS Trust
Bristol, Great Britain

Emily Hotton, MBChB, BSc
Women's and Children's Research
Southmead Hospital
Bristol, Great Britain

Lorna Hutchison, MBChB, MRCOG
Consultant in Obstetrics & Gynaecology
Obstetrics & Gynaecology
Royal Alexandra Hospital
Paisley, Great Britain

Stamatina Iliodromiti, PhD, MD, MSc, MRCOG
Reader
Queen Mary University London
Honorary Consultant in Obstetrics and Gynaecology
Royal London Hospital
Lead for the Women's Health Research Unit
Wolfson Institute of Population Health, QMUL
Deputy Lead for the Centre for Public Health
Wolfson Institute of Population Health, QMUL
Research Lead for Women's Health
Barts Health NHS Trust
London, Great Britain

Rod Kelly, BSc (Hons), MBChB, MRCPCH
Registrar
Neonatal Unit
Simpson Centre for Reproductive Health
Royal Infirmary of Edinburgh
Edinburgh, Great Britain

Michelle Kent, MBChB, MRCS, MRCOG, PhD
Consultant Gynaecological Oncologist
Glasgow Royal Infirmary
Glasgow, Great Britain

Mark D. Kilby, MD, FRCOG
Professor of Fetal Medicine
School of Clinical & Experimental Medicine
University of Birmingham
Birmingham, Great Britain

Lindsay Kindinger, BMedSci, BMBS, MRCOG, PhD
Doctor
Fetal Medicine Unit
University College London Hospital
London, Great Britain

Anna King, BMSc (Hons), MBChB, DFSRH
O&G Specialty Registrar
Royal Infirmary of Edinburgh
Edinburgh, Great Britain

Geeta Kumar, MBBS, MD, FRCOG
Doctor
Obstetrics & Gynaecology
Wrexham Maelor Hospital, BCUHB
North Wales, Great Britain

Marie-Anne Ledingham, MD, FRCOG
Maternal Fetal Medicine Consultant
Queen Elizabeth University Hospital
Glasgow, Great Britain

Sophie Mackay, MBChB
Specialty Trainee
Simpson Centre for Reproductive Health
Royal Infirmary of Edinburgh
Edinburgh, Great Britain

Alice Main, MBChB, BSc (Hons), DRCOG
Registrar in Obstetrics and Gynaecology
Simpson Centre for Reproductive Health
Royal Infirmary of Edinburgh
Edinburgh, Great Britain

Kay McAllister, MRCOG, DFFP
Consultant Gynaecologist in Sexual and Reproductive
    Healthcare
NHS Greater Glasgow and Clyde
Glasgow, Great Britain

Katie McBride, MBBCh , MRCOG
Consultant Obstetrician
Princess Royal Maternity Hospital
Glasgow, Great Britain

Alastair McKelvey, MB BCh, BAO, MRCOG
Consultant Obstetrician and Subspecialist in
    Maternal-Fetal Medicine
Norfolk and Norwich University Hospitals NHS
    Foundation Trust
Norwich, Great Britain

Lauren Megaw, MBBS, FRANZCOG
Consultant O&G
O&G Clinical Care Unit
King Edward Memorial Hospital
Perth, Western Australia, Australia

Deirdre J. Murphy, MD, MSc, FRCOG
Professor, Obstetrics & Gynaecology
Trinity College
University of Dublin
Dublin, Ireland

Scott Nelson, BSc, PhD, MRCOG
Muirhead Professor of Obstetrics & Gynaecology
University of Glasgow, Great Britain
Consultant Gynaecologist
NHS Greater Glasgow and Clyde
Glasgow, Great Britain

Catherine Nelson-Piercy, MBBS, MA, FRCP, FRCOG
Professor of Obstetric Medicine
Women's Health Academic Centre
King's Health Partners
London, Great Britain

Christina Neophytou, MBBS, BSc, MRCOG
Specialty Trainee in Obstetrics and Gynaecology
Barts Health NHS Trust
London, Great Britain

Fiona Nugent, BSc, MBChB, MRCOG
Specialty Trainee in Obstetrics and Gynaecology
NHS Scotland
Glasgow, Great Britain

David Obree, BDS, BA (Hons), MSc, MGCDent
Archie Duncan Fellow in Medical Ethics and Fellow
    in Medical Education
The Usher Institute
University of Edinburgh
Edinburgh, Great Britain

Nancy O'Hanrahan, MBBCh, BAO, MRCPI (Paediatrics)
Paediatric Specialist Registrar
General Paediatrics
Our Lady of Lourdes Hospital
Drogheda, Ireland

Judy Ormandy, MBChB, Dip Obs (Dist), FRANZCOG, MClinEd (Hons)
Senior Lecturer
Obstetrics, Gynaecology & Women's Health
University of Otago, Wellington
Te Whare Wānanga o Otāgo ki Te Whanga-Nui-a-Tara
Wellington, New Zealand

Nick Panay, BSc, MBBS, FRCOG, MFSRH
Consultant Gynaecologist
Queen Charlotte's & Chelsea Hospital and Chelsea &
    Westminster Hospital
London, Great Britain
Honorary Senior Lecturer
Imperial College London
London, Great Britain

Pranav P. Pandya, BSc, MBBS, MD, FRCOG
Director of Fetal Medicine
Fetal Medicine
University College London Hospitals
London, Great Britain

Neelam Potdar, MD, MSc, FRCOG
Consultant Gynaecologist
University Hospitals of Leicester, Great Britain
Honorary Senior Lecturer
University of Leicester, Great Britain

Katharine Rankin, MBChB, BMSc, MRCOG
Consultant in Obstetrics and Gynaecology
NHS Fife
Victoria Hospital
Kirkcaldy, Great Britain

Sophie Renwick, MBChB
Doctor
Obstetrics and Gynaecology
Southmead Hospital
Bristol, Great Britain

Jenifer Sassarini, MBChB, PhD
Doctor, Obstetrics and Gynaecology
NHS Greater Glasgow and Clyde
Glasgow, Great Britain

**Janine Dorothea Simpson, MBChB, MFSRH, DiPGUM,
PGA, HPE**
Specialty Registrar Community Sexual and
    Reproductive Healthcare
Sexual and Reproductive Health
Sandyford, NHS Greater Glasgow & Clyde
Glasgow, Great Britain

Laura I. Stirrat, MBChB, MRCOG, PhD
Specialty Registrar in Obstetrics & Gynaecology
NHS Fife
Kirkcaldy, Great Britain

Sarah Stock, BSc, MBChB, MRCOG, PhD
Reader in Maternal and Fetal Health
University of Edinburgh, Great Britain
Honorary Consultant and Subspecialist in Maternal
    and Fetal Medicine
NHS Lothian
Edinburgh, Great Britain

Claire Thompson, MBBCh, BAO, MRCOG, MRCPI
Consultant Gynaecological Oncologist
Gynaecological Oncology
Mater Misericordiae University Hospital
Dublin, Ireland

John Tidy, BSc, MBBS, MD, FRCOG
Professor of Gynaecological Oncology
University of Sheffield
Sheffield, Great Britain
Consultant
Sheffield Trophoblastic Disease Centre
Sheffield, Great Britain

Paul Timmons, MBChB, MRCOG
Senior Registrar
Obstetrics and Gynaecology
Norfolk and Norwich University Hospitals
NHS Foundation Trust
Norwich, Great Britain

Veenu Tyagi, MBBS, MRCOG
Consultant Urogynaecologist
NHS Greater Glasgow and Clyde
Glasgow, Great Britain

Cara Williams, MBChB, MRCOG
Consultant Gynaecologist
Gynaecology
Liverpool Women's Hospital
Liverpool, Great Britain

Language Statement

For simplicity of language, this textbook uses the term women throughout; this should be taken to include people who do not identify as women but who are pregnant or have gynaecological conditions.

Contents

Section 5
ONLINE-ONLY CHAPTERS

Section 6
SELF-ASSESSMENT

FUNDAMENTALS

Section Outline

Chapter 1

Clinical Pelvic Anatomy

Brian A. Magowan

Chapter Outline

Introduction

A thorough understanding of pelvic anatomy is essential for clinical practice. Not only does it facilitate an understanding of the process of labour, it also allows an appreciation of the mechanisms of sexual function and reproduction, and establishes a background to the understanding of gynaecological pathology. Congenital abnormalities are discussed in Chapters 3, 25, and 40.

Obstetric Anatomy

THE BONY PELVIS

The girdle of bones formed by the sacrum and the two innominate bones has several important functions (Fig. 1.1). It supports the weight of the upper body and transmits the stresses of weight bearing to the lower limbs via the acetabulae. It provides firm attachments for the supporting tissues of the pelvic floor, including the sphincters of the lower bowel and

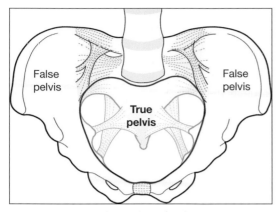

Fig. 1.1 The 'true' and 'false' pelvis.

bladder, and forms the bony margins of the birth canal, accommodating the passage of the fetus during labour.

The birth canal is bounded by the true pelvis, that is, the part of the bony girdle which lies below the pelvic brim – the lower parts of the two innominate bones and the sacrum. These bones are bound together at the sacroiliac joints and at the symphysis pubis anteriorly. The brim is outlined by the promontory of the sacrum, the sacral alae, the iliopectineal lines, and the symphysis. The pelvic outlet is bounded by bone and ligament, including the tip of the sacrum, the sacrotuberous ligaments, the ischial tuberosities, and the subpubic arch (of rounded 'Norman' shape) formed by the fused rami of the ischial and pubic bones. In the erect posture, the pelvic brim is inclined at an angle of 65 to 70 degrees to the horizontal. Because of the curvature of the sacrum, the axis of the pelvis (the pathway of descent of the fetal head in labour) is a J-shaped curve (Fig. 1.2).

The change in the cross-sectional shape of the birth canal at different levels is fundamentally important in understanding the mechanics of labour. The canal can be envisaged initially as a sector of a curved cylinder of about 12 cm in diameter (see Fig. 1.2). The stresses of weight bearing at the brim level in the average woman tend to flatten the inlet a little, reducing the anteroposterior diameter but increasing the transverse diameter. In the lower pelvis, the counterpressure through the necks of the femora tends to compress the pelvis from the sides, reducing the transverse diameters of this part of the pelvis (see Fig. 1.1). At an intermediate level, opposite the third segment of the sacrum, the canal retains a circular cross-section. With this picture in mind, the 'average' diameters of the pelvis at brim,

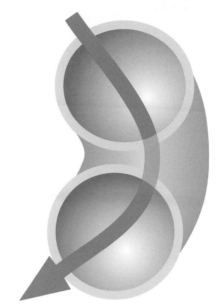

Fig. 1.2 The birth canal resembles a curved cylinder.

cavity, and outlet levels can be readily understood (Table 1.1).

The distortions from a circular cross-section, however, are very modest. If, in circumstances of malnutrition or metabolic bone disease, the consolidation of bone is impaired, more gross distortion of the pelvic shape is liable to occur and labour is likely to involve mechanical difficulty. This is termed 'cephalopelvic disproportion'. The changing cross-sectional shape of the true pelvis at different levels – transverse oval at the brim and anteroposterior oval at the outlet – usually determines a fundamental feature of labour, that is, that the ovoid fetal head enters the brim with its longer (anteroposterior) diameter in a transverse or oblique position but rotates during descent to bring the longer head diameter into the longer anteroposterior

TABLE 1.1	**Average Pelvic Diameters**	
	Diameter	
Level	**Direction**	**Size (cm)**
Inlet	Anteroposterior	11.5
	Transverse	13
Cavity	All diameters	12
Outlet	Anteroposterior	12.5
	Transverse intertuberous	11
	Interspinous	10.5

diameter of the outlet before the time of birth. This rotation is necessary because of the relatively large size of the human fetal head at term, which reflects the unique size and development of the fetal brain.

In most high-resource countries, marked pelvic deformation is rare. Pelvimetry using X-rays, computed tomography, or magnetic resonance imaging scans can be used to measure the pelvic diameters but is of limited clinical value in predicting the likelihood of a successful vaginal delivery. Mechanical difficulty in labour is assessed by close observation of the progress of dilatation of the cervix and of descent, assessed by both abdominal and vaginal examination.

The Pelvic Organs During Pregnancy

THE UTERUS

The uterus is a remarkable organ, composed largely of smooth muscle (the myometrium), which increases in weight during pregnancy from about 40 g to around 1000 g as the myometrial muscle fibres undergo both hyperplasia and hypertrophy (Fig. 1.3). It provides a 'protected' implantation site for the genetically 'foreign' fertilized ovum, accommodates the developing fetus as it grows and, finally, expels it into the outside world during labour.

Whereas the body of the uterus is formed from a thick layer of plain muscle, the cervix, which communicates with the upper vagina, is largely composed of denser collagenous tissue. This forms a rigid collar,

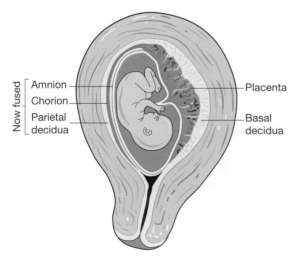

Fig. 1.3 The uterus and developing fetus at 12 weeks' gestation.

Labels: Now fused [Amnion, Chorion, Parietal decidua]; Placenta; Basal decidua

retaining the fetus in utero as the myometrium hypertrophies and stretches. The junctional area between the body and cervix is known as the isthmus, which, in late pregnancy and labour, undergoes dilatation and thinning, forming the lower segment of the uterus. It is through this thinned area that the uterine wall is incised during caesarean section.

The uterine arteries, branches of the anterior division of the internal iliac arteries, become tortuous and coiled within the uterine wall (Fig. 1.4). Innervation of the uterus is derived from both sympathetic and parasympathetic systems, and the functional significance of the motor pathways is incompletely understood. Drugs that stimulate alpha-adrenergic receptors activate the myometrium, whereas beta-adrenergic drugs have an inhibitory effect, and both beta-agonists and alpha-antagonists have been used in attempts to inhibit premature labour. Afferent fibres from the cervix enter the spinal cord via the pelvic splanchnic (parasympathetic) nerves (S2,3,4). Pain stimuli during labour from the fundus and body of the uterus travel via the hypogastric (sympathetic) plexus and enter the spinal cord at the level of the lower thoracic segments.

THE CERVIX

The cervix becomes more vascular and softens in early pregnancy. The mucous secretion from the endocervical glands becomes thick and tenacious, forming a mechanical barrier to ascending infection. In late pregnancy, the cervix 'ripens' – the dense mesh of collagen fibres loosens, as fluid is taken up by the hydrophilic mucopolysaccharides that occupy the interstices between the collagen bundles. This allows the cervix to become shorter as its upper part expands.

ADDITIONAL CHANGES

The ligaments of the sacroiliac and symphyseal joints become more extensible under the influence of pregnancy hormones. As a result, the pelvic girdle has more 'give' during labour. The increased mobility of the joints may result in backache or symphyseal pain.

THE URINARY TRACT IN PREGNANCY

Frequency of micturition is often noticed in early pregnancy. As pregnancy advances, the ureters become dilated, probably due to the relaxing effect of progesterone on the smooth muscle wall but also in part due to

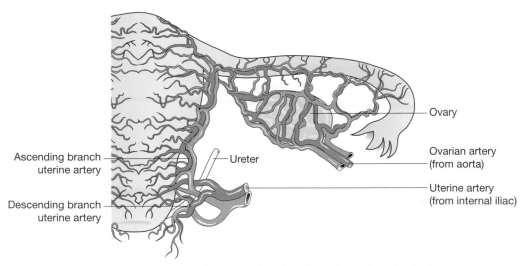

Fig. 1.4 The blood supply of the uterus, fallopian tube, and ovary (posterior view).

the mechanical effects of the gravid uterus. The urinary tract is therefore more vulnerable to ascending infection (acute pyelonephritis) in comparison to non-pregnancy.

THE PERINEUM

This term usually refers to the area of skin between the vaginal orifice and the anus. The underlying musculature at the outlet of the pelvis, surrounding the lower vagina and the anal canal, is important in the maintenance of bowel and urinary continence, and in sexual response. The muscles intermesh to form a firm pyramidal support, the perineal body, between the lower third of the posterior vaginal wall and the anal canal (Fig. 1.5). The tissues of the perineal body are often markedly stretched during the expulsive second stage of labour and may be torn as the head is delivered. Injury to the anal sphincters may lead to impaired anal continence of faeces and/or flatus. Poor healing of an episiotomy or tear is liable to result in scarring, which may cause dyspareunia (pain during intercourse).

Anatomical Points for Obstetric Analgesia

PUDENDAL NERVE BLOCK

Knowledge of the pudendal nerves is important in obstetrics because they may be blocked to minimize pain during instrumental delivery and because their integrity is vital for visceral muscular support and sphincter function. These nerves, which innervate the vulva and perineum, are derived from the second, third, and fourth sacral roots (see Fig. 31.13). On each side the nerve passes behind the sacrospinous ligament close to the tip of the ischial spine and re-enters the pelvis, along with the pudendal blood vessels, in the pudendal canal. After giving off an inferior rectal branch, they divide into the perineal nerves and dorsal nerves of the clitoris. Motor fibres of the pudendal nerve supply the levator ani, the superficial and deep perineal muscles, and the voluntary urethral sphincter. Sensory fibres innervate the central areas of the vulva and perineum. The peripheral skin areas are supplied by branches of the ilioinguinal nerve, the genitofemoral nerve, and the posterior femoral cutaneous nerve (Fig. 1.6). The pudendal nerve can be blocked by an injection of local anaesthetic just below the tip of the ischial spine, as described in Fig. 31.13.

SPINAL BLOCK

The spinal cord ends at the level of L1–2. A spinal injection at the level of the L3–4 space will produce excellent analgesia up to around the level of the T10 nerve root or above, depending on the position of the patient and the volume of local anaesthetic used.

EPIDURAL BLOCK

The epidural space, between the dura and the periosteum and ligaments of the spinal canal, is about

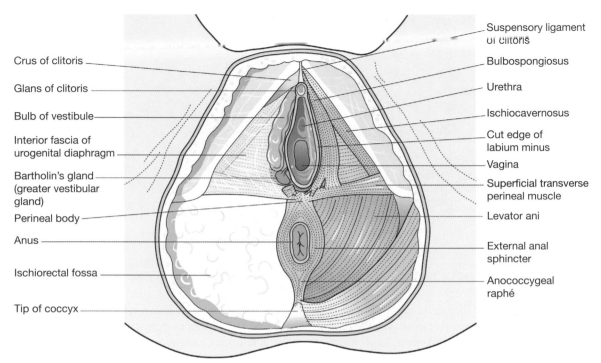

Crus of clitoris

Glans of clitoris

Bulb of vestibule

Interior fascia of
urogenital diaphragm

Bartholin's gland
(greater vestibular
gland)

Perineal body

Anus

Ischiorectal fossa

Tip of coccyx

Suspensory ligament
of clitoris

Bulbospongiosus

Urethra

Ischiocavernosus

Cut edge of
labium minus

Vagina

Superficial transverse
perineal muscle

Levator ani

External anal
sphincter

Anococcygeal
raphé

Fig. 1.5 The perineum: a view from below the pelvic outlet, showing the intermeshing muscles.

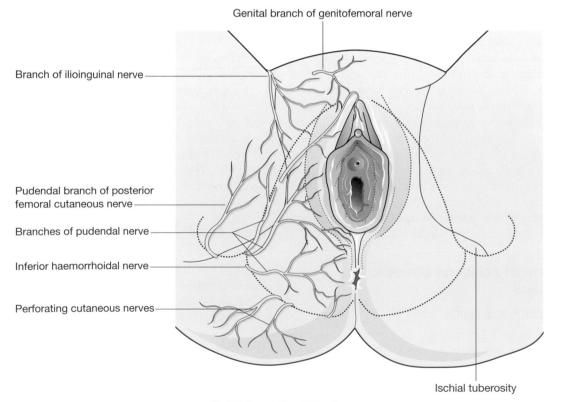

Genital branch of genitofemoral nerve

Branch of ilioinguinal nerve

Pudendal branch of posterior
femoral cutaneous nerve

Branches of pudendal nerve

Inferior haemorrhoidal nerve

Perforating cutaneous nerves

Ischial tuberosity

Fig. 1.6 Innervation of the vulva.

4 mm deep. Epidural injection of local anaesthetic blocks the spinal nerve roots as they traverse the space.

Gynaecological Anatomy

THE UTERUS

The uterus has the shape of a slightly flattened pear and measures, on average, 7.5 × 5.0 × 2.5 cm. Its principal named parts are the fundus, the cornua, the body, and the cervix (Fig. 1.7).

It forms part of the genital tract, lying in close proximity to the urinary tract anteriorly and the lower bowel behind. All three tracts traverse the pelvic floor in the hiatus between the two bellies of the levator ani muscle. Clinically, this means that a problem in one tract can readily affect another (Fig. 1.8).

The uterine cavity is around 6 or 7 cm in length and forms a flattened slit, with the anterior and posterior walls in virtual contact. The wall has three layers: the endometrium (innermost), myometrium, and peritoneum (outermost).

Endometrium

The endometrium is the epithelial lining of the cavity. The surface consists of a single layer of columnar ciliated cells, with invaginations forming uterine mucus-secreting glands within a cellular stroma. It undergoes cyclical changes in both the glands and stroma, leading to shedding and renewal about every 28 days.

There are two layers: a superficial functional layer which is shed monthly and a basal layer which is not shed, from which the new functional layer is regenerated. The epithelium of the functional layer shows active proliferative changes after a menstrual period until ovulation occurs, when the endometrial glands undergo secretory changes. Permanent destruction of the basal layer will result in amenorrhoea. This fact forms the basis for ablative techniques for the treatment of heavy menstrual bleeding.

The normal changes in endometrial histology during the menstrual cycle are determined by changing secretion of ovarian steroid hormones. If the endometrium is exposed to sustained estrogenic stimulation,

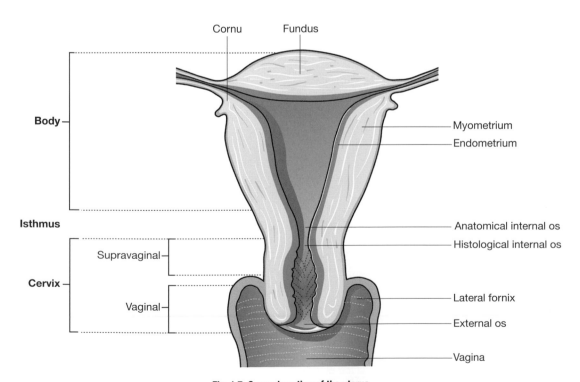

Fig. 1.7 Coronal section of the uterus.

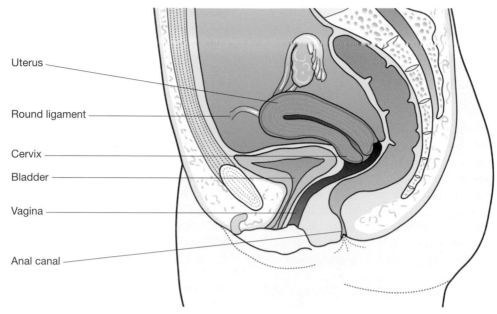

Fig. 1.8 Female pelvic organs: sagittal view.

whether endogenous or exogenous, it may become hyperplastic. Benign hyperplasia may precede malignant change.

Myometrium

The smooth muscle fibres of the uterine wall do not form distinct layers. While the outermost fibres are predominantly longitudinal, continuous with the musculature of the uterine tubes above and the vaginal wall below, the main thickness of the uterine wall is formed from a mesh of criss-crossing spiral strands. The individual muscle cells contain filaments of actin and myosin, which interact to generate contractions. During labour, the propagation of contractile excitation throughout the uterine wall is facilitated by the formation of 'gap junctions' between adjacent muscle cells. As a result, the spread of excitation resembles that in a syncytium.

Peritoneum

The posterior surface of the uterus is completely covered by peritoneum, which passes down over the posterior fornix of the vagina into the pouch of Douglas. Anteriorly, the peritoneum is reflected off the uterus at a much higher level onto the superior surface of the bladder.

THE CERVIX

The cervix connects the uterus and vagina, and projects into the upper vagina. The 'gutter' surrounding this projection comprises the vaginal fornices – lateral, anterior, and posterior. The cervix is about 2.5 cm long. The shorter part of it, which lies above the fornices, is termed the 'supravaginal part'. The endocervical canal is fusiform in shape between the external and internal os. After childbirth, the external os loses its circular shape and resembles a transverse slit. The epithelial lining of the canal is a columnar mucous membrane with an anterior and posterior longitudinal ridge from which shallow palmate folds extend – hence, the name 'arbor vitae'.

There are numerous glands secreting mucus that becomes more abundant and less viscous at the time of ovulation in mid-cycle. The vaginal surface of the cervix is covered with stratified squamous epithelium, similar to that lining the vagina. The squamocolumnar junction (histological external os) commonly does not correspond to the anatomical os but may lie either above or external to the anatomical os. This 'tidal zone', within which the epithelial junction migrates at different stages of life, is termed the 'transformation zone'. The ebb and flow of the squamocolumnar junction is influenced by estrogenic stimulation. In the newborn female, and in pregnancy particularly, outgrowth of the columnar epithelium is very common, forming a bright pink 'rosette' around the external os. This appearance has been misnamed an 'erosion'. In fact, the epithelial covering, though delicate, is intact and is more correctly termed 'ectropion'. In cases in which the cervix has undergone deep bilateral laceration during childbirth, the resulting anterior and posterior lips tend to evert, exposing the glandular epithelium of the canal widely.

Clinical Aspects

The transformation zone is typically the area where precancerous change occurs. This can be detected by microscopic assessment of a cervical cytological smear. If the duct of a cervical gland becomes occluded, the gland distends with mucus to form a retention cyst (or Nabothian follicle). Multiple follicles are not uncommon, giving the cervix an irregular nodular feel and appearance. The body of the uterus is usually angled forward in relation to the cervix (anteflexion), while the uterus and cervix as a whole lean forward from the upper vagina (anteversion). In about 15% of women, the uterus leans backwards towards the sacrum, and is described as retroverted. The cervical os then faces down the long axis of the vagina rather than at right angles to it. In most instances, retroversion is an asymptomatic variant of normality.

It is especially important to distinguish retroversion from anteversion before introducing a sound or similar instrument into the uterine cavity, to avoid perforation of the uterine wall. After menopause, the uterus and cervix gradually become atrophic, and cervical mucus is scanty. The amount of cervix projecting into the vagina also diminishes.

Because the uterus lies immediately behind the bladder and between the lower parts of the ureters, particular care must be taken not to damage these structures during hysterectomy (Fig. 1.9). The endometrium and uterine cavity can be examined by hysteroscopy. The tubal ostia can be seen (Fig. 1.10). Because the anterior and posterior walls are normally in contact, the cavity must be inflated with gas or fluid to obtain an adequate view of the surfaces.

THE UTERINE ATTACHMENTS AND SUPPORTS

Structures attached to the uterus include (Fig. 1.11):
- Round ligament
- Ovarian ligament

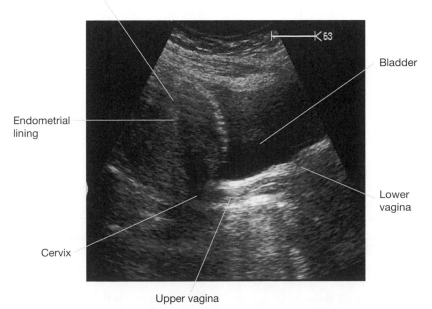

Fundus of anteverted uterus

Bladder

Endometrial lining

Lower vagina

Cervix

Upper vagina

Fig. 1.9 Transabdominal scan of the bladder, uterus, and vagina.

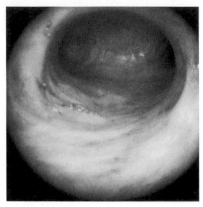

Fig. 1.10 Normal hysteroscopic view of the endometrial cavity, showing both tubal ostia.

- Uterosacral ligament or fold
- Cardinal ligament/transverse cervical ligament (of Mackenrodt).

The broad ligament is merely a double fold of peritoneum extending laterally from the uterus towards the pelvic sidewall. The hilum of the ovary arises from its posterior surface. The portion of the fold lateral to the ovary and tube is termed the infundibulopelvic ligament. Between the leaves of this fold, the uterine and ovarian blood vessels form an anastomotic loop. The ovarian ligament forms a ridge on the posterior leaf of the broad ligament, from the cornu of the uterus to the medial pole of the ovary. Developmentally, it is part of the gubernaculum of the ovary, in continuity with the round ligament, which curves round anteriorly from the cornu towards the inguinal canal, through which it passes. The uterosacral ligaments pass upwards and backwards from the posterior aspect of the cervix towards the lateral part of the second piece of the sacrum. In their lower part, they contain plain muscle along with fibrous tissue and autonomic nerve fibres. In their upper part, they dwindle to shallow peritoneal folds. The ligaments divide the pouch of Douglas from the pararectal fossa on each side.

The main ligaments providing support to the internal genital organs are the cardinal ligaments. The traditional name 'transverse cervical ligaments' is a misnomer. The cardinal ligaments are essentially dense condensations of connective tissue around the venous and nerve plexuses and arterial vessels, which extend from the pelvic sidewall towards the genital tract. Medially, they are firmly fused with the fascia surrounding the cervix and upper part of the vagina. They pass upwards and backwards towards the root of the internal iliac vessels. These condensations of fibrous and elastic tissue, together with plain muscle fibres, are sometimes referred to as the 'parametrium'. They support the upper vagina and cervix, helping to maintain the angle between the axis of the vagina and that of the anteverted uterus. Inferiorly, they are continuous with the fascia on the upper surface of the levator muscles.

THE PELVIC DIAPHRAGM

Below the level of the cardinal ligaments, the pelvic organs are supported by a sloping shelf of muscle on each side, formed by the levator ani muscle (Fig. 1.12). The disposition of the muscle bundles is comparable with that of the abdominal musculature. Near to the midline, there is a longitudinal muscle bundle, the puborectalis (cf. the rectus abdominis). Laterally, the muscle sheets (iliococcygeus and ischiococcygeus) are oblique/transverse. The most medial fibres of puborectalis are inserted into the upper part of the perineal body. The succeeding fibres turn medially behind the anorectal flexure and are inserted into the anococcygeal raphe and the tip of the coccyx along with the fibres of ilio- and ischiococcygeus. Thus, all three visceral tubes reach the body surface via a hiatus between the medial margins of puborectalis, and all are supported from behind by the sling action of the muscle when it contracts. Innervation is from the pudendal nerve (S2,3,4). The fascia on the upper surface of the pelvic diaphragm blends with the lower part of the cardinal ligaments. The fascia on the inferior surface of levator ani forms the roof of the ischiorectal fossa.

The main blood supply of the uterus is from the uterine arteries, which are branches of the internal iliac vessels (Fig. 1.13). Each passes medially in the base of the broad ligament above the ureter and ascends along the lateral aspect of the uterus, forming an anastomotic loop in the broad ligament with the ovarian artery (see Fig. 1.4). The uterine veins form a plexus in the parametrium below the uterine arteries, draining into the internal iliac veins. The principal lymph drainage is to the iliac and obturator glands on the pelvic sidewall. From the fundus and cornua, lymph drains via the ovarian pathway to aortic nodes, while a few lymphatics in the round ligaments drain

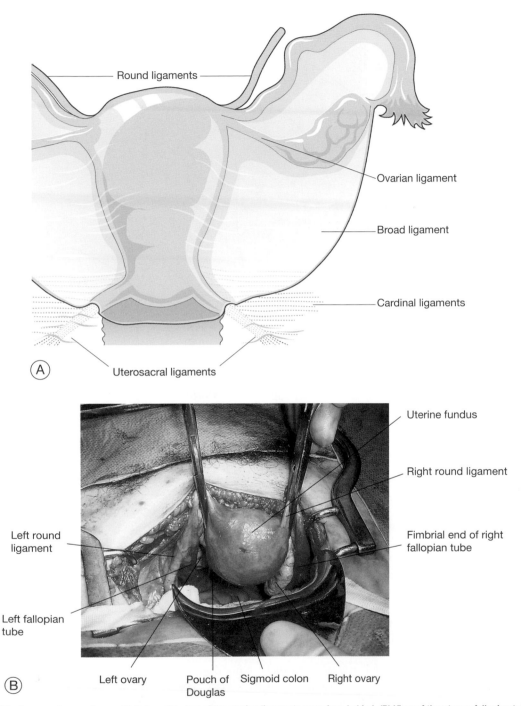

Fig. 1.11 The uterus and appendages. (A) Schematic view of the uterine ligaments seen from behind. **(B)** View of the uterus, fallopian tubes, and ovaries at abdominal hysterectomy.

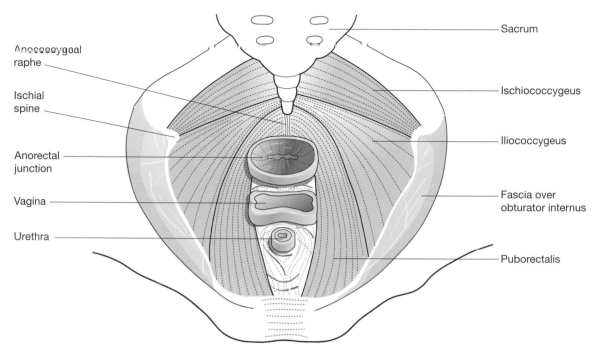

Anococcygeal raphe

Ischial spine

Anorectal junction

Vagina

Urethra

Sacrum

Ischiococcygeus

Iliococcygeus

Fascia over obturator internus

Puborectalis

Fig. 1.12 The urogenital diaphragm from above.

into the inguinal nodes (Fig. 1.14). The uterus is supplied by sympathetic and parasympathetic nerves, the exact functional significance of which is uncertain.

CONGENITAL ABNORMALITIES OF THE UTERUS

Most of the female genital tract develops from the two paramesonephric (Müllerian) ducts, the caudal portions of which approximate in the midline and fuse to form the uterus, cervix, and upper part of the vagina. The upper divergent portions of the ducts form the uterine tubes.

Congenital abnormality can result from:
- Failure of or incomplete fusion
- Failure of canalization
- Asymmetrical maldevelopment.

The diagrams in Fig. 3.9 illustrate some of abnormalities that may be encountered. Failures of canalization are likely to present at puberty, as menstrual blood has no way to escape. Incomplete fusion is associated with late miscarriage, pre-term labour and malpresentation. Because of the intimate association during development, congenital abnormality of the female genital tract is commonly associated with abnormality of the urinary tract.

THE VULVA

The term 'vulva' generally encompasses all of the external female genitalia, that is, the mons pubis, labia majora and minora, clitoris, and structures within the vestibule – the external urinary meatus and hymen. The mons pubis is a thickened pad of fat, cushioning the pubic bones anteriorly. The labia majora contain fatty tissue overlying the vascular bulbs of the vestibule and the bulbospongiosus muscles. The skin of the labia majora bears secondary sexual hair on the lateral surfaces only. There are abundant sebaceous, sweat, and apocrine glands. The folds of the labia minora vary considerably in size and may be concealed by the labia majora or may project between them. They contain no fat but are vascular and erectile during sexual arousal; the skin contains many sebaceous glands. Anteriorly, the folds bifurcate before uniting to form a hood above the clitoris and a frenulum along its dorsal surface. Posteriorly, the labia minora are linked by a fine ridge of skin, the 'fourchette'.

The labia minora and the fourchette form the boundaries of the vestibule. Between the fourchette and the posterior part of the hymen, there is a crescentic furrow termed the 'navicular fossa'. The urethral meatus lies

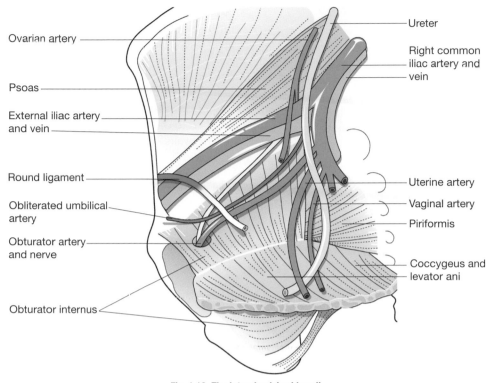

Ovarian artery

Psoas

External iliac artery and vein

Round ligament

Obliterated umbilical artery

Obturator artery and nerve

Obturator internus

Ureter

Right common iliac artery and vein

Uterine artery

Vaginal artery

Piriformis

Coccygeus and levator ani

Fig. 1.13 The lateral pelvic sidewall.

within the vestibule, close to the anterior margin of the vaginal orifice. There are pairs of small mucus-secreting paraurethral glands in the lower part of the posterior wall of the urethra. These rudimentary tubules are homologous with the glands in the male prostate. If they become infected and blocked, they may form a paraurethral abscess, cyst, or urethral diverticulum. Two mucus-secreting glands, known as 'Bartholin's glands' (or 'greater vestibular glands'), lie posterolateral to the vaginal orifice on each side, embedded in the posterior pole of the vascular vestibular bulb (see Fig. 1.5). Their ducts open near the lateral limits of the navicular fossa. The glands become palpable and the duct orifices become visible only if the ducts are occluded, resulting in a cyst, or if infection is present.

Blood Supply

The main sources of the vascularity of the vulva are branches of the internal pudendal arteries. There are also branches from the superficial and deep external pudendal arteries.

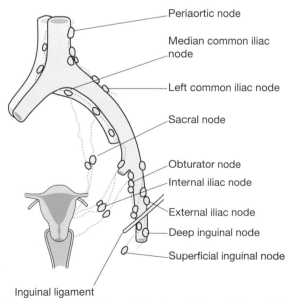

Periaortic node

Median common iliac node

Left common iliac node

Sacral node

Obturator node

Internal iliac node

External iliac node

Deep inguinal node

Superficial inguinal node

Inguinal ligament

Fig. 1.14 Lymphatic drainage of the uterus. The lymph channels follow the blood supply.

Nerve Supply

The main sensory supply to the vulva is via the pudendal nerves. Peripheral parts of the vulvar skin are supplied by filaments from the iliohypogastric and ilio-inguinal nerves, and from the perineal branches of the posterior cutaneous nerves of the thigh (see Fig. 1.6). The pudendal nerve provides motor fibres to all of the muscles of the perineum, including the voluntary urinary and bowel sphincters, as well as the levator ani.

Lymph Drainage

The main pathway of drainage is to the superficial inguinal glands and on through the deep inguinal to the external iliac glands. Some lymphatics from the deeper structures of the vulva pass with vaginal lymphatics to the internal iliac nodes.

THE FALLOPIAN TUBES

The tubes extend on each side from the cornu of the uterus, within the upper border of the broad ligament, for about 10 cm. The tubes and ovaries together are commonly described as the uterine appendages, or adnexa (Fig. 1.15).

The tube can be divided into four parts (Fig. 1.16). The interstitial (intramural) part forms a narrow passage through the thickness of the myometrium. The isthmus, extending out from the cornu for about 3 cm, is also narrow. The ampulla is thin walled, 'baggy', and tortuous. Its lateral portion is free from the broad ligament and droops down behind it towards the ovary. Near its lateral limit, the abdominal ostium is constricted, but opens out again to form the infundibulum. This trumpet-shaped expansion is fringed by a ring of delicate fronds (or fimbriae), one of which is attached to the surface of the ovary.

The walls of the tubes include outer longitudinal and inner circular layers of smooth muscle. The delicate lining (endosalpinx), containing columnar ciliated and secretory cells, has longitudinal folds in the isthmic segment, which change into a highly intricate branching pattern in the ampulla.

Tubal Function

At the time of ovulation, the fimbriae clasp the ovary in the area where the stigma (or point of follicular rupture) is forming. Usually, therefore, the ovum is discharged into the infundibulum (funnel) and is carried by tubal peristalsis into the ampulla of the tube, which is where fertilization occurs. Transit of the zygote to the site of implantation in the uterus takes several days.

Sterilization is effected by occluding both tubes, preferably in the narrow isthmic portion, using clips, sutures, rings, or diathermy.

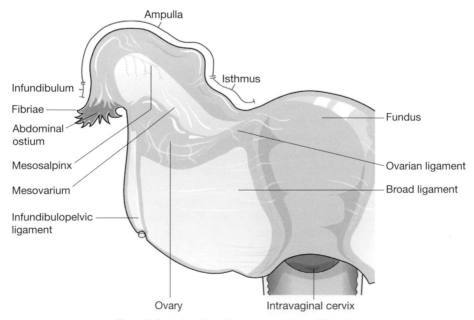

Fig. 1.15 Posterior view of the uterus and broad ligament.

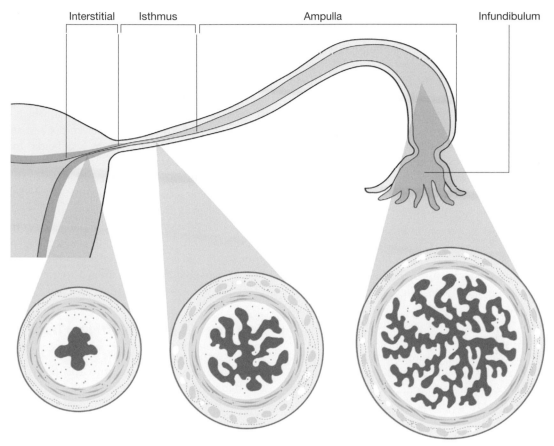

Interstitial　Isthmus　Ampulla　Infundibulum

Fig. 1.16 The oviduct, showing the structure of the mucosal layer.

Patency of the tubes can be tested by injecting a watery dye (methylthioninium chloride – methylene blue) through the cervix and observing spill from the abdominal ostia by laparoscopy. The contours of the uterine cavity and tubal lumen may also be demonstrated with radio-opaque fluid during a hysterosalpingogram.

THE VAGINA

The vagina, which links the external and internal parts of the female genital tract, has a dual function. It forms the coital canal, affording access for spermatozoa to reach the cervix and, with the cervix, it forms the soft-tissue birth canal. It lies in close proximity to the urethra and bladder anteriorly, and to the anal canal and rectum posteriorly. All three canals traverse the pelvic floor, passing between the medial (puborectalis) portions of the levator ani muscles. The insertion of these muscle fibres into the anococcygeal raphe creates a sling behind the bowel so that a sharp angle is created at the junction of the lower rectum and the anal canal, which is opened when the muscle relaxes. Other muscle fibres are inserted into the perineal body near its apex, creating a similar sling which angulates the axis of the vagina at that level. In turn, the anterior vaginal wall in the area of the bladder neck receives support.

There are differences in the anatomy of the vagina above and below this level. The lower third of the vagina is closely invested by the superficial and deep muscles of the perineum. It:

- Incorporates the urethra in its anterior wall
- Is separated from the bowel by the perineal body
- Has a rich arterial blood supply from branches of the vaginal arteries and from both external and internal pudendal vessels.

The upper two-thirds of the vagina, above the levator shelf:

- Is not invested by muscles – rather, it is wide and capacious
- Is in apposition with the bladder base anteriorly and with the rectum (and, above that, the pouch of Douglas) posteriorly
- Is supported laterally and at the vault by the parametrium (cardinal and uterosacral ligaments). During sexual arousal, the smooth muscle fibres within the parametrium elevate the vaginal vault and cervix, thereby elongating the vagina and straightening its long axis.

Vaginal Structure

The vaginal walls form an elastic fibromuscular tube with a multilayered structure. The lining of stratified squamous epithelium is corrugated into transverse folds (or rugae), which facilitates stretching during childbirth. The epithelium contains no glands, but during the reproductive years the more superficial cells contain abundant glycogen. This polysaccharide is broken down by lactobacilli, which form the normal flora of the vagina, producing lactic acid. This accounts for the low pH in the vaginal lumen (average pH, 4.5).

Between the epithelium and the muscle, there is a layer of areolar tissue containing an extensive venous plexus. Vascular engorgement during sexual arousal, analogous to erection in the male, is most marked in the lower part of the vagina, encroaching on the vaginal lumen as the rugae distend. The vasocongestive response also results in increased transudation into the vaginal lumen.

The smooth muscle layers (outer longitudinal, inner circular) are not distinct, and an interlacing pattern is usual. Deep to the muscle, there is another extensive plexus of veins within the outer vaginal fascia.

THE OVARY

The ovaries are attached on each side to the posterior surface of the broad ligaments through a narrowed base, termed the 'hilum'. The ovaries are also attached to the cornua of the uterus by the ovarian ligaments. Developmentally, these are the upper portions of the gubernacula ovarii. They are responsible for drawing the ovaries down into the pelvis from the posterior wall of the abdominal cavity. Typically, each ovary lies in an ovarian fossa, a shallow peritoneal depression lateral to the ureter, near the pelvic sidewall. However, the position may vary; when the uterus is retroverted, one or both ovaries may lie in the pouch of Douglas.

The ovaries are ovoid in shape, with an irregular surface and a firm, largely solid, stroma, which can be divided indistinctly into an outer cortex and an inner medulla. The surface epithelium of cuboidal coelomic cells forms an incomplete layer, beneath which is a fibrous investment – the 'tunica albuginea'. The germ cells from which the ova are derived are embedded in the substance of the ovaries.

The ovarian blood vessels and nerves enter through the hilum from the broad ligament. The ovarian arteries are direct branches of the aorta. Within the broad ligaments, they form an anastomotic loop with branches of the uterine arteries.

Anatomy of the Lower Urinary Tract

The descending ureters are narrow, thick-walled muscular tubes that cross into the pelvis close to the bifurcation of the common iliac arteries. They lie immediately under the peritoneum of the pelvic sidewall, behind the lateral attachment of the broad ligaments. Curving medially and forwards, they pass through the base of the broad ligaments below the uterine arteries, about 2 cm lateral to the supravaginal part of the cervix, a short distance above the lateral fornices of the vagina.

Approaching the bladder, the ureters pass medially in front of the upper vagina and enter the bladder base obliquely at the upper angles of the trigone.

The wall of the ureter is composed of three elements: an external fibrous sheath, layers of smooth muscle, and a lining of transitional epithelium. There may be partial or complete duplication of one or both ureters. An ectopic ureter is one that opens anywhere but the trigone of the bladder; this may even be into the vagina or the vestibule. Urinary incontinence inevitably results.

THE BLADDER

The urinary reservoir, lined with transitional epithelium, has the shape of a tetrahedron when empty. However, the mesh of smooth muscle in the bladder wall can readily distend to contain a volume of half a litre or more. This muscle coat (the detrusor muscle) is thus normally relaxed and capable of considerable stretching without a contractile response. If urinary outflow during micturition is chronically impeded, however, the detrusor muscle becomes irritable and ultimately hypertrophic, producing prominent trabecular bands visible at cystoscopy.

The bladder is covered with peritoneum on its superior surface only. The peritoneum is reflected onto the anterior abdominal wall at varying levels dependent on the degree of bladder filling. The oblique passage of the terminal part of each ureter through the bladder wall creates a one-way valve, which normally prevents urinary backflow from the bladder. This protects the kidneys from ascending infection. The triangular area within the bladder base defined by the two ureteric orifices and the internal urethral orifice is termed the 'trigone'. Over this area, the epithelium remains smooth even when the bladder is empty.

THE URETHRA

The female urethra is about 4 cm long. Below the bladder neck, it is embedded in the anterior vaginal wall, and the smooth muscle layers of the two structures intermingle. The urethral tissues also reflect the vascularity and turgidity of the vagina itself. Many of the urethral muscle fibres near the bladder neck are longitudinal and continuous with those of the bladder above, forming a funnel that opens out when these fibres contract, flattening the angle between the bladder base and the upper urethra. There are also abundant elastic fibres at this level, whose action helps to restore urethral closure after micturition. Around the lower part of the urethra, there is a fusiform collar of voluntary muscle – 'the external urethral sphincter'. This segment of the urethra passes through the perineal membrane, which keeps it in a stable position. The upper urethra, on the other hand, shares the mobility of the bladder neck. The urethra is lined by transitional epithelium in its upper part, and by squamous epithelium below.

NERVE SUPPLY

Apart from the external sphincter, the efferent nerve supply controlling bladder function is from the pelvic parasympathetic system (S2,3,4), which provides the main motor fibres to the detrusor muscle. Afferent fibres conveying the normal sensations of bladder filling also return through the parasympathetic pathway, though some sympathetic sensory fibres convey the feelings of bladder overdistension via the hypogastric plexus. At the level of the second, third, and fourth sacral segments of the spinal cord, the sensory and motor parasympathetic nerves form spinal reflex arcs, which are moderated by interaction with higher centres in the brain. Urinary continence depends upon a variety of factors. These include the elastic fibres surrounding the bladder neck, which normally maintain urethral closure, and the tone or reflex contraction of the levator ani muscles, which, through their insertion into the perineal body, elevate the urethrovesical junction, creating an angulation at the junction of the mobile (upper) and fixed (lower) portions of the urethra. The turgidity of spongy tissue underlying the urethral epithelium also assists in occluding the urethra, as does the action of the voluntary sphincter.

Key Points

- Without understanding the anatomy of the pelvis, it is impossible to understand the mechanisms of labour.
- The cross-sectional shape of the birth canal is different at different levels. At the pelvic brim, it is oval in shape; the widest part of this oval is in the lateral plane from one side to the other. The outlet is also oval, with the widest part in the anteroposterior plane. The head enters the pelvic brim in the transverse position, as the inlet is widest in this plane, but rotates 90 degrees at the pelvic floor to the anteroposterior plane before delivery. The shoulders also follow the same rotation.

Chapter 2

History and Examination

Kate Darlow

Chapter Outline

Introduction

In general, history and examination cannot be divided neatly into different specialties, and questions relating to obstetrics and gynaecology should form part of the assessment of any woman presenting to any specialty. There may be embarrassment and recrimination, for example, when a suspected appendicitis turns out to be a pelvic infection secondary to an unsuspected intrauterine contraceptive device (IUCD). Similarly, not all problems presenting to obstetricians and gynaecologists are obstetrical or gynaecological in nature. It is therefore important to take a full history and perform an appropriate examination in all cases. The key points of gynaecological and obstetrical history and examination are emphasised in the next sections.

Gynaecological History

A gynaecological history should follow the usual model for history taking, with questions about the presenting complaint, its history and associated problems. It should include a past medical history and information about prescription and non-prescription drugs used, and any known allergies. After questions about social circumstances and activities, plus family history, the history is completed with a general systemic enquiry. However, during a gynaecological history, there are specific key areas to be expanded upon. These include menstrual, fertility, pelvic pain, urogynaecological and obstetrical histories.

MENSTRUAL HISTORY

The Pattern of Bleeding

The simple phrase 'tell me about your periods' often elicits all the information required. The bleeding pattern of the menstrual cycle is expressed as a fraction, such that a cycle of 4/28 means the woman bleeds for 4 days every 28 days. A cycle of 4 to 10/21 to 42 means the woman bleeds between 4 and 10 days every 21 to 42 days. Asking the shortest time between the start of successive periods, the longest time between periods, and the average time between periods helps determine the cycle characteristics.

Bleeding Too Little

Amenorrhoea is the absence of periods. Primary amenorrhoea is when someone has not started menstruating by the age of 16 years. Secondary amenorrhoea means that periods have been absent for longer than 6 months. Oligomenorrhoea means that the periods are infrequent, with a cycle of 42 days or more.

Climacteric is the perimenopausal time when periods become less regular and are accompanied by increasing menopausal symptoms. Menopause is the time after the last ever period; therefore, it can only be assessed retrospectively.

Irregular periods, oligomenorrhoea or amenorrhoea, suggest anovulation or irregular ovulation. Specific

questions about weight, weight change, acne, greasy skin, hirsutism, flushes or galactorrhoea may help identify the nature of the patient's ovarian dysfunction.

Bleeding Too Much

It is very difficult to find out how heavy someone's periods are. If menstrual blood loss is accurately measured, an average of 35 mL of blood is lost each month. Heavy menstrual bleeding (previously known as 'menorrhagia') is defined as loss of more than 80 mL during regular menstruation. Some women will complain of very heavy periods with a normal blood loss, while others will not complain in the presence of heavy menstrual bleeding. Asking how often pads or tampons have to be changed and using pictorial charts can provide more objective information. Whether menstrual loss is excessive, however, is a largely subjective assessment.

Specific symptoms can indicate abnormally heavy menstruation. Although small pieces of tissue are normal, blood clots are not. 'Flooding' is when menstrual blood soaks through all protection. It is both abnormal and distressing. Symptoms of anaemia may also be present. A history of the menstrual cycle since menarche (the first period) can reveal changes in the bleeding pattern. However, an emphasis on the effect on lifestyle and treatments tried previously is particularly important.

Bleeding at the Wrong Time

It is important to ask specifically about bleeding, brown or bloody discharge between periods (intermenstrual bleeding), or after intercourse (post-coital bleeding). These symptoms can point to abnormalities of the cervix or uterine cavity. Postmenopausal bleeding is defined as bleeding more than 1 year after the last period. Undiagnosed abnormal bleeding requires further investigation. If a woman is postmenopausal, enquiry should be made about past or current use of hormone replacement therapy.

FERTILITY HISTORY

Last Menstrual Period (LMP)

This question is vital and should be followed with whether that period came at the expected time and was of normal character. As well as alerting to the possibility of pregnancy, the information is important because some investigations need to be performed at specific times of the menstrual cycle.

OONTRACEPTIION

It is useful to establish whether the woman is sexually active, perhaps with something like, 'Are you currently in a physical sexual relationship?' and then, 'Are you using any contraception at present?' A further discussion about fertility issues, unprotected intercourse, and risk factors for certain diseases may be appropriate. A contraceptive history should include any problems with chosen contraceptives and why they were stopped. Questions may be followed-up with 'Are you hoping for a pregnancy?' if the situation is not clear.

If there are any infertility issues, their duration and the results of any investigation or treatment may be of relevance.

CERVICAL SMEARS

Cervical screening programmes vary in different countries but, generally, women between the ages of 20 to 25 and 60 to 64 years are invited to participate every 3 to 5 years. The date of the woman's last smear should be noted and when it was recommended that she have her next smear. Any previous abnormalities or vaccination should also be noted and whether she has had any colposcopic investigation or treatment. If she is over 50 years of age, it may be relevant to discuss breast screening.

PELVIC PAIN HISTORY
Painful Periods

Dysmenorrhoea is a common problem and its effects on lifestyle are important. The cramping pain of primary dysmenorrhoea is at its most intense just before and during the early stages of a period. Young women are particularly affected, and the pain has usually been present from the time of the first period. It is not usually associated with structural abnormalities and may improve with age or after a pregnancy. Secondary dysmenorrhoea is when menstruation has not tended to be painful in the past; it is more likely to indicate pelvic pathology. In particular, progressive dysmenorrhoea, in which the intensity of the pain increases throughout menstruation, may suggest endometriosis.

Pelvic Pain

The relationship of pelvic pain to the menstrual cycle is important. Pain immediately prior to or during periods is more likely to be of gynaecological origin. 'Mittelschmerz' is a cramping pelvic pain that can be midline or unilateral. It occurs 2 weeks before a period and is caused by ovulation. Intermittent discomfort may suggest some scarring or ovarian pathology, but it is more commonly non-gynaecological. It is vital to take a urinary and lower gastrointestinal history, as urinary tract infection or irritable bowel syndrome may present with pelvic pain. Any pain is likely to be worse if the person is anxious, stressed or depressed. Chronic pelvic pain is particularly affected by psychosomatic factors – recognising this during history taking is important.

Pain With Intercourse

There are two main types of dyspareunia: superficial and deep. They can be differentiated by asking, 'Is it painful just as he begins to enter or when he is deep inside?' Deep dyspareunia is associated with pelvic pathology, such as scarring, adhesions, endometriosis or masses that restrict uterine mobility. Superficial dyspareunia can arise from local abnormalities at the introitus or from inadequate lubrication. It can also be due to a voluntary or involuntary contraction of the muscles of the pelvic floor referred to as 'vaginismus' (see Chapter 19).

VAGINAL DISCHARGE

Discharge can be normal or associated with cervical ectopy and, particularly if offensive or irritant, can indicate infection. It can also suggest neoplasia of the cervix or endometrium. Enquire about the duration, amount, colour, smell and relationship to cycle.

UROGYNAECOLOGICAL HISTORY
Urinary Symptoms

A good initial question to ask is, 'Do you ever leak urine when you don't intend to?' If so, find out what provokes it, how it affects her quality of life and how troublesome her symptoms are. Symptoms suggestive of an overactive bladder include frequency, urgency and nocturia. Incontinence after exercise, coughing, laughing or straining can suggest stress incontinence. It can be difficult to differentiate stress incontinence and urge incontinence, however, as there is often a mixed picture. It is important to ask about fluid intake, in particular about caffeine and alcohol, which can exacerbate urinary symptoms.

A history of dysuria or haematuria may suggest bladder infection or pathology. 'Strangury' is the constant desire to pass urine and suggests urinary tract inflammation.

Prolapse

Prolapse may be associated with vaginal discomfort, a dragging sensation, the feeling of something 'coming down', and possibly backache. Although the uterus, anterior vaginal wall and posterior vaginal wall can prolapse, it is difficult to separate these by history. Bladder and bowel function should be explored, including a question about the need to digitally manipulate the vagina in order to be able to void.

Gynaecological Examination

Signs of gynaecological disease are not limited to the pelvis. A full examination may reveal anaemia, pleural effusions, visual field defects or lymphadenopathy in gynaecological conditions. However, passing a speculum, taking a cervical smear and performing a bimanual pelvic examination are the key skills to acquire. A great deal of sensitivity is required in their use.

PASSING A SPECULUM

Preparation

The woman should empty her bladder and remove sanitary protection. The examination room should be quiet and have a private area for the woman to undress. It should contain an examination couch with a modesty sheet and good adjustable lighting. A chaperone should always be present. The examination requires full explanation and verbal consent.

Stand on the right side of the woman with gloves, speculum and lubricating gel immediately to hand. The woman should be asked to lie back, bend her knees, put her heels together and let her knees fall apart. The light should be adjusted to give a good view of the vulva and perineum; the modesty sheet should cover the woman's abdomen and thighs.

Inspection

Inspect the hair distribution and vulval skin. Hair extending towards the umbilicus and onto the inner thighs can be associated with disorders of androgen excess, as can clitoromegaly. The vulva can be a site of chronic skin conditions such as eczema and psoriasis, specific conditions such as lichen sclerosis and warts, cysts of the Bartholin glands and cancers. Ulceration may imply herpes, syphilis, trauma or malignancy.

Look at the perineum (Fig. 2.1) and gently part the labia to inspect the introitus. Perineal scars are usually secondary to tears or episiotomy during childbirth. A red papule around the urethral opening is usually a prolapsed area of urethral mucosa. A white, plaque-like discharge may suggest thrush, and pale skin with punctate red areas implies atrophic vaginitis. Asking the woman to cough may reveal demonstrable stress incontinence or the bulge of a prolapse.

Speculum Examination

Disposable speculums come in different sizes. Ensure that the speculum is working normally and lubricated with gel. Hold the speculum so that its blades are oriented in the same direction as the vaginal opening. Part the labia and slowly insert the speculum, rotating it gently until the blades are horizontal (Fig. 2.2).

If the woman is in the lithotomy position at the edge of the couch, the speculum can be turned downwards to avoid pressure on the clitoris. If the woman is lying on the couch itself, it is usually easier to rotate the speculum upwards. It should be inserted fully in a slightly posterior direction, before firmly, but gently, opening to visualize the cervix (Fig. 2.3). The speculum can be closed a little when the cervix pops into view.

If the cervix is not visible, it is often because the speculum has not been inserted far enough before opening. If this is not the case, the cervix is either above or below the blades. As most uteri are anteverted, it is usually below the blades, and the speculum should be angled more posteriorly before reopening. Otherwise, gently insert a finger to determine its position. For removal, the speculum should be opened further and withdrawn beyond the cervix before rotation back again, closure and removal.

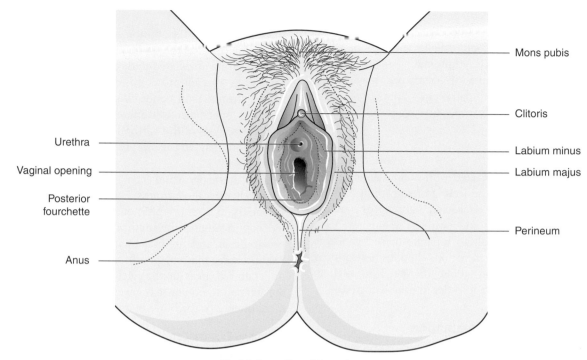

Fig. 2.1 Inspection of the perineum.

Labels on figure:
- Mons pubis
- Clitoris
- Labium minus
- Labium majus
- Perineum
- Urethra
- Vaginal opening
- Posterior fourchette
- Anus

Inspect the vagina for atrophic vaginitis and discharge. A creamy or mucousy discharge is normal. A yellow-greenish frothy discharge is seen with *Trichomonas vaginalis* and a grey-green fishy discharge suggests bacterial vaginosis. There may be a purulent cervical discharge with gonorrhoea, and an increased mucousy discharge may occur with chlamydial cervicitis. Swabs, if required, should be taken from the vaginal fornices (high vaginal) or the cervical canal (endocervical).

The cervical os is small and round in the nulliparous and bigger and more slit-like in parous women. Threads from an IUCD may be present. Translucent lumps or cysts around the os are Nabothian follicles, but warts and tumours can sometimes be seen. An ectopy is red, as the epithelium of the cervical canal extends onto the surface of the paler outer cervical epithelium. It varies across the cycle and should be considered as normal, although it may be associated with contact bleeding or increased discharge.

A bivalve speculum holds open the vaginal walls and obscures any cystocele or rectocele, but a univalve speculum can demonstrate these well. For this, a woman lies in the left-lateral position with her knees drawn up and the lubricated blade of the speculum is used to hold back the anterior vaginal wall. Coughing will show a bulge of the posterior wall if a rectocele is present. When the posterior wall is held back, coughing will demonstrate the bulge of a cystocele and/or uterine descent (Figs 2.4 and 2.5).

TAKING A CERVICAL SMEAR

Smears should ideally be performed in the mid- to late follicular phase, not during menstruation, and only as part of the screening programme. Confirm the woman's details and ensure that you have ascertained all of the information required for the request form. Run the speculum under warm water to provide appropriate lubrication and then visualize the cervix.

The most commonly used technique involves liquid-based cytology and a broom-type sampling device. Insert the central bristles of the broom-like device into the endocervical canal deep enough to allow the shorter bristles to fully contact the ectocervix. Push

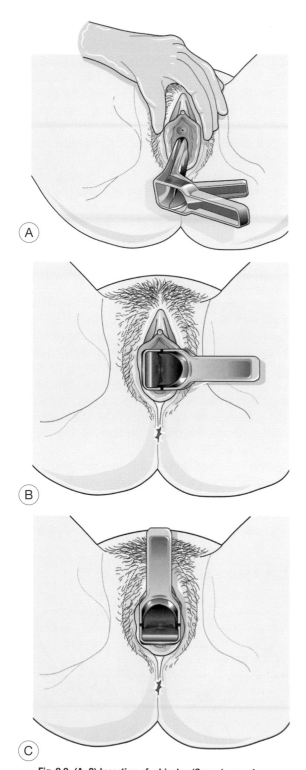

Fig. 2.2 (A–C) Insertion of a bivalve (Cusco) speculum.

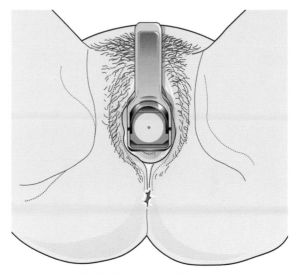

Fig. 2.3 Visualization of the cervix.

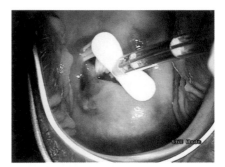

Fig. 2.4 Taking a cervical smear.

gently and rotate the broom in a clockwise direction five times (Fig. 2.6).

Immediately put the broom into the container of preserving solution and rotate 10 times while pushing against the side of the container. Discard the broom, tighten the lid and label the container with the woman's details. Complete and check the cytology request form, ensuring that all of the information required is provided, and match this, or the computer-generated barcode if the form is completed electronically, to the container for transport to the laboratory. Inform the woman of how long the result will take and how it will be delivered.

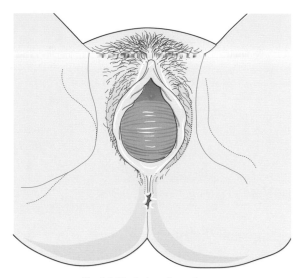

Fig. 2.5 **The bulge of a prolapse.**

PELVIC EXAMINATION

Apply lubricating gel to the gloved fingers of the right hand. Part the labia with the index and middle fingers of the left hand. Gently insert the right index finger into the vagina. If comfortable for the woman, insert the middle finger in below the index finger, making room posteriorly to avoid the sensitive urethra. The cervix feels like the tip of a nose and protrudes into the top of the vagina (Fig. 2.7).

Feel the cervix and record irregularities or discomfort. 'Cervical excitation' is when touching the cervix causes intense pain, which implies active pelvic inflammation. The dimple of the os can be felt and the firmness of the uterine body lies above or below the cervix. A vaginal cyst may be an embryological duct remnant, and vaginal nodules may represent endometriosis.

Assess the position of the uterus. It is usually ante-verted, with the cervix posterior and the uterine body anterior. If the uterus is retroverted, the cervix is ante-rior and the uterine body lies posteriorly. The fingers should be manipulated behind the cervix to lift the uterus. With the left hand above the umbilicus, feel through the abdomen for the moving uterus (Fig. 2.8). If the uterus cannot be palpated, the hand should be moved gradually down until the uterus is between the fingers (Fig. 2.9A).

Assess the mobility, regularity and size of the uterus. The adhesions of endometriosis, infection, sur-gery or malignancy fix the uterus and make bimanual examination more uncomfortable. Asymmetry of the uterus may imply fibroids. Uterine size is often related

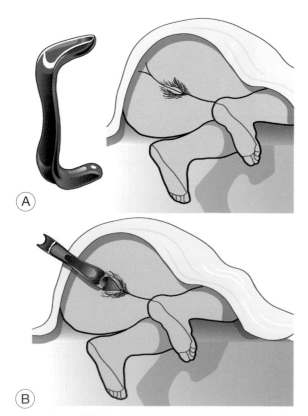

Fig. 2.6 **(A,B) Examination with a univalve speculum.**

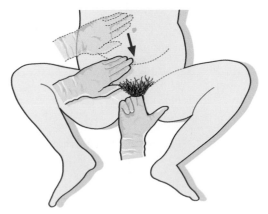

Fig. 2.7 **Digital pelvic examination.**

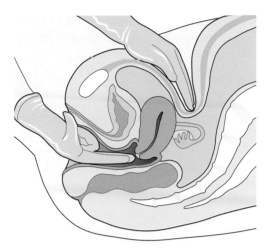

Fig. 2.8 Bimanual examination.

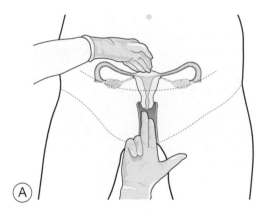

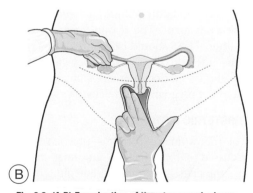

Fig. 2.9 (A,B) Examination of the uterus and adnexa.

to stage of pregnancy. A normally sized uterus feels like a plum. At 6 weeks, a pregnant uterus feels like a tangerine, at 8 weeks an apple, at 10 weeks an orange,

and at 12 weeks a grapefruit. At 14 weeks, the uterus can be felt on abdominal palpation alone.

Feel for adnexal masses in the vaginal fornices lateral to the cervix on each side. Push up the tissues in the adnexa and, starting with the left hand above the umbilicus, bring it down to the appropriate iliac fossa, trying to feel a mass bimanually (Fig. 2.9B). In thin women, the ovaries can just be felt, but a definite adnexal mass is abnormal and should be investigated further. As large adnexal masses tend to move to the midline, it can be difficult to differentiate a large ovarian cyst from a large uterus.

Obstetrical History

An obstetrical history follows the usual model for history taking. However, as with gynaecological histories, there are several unique things to be covered. A history from a pregnant woman starts with calculating the gestation and putting this pregnancy in the context of previous pregnancies. The presenting complaint is next, which encompasses a record of what is happening now, risk factors and symptom progression. It is followed by a complete history of this pregnancy and previous pregnancies. After this, medical, gynaecological, drug, social and family histories are expanded. However, these are often straightforward, as pregnant women are usually young and healthy.

ESTABLISHMENT OF THE ESTIMATED DAY OF DELIVERY (EDD)

Term is between 37 and 42 weeks' gestation, but the actual EDD is 40 weeks after day 1 of the LMP. This can cause confusion, as gestation is calculated from the LMP, not conception. When someone is 12 weeks' pregnant, she conceived 10 weeks ago. Phone-based apps or gestational wheel calculators allow the easy calculation of EDD and current gestation from the LMP (Fig. 2.10). In their absence, Naegele's rule can be used. To calculate the EDD, subtract 3 months from the LMP and add 10 days.

These methods assume a regular 4-week cycle. If this is not the case, the EDD may require adjustment. With a regular 5-week cycle, the true EDD will be 1 week later than calculated. An ultrasound scan (USS) is used to confirm the final EDD. However,

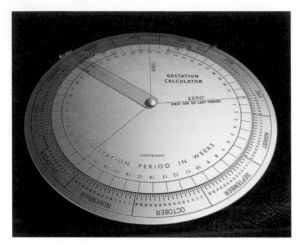

Fig. 2.10 Gestational wheel.

scans have an associated error that increases with gestation. In the early second trimester, this is approximately plus or minus 1 week. In general, the EDD from the LMP is used unless the USS date differs by more than a week.

OBSTETRICAL SUMMARY

Parity is a summary of a woman's obstetrical history; two numbers are used to document this. Added together, the numbers give the number of previous pregnancies. Someone who is para 0 + 0 has not been pregnant before. The first number is the total number of live births, plus the number of stillbirths after 24 weeks' gestation. The second number is the number of pregnancies before 24 weeks, in which the baby was not born alive.

A woman who is para 3 + 3 has been pregnant six times. The first '3' might represent a normal-term delivery, a live birth at 23 weeks after which the baby died and a stillbirth at 25 weeks' gestation. The other three pregnancies may have been a spontaneous miscarriage at 23 weeks, an early ectopic pregnancy and a first-trimester termination. The numbers relate to pregnancies rather than babies, so that the mother of twins would be para 1 + 0. A woman who is primiparous is 'pregnant and para 0'. A parous woman is 'pregnant and para 1' (or more).

Gravidity is the number of times a woman has been pregnant, including the current pregnancy. A woman who is currently pregnant and has had two previous pregnancies resulting in one live birth and one miscarriage is 'gravida 3, para 1' (or 'G3 P1').

WHAT IS HAPPENING NOW?

The next stage is the presenting complaint and its history. Assuming that there is a specific problem, the history should include when it was first noticed, its progress, treatment and associated symptoms. It may also be useful to ask about important risk factors, for example, a past history of placental abruption, chronic hypertension, smoking or pre-eclampsia.

Remember that there are two patients. The fetus should be assessed by asking about movements and any recent tests of fetal well-being. Fetal movements are first felt around 20 weeks, a time referred to as the 'quickening', but can be as early as 16 weeks. Concerns about fetal well-being may be established by a reduction in the frequency or change in pattern of fetal movements.

HISTORY OF THIS PREGNANCY

This pregnancy should now be covered in detail. The first thing to ask about is pre-conceptual folic acid, followed by the diagnosis of pregnancy and problems such as bleeding and vomiting or pain in the first trimester. The next thing to ask about is the booking appointment, results of investigations, including dating and anomaly USS and additional prenatal screening tests. Then, cover subsequent antenatal care, including clinics, parentcraft, and any day unit assessment. The reason for and outcome of any additional USS should be reported. Any concerns, problems identified or emergency attendance at hospital should be documented, along with plans for the rest of the pregnancy and delivery.

PAST OBSTETRIC HISTORY

Each of the woman's previous pregnancies should be discussed chronologically. Information required includes the date, gestation and outcome. If the pregnancy ended in the first or second trimester, the diagnosis and management, including any operative procedures, should be recorded. For other pregnancies, information about the method of delivery, the reason for an operative delivery, the sex, weight, health and method of feeding of the baby should be obtained. In particular, any pregnancy and postnatal complication should be highlighted.

MEDICAL HISTORY

The medical history should include previous operations, hospitalizations and medical problems. Continuing medical problems are of great importance because they may have an effect on the pregnancy and make complications more likely or complex. In addition, pregnancy may have an effect on medical problems, resulting in their deterioration, improvement or an alteration in recommended care.

GYNAECOLOGICAL HISTORY

All or some of the gynaecological topics may be important in the history. Infertility treatment, particularly the use of assisted reproductive technologies (such as egg donation, pre-gestational diagnosis or screening), may suggest the need to modify counselling and tests. The date of the last cervical smear is relevant.

DRUG HISTORY

It is important to record drugs taken, both over-the-counter and prescribed, and the reasons for their use. The need to continue the drug or change its dose, as well as any possible teratogenic effects, should be considered.

FAMILY HISTORY

In a pregnant woman, a family history of fetal abnormalities, genetic conditions or consanguinity is particularly important. Some obstetrical conditions – such as twins, pre-eclampsia, gestational diabetes and obstetric cholestasis – may also have a familial element.

SOCIAL HISTORY

It is important to assess the facilities for the forthcoming baby and determine whether further support is required. The risk of intimate partner violence (IPV) increases during pregnancy and is associated with poorer maternal and perinatal outcomes. Therefore, all pregnant women should be routinely asked if they have experienced IPV. A woman's occupation and her plans for working during the pregnancy should be noted. It is also important to ask about smoking, drinking alcoholic beverages and other drugs of misuse.

SYSTEMIC ENQUIRY

Often, the systemic enquiry will be covered in the history of the presenting complaint. However, remember that many symptoms are more common in pregnancy, including urinary frequency, shortness of breath, tiredness, headache, nausea and breast tenderness.

LOW-RISK VERSUS HIGH-RISK PREGNANCY

The key to good antenatal care is to recognise which women are more likely to develop problems in pregnancy before they happen. Clearly, all women can develop problems, but women at extremes of age and weight; those with pre-existing medical conditions such as diabetes, hypertension and epilepsy; those with significant past or family histories of obstetric problems; and those who smoke heavily, misuse drugs or have poor social circumstances are all more likely to develop problems. In these 'high-risk' pregnancies, antenatal care should be tailored to meet the increased needs of the woman and her baby.

Obstetrical Examination

In an obstetrical examination, the areas to focus on should be guided by the clinical history. It is only by becoming familiar with examination findings in normal pregnancy that deviations from normal can be fully appreciated. In the hyperdynamic circulation of pregnancy, for example, cardiac murmurs are common. The vast majority of these are flow murmurs, but previously unrecognised pathological murmurs occasionally become apparent. Likewise, in normal pregnancy, skin changes and increasing oedema are common.

A systematic approach is preferable. Starting with the hands and working up to the head and down to the abdomen and legs will avoid missing important signs. Examination of the skin, sclera, conjunctiva, retina, thyroid, liver and tendon reflexes may reveal important abnormalities that may otherwise be missed. There are three elements of obstetrical examination that are particularly important: blood pressure assessment, abdominal palpation and vaginal examination if indicated.

BLOOD PRESSURE ASSESSMENT

The pregnant woman should lie in a semi-recumbent position at an approximately 30-degree angle and

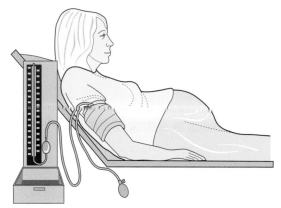

Fig. 2.11 Blood pressure measurement.

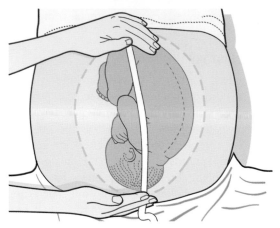

Fig. 2.12 Measurement of symphysis fundal height.

time should be taken to ensure that she is relaxed. The room should be quiet and any tight clothing on her arm removed. The blood pressure should be taken from her right arm, supported at the level of the heart (Fig. 2.11).

An appropriately sized cuff should be used, as too small a cuff will overestimate the blood pressure. The best cuffs have an indication of acceptable arm circumference on them. Ideally, the cuff bladder should cover 80% of the arm circumference and the width of the bladder should be 40% of the arm circumference. Problems occur if the bladder length is <67% (this usually means the arm circumference is >34 cm). In such cases, a large or thigh cuff should be used.

ABDOMINAL PALPATION

Ensure that the woman has privacy and is comfortable and relaxed. Although pregnant women should avoid lying flat on their back for any period of time as this can compress major vessels, the woman should be examined in the recumbent position.

Initially, the abdomen is inspected. During inspection, look for the distended abdomen of pregnancy and note asymmetry, fetal movements and tense stretching. The skin may reveal old or fresh striae gravidarum, a midline pigmented linea nigra and any scars from previous surgery. The most common scars to note are the Pfannenstiel scars of previous pelvic surgery, the small subumbilical and suprapubic scars of laparoscopy, and the gridiron incision of a previous appendicectomy.

The next stage is palpation. This begins with the symphysis fundal height (SFH; Fig. 2.12). The uterus is palpated with the palm of the left hand, moving it upwards and pressing with the lateral border. There is a 'give' at the fundus. Hold the end of a tape measure, measuring side (i.e., centimetre side) down, at the fundus and mark the tape at the upper border of the pubic symphysis.

At 20 weeks' gestation, the uterus comes up to around the umbilicus and the SFH is ~20 cm. Each week, the uterus grows 1 cm so that at 28 weeks it is ~28 ± 2 cm and at 32 weeks it is ~32 ± 2 cm. Metric measurement is therefore a reasonable guide to size for gestation and is useful in identifying those that are large- or small-for-dates.

The next stage is to feel the uterus using gentle pressure with both hands, noting any irregularities, any tender areas, and the two fetal 'poles', head and bottom. The 'lie' of the fetus refers to the axis of the poles in relation to the mother. It is usually longitudinal but can be transverse or oblique. The presentation refers to the part of the baby that is entering the pelvis. Generally, it is the head (cephalic) or the bottom (breech), but it can be the back or limbs (Figs 2.13–2.16). In twins, it should be possible to feel at least three fetal poles.

The 'engagement' of the head refers to how far into the pelvis it has moved (Figs 2.17–2.21). This may be palpated by turning to face the woman's feet and pushing suprapubically, trying to ballot the head between the fingers. The descent can be likened to a setting sun and is recorded as 'fifths palpable'. It is 'engaged'

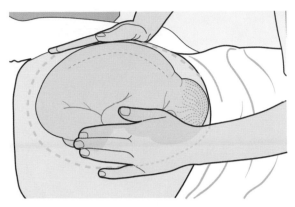

Fig. 2.13 Palpation of the lie and liquor volume.

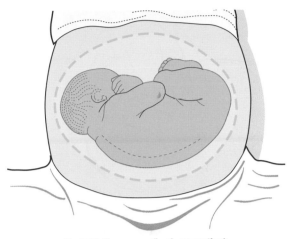

Fig. 2.16 Transverse (back presenting).

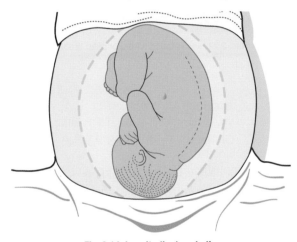

Fig. 2.14 Longitudinal cephalic.

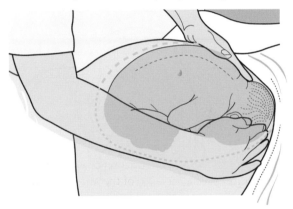

Fig. 2.17 Palpation of the descent of the fetal head.

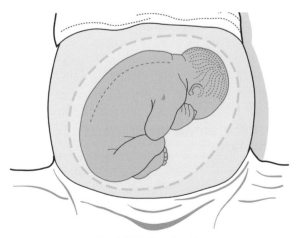

Fig. 2.15 Oblique breech.

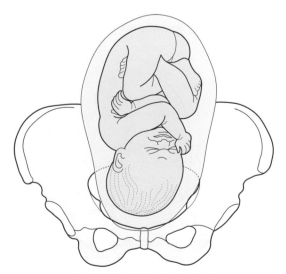

Fig. 2.18 Head 5/5 palpable (free).

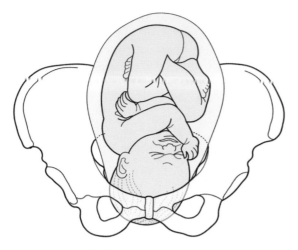

Fig. 2.19 Head 4/5 palpable.

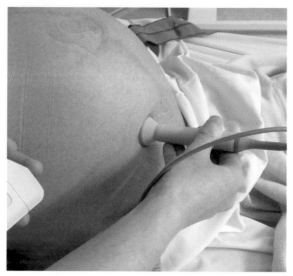

Fig. 2.22 Auscultation with a Doppler probe.

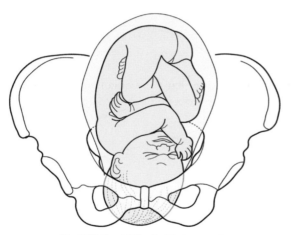

Fig. 2.20 Head 2/5 palpable (engaged).

when the maximum diameter of the fetal head has passed through the pelvic brim. Therefore, at three-fifths (3/5) palpable, it is not engaged but at two-fifths (2/5) palpable, it is.

An attempt should be made to get an impression of the liquor volume, particularly if the SFH is abnormal. In oligohydramnios, fetal parts can often be felt easily; in polyhydramnios, the uterus is usually tense and fetal parts are difficult to feel. Also, feel for the back of the fetus. It is firmer than the limbs (the side of most movements) and lies to one side. This helps work out the position of the fetus and where to pick up the fetal heart. To hear the fetal heart, place a USS transducer over the anterior shoulder of the fetus (Fig. 2.22). The rate should be between 100 and 160 bpm and differentiated clearly from the mother's pulse. At the end of the examination, ensure that the woman is comfortable, cover her abdomen and help her to sit up.

OBSTETRICAL VAGINAL AND SPECULUM EXAMINATION

Speculum and vaginal examination in a pregnant woman should only be performed with a clear clinical indication. Vaginal examination is the cornerstone of intrapartum care. A speculum is used in the diagnosis of antepartum haemorrhage, pre-labour rupture of membranes and to assess pre-labour cervical change.

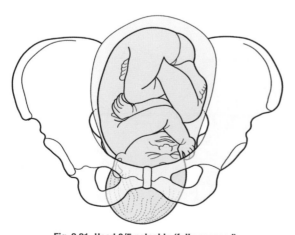

Fig. 2.21 Head 0/5 palpable (fully engaged).

If the diagnosis of pre-term labour or membrane rupture is suspected from the clinical history, a speculum examination is important for three reasons. The first is to look for evidence of liquor in the vagina. The technique is similar to gynaecological speculum examination, with careful aseptic technique. A pool of fluid, sometimes containing white flecks of vernix, can usually be seen in the posterior vagina or coming from the cervix on coughing. The second is to allow swabs to be taken – either looking for pathogenic bacteria – in particular, group B beta-haemolytic streptococci – or to test for fetal fibronectin as part of pre-term labour assessment. The third is to allow a visual inspection of the cervix. Digital examination is used to assess the cervical length/effacement (shortening of the cervix), cervical dilatation and descent and position of the presenting part. Feel for the cervix and note its position. Is it anterior or posterior and difficult to reach? Note its length. The cervix shortens from 3 to 4 cm until it is flush with the fetal head and does not protrude into the vagina. This is called 'effacement'. What is its consistency? Is it soft like a cheek or hard like a nose? Feel for the os and how much it is dilated, as determined by how far the fingers can stretch inside it. This may be only 1 to 2 cm or up to 10 cm at full dilatation. The station of the presenting part is determined relative to the mother's ischial spines. When the biparietal diameter of the fetal head is level with the ischial spines, this is described as station 0. Above this point is −1, −2, etc. When the head is below the ischial spines, it is +1 or +2.

In the early stages of labour and during the induction process, the findings of the cervix can be described using the modified Bishop score (see Table 33.1). As the cervix ripens, it becomes softer, shorter, more anterior and more dilated, and the fetal head descends. As the onset of spontaneous labour approaches, the Bishop score increases.

Key Points

- **Taking a history is never the same for any two women, and many questions will follow from previous answers.**
- **Always ensure that the woman is comfortable and an appropriate chaperone is present during the examination.**

GYNAECOLOGY

Section Outline

Chapter 3

Paediatric Gynaecology and Differences in Sex Development

Cara Williams

Chapter Outline

Introduction

Puberty should transform a girl into a fertile woman. Its social importance is so great that any deviation from normality may be the cause of considerable embarrassment and anxiety. This chapter describes normal puberty and outlines the management of both precocious and delayed puberty. It will also cover some of the gynaecological conditions which may affect pre- and post-pubertal girls.

Normal Puberty

PATHOPHYSIOLOGY OF NORMAL PUBERTY

The onset of pubertal development is heralded by an increase in pulsatile release of gonadotrophin-releasing hormone (GnRH) from the hypothalamus. Following brief activation of the GnRH neurons in the neonatal period, they remain in a dormant state until the onset of puberty. Initially, the pulsatile release of GnRH occurs only at night. However, as puberty progresses, it occurs throughout the day and night. Pulsatile GnRH release causes gonadotropic cells of the anterior pituitary to release luteinizing hormone (LH) and follicle-stimulating hormone (FSH). These gonadotrophins lead to the production of ovarian estrogen, which initiates the physical changes of puberty.

PUBERTAL DEVELOPMENT

The external signs of puberty usually (but not always) occur in a specific order (Fig. 3.1) and are described in five Tanner stages (Figs. 3.2 and 3.3). Breast development (thelarche) is usually the first sign of puberty. Pubic and axillary hair (pubarche) normally develops about 6 months later, although in one-third of girls' pubic hair may appear before breast development. Breast development occurs as a result of rising estradiol levels, and pubic and axillary hair by adrenal androgen secretion. Menarche occurs late in puberty, normally corresponding to the end of the growth spurt. Maximal growth velocity usually occurs after the start of breast and pubic and axillary hair development. However, in some girls, the growth spurt may be the first sign of puberty. The complete process of puberty is usually a slow progression, taking a minimum of 18 months.

During puberty, the ovaries enlarge and develop multifollicular cysts under the influence of pulsatile gonadotrophin secretion. The uterus also grows steadily through puberty. Due to the relative immaturity of the hypothalamic–pituitary–ovarian axis in the first 2 years following menarche, more than half of menstrual cycles are anovulatory, resulting in irregular cycles. After the first 1 to 2 years, the capacity for estrogen-positive feedback on the anterior pituitary develops with the subsequent mid-cycle LH surge and ovulation, resulting in regulation of the menstrual cycle. Anovulatory cycles are often heavy and prolonged, with some girls bleeding for several weeks at a time. This can lead to iron-deficiency anaemia and, in very rare cases, cardiovascular collapse requiring admission and blood transfusion. Initial anovulatory cycles tend to be pain free, although heavy menstrual loss can result in an element of dysmenorrhoea. When regular ovulatory cycles commence, the periods often become more painful due to the increased levels of circulating prostaglandins.

AGE OF MENARCHE

Since the late 19th century, there has been a gradual decline in the age of menarche. In the United Kingdom, the average age of menarche has fallen from 15 years in 1860 to the current average age of 12.3 years. The onset of puberty will range between individuals, with 95% of girls showing signs of secondary sexual characteristics between the ages of 8.5 and 13 years.

Energy reserves and metabolic conditions play an important role in the timing of pubertal development. Leptin, a hormone released by adipose cells, is known to play a critical role in body weight homeostasis and the metabolic control of puberty. Childhood obesity is consistently associated with an early onset of puberty. Factors which delay the attainment of a critical body weight may delay puberty. These include malnutrition, eating disorders, and excessive exercise.

Variations of Normal Puberty

Premature adrenarche is the secretion of adrenal androgens resulting in the appearance of pubic hair before the age of 8 years. Axillary hair, body odour and acne may occur, but other secondary sexual characteristics do not. It can be slowly progressive or stay stable, and puberty usually begins at the normal time. Serum androgen concentrations may be slightly raised or normal. Gonadotrophin levels are pre-pubertal and bone age is normal.

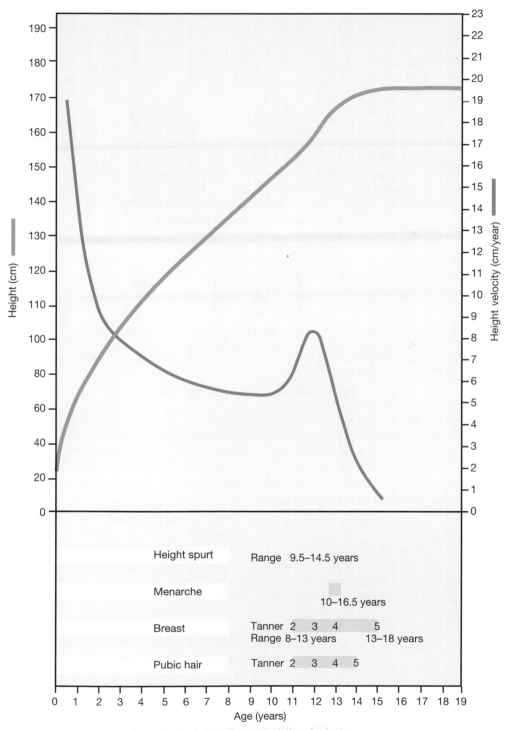

Fig. 3.1 Schematic representation of puberty.

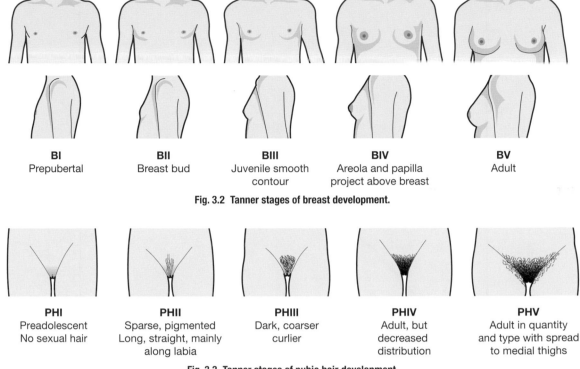

| **BI**
Prepubertal | **BII**
Breast bud | **BIII**
Juvenile smooth
contour | **BIV**
Areola and papilla
project above breast | **BV**
Adult |

Fig. 3.2 Tanner stages of breast development.

| **PHI**
Preadolescent
No sexual hair | **PHII**
Sparse, pigmented
Long, straight, mainly
along labia | **PHIII**
Dark, coarser
curlier | **PHIV**
Adult, but
decreased
distribution | **PHV**
Adult in quantity
and type with spread
to medial thighs |

Fig. 3.3 Tanner stages of pubic hair development.

Premature thelarche is defined as the premature development of breast tissue in the absence of other secondary sexual characteristics before the age of 8 years. The most common age of onset is within the first 2 years of life but can occur at any age. Progression to precocious puberty can occur in up to a third of girls.

Isolated premature menarche is the occurrence of vaginal bleeding in the absence of other secondary sexual characteristics. It is a diagnosis of exclusion after vaginal and uterine pathology, foreign body, and precocious puberty have been ruled out. It can be an isolated event or it can recur. Puberty will be expected to start at the normal time and final adult height will not be affected.

Precocious Puberty

The development of secondary sexual characteristics prior to the age of 8 years in girls constitutes precocious puberty and must be investigated. Central (gonadotrophin-dependent) precocious puberty occurs when there is a pituitary or hypothalamic cause. Peripheral (gonadotrophin-independent) precocious puberty occurs when puberty is induced by sex steroids from other causes, such as a hormone-secreting tumour. The growth spurt is a striking feature, but frequently it is the occurrence of menstruation which brings the girl to medical attention. In the event of vaginal bleeding, a local cause—such as a foreign body or malignancy—should always be ruled out. Children with precocious puberty should be under the care of a paediatric endocrinologist.

CAUSES OF PRECOCIOUS PUBERTY

Gonadotrophic-Dependent Precocious Puberty (GDPP)

In 90% of girls with GDPP, no cause is found. In the remaining 10%, causes are intracranial and include encephalitis, meningitis, cranial radiation, hydrocephaly, and space-occupying neoplasms, such as optic nerve gliomas. Sexual abuse has been reported as a precipitating cause.

Gonadotrophic-Independent Precocious Puberty (GIPP)

Causes of GIPP include feminising tumours of the ovary or adrenal, which may give rise to vaginal bleeding without signs of pubertal development. Other causes include hypothyroidism, and the very rare McCune–Albright syndrome, in which cystic cavities develop in the long bones (polyostotic fibrous dysplasia) and café-au-lait skin pigmentation is evident. Estrogen-secreting cysts are found in the ovaries on ultrasound. Other rare causes include ingestion of exogenous estrogens.

INVESTIGATION OF PRECOCIOUS PUBERTY

1. Plasma FSH, LH, estradiol, and thyroid function tests
2. X-ray of the hand to determine bone age, which may be advanced
3. Ultrasound scan of the abdomen and pelvis
4. Radiological skeletal survey of the long bones if McCune–Albright syndrome is suspected
5. Cranial magnetic resonance imaging (MRI) scan.

In the constitutional and cerebral forms, the ovaries may show a multicystic appearance on ultrasound as seen in normal puberty. Ultrasound will also distinguish between a follicular cyst, which will be expected to subside spontaneously, and a predominantly solid estrogen-secreting granulosa/theca cell tumour of the ovary, which will require surgical removal.

CARE OF CHILDREN WITH PRECOCIOUS PUBERTY

With precocious puberty the aims of treatment are to:
1. Suppress menstruation and prevent progression of puberty
2. Maximise growth potential and
3. Achieve psychological well-being.

Not all children need treatment, as symptoms may only be slowly progressive. Treatment prevents progression but does not usually reverse changes that have already happened. If an underlying aetiology is found, this should be treated.

GnRH agonists suppress gonadotrophin secretion. Depot injections are given every 3 months and treatment can be continued for 2 to 3 years without significant side effects. Treatment is stopped when an acceptable age for puberty is reached.

Delayed Puberty

Delayed puberty in girls is defined as the absence of physical manifestations of puberty by the age of 13 years. Primary amenorrhoea is the absence of menarche and needs to be evaluated in the context of secondary sexual characteristics. The diagnosis may be made by age 15 years if a patient has normal secondary sexual characteristics or if menarche has failed to occur by 2 years post breast budding. In some instances, a girl may enter puberty but the normal progression is not maintained. This is described as 'arrested puberty'.

CAUSES OF DELAYED PUBERTY

These features of delayed puberty fall into three main categories (Table 3.1).

Constitutional Delay

Constitutional delay is the most common cause of delayed puberty. These girls are normal but just inherently late at entering puberty. They are usually of short stature, but their height is generally appropriate for their bone age. All stages of development are delayed. They may be considered to be physiologically immature, with a functional deficiency of GnRH for their chronological age but not for their stage of physiological development. There is frequently a history of delayed menarche in their mothers.

In these patients, bone age shows a better correlation with the onset and progression of puberty than does chronological age. On attaining a bone age of 11 to 13 years, they can be expected to enter puberty.

TABLE 3.1 **Differential Features of Delayed Puberty**				
	Stature	Gonadotrophins	Gonadal steroids	Karyotype
Constitutional delay	Short	Pre-pubertal	Low	Normal
Hypogonadotrophic hypogonadism	Normal	Low	Low	Normal
Primary gonadal failure:				
Turner syndrome and variants	Short	High	Low	XO and variants
Gonadal dysgenesis	Normal/tall	High	Low	XX or XY

Hypogonadotrophic Hypogonadism

This is caused by the deficient production, secretion, or action of GnRH. It may be associated with:

- Conditions affecting body weight, such as chronic systemic disease, malnutrition or anorexia nervosa.
- Central nervous system tumours—the most common of these rare conditions is craniopharyngioma. Girls may also have associated growth hormone deficiency and, therefore, short stature.
- Isolated gonadotrophin deficiency. Such patients are generally of appropriate height for chronological age. The association of hypogonadotrophic hypogonadism with anosmia or hyposmia is called Kallmann syndrome, which results from incomplete embryonic migration of GnRH-synthesising neurons. This occurs in 50% of cases.

Premature Ovarian Insufficiency (POI)

POI is defined by the loss of ovarian activity before the age of 40 years. If this happens at a young age, puberty will not occur. There are various different causes of POI, including:

- Autoimmune disease (this may also be associated with autoimmune thyroid and adrenal disease)
- Chromosomal disorders (Turner syndrome and Fragile X carrier status)
- Chemotherapy or radiotherapy for a childhood malignancy, as a result of germ cell damage
- Metabolic disorders, such as galactossaemia
- Surgical—bilateral oophorectomy.

Other Causes

These include hyperprolactinaemia and hypothyroidism. Differences in sex development may also present with delayed puberty. This is discussed in more detail later.

INVESTIGATION OF DELAYED OR ARRESTED PUBERTY

The scheme of investigation follows logically from the differential diagnosis discussed previously:

1. Plasma FSH, LH, estradiol, prolactin, and thyroid function tests
2. Karyotype
3. X-ray for bone age
4. Pelvic ultrasound scan
5. Cranial MRI scan.

Care of Children with Delayed Puberty

Constitutional Delay

Often, reassurance and continued observation are sufficient. It is important to reassure the parents as well as the girl herself. Where psychological problems arise as a result of comparison with her peers, induction of puberty may be indicated.

Hypogonadotrophic Hypogonadism

In those with low weight, restoration of weight may result in spontaneous onset of puberty. Those with central nervous system tumours require appropriate neurosurgical treatment. Induction of puberty is required, and treatment with hormone replacement is continued until approximately age 50 years, although 10% to 20% will have spontaneous return of reproductive function.

Premature Ovarian Insufficiency (POI)

Induction of puberty is required, and hormone replacement is continued until approximately age 50 years. Pregnancy can be achieved through in vitro fertilization (IVF) with ovum donation.

Spontaneous ovulation can occur in this group, with a pregnancy risk of approximately 5%.

Induction of Puberty

The aim is to ensure normal progress through puberty. This is achieved by incremental doses of estrogen, preferably transdermal 17β-estradiol. A low dose of estrogen is commenced and increased gradually over approximately 2 to 3 years in order to maximise breast development. After 2 to 3 years of estrogen therapy, or after the first menstrual bleed, a progestogen is added to avoid unopposed estrogenic stimulation of the endometrium. Commonly, hormone replacement therapy is used, but the combined contraceptive pill is an alternative, preferably on a continuous basis to maximise estrogen replacement. Bone mineral density should be assessed every 3 to 5 years. Vitamin D and calcium levels should also be optimised.

Pre-Pubertal Conditions

VAGINAL DISCHARGE

Vaginal discharge is one of the most common reasons for referral to a paediatric gynaecology clinic. The most frequent age of referral is 3 to 10 years. Non-specific vulvovaginitis is the most common cause. Positive low vaginal swabs are only found in approximately 20%. Vaginal cultures are often non-specific, but organisms commonly found in the rectum or upper respiratory tract are often found, such as group A *Streptococcus* or *Haemophilus influenzae*. Symptoms include discharge, soreness, and itching, all of which can be chronic and distressing.

Contributory aetiological factors include the hypo-estrogenic state and neutral pH of the pre-pubertal vagina, proximity of the vagina and anus, under-developed flat labia, and hygiene. Rarer causes, such as a foreign body or tumour, must be excluded if symptoms are persistent. Sexual abuse should always be considered but is not the cause in the majority of cases. Vulval hygiene, with the avoidance of soaps in the genital area and the use of emollients, is the cornerstone of successful management. Threadworms can lead to genital irritation, particularly at night; thus, empirical treatment could also be tried.

VAGINAL BLEEDING

Vaginal bleeding in the pre-pubertal girl always needs specialist referral and may require examination under anaesthesia (vaginoscopy and cystoscopy) to rule out local causes such as a foreign body or malignancy. Hormone profile, bone age, and pelvic ultrasound should also be performed to look for precocious puberty.

LABIAL ADHESIONS

Labial adhesions occur due to the hypo-estrogenic state of the pre-pubertal genitalia. The labia minora fuse together in the midline. There may be a small opening or there may be no visible opening (Fig. 3.4). Typically, the labia are apart at birth due to the effect of maternal estrogens. They then fuse after a few months. Usually, they are asymptomatic, but occasionally urine can get trapped behind them, causing post-void dribbling or even urinary tract infections. In most cases, no treatment other than emollients is required and the parents can be reassured that the adhesions will open up as the girl progresses through puberty. In cases in which there are significant urinary symptoms or for maternal reassurance, a low-dose estrogen ointment can be applied to the adhesions twice daily for 6 weeks. This can cause some breast budding, which will usually disappear after treatment finishes,

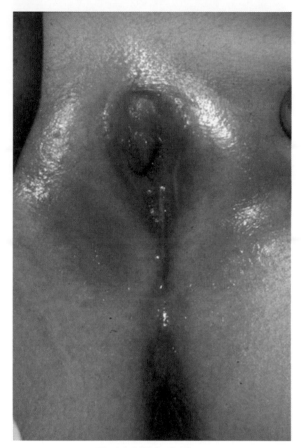

Fig. 3.4 Labial adhesions.

and the labial adhesions often reoccur. Good hygiene and use of emollients can help to prevent recurrence. In very rare cases, the labia may need to be separated under general anaesthetic.

LICHEN SCLEROSUS

Lichen sclerosus is an inflammatory skin condition that occurs in postmenopausal women and pre-pubertal girls. It can affect any part of the body, but it most frequently occurs on the genitalia. It can cause itching and discomfort, which can be quite severe. White plaques occur typically in a figure-of-eight pattern around the vulva and anus. There may also be areas of superficial haemorrhage, thickening of the skin, and fissures (Fig. 3.5). Diagnosis is usually made by the typical appearance, and biopsies are rarely required. Treatment is with a potent steroid ointment in a reducing regime over 3 months. Once it clears

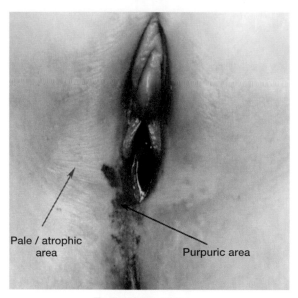

Pale / atrophic area

Purpuric area

Fig. 3.5 Lichen sclerosus.

up, it may not recur or it may flare intermittently; it will usually (but not always) resolve when the girl goes through puberty. If there are frequent recurrences, the steroid-sparing agent tacrolimus may be required. In severe cases, systemic immunosuppressant treatment may be required. Unlike lichen sclerosus in postmenopausal women, parents can be reassured that the risk of malignancy is extremely low.

Post-Pubertal Conditions

ADOLESCENT MENSTRUAL DYSFUNCTION

Menstrual disorders are common in adolescent girls. In up to 25% of girls, this can be quite significant, affecting daily life and resulting in school absence. However, serious pathology is rare. Periods can be irregular, heavy, and/or painful, especially in the first few years following menarche. There are many treatment options that are safe to use in adolescents, although the evidence for their use is extrapolated from adult data.

- Tranexamic acid. This is an antifibrinolytic taken during menstruation, which can reduce blood loss by up to 50%.
- Mefenamic acid. This is a non-steroidal anti-inflammatory that inhibits prostaglandin synthetase. It should be taken regularly, starting the day before menstruation, and can be very effective for dysmenorrhea. It can also reduce blood flow by up to 20%.
- Contraceptive pill. This can be used as first-line management of irregular, heavy, and painful periods. It can reduce blood loss by over 40% and reduce menstrual cramping by 50%. The combined contraceptive pill tends to give the best cycle control. However, the progestogen-only contraceptive pill can also be used, although this can result in irregular bleeding. The combined pill can be used cyclically, tri-cyclically or on a continuous basis. For girls who are troubled with acne, a more anti-androgenic pill would be appropriate.
- Oral progestogens. These are commonly used for adolescent menstrual dysfunction. They can be taken continuously to defer or delay menstruation or cyclically to improve irregular and heavy periods. They should be taken for 21 days, with a 1-week break for menstruation. They have been found to reduce blood loss by over 80%.
- Levonorgestrel-releasing intrauterine system (e.g., Mirena). This is a T-shaped plastic frame that sits in the uterine cavity and releases a small amount of progestogen each day. It can be very useful when first-line treatments have failed or when there are medical contraindications to the use of the contraceptive pill. It can be safely used from menarche onwards and lasts for 5 years. In girls who have never been sexually active, it needs to be inserted and removed under general anaesthetic. It is very effective for both heavy and painful periods. Bleeding can be irregular for the first 3 to 6 months, but by 12 months the majority will be amenorrhoeic.

Müllerian Duct Anomalies

DEVELOPMENT OF THE GENITAL TRACT

The Müllerian ducts begin to develop during the sixth week of embryonic development. The two ducts develop caudally and medially; they then fuse in the midline to create the fallopian tubes, uterus, cervix, and upper vagina. The Wolffian ducts regress at around 10 weeks' gestation due to the absence of testosterone. The urogenital sinus forms by week 7. Cells proliferate from the upper portion of the urogenital sinus to form sinovaginal bulbs. These fuse to form the vaginal plate, which extends from the Müllerian ducts to the urogenital sinus. This plate begins to canalize, starting at the hymen, and proceeds upwards to the cervix. This process is complete by 21 weeks' gestation. (See Chapter 40, Human Embryology, for more details.) The Müllerian duct develops in close proximity to the kidneys. Therefore, if a Müllerian anomaly is identified, the renal tract should always be assessed.

Imperforate Hymen

The hymen is a thin membrane that covers the vaginal opening until late fetal life. It becomes perforate towards term. The incidence of imperforate hymen is approximately 1:1000 live female births. Presentation is usually with increasing cyclical abdominal pain in the absence of menstruation, towards the end of puberty. There may be a palpable abdominal mass and, on gently parting the labia, there may be a visible blue bulging membrane (Fig. 3.6). Ultrasound will show a large haematocolpos, where the vagina is filled with blood. Treatment is with incision and resection of the hymen. If the hymen is not resected, there is a risk of re-obstruction. However, care must be taken not to resect too close to the vaginal mucosa, which may lead to scarring and stenosis at the vaginal introitus.

Transverse Vaginal Septa

A transverse vaginal septum (Fig. 3.7) results from a failure of canalization of the vaginal plate where the urogenital sinus meets the Müllerian duct. They can be perforate and present difficulties with tampons or sex, or they can be imperforate and present with obstructed menstruation. They can vary in thickness and location within the vagina. On external genital examination, the vaginal opening may look normal. An ultrasound will reveal a haematocolpos. MRI of the pelvis is essential in order to assess location and thickness of the septum for preoperative planning. Transverse vaginal septa should be referred to a specialist surgeon. Treatment involves surgical resection of the septum with anastomosis of the proximal and distal vaginas. Septa can be resected vaginally, laparoscopically, or via an abdomino-perineal approach depending on the classification of the septum. Pregnancy outcomes for low, thin septa are very good. Abdomino-perineal procedures often involve complex reconstructive surgery. Therefore, long-term complications are more common and pregnancy outcomes are poor.

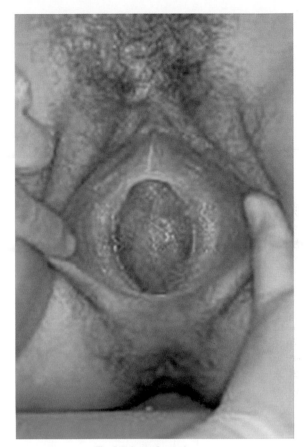

Fig. 3.6 Imperforate hymen.

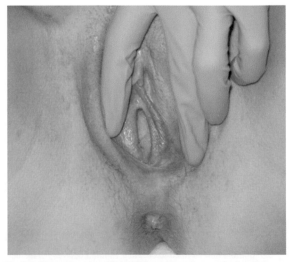

Fig. 3.7 Haematometrocolpos with a transverse vaginal septum.

Longitudinal Vaginal Septa

Longitudinal vaginal septa result from a failure of canalization of the vaginal plate. Septa can be complete, extending from the cervix to the introitus, or they can be partial, involving any part of the vagina. They often present with dyspareunia, difficulty with tampons, or they may be diagnosed during labour. Over 85% of longitudinal vaginal septa are associated with a uterine anomaly, most commonly a complete septate uterus or uterus didelphys. When there are two separate uteri, one hemivagina can be obstructed, resulting in increasing pain despite normal menstruation. This can be associated with renal anomalies, as in obstructed hemivagina and ipsilateral renal anomaly syndrome (OHVIRA). Longitudinal vaginal septa can be resected vaginally.

Mayer-Rokitansky-Küster-Hauser (MRKH) Syndrome

This results from interrupted development and failure of fusion of the Müllerian ducts. There is an absent uterus or rudimentary uterine buds, with vaginal agenesis. It affects 1 in 4500 females. Ovarian function is normal; thus, it presents with primary amenorrhoea with normal secondary sexual characteristics. Diagnosis is usually made by clinical examination and ultrasound assessment. MRI can be used if there is diagnostic uncertainty. It is possible to create a vagina with regular use of vaginal dilators (Fig. 3.8). This is successful in approximately 85% of cases. If dilation is unsuccessful, vaginas can be created surgically with a laparoscopic Vecchietti procedure (traction vaginoplasty) or with the use of extravaginal tissues such as bowel. Options for fertility include surrogacy (using their own eggs through IVF) and adoption. Uterine transplants are being trialled in several countries; although they are still experimental, they are an exciting possibility for the future. Psychological input is essential in the management of girls with MRKH syndrome.

UTERINE ANOMALIES

Abnormal uterine shapes (Fig. 3.9) are usually asymptomatic but may present with menorrhagia, primary infertility, recurrent pregnancy loss, pre-term

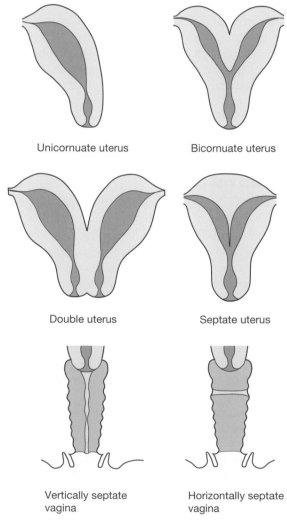

Unicornuate uterus   Bicornuate uterus

Double uterus   Septate uterus

Vertically septate vagina   Horizontally septate vagina

Fig. 3.9 Common genital tract anomalies.

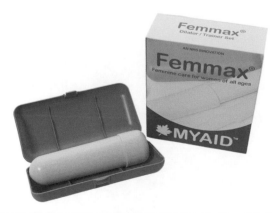

Fig. 3.8 Dilators can be used to create a vagina. (Courtesy of Medical Devices Technology International Ltd.)

labour, or abnormal fetal lie. There is no place for surgery with a unicornuate uterus, bicornuate uterus, or uterus didelphys. If there is a non-communicating obstructed horn, this will need to be removed laparoscopically. Pregnancy in a rudimentary horn carries a risk of rupture and significant haemorrhage. If a uterine septum is associated with infertility or recurrent pregnancy loss, surgical resection can be considered. Cervical agenesis is a very rare anomaly, which presents with obstructed menstruation. Management is with laparoscopic uterovaginal anastomosis.

Differences in Sex Development (DSD)

DSD are a group of conditions in which the development of chromosomal, gonadal, or anatomical sex is atypical. The incidence of DSD is estimated to be in the region of 1 in 4500 births. Presentation can vary from atypical genitalia at birth, discordance between prenatal karyotype and phenotype at birth, inguinal hernias in childhood, delayed puberty, primary amenorrhoea or virilisation at puberty, or it may be diagnosed following a diagnosis in a sibling. The term 'disorders of sex development' was adopted at a consensus conference in 2006. However, it has not been universally accepted by some patients and support groups. Negative aspects of the term DSD include the stigma of having a 'disorder', and the perception that 'sex' implies sexual behaviour. The terms 'differences in sex development' and 'diverse sex development' are now preferred.

NORMAL GONADAL AND GENITAL TRACT DEVELOPMENT

The primordial gonads appear during the sixth week of development. Müllerian and Wolffian ducts also begin to develop at this stage. Presence of the SRY gene (sex-determining region of the Y chromosome) in XY embryos stimulates testicular development. Testes produce testosterone, which results in development of the Wolffian structures (the vas deferens, seminal vesicles and epididymis). Peripheral conversion of testosterone to dihydrotestosterone (DHT) requires the enzyme 5-alpha-reductase and causes virilisation of the external genitalia. At 12 weeks, the fetus is recognisably male and masculinization of the genitalia is said to be complete by 14 weeks. The penis, similar in size to the clitoris at 14 weeks, enlarges from

around 20 weeks until birth. The testes also produce anti-Müllerian hormone (AMH), which causes regression of the Müllerian ducts. Ovarian development was previously considered a 'default' development due to the absence of SRY. However, regulatory gene networks are now known to be involved. In the XX gonad, ovarian development is promoted and testicular development inhibited by the expression of specific embryonic genes. The ovarian cortex develops at 12 weeks and by 13.5 weeks primordial follicles are present. The Wolffian structures regress at around 10 weeks due to the absence of testosterone. As AMH is not produced, the Müllerian ducts develop and, in the absence of testosterone, female external genitalia develop, as previously described. (See also Chapter 40, Human Embryology.)

TURNER SYNDROME

Turner syndrome results from a complete or partial absence of one X chromosome. It is the most common chromosomal anomaly in females, occurring in 1 out of 2500 female births. Clinical features associated with Turner syndrome include:

- Short stature
- POI and infertility
- Autoimmune thyroid disease (hypothyroidism)
- Diabetes
- Inflammatory bowel disease
- Sensorineural and conduction deafness
- Renal anomalies
- Cardiovascular disease, both structural (e.g., aortic root dilatation, bicuspid aortic valve, and coarctation) and atherosclerosis
- Hypertension
- Osteoporosis.

The most common chromosome complement in Turner syndrome is monosomy 45,X or the presence of an abnormal X chromosome such as isochromosome X, a partial deletion, or a ring X. Mosaicism is also common and includes 45,X/46,XX, 45,X/46,XY, and 45XO/47XXX. An accurate karyotype is important, as it allows some prediction of clinical severity. Ring karyotype is associated with a more severe phenotype; mosaics generally have a milder phenotype, with up to 40% entering spontaneous puberty. If there is a Y chromosome or fragment of a Y chromosome present, then there is a higher incidence of gonadal tumours and the streak gonads should be removed prophylactically. This can be done laparoscopically.

Although the majority of individuals with Turner syndrome are diagnosed during childhood or adolescence, about 10% are not diagnosed until adulthood. The focus of paediatric care is on short stature, whereas adult women are generally more concerned with estrogen replacement and fertility prospects. Pregnancy is possible; however, in general, ovum donation and IVF are required. Pre-pregnancy counselling is essential and women should be looked after in a high-risk antenatal clinic. Aortic root dissection can be catastrophic in pregnant women with Turner syndrome.

Women with Turner syndrome should be looked after by clinicians experienced in this condition and regular monitoring for associated problems is essential.

46,XX DSD

Congenital Adrenal Hyperplasia (CAH)

CAH is the most common DSD, with an incidence of 1 in 14,000 worldwide. It usually presents with atypical genitalia in the neonate. The name is derived from hyperplasia in the adrenal gland, which arises from the overproduction of steroids (Fig. 3.10). Affected individuals have an enzyme block in the steroidogenic pathway in the adrenal gland, with over 90% being a deficiency in 21-hydroxylase. This enzyme converts progesterone to deoxycorticosterone in the aldosterone biosynthetic pathway, and 17-hydroxyprogesterone (17-OHP) to deoxycortisol in the cortisol biosynthetic pathway. The resultant low levels of cortisol continue to drive the negative feedback loop, leading to increased levels of androgen precursors and, in turn, to elevated testosterone production. 17-OHP levels can be used in the diagnosis and in monitoring control.

Excessive testosterone levels in a female fetus will lead to virilization of the external genitalia. The clitoris is enlarged and the labia are fused and scrotal in appearance. The upper vagina joins the male-type urethra and opens as one common channel onto the perineum. The chromosomes are XX and the ovaries are normal, as are the internal structures, including the fallopian tubes, uterus, and upper vagina.

Approximately 75% of children with 21-hydroxylase deficiency CAH will have a 'salt-losing' variety, which affects the ability to produce aldosterone. This represents a life-threatening situation—those children who are salt-losers often become dangerously unwell within a few days of birth. Affected individuals require lifelong steroid replacement, such as hydrocortisone, along with fludrocortisone for salt-losers. Both under- and over-treatment may result in short stature, and girls may have oligomenorrhoea or amenorrhoea, leading to fertility difficulties.

Traditional management was with feminising genital surgery during the first year of life to reduce the size of the clitoris and open up the lower vagina. However, childhood clitoral surgery can reduce clitoral sensation and be detrimental to adult sexual function. In addition, vaginal surgery usually needs revising at adolescence, often involving very complex surgery with associated risks. Vaginal surgery is much more successful when performed after puberty, when

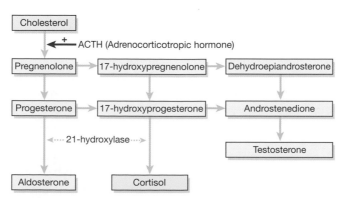

Fig. 3.10 Synthesis of steroid hormones. Deficiency of the enzyme 21-hydroxylase leads to a build-up of precursors, particularly the weak androgens dehydroepiandrosterone and androstenedione.

the tissues are estrogenised. Delaying genital surgery until adolescence or adulthood also allows the girl to be fully informed and involved in the decision-making process. Psychological support for the parents and child is imperative.

CAH is an autosomal-recessive condition and molecular genetics now allows prenatal diagnosis in families where an affected child has already been born. Prenatal therapy is possible with dexamethasone, as this crosses the placenta and should reduce the drive mediated by low cortisol levels. However, there are concerns about the effect of antenatal steroid treatment on the neurodevelopment of the child; research into this is ongoing.

46,XY DSD

Complete Androgen Insensitivity Syndrome (CAIS)

CAIS is the most frequently occurring 46,XY DSD, with an incidence of 1 in 40,000 births. CAIS is due to an abnormality of the androgen receptor, which is completely or partially unable to respond to androgen stimulation. In a fetus with CAIS, testes form normally due to the action of the SRY gene. These testes secrete AMH, leading to regression of the Müllerian ducts. CAIS women, therefore, do not have a uterus. Testosterone is also produced; however, due to the inability of the androgen receptor to respond, the external genitalia do not virilise and instead undergo female development. The result is a female (both physically and psychologically) with no uterus, and testes are found at some point in their line of descent through the abdomen from the pelvis to the inguinal canal. During puberty, breast development will be normal due to the aromatisation of testosterone to estrogen. However, the effects of androgens are not seen, and pubic and axillary hair growth is minimal. Around two-thirds of women with CAIS have inherited the androgen receptor gene mutation from their mother (i.e., X-linked inheritance), with the remaining one-third thought to be new mutations.

The most common presentation is with primary amenorrhoea, although children can also present before puberty with an inguinal hernia found to contain a testis. The diagnosis is made on clinical examination, with typical findings in association with an XY karyotype, and a pathogenic variant in the androgen receptor (AR) gene on a DSD panel. Psychological support is the initial mainstay of treatment, with full disclosure of diagnosis, including karyotype. Well-organised patient peer support groups have a valuable role.

Gonadectomy is usually recommended post-puberty due to the small risk of malignancy associated with intra-abdominal testes. After gonadectomy, estrogen replacement is necessary to maintain bone mineral density and general well-being. The vagina is blind-ending and usually short. Vaginal dilation has good success rates in creating a vagina adequate for intercourse and reconstructive vaginal surgery is rarely required.

Ongoing psychological input from a suitably trained professional who has clinical experience with DSD is a vital part of long-term management.

Partial forms of androgen insensitivity also occur, leading to a spectrum of clinical features. Presentation in this situation is often at birth with atypical genitalia; careful assessment by a specialist multidisciplinary team is required to determine the most appropriate sex of rearing. Due to the spectrum of clinical features, partial androgen insensitivity is a genetic diagnosis. Therefore, a full genetic workup with a DSD panel showing a pathogenic variant in the AR gene is required.

Disorders of Testosterone Biosynthesis

Rarer DSDs include those resulting from a deficiency in any enzyme required in the biosynthesis or metabolism of testosterone. 5-Alpha-reductase converts testosterone to the more active metabolite dihydrotestosterone. Deficiency leads to the development of an undervirilised male (46,XY). The condition is autosomal recessive, and individuals have normal testes. The external genitalia may be atypical or phenotypically female. The majority of individuals are reared as female, although subsequent virilisation may occur at puberty if the gonads have not been removed. Virilisation can often be quite profound and irreversible. Fertility has been reported in those reared as male, but they are generally considered infertile.

17-Beta hydroxysteroid dehydrogenase deficiency occurs when there is an absence or reduction of the enzyme converting androstenedione to testosterone. This condition is autosomal recessive, and results in a 46,XY individual with atypical or phenotypically female genitalia. Virilisation occurs at puberty.

In both of these conditions, the girl can decide to stay in the female gender, change to the male gender, or stay gender neutral. Initial management is with GnRH analogues to suppress pubertal development until they can make fully informed decisions about their management. Psychological support along with multidisciplinary team involvement is imperative in helping them to make these difficult decisions.

Ovotesticular DSD

Ovotesticular DSD is the **rarest** DSD, with an incidence of less than 1:20,000. It refers to the presence of both ovarian and testicular tissue in the same individual. The karyotype is 46,XX in over 70% of cases and the gonads may be a separate ovary and/or testes, and/or an ovotestis. The external genital appearance may be atypical, with Müllerian and Wolffian structures present internally. Asymmetry of gonads and subsequent reproductive tracts and external genitalia may occur. Fertility may be possible depending upon karyotype and phenotype. Ovotesticular DSD is diagnosed via a combination of karyotype, DSD panel, hormone profile, ultrasound, or MRI and sometimes gonadal biopsy.

Complete Gonadal Dysgenesis

This condition is also known as Swyer syndrome. The chromosomes are XY but the gonads are streak and do not function. A total of 10% to 20% of women with this syndrome have a deletion in the DNA-binding region of the *SRY* gene. Nevertheless, in approximately 80% to 90% of cases, the *SRY* gene is normal and mutations in other testis-determining factors are probably implicated. As the gonads are dysgenetic, no testosterone or AMH is produced and development is phenotypically female. The external genitalia are unambiguously female at birth and the uterus, vagina, and fallopian tubes are normal. The condition usually first becomes apparent in adolescence with delayed puberty and amenorrhoea. Women are often taller than may have been expected. A high incidence of gonadoblastoma and germ cell malignancies in the dysgenetic gonad has been reported. Current practice is to proceed to a gonadectomy once the diagnosis is made. Management is otherwise in line with other cases of POI and involves induction of puberty with estrogen in order to develop secondary sexual characteristics and long-term combined hormone replacement therapy with estrogen and progestogen. Pregnancy is possible with ovum donation and IVF.

Summary

All individuals with a DSD should be managed by a multidisciplinary team, including an endocrinologist, psychologist, urologist, gynaecologist, and geneticist. Careful clinical assessment is essential and is supported by specialist imaging as well as biochemical and genetic investigation. For newborns with DSD, the decision must be taken as to the most appropriate sex of rearing. Factors taken into consideration will include diagnosis, clinical findings, future fertility potential, and the opinions of the family. If the diagnosis is made later in childhood or at adolescence, the sex of rearing is already determined and is not usually reassigned, unless there is virilisation at puberty. The diagnosis of CAH in a neonate is a medical emergency due to the risk of a salt-losing crisis. However, the allocation of sex of rearing should not be rushed into and birth registration can be deferred until a decision has been made.

Early psychological input provided by a specialist clinical psychologist with experience in supporting people with DSD conditions and their parents is essential. This will enable them to explore their emotions and concerns, manage the period of uncertainty during the diagnostic process, facilitate informed decision-making and help with disclosure at an age-appropriate level. All adolescents with a newly diagnosed DSD or existing DSD requiring medical or surgical attention should also be routinely offered clinical psychology input.

CONTROVERSIES

The most controversial aspect of management is the role of feminising genital surgery in children with atypical genitalia assigned to a female sex of rearing. Parents can be very worried about the immediate appearance and find it difficult to look at the long-term issues. It is important that parents and clinicians are aware of the impact on future sexual function when making a decision about irreversible genital surgery for the child. As previously discussed, surgical decisions must be made in the context of a multidisciplinary team. Psychological support throughout this decision-making process for both the parents and child is imperative.

Key points

- Delayed puberty, the absence of physical manifestations of puberty by the age of 13 years, is most commonly a variant of normality referred to as 'constitutional delay'. It may, however, be caused by hypogonadotrophic hypogonadism, Turner syndrome, or gonadal dysgenesis. Gonadotrophin levels and a karyotype should be performed.
- Precocious puberty, the appearance of signs of sexual maturation prior to the age of 8 years, may be idiopathic but is also associated with intracranial lesions, feminising tumours, and the very rare McCune–Albright syndrome. Vaginal bleeding in a pre-pubertal girl should always be investigated.
- Adolescent menstrual dysfunction is common and can be severe enough to affect daily life, but serious pathology is rare.
- If an adolescent girl presents with obstructed menstruation and haematocolpos, and there is not a blue bulge on examination, it is likely to be a transverse vaginal septum. In this case, further imaging with MRI and specialist referral is required.
- If a Müllerian anomaly is found, always assess the renal tract.
- Development of a male requires a Y chromosome, testosterone production, and functioning androgen receptors.
- DSD are a group of conditions in which the development of chromosomal, gonadal, or anatomical sex is atypical.
- Presentation of a DSD can be at birth or during childhood or adolescence.
- Management of DSD should be undertaken by a multidisciplinary specialist team.

Chapter 4

Menstruation and Amenorrhoea

Sharon Cameron

Chapter Outline

The Menstrual Cycle

OVERVIEW OF THE CYCLE

The endometrial cycle results from the growth and shedding of the uterine lining – the endometrium. This cycle, the average duration of which is 28 days, is controlled by the hormones from the ovary and consists of a follicular phase, ovulation, and a post-ovulatory (or luteal) phase. During the follicular phase, the endometrium thickens (proliferative phase of the endometrium). After ovulation, endometrial growth stops and the endometrial glands become active and full of secretions (the secretory phase of the endometrium). If the cycle is prolonged, the follicular phase lengthens (longer time to ovulation), but the luteal phase remains constant at 14 days. Fundamental to the menstrual cycle are:

- An intact hypothalamic–pituitary–ovarian endocrine axis
- The presence of responsive follicles in the ovaries
- The presence of a responsive endometrium in the uterus.

Endocrine Control of the Menstrual Cycle

The hypothalamic–pituitary–ovarian axis controls follicular maturation and ovulation (Fig. 4.1). The hypothalamus controls the cycle, but it can itself be influenced by higher centres in the brain, allowing

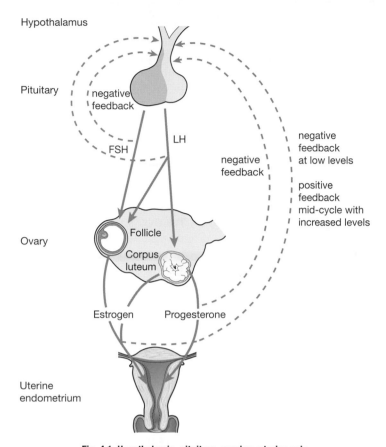

Fig. 4.1 Hypothalamic–pituitary–ovarian–uterine axis.

factors such as anxiety or stress to affect the cycle. The hypothalamus acts on the pituitary gland by secreting gonadotrophin-releasing hormone (GnRH), a decapeptide that is secreted in a pulsatile manner approximately every 90 minutes. GnRH travels through the small blood vessels of the pituitary portal system to the anterior pituitary, where it acts on the pituitary gonadotrophs to stimulate the synthesis and release of follicle-stimulating hormone (FSH) and luteinizing hormone (LH). Although there are two gonadotrophins, there is just a single releasing hormone for both.

FSH is a glycoprotein that stimulates growth of follicles during the 'follicular phase' of the cycle. FSH also stimulates sex hormone secretion, predominantly of estradiol, by the granulosa cells of the mature ovarian follicle.

LH is also a glycoprotein, and it also stimulates sex hormone production (mainly testosterone, which is subsequently converted by the action of FSH into estradiol). LH plays an essential role in ovulation. It is the mid-cycle surge of LH that triggers rupture of the mature follicle with release of the oocyte. Post-ovulatory production of progesterone by the corpus luteum is also under the influence of LH.

The cyclical activity within the ovary which constitutes the ovarian cycle is maintained by the feedback mechanisms that operate between the ovary, hypothalamus, and pituitary. These are described in the next section.

The Ovarian Cycle

FOLLICULAR PHASE

Days 1 to 8

At the start of the cycle, levels of FSH and LH rise in response to the fall of estradiol and progesterone at menstruation. This stimulates development of 10 to

20 follicles. The follicle that is most sensitive to FSH is the 'dominant' follicle and is the one destined to reach full maturation and ovulation. This dominant follicle appears during the mid-follicular phase, while the remainder undergo atresia. With growth of the dominant follicle, estradiol levels increase.

Days 9 to 14

As the follicle increases in size, localized accumulations of fluid appear among the granulosa cells that surround the oocyte and become confluent, giving rise to a fluid-filled central cavity called the 'antrum' (Fig. 4.2). This transforms the dominant follicle into a Graafian follicle, in which the oocyte occupies an eccentric position, surrounded by two to three layers of granulosa cells termed the 'cumulus oophorus'.

Associated with follicular maturation, there is a progressive increase in the production of estrogen (mainly estradiol) by the granulosa cells of the developing follicle. As the estradiol level rises, the release of both gonadotrophins is suppressed (negative feedback), which serves to prevent the maturation of multiple follicles simultaneously.

The granulosa cells also produce anti-Müllerian hormone (AMH) which regulates folliculogenesis by restricting of the number of follicles undergoing maturation in order to select the dominant follicle. AMH production is highest in small pre-antral and antral follicles. Thus, AMH levels are sometimes used as a marker of ovarian reserve (egg supply), since levels decline as the woman approaches menopause. Women with many small follicles, such as those with polycystic ovary syndrome (PCOS), have high AMH levels.

OVULATION

Day 14

Ovulation is associated with rapid enlargement of the follicle, followed by protrusion from the surface of the ovarian cortex and rupture of the follicle, with extrusion of the oocyte and adherent cumulus oophorus (Fig. 4.3). Some women can identify the time of ovulation because they experience a short-lived pain in one or other iliac fossa. Ultrasound studies have shown that this mid-cycle pain—known as 'mittelschmerz' (German for 'middle pain')—actually occurs just before follicular rupture.

The final rise in estradiol concentration is thought to be responsible for the subsequent mid-cycle surge of LH and, to a lesser extent, of FSH—positive feedback. Immediately before ovulation, there is a precipitous fall in estradiol levels and an increase in progesterone production. Ovulation follows within 18 hours of the mid-cycle surge of LH.

LUTEAL PHASE

Days 15 to 28

The remainder of the Graafian follicle, which is retained in the ovary, is penetrated by capillaries and fibroblasts from the theca, which are the cells that surround the follicles. The granulosa cells undergo luteinization; these structures collectively form the corpus luteum (Fig. 4.4). This is the major source of the sex steroid hormones estradiol and progesterone, which are secreted by the ovary in the post-ovulatory phase.

Establishment of the corpus luteum results in a marked increase in progesterone secretion and a second rise in estradiol levels. Progesterone levels peak 1 week after ovulation (day 21 of the 28-day cycle). Tests of serum progesterone at this time may be used in fertility investigations to confirm the development of a corpus luteum, implying that ovulation has occurred.

During the luteal phase, gonadotrophin levels reach a nadir and remain low until the regression of the corpus luteum, which occurs at days 26 to 28. If conception and implantation occur, the corpus luteum does

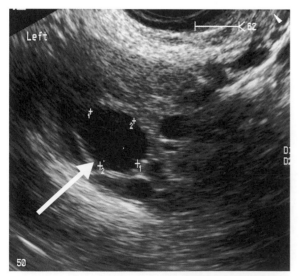

Fig. 4.2 A dominant follicle on transvaginal ultrasound scan.

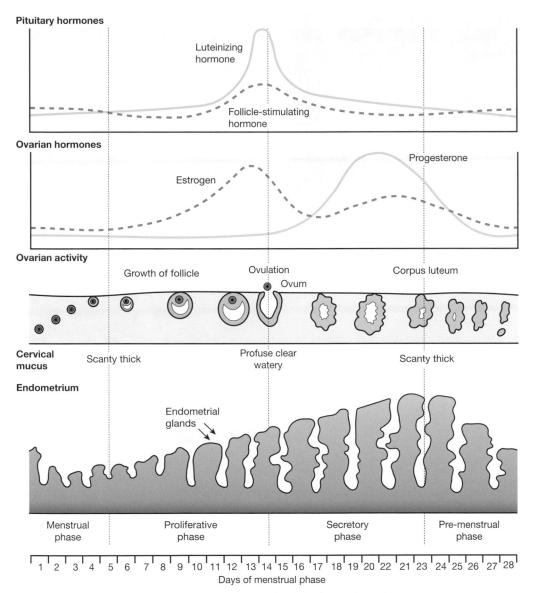

Fig. 4.3 Schematic diagram of ovulation in a 28-day cycle.

not regress because it is maintained by human chorionic gonadotrophin (hCG) secreted by the trophoblast. The detection of the presence of hCG in a sample of urine or blood forms the basis of pregnancy testing. If conception and implantation have not occurred, which is the case for the majority of menstrual cycles, the corpus luteum regresses. Then, progesterone levels fall and menstruation is triggered. The consequent fall in the levels of sex hormones allows the FSH and LH levels to rise and initiate the next cycle.

The Uterine Cycle

The cyclical production of sex hormones by the ovary induces important changes in the uterus. These involve the endometrium and cervical mucus.

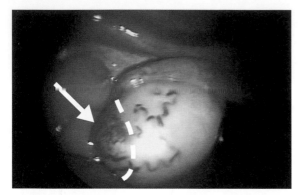

Fig. 4.4 Laparoscopic view of ovary with corpus luteum.

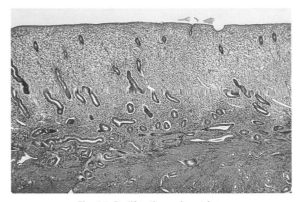

Fig. 4.5 Proliferative endometrium.

THE ENDOMETRIUM

The endometrium is composed of two layers: a superficial layer, which is shed in the course of menstruation, and a basal layer, which does not take part in this process but which regenerates the superficial layer during the subsequent cycle.

The junction between these layers is marked by a change in the character of the arterioles supplying the endometrium. The arterioles traverse the basal endometrium straight, but thereafter their course becomes convoluted, giving rise to the spiral section of the arteriole. This anatomical configuration assumes importance in the physiological shedding of the superficial layers of the endometrium.

Proliferative Phase

During the follicular phase in the ovary, the endometrium is exposed to estrogen. After menstruation, the secretion of estradiol from the ovary brings about repair and regeneration of the endometrium. With ongoing exposure to estradiol, there is ongoing growth and proliferation of glands and blood vessels. At this stage—the 'proliferative' phase—the glands are tubular and arranged in a regular pattern, parallel to each other (Fig. 4.5).

Secretory Phase

After ovulation, progesterone production induces secretory changes in the endometrial glands, preparing the endometrium for implantation (Fig. 4.6). This is first evident as the appearance of secretory vacuoles in the glandular epithelium below the nuclei. This swiftly progresses to secretion of material into the lumen of the glands, which become tortuous and their margins appear serrated.

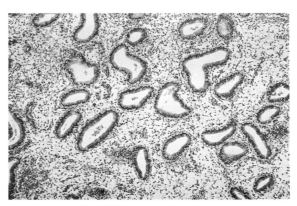

Fig. 4.6 Secretory endometrium.

Menstrual Phase

Normally, the luteal phase of the ovary lasts for 14 days, at the end of which regression of the corpus luteum is associated with a decline in ovarian estradiol and progesterone production. This fall is followed by intense spasmodic contraction of the spiral section of the endometrial arterioles, resulting in ischaemic necrosis, then shedding of the superficial layer of the endometrium and, finally, bleeding.

The vasospasm appears to be due to local production of prostaglandins. Prostaglandins may also account for the increased uterine contractions at the time of the menstrual flow.

CERVICAL MUCUS

The glands of the cervix secrete mucus. This changes in quantity and character throughout the cycle in response to sex hormones from the ovary:

- Early in the follicular phase, the cervical mucus is scant.
- Later in the follicular phase, the increasing estradiol levels induce changes in the composition of the mucus (becomes more stretchy). This change is described by the term 'spinnbarkheit' (German for 'the ability to be spun'). The water content increases progressively so that just before ovulation occurs the mucus has become watery and is easily penetrated by the spermatozoa. This mid-cycle mucus has a characteristic fern-like pattern when examined microscopically (Fig. 4.7).
- After ovulation, progesterone secreted by the corpus luteum counteracts the effect of estradiol and the mucus becomes thick and impermeable. This prevents entry of further spermatozoa. This effect on mucus is one of the ways by which the progestogen-only methods of contraception have their contraceptive effect.

These changes can be monitored by the woman herself if she is using a fertility awareness–based method (also known as 'natural family planning') for contraception.

Other Cyclical Changes

Although cyclical changes in ovarian hormones affect the genital tract, these hormones also circulate throughout the body and can affect other organs.

BASAL BODY TEMPERATURE

A rise in basal body temperature of approximately 0.5°C occurs following ovulation and is sustained until the onset of menstruation. This is due to the thermogenic effect of progesterone acting upon the hypothalamus. Should conception occur, the elevation in basal body temperature is maintained throughout pregnancy. A similar effect is caused by the administration of progestogens.

BREAST CHANGES

The human mammary gland is very sensitive to estrogen and progesterone. Breast swelling is often the first sign of puberty in response to the small increase in ovarian estrogens. Estradiol and progesterone act synergistically on the breast, and, during the normal cycle, breast swelling occurs in the luteal phase, apparently in response to increasing progesterone levels. The swelling is probably due to vascular changes and not to changes in the glandular tissue.

PSYCHOLOGICAL CHANGES

Some women notice changes in mood during the menstrual cycle, with an increase in emotional lability in the late luteal phase. Such changes may be directly due to falling levels of progesterone, although mood changes are not always closely synchronised with hormonal fluctuations.

Amenorrhoea

Amenorrhoea may be defined as the failure of menstruation to occur at the expected time. It can be considered in two categories:

1. Primary amenorrhoea, when menstruation has never occurred
2. Secondary amenorrhoea, when established menstruation ceases for 6 months or more.

Primary Amenorrhoea

Failure to menstruate by the age of 16 years is referred to as 'primary amenorrhoea'. The likely cause of primary amenorrhoea depends on whether secondary sexual characteristics are present. If secondary sexual characteristics are absent, then the cause is most likely delayed puberty (see pp. 37). If pubertal development is normal, then an anatomical cause should be suspected. The main 'anatomical' causes are:

- Congenital absence of the uterus, due to a failure of the Müllerian ducts to develop

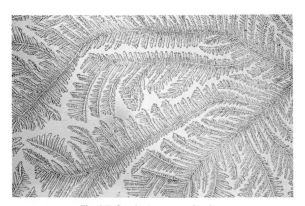

Fig. 4.7 Cervical mucus—ferning.

• Imperforate hymen—the menstrual blood is trapped behind the hymen, within the vagina (haematocolpos), causing cyclical lower abdominal pain each month at the time of menstruation (cryptomenorrhoea). Inspection of the vulva reveals a distended hymenal membrane through which dark blood may be seen. Treatment by incision of the hymen is required, usually under anaesthesia (Fig. 4.8).

Failure to menstruate may also be a physiological delay; in other words, the development is normal but there is an inherent delay in the onset of menstruation. There is often a family history of the same delay in the mother. A progestogen challenge test is useful to identify constitutional menstrual delay. A progestogen (e.g., medroxyprogesterone acetate) is given orally for 5 days; if the endometrium has been stimulated from endogenous estradiol, then withdrawal of progestogen should lead to a vaginal bleed. If such a bleed occurs, it is reasonable to offer reassurance that spontaneous menstruation is likely to occur. An abdominal ultrasound may be reassuring to confirm that the uterus and ovaries are normal.

Low body weight and excessive exercise are also associated with primary amenorrhoea. The other causes listed in Table 4.1 are rare, although a few are outlined in the next section, 'Secondary amenorrhoea' (see also Chapter 5).

Secondary Amenorrhoea

Secondary amenorrhoea means the cessation of established menstruation. It is defined as no menstruation for 6 months in the absence of pregnancy. A full list of causes is given in Table 4.2, but the most common clinical causes are weight loss, low body weight,

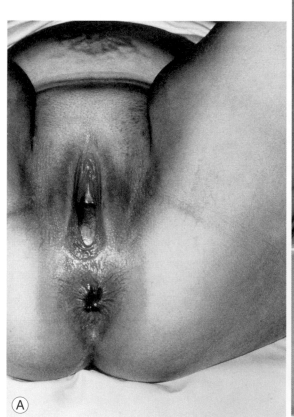
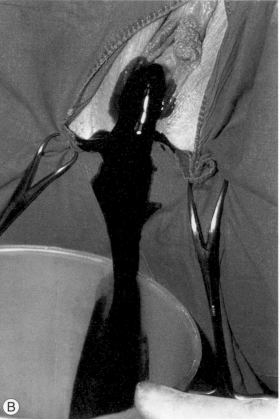

Fig. 4.8 Imperforate hymen (A) before and (B) after incision.

TABLE 4.1 Causes of Primary Amenorrhoea

System	Problem	Incidence
Chromosomal	XO—Turner syndrome	Rare
	46,XY disorders of sex development (DSD)	Rare
	Ovotesticular DSD	Rare
Hypothalamic	Physiological delay	Common
	Weight loss/anorexia/ excessive exercise	Common
	Isolated gonadotrophin-releasing hormone deficiency	Rare
	Congenital central nervous system defects	Rare
	Intracranial tumours	Rare
Pituitary	Partial/total hypopituitarism	Rare
	Hyperprolactinaemia	Rare
	Pituitary adenoma	Rare
	Empty sella syndrome	Rare
	Trauma/surgery	Rare
Ovarian	True agenesis	Rare
	Premature ovarian insufficiency	Rare
	Radiation/chemotherapy/ autoimmune	Rare
	Polycystic ovary syndrome	Common
	Virilising ovarian tumours	Rare
Other endocrine	Primary hypothyroidism	Rare
	Adrenal hyperplasia	Rare
	Adrenal tumour	Rare
Uterine/ vaginal	Imperforate hymen	Less rare
	Uterovaginal agenesis	Rare

TABLE 4.2 Causes of Secondary Amenorrhoea

System	Problem	Incidence
Physiological	Pregnancy	Common
	Lactation	Common
	Menopause	Common
Hypothalamic	Weight loss/ anorexia	Common
	Excessive exercise	Common
	Stress	Common
Pituitary	Hyperprolactinaemia	Less rare
	Partial/total hypopituitarism	Rare
	Trauma/surgery	Rare
Ovarian	Polycystic ovary syndrome	Common
	Premature ovarian insufficiency	Uncommon
	Surgery/radiotherapy/ chemotherapy	Uncommon
	Resistant ovary syndrome	Rare
	Virilising ovarian tumours	Rare
Other endocrine	Primary hypothyroidism	Rare
	Adrenal hyperplasia	Rare
	Adrenal tumour	Rare
Uterine/vaginal	Surgery— hysterectomy	Common
	Endometrial ablation	Common
	Progestogen intrauterine device	Common
	Asherman syndrome	Rare

PCOS, and hyperprolactinaemia, all of which are discussed in the next section.

CAUSES

Physiological

The most common causes of amenorrhoea during the reproductive phase of life are physiological—pregnancy and lactation. A pregnancy test should be administered to all sexually active women presenting with amenorrhoea.

The high postpartum level of prolactin associated with breastfeeding suppresses ovulation and gives rise to lactational amenorrhoea. Amenorrhoea usually persists throughout the time that the infant is fully breastfed, but with the reduction in the frequency of suckling, prolactin levels fall and ovarian activity is resumed. Lactational amenorrhoea is a hypo-estrogenic state which may lead to atrophic vaginitis and, occasionally, to painful intercourse.

Hypothalamic

Hypothalamic amenorrhoea ('hypogonadotrophic hypogonadism') is frequently associated with stress. In such cases, the condition usually resolves spontaneously. Physical stress in the form of athletic training can also result in suppression of the hypothalamic–pituitary–ovarian axis:

there are low levels of pituitary gonadotrophins in association with low levels of prolactin and estradiol.

The hypothalamus is also sensitive to changes in body weight; weight loss, even to only 10% to 15% below the ideal, may be associated with amenorrhoea. Anorexia nervosa and other eating disorders should be considered. Restoration of body weight results in the return of ovulatory function, although there may be a significant time interval between the attainment of the ideal body weight and the resumption of ovarian activity. Ovulation induction therapy is not recommended until the restoration of body weight, as pregnancy, if it occurs, carries the risk of growth restriction of the fetus and increased perinatal mortality.

If hypothalamic amenorrhoea is not related to low body weight, treatment will depend upon whether the woman wants to conceive. If pregnancy is not desired, estrogen replacement therapy is advisable. This can also be conveniently provided in the form of the combined oral contraceptive pill. If the woman wishes to become pregnant, ovulation may be induced with pulsatile GnRH therapy or exogenous gonadotrophins.

Pituitary

Prolactin stimulates breast development and subsequent lactation. The secretion of prolactin, a polypeptide hormone produced by the lactotrophs of the anterior pituitary, is inhibited by dopamine from the hypothalamus. High levels of prolactin, which may be either physiological (during lactation) or pathological (see later discussion), in turn suppress ovarian activity by interfering with the secretion of gonadotrophins.

Mildly elevated prolactin levels are common and can be due to stress (e.g., of venepuncture). Sustained higher levels can result in galactorrhoea (production and release of breast milk) and amenorrhoea unrelated to pregnancy. Galactorrhoea occurs in less than half of those with hyperprolactinaemia, and less than half of those with galactorrhoea have an elevated prolactin level. The causes of hyperprolactinaemia are given in Box 4.1.

Adenomas can occur in the lateral wings of the anterior pituitary. They are usually soft and discrete, with a pseudocapsule of compressed tissue (Fig. 4.9). If the prolactin level is more than 1000 mU/L, then imaging with magnetic resonance imaging (MRI) should be carried out. A microadenoma is <10 mm in

BOX 4.1 CAUSES OF HYPERPROLACTINAEMIA

Pituitary adenoma
- Microadenomas
- Macroadenomas

Secondary to other causes
- Primary hypothyroidism
- Chronic renal failure
- Pituitary stalk compression
- Polycystic ovarian syndrome
- Drugs (phenothiazines, haloperidol, metoclopramide, cimetidine, methyldopa, antihistamines, and morphine)
- Idiopathic

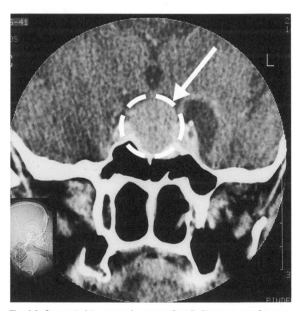

Fig. 4.9 Computed tomography scan of a pituitary macroadenoma.

diameter and a macroadenoma is >10 mm. Visual fields should be checked, as optic chiasma compression may lead to bitemporal hemianopia. One-third of adenomas regress spontaneously and fewer than 5% of microadenomas become macroadenomas. Serum levels correlate well with tumour size so that if the adenoma is relatively large and the prolactin level only modestly elevated, then pituitary stalk compression from a non-secreting macroadenoma or other tumour (e.g., a craniopharyngioma) is possible. It is possible that apparently idiopathic hyperprolactinaemia may be caused by microadenomas that are too small to be picked up by an MRI scan.

All women should have pituitary imaging before treatment. This treatment is usually with a dopamine agonist, either bromocriptine or cabergoline, which suppresses the prolactin level and induces regression of the prolactinoma. Surgical excision of an adenoma is only rarely required and would be performed trans-sphenoidally.

Ovarian

Premature Ovarian Insufficiency

Menopause (with cessation of ovarian function) normally occurs around the age of 50 years. The term 'premature ovarian insufficiency' is commonly used to describe cessation of ovarian function before the age of 40 years. As in natural menopause, this is due to depletion of primordial follicles in the ovaries.

Premature ovarian insufficiency occurs in 1% of women and may be due to surgery, viral infections (e.g., mumps), cytotoxic drugs, or radiotherapy. It may also be idiopathic and is occasionally associated with chromosomal abnormality (XO mosaicism or XXX). A low estradiol level, very high FSH, and the absence of any menstrual activity are poor prognostic signs for recovery. Pregnancy by in vitro fertilization with donor oocytes may be possible. There is an association with other autoimmune disorders. Hormone replacement therapy is required to minimise the risk of osteoporosis and address any postmenopausal symptoms (see Chapter 9).

Polycystic Ovary Syndrome (PCOS)

PCOS is associated with menstrual disturbance and is the most common form of anovulatory subfertility. It is estimated to affect up to 20% of women in the United Kingdom. It is characterised by the presence of at least two out of the following three criteria:

- Oligomenorrhoea or amenorrhoea
- Ultrasound appearance of either or both ovaries with a volume of >10 cm³ and/or multiple small follicles (12 or more <10 mm; Fig. 4.10)
- Clinical evidence of excess androgens (acne, hirsutism) or biochemical evidence (raised serum testosterone).

The aetiology of the condition is unknown. However, evidence suggests that the principal underlying disorder is one of insulin resistance, with the resultant hyperinsulinaemia stimulating excess

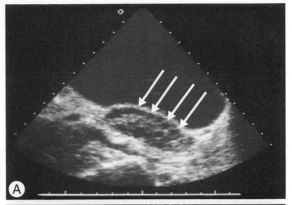
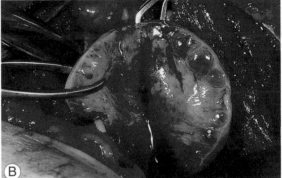
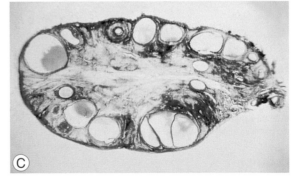

Fig. 4.10 Polycystic ovaries. These are classically bilaterally enlarged with multiple peripherally situated cysts 'like a ring of pearls' in a dense stroma: **(A)** ultrasound scan; **(B)** during surgery; **(C)** pathological preparation.

ovarian androgen production. Associated with the prevalent insulin resistance, there is a characteristic dyslipidaemia and a predisposition to diabetes and cardiovascular disease in later life. Therefore, PCOS may be considered to be a systemic metabolic condition rather than one primarily of gynaecological origin (Fig. 4.11).

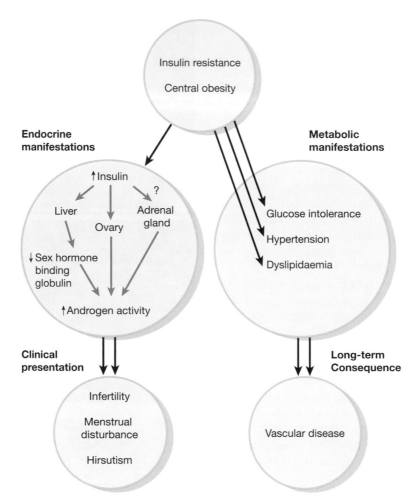

Fig. 4.11 Pathogenesis of polycystic ovary syndrome (PCOS). PCOS can be considered to be a disorder primarily of insulin resistance, with the resultant hyperinsulinaemia stimulating excess ovarian androgen production. There may also be dyslipidaemia and a predisposition to later diabetes and cardiovascular disease. *?* = Uncertain relationship between insulin and the adrenal gland.

Treatment depends on whether the presenting problem has been menstrual irregularity, hirsutism, or subfertility. The combined oral contraceptive pill has been used to regulate menstruation. Hirsutism may be treated by cosmetic measures, such as waxing or laser treatment. Hirsutism may also be treated with the combined oral contraceptive pill, as it suppresses ovarian androgen production, or with the antiandrogen cyproterone acetate. Women taking an antiandrogen should use effective contraception during, and for at least 3 months after, treatment due to the potential risk of teratogenicity (feminisation of a male fetus) with antiandrogen therapy. Clomifene is used to induce ovulation in women with anovulatory subfertility (see p. 68). If clomifene does not work, ovulation may be induced by gonadotrophin injections or by laparoscopic diathermy to the ovary (see Chapter 5).

Individuals may gain benefit from early screening for cardiovascular risk factors, particularly hypertension and glucose intolerance. There is also a longer-term increased risk of endometrial hyperplasia and endometrial carcinoma as a consequence of the effects of estrogen stimulation of the endometrium not counteracted by the regular shedding associated with progesterone withdrawal and ovulation.

Other Endocrine Causes

These are rare. Women with thyrotoxicosis may have amenorrhoea. Primary hypothyroidism is also associated with amenorrhoea, as thyrotrophin-releasing hormone stimulates prolactin secretion. The most common of the rarer adrenal problems is late-onset congenital adrenal hyperplasia. This is usually due to a deficiency of the enzyme 21-hydroxylase; treatment with a low dose of corticosteroids is usually sufficient to re-establish ovulatory function by suppressing adrenal function. Androgen-secreting adrenal tumours can also occur.

Uterine

Excessive uterine curettage—usually at the time of miscarriage, termination of pregnancy, or secondary postpartum haemorrhage—may remove the basal layer of the endometrium and result in the formation of uterine adhesions (synechiae), a condition known as Asherman syndrome (Fig. 4.12). It may rarely also result from severe postpartum infection. Treatment involves breaking down the adhesions through a hysteroscope and inserting an intrauterine contraceptive device for 3 to 6 months. This will deter re-formation of adhesions, and the resumption of menstruation will signal that regrowth of the endometrium has occurred.

Care of Women With Secondary Amenorrhoea

Initial care:
- Check pregnancy test
- Ask about perimenopausal symptoms (e.g., flushing, vaginal dryness)

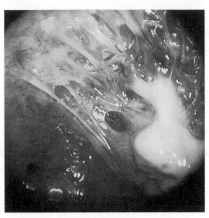

Fig. 4.12 Adhesions can form within the uterine cavity following surgery, pregnancy, or infection: Asherman syndrome.

- Take a history, including weight changes, drugs, medical disorders, and thyroid symptoms
- Carry out an examination, looking particularly at height, weight, visual fields, and the presence of hirsutism or virilisation; also, carry out a pelvic examination unless contraindicated
- Check serum for LH, FSH, prolactin, testosterone, thyroxine, and thyroid-stimulating hormone (TSH)
- Arrange for a transvaginal ultrasound scan, looking for polycystic ovaries
- Review with the results (Table 4.3).

If the tests listed in Table 4.3 are normal, consider the following causes:
- Weight loss
- Depression, emotional disturbance, or extreme exercise

TABLE 4.3	Further Management Based on Test Results	
Ultrasound scan	A scan showing either or both large-volume ovaries (>10 cm³) and/or multiple small follicles (12 or more <10 mm diameter)	If pregnancy desired, clomifene or gonadotrophins. If pregnancy not desired, consider the combined oral contraceptive pill.
Elevated PRL level	If PRL >1000 mU/L on at least two occasions, the diagnosis is hyperprolactinaemia.	Arrange for MRI of the pituitary. Treat with dopamine antagonist.
Elevated FSH	If FSH >30 IU/L, repeat 4–6 weeks later. If still elevated and the woman >40 years old, the woman is likely menopausal. If less than 40 years, then diagnosis is likely premature ovarian insufficiency.	Consider HRT. Pregnancy with oocyte donation is possible.
Abnormal TFTs	If the TFTs are abnormal, treat as appropriate.	

FSH, Follicle-stimulating hormone; *HRT,* hormone replacement therapy; *LH,* luteinizing hormone; *MRI,* magnetic resonance imaging; *PRL,* prolactin; *TFTs,* thyroid function tests.

- Asherman syndrome
- Idiopathic amenorrhoea.

In the majority of women who present with secondary amenorrhoea, investigations will fail to demonstrate any significant endocrine abnormality—known as idiopathic amenorrhoea. It is probable that there is a disturbance of the normal feedback mechanisms of control. Undue sensitivity of the hypothalamus and pituitary to the negative feedback suppression of endogenous estrogen may result in impaired gonadotrophin secretion, which is inadequate to stimulate follicular development and results in cycle initiation failure. Those requiring ovulation usually respond well to an anti-estrogen such as clomifene. This affects the negative feedback and results in higher FSH levels, stimulating the ovaries.

Key Points

- At the start of the cycle, levels of FSH and LH rise, which stimulate the development of 10 to 20 follicles. A single dominant follicle matures, secreting estradiol, and the remainder undergo atresia. As the estradiol level rises, the release of both gonadotrophins is suppressed (negative feedback), which serves to prevent multiple follicles from maturing and ovulating.
- The very high preovulatory estradiol level stimulates a positive-feedback mid-cycle surge of LH, which triggers ovulation. The remainder of the ruptured follicle becomes the corpus luteum and secretes progesterone.
- Progesterone brings about secretory changes in the endometrium that are necessary for successful implantation.
- If conception and implantation occur, the corpus luteum is maintained by hCG secreted by the trophoblast. If conception and implantation have not occurred successfully, the corpus luteum regresses, the levels of sex hormones fall, and menstruation ensues.
- The most common causes of primary amenorrhoea (when menstruation has never occurred) are physiological delay, weight loss, heavy exercise, and an imperforate hymen.
- Secondary amenorrhoea is said to have occurred when established menstruation ceases for 6 months or more. Outside pregnancy, lactation, and menopause, the most common causes are PCOS, stress, weight loss, and hyperprolactinaemia.
- PCOS is the most common cause of anovulatory subfertility.

Chapter 5

Subfertility

Scott Nelson, Karema Al Rashid

Chapter Outline

Introduction

Subfertility is a condition that affects approximately one in six couples. The cause may be related to a problem with the man, woman or both. In view of the intimate nature of the problem, subfertility is often associated with personal distress and embarrassment; effective treatment is available to help an increasing proportion of these couples.

Definitions

Subfertility is formally recognized as a disease by the World Health Organization (WHO) and is defined as the inability of a couple to achieve a clinical pregnancy within 12 months of beginning regular unprotected sexual intercourse. A couple can have primary subfertility – no previous pregnancies within the relationship – or secondary subfertility, in which the couple have achieved at least one pregnancy.

Subfertility is rarely absolute (infertility). Around 84% of the normal fertile population will conceive within 1 year and 92% by the end of 2 years. However, this is strongly age dependent and the older the couple are when they start trying to conceive, the lower the chance of pregnancy. Age factors into when, even in the absence of critical history or physical findings, investigations and treatment may be initiated; at 12 months in women under 35 years of age; at 6 months in women aged 35 or older; and in women over 40 years, more immediate evaluation and treatment may be warranted.

'Cumulative pregnancy rates' and 'live birth rates' are the terms used to express the chance of conception within a given time interval. Fig. 5.1 illustrates the relationship between female age at which couples start building a family and their chance of realizing a family with one child, with and without use of in vitro fertilization (IVF).

Fecundability is the percentage of women exposed to the chance of a pregnancy for one menstrual cycle who will subsequently produce a live-born infant (normal range 15% – 28%). Fecundability decreases with increasing age, and hence diminishes slightly with each passing month of not conceiving.

Age and Fertility

Fertility declines as the woman's age increases, reflecting the decrease in oocyte quantity and quality. A woman is born with a finite number of oocytes; around 1 million. This falls to approximately 250,000 at puberty; by the time menopause is reached, the number of oocytes has fallen to below 1000. During her reproductive life, a woman will release around 500 mature oocytes – a form of pre-conceptual natural selection – while the remaining oocytes undergo atresia or apoptosis. At menopause, which occurs at an average age of 51 years, there are in effect no functioning oocytes.

The decline in fertility is directly related to the declining oocyte population and the eggs' inherent quality. There is a small fall in monthly pregnancy rates from the age of 31 years, a more pronounced decrease from the age of 36 years and a very steep decline from the age of 40 years. In assisted-conception procedures, this decline is also observed with a gradual decline in success rates from age 34 years. In addition, in both natural and assisted-conception pregnancies, there is a substantial increase in rates of miscarriage with advancing maternal age. Although older men become less fertile, the effect of age on men's fertility is much less pronounced than for women.

Causes of Subfertility

The causes of subfertility can be categorized in a simple manner. In reality, however, more than one problem is often identified in a couple. Causes include ovulation disorders (25%), male factor (30%), unexplained (25%) and tubal factors (10%). Remaining causes include uterine or peritoneal disorders, such as endometriosis-related subfertility.

Diagnosis

The diagnosis of subfertility is a process of exclusion, identifying couples in whom the cause is clear, those in

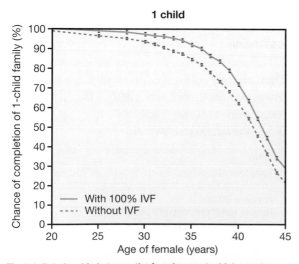

Fig. 5.1 Relationship between the female age at which couples start building a family and the chance of realizing a family with one child, with and without use of in vitro fertilization (IVF). (From Habbema JDF, Eijkemans JC, Leridon H, te Velde ER. Realizing a desired family size: when should couples start? *Hum Reprod.* 2015;30(9): 2215–2221.)

whom there is a possible cause and those in whom the cause is unexplained. The aim of investigation should be to reach a diagnosis as soon as possible, using only tests that are of proven value.

History and Examination

Factors that provide clues to the aetiology are outlined in Tables 5.1 and 5.2. Other important factors to be noted are the woman's age and the duration of subfertility – generally, the older the woman is and the longer the period of subfertility, the poorer the prognosis. The order in which the investigations are performed varies depending on whether the couple has primary or secondary subfertility, with an earlier assessment of tubal patency in the latter. Early assessment is also indicated if a specific abnormality is suspected from the history and for an older patient.

EXAMINATION OF THE WOMAN

Height and weight should be recorded and used to calculate the body mass index (BMI). The normal BMI range is between 19 and 25 kg/m^2. A change of weight of >10% in the preceding year may cause a disturbance of the menstrual pattern and anovulation. A BMI at either extreme is detrimental to fertility (see later discussion).

Increased body hair is associated with hyperandrogenism, most commonly due to polycystic ovary syndrome (PCOS). Breast examination may demonstrate galactorrhoea, which is associated with hyperprolactinaemia. Pelvic examination is important to look for signs of structural abnormalities, infection and pathological processes, such as endometriosis or pelvic inflammatory disease. More detailed information regarding structural abnormalities of the pelvic organs is obtained by augmenting clinical examination with transvaginal ultrasound.

EXAMINATION OF THE MAN

Examination of the man is frequently omitted in the absence of a relevant history. However, if the semen analysis is abnormal, examination of the genitalia may be helpful, looking specifically at size (volume); consistency and position of the testes; the outline of the epididymis (for the presence of the vas deferens); and, finally, the scrotum, for evidence of swellings.

Investigations and Their Interpretation

Investigations should be arranged in a logical manner with reference to the history, along with appropriate general health screening (Box 5.1). Additional tests may be necessary depending on the circumstances (Box 5.2).

MALE FACTORS

Classification

Male factor subfertility can be a problem of sperm production, sperm function or sperm delivery. Sperm production may be completely absent (azoospermia) in

TABLE 5.1 Examination of a Woman

Examination	Reason
Height and weight to calculate body mass index (BMI)	High or low BMI associated with lower fertility
Body hair distribution	Hyperandrogenism
Galactorrhoea	Hyperprolactinaemia
Uterine structural abnormalities (most usefully determined by transvaginal ultrasound)	May be associated with subfertility
Immobile and/or tender uterus	Endometriosis or pelvic inflammatory disease

TABLE 5.2 Examination of a Man

Examination	Reason
Scrotum	Varicocele
Size (volume) of the testes	Small testes associated with oligospermia
Position of the testes	Undescended testes
Prostate	Chronic infection

BOX 5.1 INITIAL INVESTIGATIONS

Female
- Early follicular phase: luteinizing hormone (LH), follicle-stimulating hormone (FSH), estradiol, anti-Müllerian hormone (AMH)
- Rubella (offer vaccination if not immune)
- Luteal phase: serum progesterone (to determine whether ovulation has occurred)
- Test of tubal patency (laparoscopic hydrotubation, hysterosalpingo-contrast sonography [HyCoSy], or hysterosalpingography [HSG])

Male
- Semen analysis × 2

BOX 5.2 ADDITIONAL INVESTIGATIONS TO BE PERFORMED SELECTIVELY

Female
- Pelvic ultrasound scan for ovarian morphology and uterine abnormalities
- Laparoscopy for diagnosis of endometriosis – may be combined with tubal patency test
- Hysteroscopy for intrauterine anomalies
- Prolactin and thyroid function tests
- Testosterone, androstenedione, 17-hydroxyprogesterone and sex hormone-binding globulin (SHBG; in order to calculate the Free Androgen Index – when raised, is an indicator of hyperandrogenism)

Male
- Sperm function tests (see text), if initial test is consistently abnormal
- Mixed agglutination reaction test or immunobead test for antisperm antibodies
- FSH, LH, testosterone if low sperm count (oligospermia) (raised FSH if testicular failure, low if central nervous system cause)
- Transrectal ultrasound for suspected abnormalities of the seminal vesicles and prostate

FSH, Follicle-stimulating hormone; *LH,* luteinizing hormone.

testicular failure, for example. More commonly, there is a reduced count of sperm of normal appearance (oligospermia). Additionally, a high proportion of the sperm may demonstrate poor motility, lacking the normal forward progressive movement (asthenospermia) or may appear morphologically defective (teratospermia) with abnormalities of the head, midpiece or tail.

Normal sperm function – the ability of the sperm to reach, bind and fertilize the oocyte – is more difficult to demonstrate. At present, there are no reliable methods of measuring sperm function other than monitoring the proportion of sperm moving and assessing the speed of their progress. Antisperm antibodies can impair sperm motility.

Problems with sperm delivery may be caused by absence or blockage of the vas deferens or epididymis. It may also be related to impotence, premature ejaculation or a physical inability to have normal sexual intercourse.

Semen Analysis

Semen analysis is the cornerstone of the laboratory evaluation of the subfertile man and helps to define the severity of the male factor. Patients should receive standardised instructions for semen collection, including a defined pre-test abstinence interval of 2 to 5 days. Semen can be collected by means of masturbation into a specimen cup or by intercourse with the use of special semen collection condoms that do not contain substances toxic to sperm. Ideally, the specimen should be collected at the laboratory. If collected at home, the specimen should be kept at room or body temperature during transport and examined in the laboratory within 1 hour of collection.

Clinical reference ranges have been established for sperm concentration, motility and morphology to help classify men as fertile or subfertile. The WHO has produced a normal range of values for semen, based upon semen analyses performed upon samples obtained from men with a time-to-pregnancy interval of up to 12 months (Table 5.3). The values, do not reflect a cut-off point below which pregnancy will not occur. Rather, there is an increase in probability of conception with increasing numbers of sperm and motility up to 40 million/mL and 40%, respectively, with a relative plateau thereafter.

When the initial screening evaluation reveals an abnormal male reproductive history or demonstrates abnormal semen parameters, a thorough evaluation by a urologist or other specialist in male reproduction is indicated. Additional tests and procedures may be recommended, including serial semen analyses (>3 months apart), endocrine evaluation, post-ejaculatory urinalysis, ultrasonography, specialized tests on semen and sperm and genetic screening.

TABLE 5.3	WHO Criteria for Semen Analysis (2010)	
Parameter	**Lower Limit of Reference Range**
Volume	1.5 mL
Concentration	15×10^6/mL
Total motility	40%
Progressive motility	32%
Normal forms	4%
Vitality	58%

From World Health Organization. WHO Laboratory Manual for Examination and Processing of Human Semen. 5th ed. Geneva, Switzerland: WHO; 2010.

FEMALE FACTORS

Ovulation

Ovulation is an 'all or nothing' phenomenon, with usually one oocyte released per ovulatory cycle.

Causes of Anovulation

Ovarian failure is found in about 50% of women with primary amenorrhoea and 15% of those presenting with secondary amenorrhoea. Most women with primary amenorrhoea will have an established diagnosis before presenting to a subfertility clinic. The cause may be genetic, for example, Turner syndrome (45,XO), or autoimmune. In those presenting with secondary amenorrhoea and ovarian failure, there may be an obvious cause, such as previous ovarian surgery, abdominal radiotherapy or gonadotoxic chemotherapy. There will also be a proportion of women in whom no reason can be identified, termed 'idiopathic premature ovarian insufficiency' (POI).

Weight-Related Anovulation Weight plays an important part in the control of ovulation. A minimum degree of body fat (considered to be around 22% of body weight) is needed to maintain ovulatory cycles. Substantial weight loss leads to the disappearance of the normal 24-hour secretory pattern of gonadotrophin-releasing hormone (GnRH), which reverts to the nocturnal pattern seen in pubescent girls. As a result, the ovaries develop a multifollicular appearance on ultrasound. Prolonged exercise can, by increasing muscle bulk and decreasing body fat, have the same effect. Thus, it is not uncommon for women athletes or ballerinas to be amenorrhoeic. Excessive weight can also have an adverse effect on ovulation. This probably results from excess estrone, generated in the adipose tissue by conversion from androgens, interfering with the normal feedback mechanism to the pituitary gland.

Excess weight has a profound effect on female fertility, with a significant reduction in the chance of a successful pregnancy: it reduces the chance of conception and increases the risk of miscarriage, as well as substantially increasing the risk of obstetric complications during pregnancy and at birth. The distribution of the fat is important, with central (visceral) fat having a bigger impact than peripheral fat distribution. The waist – hip ratio, which more reliably reflects visceral fat distribution, is a more reliable guide to the impact of fat on fertility, than the BMI.

Polycystic Ovary Syndrome Of the women presenting with anovulatory subfertility, 50% will have PCOS (see Chapter 4).

Luteinized Unruptured Follicle Syndrome In certain patients, the oocyte may be retained following the luteinizing hormone (LH) surge, the so-called 'luteinized unruptured follicle syndrome'. Repeated pelvic ultrasound scans fail to show the expected collapse of the follicle at ovulation, and the follicle persists into the luteal phase. As no longitudinal studies have shown this to be a persistent finding in the same woman, there is uncertainty regarding its relevance to fertility.

Hyperprolactinaemia Hyperprolactinaemia is diagnosed in 10% to 15% of cases of secondary amenorrhoea. About one-third of these women will have galactorrhoea and, occasionally, there may be some evidence of visual impairment (bitemporal hemianopia) due to pressure on the optic chiasma from a pituitary adenoma.

Tests of Ovulation

Only a pregnancy categorically confirms ovulation has occured. However, there are a number of investigations that imply that ovulation has taken place:

- History – over 90% of women with regular menstrual cycles will ovulate spontaneously. This is the basis for using tracking calendar apps.
- Urinary LH kit – this identifies the mid-cycle surge of LH that starts the cascade reaction leading to ovulation.
- Mid-luteal phase progesterone – a luteal-phase progesterone value of >28 nmol/L is found in conception cycles; as a result, this value is generally regarded as evidence of satisfactory ovulation. However, it is important to time the blood sample carefully – between 7 and 10 days before the first day of the next menstrual period. This can only be determined with some knowledge of the length of the woman's usual menstrual cycle; the information is inevitably retrospective.

Other Tests

Less commonly employed tests include serial ultrasound scans to monitor the growth and subsequent disappearance of an ovarian follicle.

Testing Ovarian Reserve

The concept of 'ovarian reserve' describes the reproductive potential as a function of the number and quality of oocytes. Decreased or diminished ovarian reserve (DOR) describes women of reproductive age having regular menses whose response to ovarian stimulation or fecundity is reduced compared with those women of comparable age. Tests utilized to assess 'ovarian reserve' include cycle-day 3 serum FSH and estradiol measurements, the clomifene citrate challenge test (CCCT), early follicular-phase antral follicle count (AFC; using transvaginal ultrasonography, the number of small developing follicles seen in the ovary is counted) and serum anti-Müllerian hormone (AMH) concentrations.

These tests may provide prognostic information in women at increased risk of DOR, such as women who (1) are over 35 years of age; (2) have a family history of early menopause; (3) have a single ovary or history of previous ovarian surgery, chemotherapy or pelvic radiation therapy; (4) have unexplained subfertility; (5) have demonstrated a poor response to gonadotropin stimulation; or (6) are planning treatment with assisted reproductive technology (ART).

Although tests of ovarian reserve may be important in identifying women who may not respond well to fertility treatment or will have a shorter reproductive lifespan, they have limited value in predicting overall natural fertility if the woman has a regular menstrual cycle and is ovulating.

Further Investigations

Pelvic ultrasound is useful in defining ovarian morphology and is more reliable than pelvic examination in identifying potentially relevant pelvic pathology, such as uterine fibroids, ovarian cysts and endometrial polyps.

Chlamydia serology was historically used as a screening test for tubal pathology. Those with a positive antibody titre are more likely to have tubal pathology because of the association between chlamydial infection and salpingitis. However, with the widespread use of nucleic acid amplification tests (NAATs), serology is now infrequently used.

Serum testosterone measurement is indicated if there is evidence of hirsutism to exclude more sinister disorders, such as androgen-secreting tumours of the ovary or adrenal gland or as part of the work-up of PCOS. In women with elevated testosterone, measurement of 17-hydroxyprogesterone is relevant in order to exclude late-onset congenital adrenal hyperplasia. Thyroid function tests are commonly performed, as approximately 7% of women in this age group will have a thyroid disorder, which may have an impact on a pregnancy if not appropriately treated

A progestogen challenge test may be useful in women with a history of amenorrhoea and normal levels of FSH and prolactin. It is used to determine whether the woman is clinically estrogenised. This acts as a guide to what would be the most appropriate medication to use to induce ovulation. If the bleeding is normal following 5 days of an oral progestogen, the woman is well estrogenised, whereas if it is absent or scanty, the woman is relatively poorly estrogenised. The presence of a withdrawal bleed also demonstrates the presence of endometrium and the patency of the cervix and vagina. The ability to visualize and measure the endometrial thickness by transvaginal scanning can also inform the progesterone challenge test, as a thick and therefore adequately estrogenised endometrium can be seen on scan.

Tubal Patency

Classification

The fallopian tube can be blocked distally – at the fimbrial end – or, less commonly, at the proximal end – the cornu. In addition, the tubo – ovarian relationship may be disrupted by peritubal adhesions. Fimbrial disease has varying degrees of severity:

- Agglutination of the fimbria to produce a narrowed opening – known as a 'phimosis'
- Complete agglutination to form a hydrosalpinx (fluid-filled tube)

Tubal damage can also involve the endosalpinx, with intraluminal adhesions and flattening of the mucosal folds. Therefore, microsurgery to relieve tubal blockage may not restore tubal function.

The important features for fertility prognosis appear to be:

- Degree of dilatation of the fallopian tube
- Extent of fibrosis of the wall of the tube
- Damage to the endosalpinx
- Whether one or both tubes are affected.

Tests of Tubal Patency

In the absence of a positive history suggestive of pelvic pathology, a negative physical examination, and negative *Chlamydia* test, the least invasive method for assessing tubal patency should be employed.

Hysterosalpingography (HSG) HSG involves inserting a cannula into the cervix and passing radio-opaque fluid into the uterine cavity and fallopian tubes, obtaining an outline of them (Fig. 5.2). The test is performed under X-ray screening on an outpatient basis. If the HSG is normal, this finding can be relied upon in 97% of cases. However, if the HSG is abnormal, the diagnosis can only be relied upon in 34% of cases (false-positive rate 66%), and a laparoscopy is required to confirm the nature of the abnormality.

Hysterosalpingo-contrast sonography (HyCoSy) This technique involves a pelvic ultrasound scan in which galactose-containing ultrasound contrast medium is inserted into the uterine cavity, outlining any abnormalities such as submucosal fibroids and endometrial polyps, before passing down the fallopian tubes to confirm tubal patency. The technique offers a similar level of diagnostic accuracy to HSG and it simultaneously allows visualization of the ovaries and uterus.

Diagnostic laparoscopy with dye hydrotubation Diagnostic laparoscopy ('lap and dye') is the gold standard investigation. It provides a direct view of the pelvic organs and offers the possibility to treat minor pathology discovered during the investigation. Methylthioninium chloride (methylene blue) dye is injected through a cannula in the cervix to demonstrate tubal patency. Hysteroscopy may be performed at the same time in order to examine the uterine cavity. The major disadvantage is that laparoscopy requires a general anaesthetic and incurs potential laparoscopy-related risks. As such, it is the most invasive and expensive investigation of tubal patency. Thus, most specialists perform HyCoSy or HSG for the first-line assessment.

Selective salpingography If HSG or laparoscopy detects a proximal blockage, further investigation may be considered. The blockage could simply be due to spasm of the muscle of the uterine cornua or represent a genuine abnormality. A fine guidewire is inserted into the internal tubal ostium under direct fluoroscopic control or by direct vision using a hysteroscope. This may dislodge a small plug of amorphous debris, restoring patency. This technique appears to increase the likelihood of pregnancy in women with proximal tubal damage.

Care of Couples With Subfertility

Early referral to assisted-conception services is generally appropriate for most couples after the initial investigations have been completed. The couple should be counselled about general health matters, such as smoking, alcohol intake, drugs, diet and optimising body weight. It is appropriate to recommend folic acid to the woman as routine prevention of neural tube defects. Where the diagnosis is established, specific treatments can be employed.

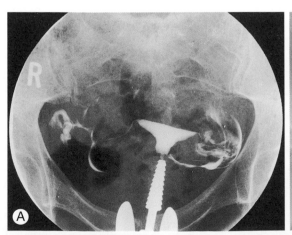 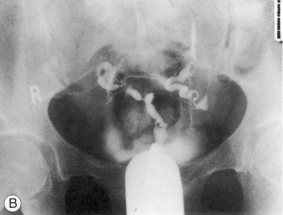

Fig. 5.2 Hysterosalpingography of normal uterus (A) and abnormal uterus (B). In (B), the radio-opaque dye does not flow through the fallopian tubes. This indicates blockage.

FEMALE FACTOR

Anovulation

There are several ways of inducing ovulation, depending on the underlying cause. Successful ovulation induction should be continued for long enough to give the optimum chance for conception – generally, 12 months. For specific disorders, such as hyperprolactinaemia and thyroid dysfunction, ovulation should recommence with successful treatment of the underlying disorder.

Anovulation in Estrogenised Patients

Most of these women have PCOS (85% of patients presenting with oligomenorrhoea and 25% of those with amenorrhoea). First-line treatment in this condition is oral anti-estrogen therapy, usually with clomifene citrate or letrozole.

Clomifene citrate's mode of action is to increase the plasma FSH concentration, mainly by competitively blocking the negative feedback effects of endogenous estradiol on the hypothalamus (FSH is the principal hormone responsible for follicular recruitment and development). Letrozole suppresses negative feedback of estrogen centrally and does not have the anti-estrogenic effects on the endometrium that are observed with clomifene.

Initially, a dose of 50 mg daily of clomifene citrate for 5 days is given at the beginning of a cycle (days 2 – 6 inclusive). If there is no response (judged by luteal-phase progesterone estimations), the dose is increased to a usual maximum of 100 mg daily for 5 days. Rarely, in obese patients, the dose may be increased to 150 mg daily for 5 days. Clomifene may induce multiple follicles; consequently, there is a 10% chance of a multiple pregnancy. The alternative approach of 2.5 mg daily of letrozole for 5 days from day 2 of the cycle, increasing to 5 mg or 7.5 mg if required, is a more successful treatment than clomifene, particularly in women with a higher BMI. However, letrozole is not currently licensed for ovulation induction in the United Kingdom.

Using these treatments, ovulation can be achieved successfully in approximately 80% of cycles, with cumulative pregnancy rates of up to 30% after 6 months' treatment.

Side effects while using clomifene citrate include vasomotor symptoms (hot flushes), pelvic discomfort, nausea and breast discomfort. These are seldom severe – explanation and reassurance are usually all that is required. More significant problems include visual disturbances (1.5%) and cholestatic jaundice (rare). In both these situations, the drug should be discontinued and not used again. Side effects of letrozole include headache, fatigue and dizziness. Some women do not respond to oral ovulation – induction agents, such as clomifene or letrozole. These patients will require treatment with exogenous gonadotrophins.

Exogenous gonadotrophins are derived from two sources: extracted from postmenopausal women's urine or, more recently, created in vitro by genetically engineered mammalian cells. Although the original urinary-derived gonadotrophins contained an equal mixture of FSH and LH, refinement of the extraction techniques has resulted in highly purified FSH compounds (>99% of protein content is FSH). The recombinant genetically engineered FSH preparations attain similar levels of purity.

All of these medications require administration by subcutaneous injection. Around 4% of women undergoing gonadotrophin treatment will develop ovarian hyperstimulation syndrome (OHSS), which will be severe in 0.5%. The incidence of multiple pregnancy with gonadotrophin treatment is around 20%, although with careful monitoring and 'step up' of the dose, this can be reduced to <5%. The aim is to achieve development of a single follicle using a low-dose regimen, starting at a low dose for 10 days and increasing the dose, if necessary, by small increments until satisfactory follicular growth occurs. Response is monitored by ovarian ultrasound, sometimes combined with serum estradiol measurement.

When the follicle reaches maturity, ovulation is induced by administering human chorionic gonadotrophin (hCG), which acts as the physiological LH surge. Gonadotrophin therapy is highly successful in restoring fertility to women with hypothalamic amenorrhoea (see later discussion) or PCOS. For women with unexplained subfertility, treatment with clomifene or exogenous gonadotrophins has not been demonstrated to improve the chance of conception. Thus, referral for IVF is appropriate in these women.

If standard ovulation – induction treatment fails in patients with PCOS, laparoscopic ovarian diathermy can be offered. The ovarian capsule is pierced four times for 5 seconds with needlepoint diathermy. Encouraging results have been reported, with spontaneous ovulation returning in up to 71% of cycles without the risk of hyperstimulation or multiple pregnancy. In women in whom spontaneous ovulation does not occur, most become more responsive to clomifene or gonadotrophin therapy. Unfortunately, the effect is time limited, with chronic anovulation returning in 50% of women within 2 years. There is the risk of iatrogenic adhesion formation and reduction in the ovarian reserve, leading to premature menopause if diathermy is used excessively.

Metformin, an oral antidiabetic drug, is of value in helping to induce ovulation in obese women with PCOS; metformin may be used either alone or in combination with clomifene, but the overall effect is inferior to letrozole.

Anovulation in Estrogen-Deficient Women

Women who have a low FSH, normal prolactin and either a low serum estradiol or negative progestogen withdrawal test (hypogonadotrophic hypogonadism), require exogenous gonadotrophins in order to ovulate (see earlier discussion).

TUBAL DISEASE

There are two treatment options in the presence of tubal disease: surgery and IVF.

Tubal Surgery

Surgery used to be the principal treatment for occlusive tubal disease. However, as the results of IVF have improved, tubal surgery is performed less frequently.

Selection of Women

Women considered for tubal surgery need to be carefully selected, taking into consideration:
- The woman's age
- The site and extent of the tubal damage
- Other factors that might influence fertility.

As with other treatments, age has an important effect on the outcome – IVF may be a better option for women in their late 30s or 40s. Distal tubal occlusion carries a poorer prognosis than proximal disease and surgery should be reserved only for cases in which damage is relatively minor. In women with minor damage, the live birth rate after surgery is around 40%

over a period of 18 months. Women with a moderate to severe distal abnormality and those with damage at more than one site on the same tube have a poor prognosis, making IVF more appropriate. With limited proximal damage, pregnancy rates of nearly 50% can be achieved after tubal surgery.

Techniques

Conventionally, tubal surgery has been performed by laparotomy through a low transverse incision, with microsurgical techniques used to restore tubal patency. However, tubal surgery is now largely performed laparoscopically. Even completely occluded tubes have been opened successfully laparoscopically, using either a CO_2 laser or electrodiathermy. In skilled hands, the results compare very favourably with conventional tubal surgery using an operating microscope.

Women who have undergone tubal surgery have a 10-fold increased risk of having an ectopic pregnancy. They are advised to undergo an ultrasound scan at around 6 weeks' gestation to assess the site of a subsequent pregnancy.

Endometriosis

Endometriosis is discussed in Chapter 8. There is no evidence that treating minimal peritoneal endometriosis with drugs improves natural fertility. Indeed, the medical treatment of endometriosis often involves creating anovulation for up to 6 months, which effectively delays the couple trying for a pregnancy. However, there is some evidence to suggest that surgery to ablate the endometriotic lesions and to divide adhesions that may have formed from endometriosis increases the chance of natural conception. Similarly, prior to IVF, treatment of endometriosis with GnRH analogues for 3 months may improve the likelihood of pregnancy.

If the endometriosis involves the ovary or fallopian tube, surgical treatment appears to be beneficial by correcting the anatomical defect. The results of surgery, even where the endometriosis is quite severe, appear to be quite encouraging. However, if pregnancy does not occur within 6 months, IVF should be considered.

MALE FACTOR

Azoospermia and a Raised Serum FSH

Azoospermia and a raised serum FSH signify spermatogenic failure (non-obstructive azoospermia). This can be confirmed by testicular biopsy. Occasionally, islands of spermatogenesis can be identified and sperm can be extracted from a testicular biopsy to be used for intracytoplasmic sperm injection (ICSI) as part of IVF treatment (see later discussion). If no sperm is identified at surgical sperm retrieval, the remaining option is the use of donor sperm.

Donor Insemination (DI)

Within the United Kingdom, sperm donors are no longer anonymous. All potential donors are screened for a family history of medical and genetic conditions and for infection, particularly human immunodeficiency virus, and hepatitis B and C. For the latter reason, semen is frozen in straws and quarantined for a minimum of 3 months prior to use. The donor is screened again for infection at the end of the period of quarantine. Only if this second screen is negative is the sperm used for treatment. Semen is inserted into the woman's uterus at the time of ovulation (see later discussion).

Azoospermia and a Normal FSH

Azoospermia in the presence of a normal FSH signifies a block of the vas deferens or epididymis. The most common group of men in this category are those who have had a vasectomy. Using microsurgical techniques, the vas can be reversed by re-anastamosis (vasovasostomy) or attached to the epididymis (vasoepididymostomy) depending on the site of the obstruction. Although good anatomical results can be achieved, pregnancy rates are often disappointing, partly because the build-up of pressure distal to the obstruction may have damaged the delicate epididymis and partly because antisperm antibodies may have formed. The time from the original vasectomy to the reversal procedure provides a useful guide to prognosis. With good surgical technique, pregnancy rates are approximately 60% but fall to 30% if the interval from vasectomy to re-anastomotic surgery is >10 years.

Men in whom spermatogenesis is normal but surgery is not possible may be suitable for epididymal sperm aspiration in combination with IVF and ICSI. The sperm can be obtained under local anaesthesia by placing a needle percutaneously into the epididymis or using more conventional microsurgical techniques under a general anaesthetic. As the sperm sample is usually of poor quality, direct ICSI into the oocytes is necessary (see later discussion).

A significant proportion of men who have congenital absence of the vas are found to carry a variant of cystic fibrosis. They have compound heterogenicity, in which each chromosome 7 carries a different mutation at the site of the transmembrane conductance regulator gene, which is responsible for cystic fibrosis. These couples are usually screened for the common cystic fibrosis mutations since if the partner is found to be a carrier of a cystic fibrosis mutations, there is a one in four chance of their child being affected with cystic fibrosis.

Hypogonadotrophic Hypogonadism

Hypogonadotrophic hypogonadism is rare but can be treated successfully with exogenous gonadotrophins (FSH and hCG) or by using an infusion pump.

Idiopathic Oligospermia

This is the most common diagnosis in male factor subfertility. A wide range of oral treatments have been employed to improve fertility but there is no firm evidence that the use of any oral medication can improve conception rates. Multivitamins have been associated with an improvement in sperm parameters and are recommended for all men whose partners are trying to conceive. The mainstay of treatment is ICSI using sperm prepared in culture medium.

Varicocele

There is ultrasound evidence of a varicocele in 15% of the general male population. Surgery to correct the defect is not justified in the absence of symptoms. Even in the presence of oligospermia, there is no evidence that the sperm count (or the conception rate) can be improved with surgery. Therefore, surgery is no longer recommended solely for subfertility reasons.

UNEXPLAINED SUBFERTILITY

If no cause can be found, then the main treatment would be to proceed to IVF, although conservative management is always an option.

Assisted Conception

'Assisted-conception' techniques are those in which gametes, either sperm or eggs, are manipulated to improve the chance of conception (Table 5.4).

TABLE 5.4 Assisted-Conception Techniques

Name	Technique	Advantages	Disadvantages
Superovulation with intrauterine insemination	Mild ovarian stimulation. Prepared sperm injected through the cervix.	For women who are not ovulating.	Chance of multiple pregnancy
In vitro fertilization (IVF)	Ovaries are superovulated, eggs retrieved and mixed with sperm before intrauterine transfer.	Effective for a number of indications, including 'unexplained' infertility.	Risks of superovulation (ovarian hyperstimulation syndrome [OHSS]) and multiple pregnancy Small increase in incidence of congenital anomalies amongst offspring Expensive
Intracytoplasmic sperm injection	Stimulation and oocyte retrieval as for IVF, but sperm injected directly into the oocyte.	Can be used to treat the majority of cases of male factor infertility.	Risks of superovulation (OHSS) and multiple pregnancy Increased incidence of genetic and developmental disorders Expensive

INTRAUTERINE INSEMINATION (IUI)

IUI was historically used to treat couples with unexplained subfertility, 'mild' male factor subfertility, and mild endometriosis. It is now mainly restricted to those with coital difficulties and couples requiring donor sperm (DI). Sperm is prepared in a culture medium, separating the seminal fluid, poorly motile sperm and other cellular debris in the ejaculate, and producing a clean sample of highly motile sperm. This is then placed directly into the uterine cavity via a fine plastic catheter. IUI is used alone, with the insemination timed to natural ovulation, or in conjunction with controlled ovarian stimulation. The latter involves ovulation – induction agents, such as clomifene or gonadotrophins, which are used to recruit up to two mature follicles. When the follicles reach an appropriate size, around 17 mm, ovulation is induced with hCG, and the prepared sperm is inserted into the uterine cavity.

In the United Kingdom, 5651 cycles of stimulated and unstimulated DI were performed in 2018. Overall, the live birth rates following unstimulated DI are 14% per cycle, very similar to the rates of 15% for stimulated DI. One complication of controlled ovarian stimulation is the high rate of multiple pregnancy. For this reason, careful dosing, monitoring and a willingness to postpone the introduction of semen due to an excessive response of the ovaries to ovulation induction, are required.

IN VITRO FERTILIZATION

The term 'in vitro fertilization' refers to the mixing of sperm and egg outside the body.

Indications

IVF was originally developed for women with tubal disease. The indications for IVF have expanded considerably and now include:
- Male factor subfertility
- Severe endometriosis
- Failed ovulation induction
- Unexplained subfertility
- Preimplantation diagnosis for genetic disease
- Surrogacy
- Egg donation

Technique
Hormonal Regimen

The aim of the treatment is to recruit, or rescue, a cohort of antral-stage follicles and support their growth through to maturity (superovulation). This is achieved by the administration of exogenous FSH, given by subcutaneous injection. To block the endogenous surge of LH that may occur with multiple follicles producing estrogen, pituitary suppression, either a GnRH agonist or an antagonist, is required. In agonist-controlled cycles, the release of LH is non-competitively blocked. Thus, hCG, which has a similar action to LH, is used as a substitute, administered approximately 36 hours before oocyte recovery. As hCG drives the risk of OHSS, in women with a higher chance of an excessive response, GnRH antagonist – based strategies are preferable with use of a GnRH agonist to trigger an endogenous LH surge and induce final oocyte maturation.

Oocyte Collection

During superovulation treatment, each ovary enlarges to the size of a tennis ball and they generally lie within 1 cm of the posterior vaginal fornix (Fig. 5.3). Whilst the woman is sedated, the oocytes are collected using

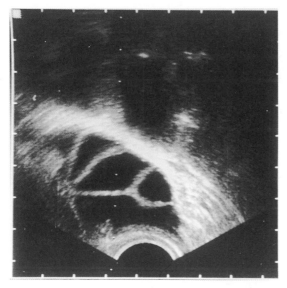

Fig. 5.3 Vaginal ultrasound illustrating superovulated ovary at egg collection.

a needle passed through the vaginal vault, guided by a vaginal ultrasound probe. The oocytes, with their cumulus cell mass, are readily identified (Fig. 5.4) and are placed in an incubator.

Fertilization and Incubation

On the morning of oocyte retrieval, the man collects a sperm sample by masturbation. After preparation in culture medium, the sperm are added to the oocytes. The tubes containing the oocytes and sperm are inspected 16 hours later for the characteristic signs of fertilization, the presence of a male and female pronucleus (Fig. 5.5). The pronucleate embryos are returned to the incubator for up to 5 days of culture (development to the blastocyst stage).

Embryo Transfer

Embryos can be transferred to the uterus at the 4- or 8-cell stage, or on day 5 at the blastocyst stage (Fig. 5.6). Transferring at the blastocyst stage appears to provide the best chance of pregnancy. An elective single embryo transfer (eSET) policy is widely employed, as it is associated with a significant reduction in the incidence of multiple pregnancies. In older women, or those with a less favourable prognosis, more than one embryo can be transferred to compensate for a lower implantation potential.

Luteal Support

As the pituitary gland has been desensitized (thus, will not be producing LH), the luteal phase has to

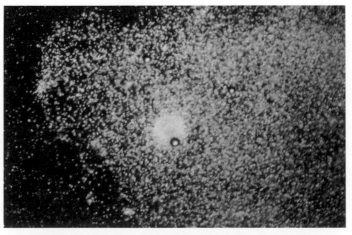

Fig. 5.4 Oocyte–cumulus cell complex identified at egg collection.

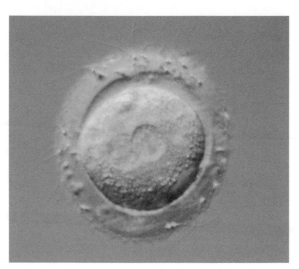

Fig. 5.5 Fertilized egg showing male and female pronucleus.

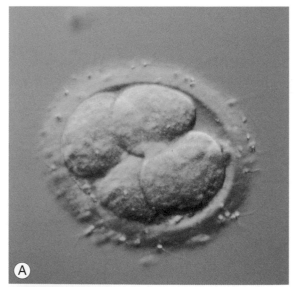

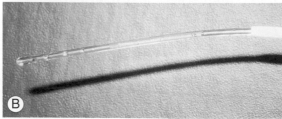

Fig. 5.6 Embryo transfer. (A) A 4-cell embryo ready for transfer into the uterus. **(B)** Loaded embryo transfer catheter.

BOX 5.3 MAIN FACTORS NEGATIVELY AFFECTING IVF SUCCESS

- Increasing age of the woman
- Increasing duration of subfertility
- Number of previous unsuccessful treatments
- Absence of previous pregnancies
- Low ovarian reserve
- Presence of hydrosalpinx (swollen and blocked fallopian tube)

be supported with progesterone pessaries for at least 14 days, until the result of the pregnancy test is known.

Results

In the United Kingdom, 68,733 cycles of IVF or ICSI were undertaken in 2018, with 86% of these using the woman's own eggs and their partner's sperm. The overall live birth rate was 26% per cycle started. However, this decreased from 32% in the women under 35 years to 12.5% in the 40- to 42-year-olds, to 1.3% in women over 44 years. The live birth rates quoted represent the chance of success in a single cycle. The first cycle of treatment gives the couple the highest chance of success (Box 5.3), but the pregnancy rate in subsequent cycles is only slightly decreased. The cumulative pregnancy rate in women under the age of 40 years is 68% after six attempts.

Embryo Freezing

Approximately 25% of couples have 'spare' embryos left over after the initial treatment. These can be frozen in liquid nitrogen ('vitrification') and replaced during a subsequent natural or artificial cycle to give a further chance of a pregnancy. With careful selection of embryos for freezing, the live birth rate following frozen embryo transfer can be equivalent to those of 'fresh' transfer.

INTRACYTOPLASMIC SPERM INJECTION (ICSI)

This technique has revolutionized the treatment of male factor subfertility. The indications for ICSI are outlined in Box 5.4. If there are no sperm in the ejaculate and none in the epididymis, sperm can still be retrieved surgically from testicular biopsies in approximately half of the men with this condition.

BOX 5.4 INDICATIONS FOR INTRACYTOPLASMIC SPERM INJECTION

- Congenital absence of the vas deferens
- Obstructive azoospermia: post-infection or post-vasectomy
- Semen analysis below reference ranges for any parameter
- Repeated failed fertilization with standard in vitro fertilization

Technique

Oocytes are collected in the standard IVF fashion and prepared for ICSI by removing their surrounding cumulus cells. A smooth-ended glass pipette is used to hold the oocyte still while a sharp ultrafine pipette pierces the egg and deposits one sperm along with a tiny amount of culture medium. Prior to injection, the selected sperm needs to be immobilized to avoid damaging the delicate structure of the oocyte. The subsequent embryo is transferred to the uterus, or frozen for potential later transfer.

Results

The pregnancy outcomes following ICSI are comparable to that of conventional IVF (live birth rate of 26% per cycle). An increased risk of genetic and developmental defects in post-ICSI pregnancies has been reported. Furthermore, a proportion of male factor subfertility has a genetic basis; by performing ICSI, the genetic abnormality may be passed on to the next generation (whereas otherwise it would not). The significance of these findings is limited, with the majority of ICSI offspring being completely healthy.

EGG DONATION

Women with primary ovarian insufficiency will require treatment involving oocyte donation (Box 5.5). This

BOX 5.5 INDICATIONS FOR EGG DONATION

- Premature ovarian insufficiency
- Gonadal dysgenesis
- Iatrogenic – surgery, radiation and chemotherapy
- Carriers of genetic disease
- Failed in vitro fertilization – poor response, inaccessible ovaries, repeated failure with woman's own eggs

treatment is also increasingly being used for 'older' women. Another indication for egg donation (or for DI when the disorder is in the male partner) is genetic disease. Egg donation is more complicated than sperm donation, as the donors have to undergo IVF treatment to the stage of oocyte collection. Some centres offer an 'egg-sharing' programme whereby an subfertile couple who cannot financially afford treatment agrees to go through an IVF cycle but donate half the harvested eggs to a recipient who funds both couples' treatment. This concept raises ethical and moral concerns, although research suggests that both parties benefit.

Results

This is a successful treatment, with pregnancy rates generally higher than conventional IVF, and maintained even in women over the age of 40 years. This is largely due to the typical age of the egg donors (on average, 25 years old) and illustrates the fact that the quality of the oocyte is the most significant factor in the age-related decline of fertility.

HOST SURROGACY

Some women have functional ovaries but no uterus due to either a congenital abnormality or previous hysterectomy. Such a woman could undergo IVF treatment, with the embryos then being transferred to another woman (a 'host surrogate') whose uterus has been suitably prepared by hormone treatment. The 'host' will carry the pregnancy and then return the baby to the subfertile ('commissioning') couple after birth. Under English law, the 'mother' is the woman who delivers the child. Therefore, the subfertile couple is required to adopt the child or have a parental order even though they are the genetic parents. This varies considerably internationally.

PREIMPLANTATION GENETIC TESTING (PGT)

Couples who have a monogenic (M) genetic disease or structural rearrangement (SR) in their chromosomes may benefit from PGT-M or PGT-SR to prevent the genetic inheritance of their condition. For couples who wish to minimize the risk of transferring aneuploid (A) embryos, PGT-A is possible. The couples undergo a conventional IVF treatment cycle, generally using ICSI as the means of fertilization. The embryos are left until

day 5, by which stage they have divided to the blastocyst stage. Generally, 5 to 10 trophectoderm cells out
of the approximately 250-cell blastocyst are removed
and analysed for specific chromosomal or genetic
abnormalities. Unaffected embryos are replaced by
embryo transfer in the usual manner. This allows the
couple to start a pregnancy knowing that the child is
unaffected by the specific genetic condition generating
the concern.

SIDE EFFECTS OF ASSISTED CONCEPTION

Globally, approximately 25% of all IVF pregnancies
are twin pregnancies; there are also some triplet pregnancies as a consequence of IVF. The introduction of
eSET has had a substantial impact on the multiple-
pregnancy rates; in the United Kingdom in 2018, the
multiple-pregnancy rate following assisted conception
was 8.2%.

OHSS is a condition in which the ovaries over-
respond to the gonadotrophin injections:

- Resulting in ovarian enlargement and abdominal
  discomfort
- Very high concentrations of estradiol and progesterone make the woman feel nauseated
- If the condition is severe, protein-rich ascites can
  accumulate and, more rarely, pleural effusion
  may result
- The sudden shift in fluid can result in hypovolaemia, with resulting renal and thrombotic
  problems; untreated, the condition can be
  fatal.

The incidence of moderate to severe OHSS is low
(<0.5%) and occurs only if the hCG injection is given
during superovulation, or if an agonist trigger is used, if
the luteal support is modified to facilitate a fresh transfer, Endogenous hCG from the implanting embryo
results in late OHSS. Women with polycystic ovaries
are the most vulnerable; they have a risk of around
5%. Once a diagnosis is made, treatment is supportive with fluid replacement, generally with protein-rich
fluids rather than crystalloid solutions. Serum electrolytes are monitored because hyperkalaemia and/or
hyponatraemia can develop. Thromboprophylaxis is
required because of the risk of venous thromboembolism. Hyperstimulation usually occurs in women
who conceive and can last throughout the early first

trimester. If the woman does not conceive, the condition is self-limiting and resolves spontaneously.

Fetal Abnormality

Approximately 3% of all infants are diagnosed with a
congenital anomaly. IVF is associated with a 30% to
40% increased risk from baseline of major congenital
anomalies compared with natural conceptions. Notably,
this risk is not attributable to the increased risk of congenital anomalies associated with multiple birth, since
the excess risk remains among singletons. It appears that
the increased risk is partly attributable to the underlying subfertility or its determinants, since couples who
take longer than 12 months to conceive naturally also
exhibit an increased risk of anomalies. The principal
anomalies which occur in IVF pregnancies include a
range of gastrointestinal, cardiovascular and musculoskeletal defects – specifically, septal heart defects, cleft
lip, oesophageal atresia and anorectal atresia. While the
relative risk of congenital anomalies amongst IVF pregnancies is increased, the absolute risk remains low.

The UK Human Fertilisation and Embryology Act

This Act, passed by the UK Parliament in 1990,
brought about the formation of a regulatory body
known as the Human Fertilisation and Embryology
Authority (HFEA). The HFEA regulates research on
human embryos, the storage of gametes and embryos
and the use in fertility treatment of donated gametes
and embryos produced outside the body. The HFEA
has the principal aims of ensuring that human embryos
and gametes are used responsibly and that subfertile couples are not exploited. Assisted-conception
treatment can be legally performed only in a centre
licenced by the HFEA. This licence is renewed on an
annual basis.

All women and men who donate gametes (either
sperm or eggs) or receive assisted-conception treatment have to be registered with the HFEA. The outcome of treatment is also recorded. The HFEA also
requires all couples considering assisted conception to
be offered counselling by a trained counsellor. Paramount in the HFEA's philosophy is the welfare of the
potential child.

Key Points

- Subfertility is defined as the inability to conceive after 12 months of regular unprotected coitus. It affects approximately one in six couples.
- The most common causes of subfertility are ovulatory problems, semen abnormalities, and blockage of fallopian tubes. However, for many, it is unexplained. Other causes include coital difficulties and endometriosis.

- Investigation involves semen analysis, tests of ovulation and tests for tubal patency.
- Treatment of anovulation may include oral anti-estrogen medications (clomifene or letrozole) or exogenous gonadotrophins administered subcutaneously.
- ICSI combined with IVF offers a treatment option to couples with male factor infertility.

Chapter 6

Early Pregnancy Care

Geeta Kumar

Chapter Outline

Introduction

Early pregnancy complications are a significant cause of maternal morbidity and mortality and a common cause for women to present to acute gynaecology services. These include miscarriage and ectopic pregnancy, and account for over 50,000 hospital admissions in the United Kingdom every year.

Miscarriage

Miscarriage is the most common early pregnancy complication, occurring in as many as 15% to 20% of all clinically recognised pregnancies. The loss of a pregnancy can be associated with significant psychological distress for women and families. Offering appropriate support in a sensitive manner during this time is vitally important.

DEFINITION

Miscarriage is defined in the UK as the spontaneous loss of an intrauterine pregnancy before 24 completed weeks of gestation, where there are no signs of life. In some countries, this is referred to as a 'spontaneous abortion'. If there are signs of life with subsequent death at any gestation, the baby is registered as a live birth and subsequent neonatal death. A baby born at or after 24 completed weeks gestation with no signs of life is registered as a stillbirth. Loss of a pregnancy in the first trimester, up to 13 completed weeks of pregnancy, is often considered an 'early pregnancy loss'.

Miscarriage can present as follows:

- *Threatened miscarriage*: presents with vaginal bleeding with or without abdominal pain, the cervix is closed on examination and ultrasound scan confirms a viable intrauterine pregnancy. It occurs in approximately 30% to 40% of pregnancies and the majority continue as healthy pregnancies without the need for intervention beyond reassurance.
- *Inevitable miscarriage*: bleeding is typically heavier, often associated with cramping-type lower abdominal pain. The cervix is open but there is no passage of pregnancy tissue yet.
- *Incomplete miscarriage*: presents with vaginal bleeding and lower abdominal pain with the passage of some, but not all, of the pregnancy tissue.
- *Complete miscarriage*: all of the pregnancy tissue has been spontaneously expelled from the uterus. In the absence of a previous scan confirming an intrauterine pregnancy, one should always be aware of the possibility of a 'pregnancy of unknown location' (see later discussion) in such situations. Women should be followed up until a definitive diagnosis is made.
- *Silent (or missed) miscarriage*: this is diagnosed by ultrasound. The pregnancy is not viable and there is an absence of pain and bleeding; 'anembryonic pregnancy' is a type of silent miscarriage in which embryo has not developed from a very early stage in the pregnancy.

INCIDENCE

The overall incidence of miscarriage is 15% to 20% with 99% of these occurring before 13 weeks' gestation. Studies of human chorionic gonadotrophin (hCG) suggest that rates of very early spontaneous pregnancy loss, soon after implantation, may be as high as 30%. After fetal heart activity is detected on an ultrasound scan, the chances of a successful pregnancy outcome are increased, with an overall risk of miscarriage of less than 5%.

The incidence of miscarriage increases with maternal age. Early pregnancy loss rates vary from 17% to 25% for women aged 35 to 40 years, rising to 33% to 50% for women aged 40 to 45 years and can be as high as 50% to 75% for women above 45 years.

AETIOLOGY

While the precise aetiology of miscarriage is not completely understood, a number of conditions have been identified as causing sporadic and/or recurrent miscarriage.

Fetal Chromosomal Abnormalities

About half of all clinically recognised first-trimester losses can be attributed to fetal chromosomal abnormalities, with 50% of these being autosomal trisomies, 20% 45XO monosomy, 20% polyploidy and 10% other abnormalities, such as structural rearrangements. Amongst pregnancies ending in second-trimester miscarriage, the incidence of chromosomal abnormality is lower, about 20% overall.

Immunological Causes

Autoimmune Disease

Approximately 15% of women investigated for recurrent miscarriage are found to be positive for antiphospholipid antibodies (lupus anticoagulants [LAs], anticardiolipin antibodies [ACAs], or both). The lupus anticoagulant is not synonymous with systemic lupus erythematosus (SLE), as it is present in only 5% to 15% of women with SLE and the majority of women who are LA or ACA positive do not have SLE.

These antibodies are also associated with arterial and venous thrombosis, fetal growth restriction and pre-eclampsia. Untreated, there is a rate of fetal loss approaching 70% to 80% in a subsequent pregnancy. Effective treatment can be provided with low-dose aspirin and low-molecular-weight heparin. Live birth rates of 54% have been seen in women receiving treatment compared with 25% in those not on any treatment.

Alloimmune Disease

It is possible that recurrent miscarriage is caused by some immunological problem at the interface between trophoblastic cells and maternal cells, although the exact nature of this interaction is unclear. There has been research and clinical interest in the role of naturally occurring uterine natural killer cells (uNK cells), which were originally thought to be the cause of miscarriage. A more recent hypothesis suggests that they might have a role in rejecting abnormal embryos and allowing normal ones to implant. It has been suggested that corticosteroids may be of benefit in women with miscarriage and high levels of uNK cells.

Endocrine Factors

In women with diabetes mellitus who have poor glycaemic control around the time of conception, the incidence of miscarriage is around 45%. Women whose blood sugar control is good are no more likely to have a miscarriage than those who do not have diabetes.

There is an association between thyroid dysfunction and miscarriage, especially recurrent miscarriage: treatment with levothyroxine is recommended in women with hypothyroidism.

Uterine Structural Anomalies

Structural uterine anomalies such as bicornuate or septate uteri may be associated with an increased risk of miscarriage, but causation remains uncertain. Uterine fibroids may interfere with early pregnancy growth, but the extent to which they cause miscarriage is difficult to determine because of other associated factors, such as the woman's age.

Cervical insufficiency is a recognised cause of midtrimester pregnancy loss (see later discussion).

Infections

Any maternal infection causing high fever may lead to pregnancy loss. Specific infectious agents – such as Zika virus, rubella virus and cytomegalovirus – can cross the placenta and may lead to miscarriage as well as to later fetal abnormality and neonatal illness. Malaria, trypanosomiasis, mycoplasma pneumonia, listeriosis and syphilis all have also been implicated in early pregnancy loss. Such infections are unlikely to cause recurrent pregnancy loss.

Environmental Pollutants

Cigarette smoking (both active and passive) and high alcohol consumption are associated with a higher chance of sporadic and recurrent miscarriage.

Unexplained

At least 50% of miscarriages, including recurrent miscarriage, have no identifiable cause.

CLINICAL PRESENTATION AND DIAGNOSIS

Presentation

There is usually a history of vaginal bleeding and lower abdominal pain. The passage of pregnancy tissue is sometimes reported. Bleeding can vary from mild to moderate blood loss to life-threateningly severe haemorrhage requiring urgent intervention. As a woman experiencing a silent miscarriage experiences no symptoms, the diagnosis is usually reached when she presents for a routine ultrasound examination.

It is seldom possible to make a reliable diagnosis of miscarriage based on clinical examination alone and management is largely based on a combination of clinical and ultrasound scan findings (Fig. 6.1). Compared

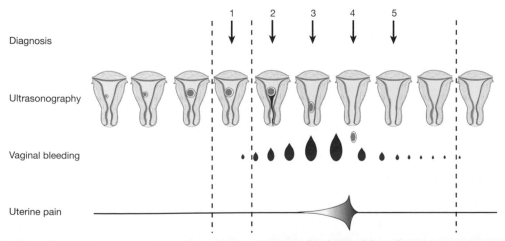

Fig. 6.1 Clinical and ultrasound features of a miscarriage. 1. Ultrasound may show fetal heart activity or the pregnancy may appear non-viable. **2.** Vaginal bleeding and pain begin. **3.** The cervical os is open – an inevitable miscarriage. **4.** The gestational sac is expelled from the uterus. **5.** Pain and bleeding usually settle rapidly.

with the transabdominal route, transvaginal scanning provides superior images.

Diagnosis

Ultrasound scans should be undertaken only after obtaining the woman's consent and be performed by appropriately experienced personnel in a systematic fashion.

The following points should be recorded for early pregnancy ultrasound scans at a minimum:

- Gestation sac number, size (mean sac diameter [MSD]), quality and location
- Presence/absence of a yolk sac
- Fetus number, size (crown-rump length [CRL]) and presence/absence of cardiac activity
- Intrauterine haematoma, if present
- Adnexal lesions, if present
- Peritoneal fluid (fluid in the pouch of Douglas), if present

Viable Intrauterine Pregnancy

If the gestation sac is within the uterus, and fetal heart activity is observed, the prognosis is good and offers reasonable reassurance (Fig. 6.2).

Empty Gestational Sac

When a transvaginal scan identifies an empty gestational sac with an MSD of 25 mm or more, the most likely diagnosis is miscarriage with an anembryonic pregnancy (Fig. 6.3). However, a second opinion should be sought and/or a repeat scan performed after

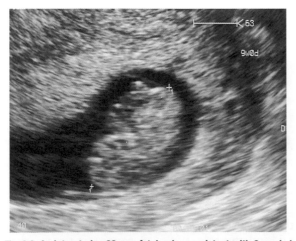

Fig. 6.2 An intrauterine 22-mm fetal pole, consistent with 9 weeks' gestation. Fetal heart activity was seen.

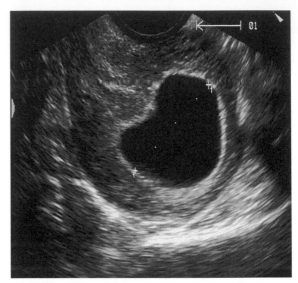

Fig. 6.3 An empty gestational sac at 8 weeks' gestation. This pregnancy was an anembryonic, sometimes referred to as a 'silent', miscarriage.

a minimum interval of 7 days to confirm the diagnosis. If the MSD is less than 25 mm and there is no visible fetal pole, a repeat scan after a minimum interval of 7 days is recommended to confirm the diagnosis. Although this time spent waiting creates anxiety, it is essential to confirm whether the pregnancy is continuing or not.

A true gestational sac should be differentiated from a 'pseudo sac', which may be present with an ectopic pregnancy (Fig. 6.4). A pseudo sac is caused by fluid secreted by the endometrium in response to the hCG produced by the ectopic pregnancy, and it lacks the characteristic 'double decidual ring' outline seen with the true gestational sac of an intrauterine pregnancy (see Figs 6.3 and 6.5).

Fetal Pole With no Fetal Heart Activity

A fetal heartbeat is usually seen on a transvaginal scan if the fetal pole is more than 2 to 3 mm and almost always seen by the time the fetal pole is 7.0 mm (see Fig. 6.5). In the absence of a visible fetal heartbeat with a CRL of more than 7.0 mm, miscarriage is the most likely diagnosis. However, a second opinion should be sought and/or re-scanning arranged in the next 7 to 10 days before confirming the diagnosis of a missed miscarriage. If the CRL is less than 7.0 mm

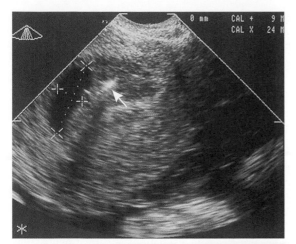

Fig. 6.4 A pseudo sac and intrauterine contraceptive device (*arrow*) in the presence of an ectopic pregnancy.

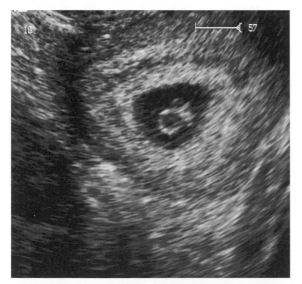

Fig. 6.5 Intrauterine gestational scan containing a 6-mm fetal pole with a yolk sac. No fetal heart activity was detected by transvaginal scan. Note the double decidual ring consistent with intrauterine pregnancy.

width and there is no heartbeat, a second scan should be performed a minimum of 7 days after the first one, before making a diagnosis.

Empty Uterus

An empty uterine cavity could mean a complete miscarriage, a very early intrauterine pregnancy, or an ectopic pregnancy. An intrauterine sac will usually be seen

on transvaginal scan if the serum hCG is >1000 IU; its absence raises the possibility of an ectopic pregnancy. The management of ectopic pregnancy and pregnancy of unknown location (PUL) is discussed later.

CARE OF WOMEN WITH EARLY PREGNANCY PROBLEMS

The care of early pregnancy problems should take place in an early pregnancy unit run by dedicated and appropriately trained healthcare professionals. Once a diagnosis of miscarriage has been made, women are usually offered a choice of treatment options.

Expectant

This is also called the 'wait and watch' approach to see if the condition will resolve naturally without intervention. It avoids medical or surgical intervention with their associated risks and is more acceptable to some women. Approximately 50% of incomplete miscarriages will resolve spontaneously within 2 weeks. Associated risks include prolonged bleeding, infection and the risk that some women may ultimately require surgical management. Expectant management can be continued for as long as the woman wishes provided there are no signs of infection. Prolonged follow-up (sometimes 6–8 weeks) yields higher success rates. If during the course of expectant management the woman changes her mind and requests medical or surgical intervention, then this can be arranged.

Medical

Medical intervention includes use of misoprostol, a synthetic prostaglandin which causes the myometrium to contract with expulsion of pregnancy tissue. This can avoid the risks associated with surgery. Success rates vary depending upon the type of miscarriage, gestational age dosage, duration and route of administration of misoprostol. Treatment for incomplete miscarriage with high-dose misoprostol administered vaginally (followed up clinically without ultrasound) is associated with higher success rates (70%–96%). Potential disadvantages include greater analgesic needs, increased vaginal bleeding, the potential requirement for surgery if unsuccessful, and the side effects of nausea, pyrexia and/or diarrhoea.

Surgical

This involves either manual vacuum aspiration (MVA) under local anaesthetic in an outpatient setting, or surgical uterine evacuation in an operating theatre under general anaesthetic. Surgery has a success rate of 95%, with the advantage of being quick and effective in most cases. The potential risks include infection, haemorrhage, cervical trauma from instrumentation, uterine perforation and the risks of anaesthesia. A surgical approach is generally recommended in the presence of heavy vaginal bleeding, infection, or haemodynamic instability.

SAFE AND SENSITIVE DISPOSAL OF FETAL TISSUE

Pregnancy products (products of conception) must be disposed of sensitively and safely in accordance with local policies and legislation, such as the Human Tissue Authority Act in England.

RECURRENT MISCARRIAGE

In the United Kingdom, recurrent miscarriage (RM) is defined as the loss of three or more consecutive pregnancies. However, the European Society of Human Reproduction and Embryology defines RM as two or more pregnancy losses, excluding ectopic pregnancies and molar pregnancies. RM affects 1% to 2% of women (depending on the definition used). Maternal age is an independent risk factor, with the risk of RM rising significantly in women over 40 years of age. Lifestyle factors such as smoking, obesity and excessive alcohol intake are associated with RM.

Recommended investigations include testing for antiphospholipid antibodies (LA-ACA), thyroid screening (thyroid-stimulating hormone levels and thyroid peroxidase antibodies) and an ultrasound for uterine anomalies. On a case-by-case basis or in research settings, further investigations may include genetic testing (genetic analysis of pregnancy tissue), immunological tests (human leukocyte antigen – antinuclear antibody [HLA-ANA]) and thrombophilia testing.

If a woman tests positive for antiphospholipid antibodies, treatment with low-dose aspirin and low molecular weight heparin is recommended. Thyroxine replacement is recommended if a woman is hypothyroid. In cases of uterine malformations, there

is insufficient evidence to recommend surgical interventions and management should be individualized. For those with identifiable genetic causes, referral for genetic counselling is appropriate.

In most women experiencing RM, these investigations do not identify a cause. Reassurance along with lifestyle advice are the mainstays of care. Preconception folic acid supplementation is routinely recommended to prevent neural tube defects but has not been shown to prevent miscarriage in women with RM. Amongst women with RM who have no apparent underlying cause, 60% to 70% will have a successful future pregnancy. Research into the aetiology and therapeutic interventions in RM continues. The use of as yet unproven investigations and treatments should be limited to research studies.

MID-TRIMESTER LOSS

Following mid-trimester loss – a pregnancy loss between 14 and 23^{+6} weeks' gestation – the possibility of cervical insufficiency should be considered. The diagnosis is suggested by a history of relatively painless cervical dilation. There may be a history of previous surgery or trauma to the cervix. Under these circumstances, women should be offered serial sonographic surveillance of cervical length in subsequent pregnancies. A cervical length of less than 25 mm prompts a discussion regarding the insertion of a cervical suture (cervical cerclage; Fig. 6.6) to reduce the risk of mid-trimester loss and preterm

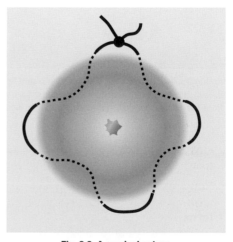

Fig. 6.6 A cervical suture.

birth. Transvaginal cerclage is usually offered but a transabdominal cerclage should be considered when a vaginal approach is not technically possible or when a vaginally placed suture has not been successful for the woman in the past. (See Chapter 29, Pre-term birth.)

Pregnancy of Unknown Location

Pregnancy of unknown location (PUL) is defined as a positive pregnancy test with no evidence of an intrauterine or ectopic pregnancy on transvaginal ultrasound scan. PUL may be managed expectantly, medically, or surgically, depending upon symptoms and serum hCG levels. As long as they remain clinically stable, all women with a PUL should be followed up until the final outcome is determined. Outcomes can be classified as a viable or non-viable intrauterine pregnancy (IUP), an ectopic pregnancy (EP), a spontaneously resolved PUL, or a persisting PUL.

Women undergoing expectant management of PUL should be given clear information about the importance of follow-up due to the risk of bleeding from an undiagnosed ectopic pregnancy. Serial serum hCG measurements should be performed until hCG levels are <5 IU/L. Medical or surgical intervention is required in 20% to 30% of cases of PUL.

Ectopic Pregnancy

An EP occurs when the fertilized egg implants anywhere other than the endometrium. The most common site for EP is the fallopian tube (95%; Fig. 6.7). However, implantation can occur in the ovary, cervix,

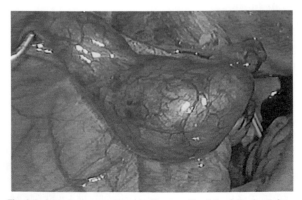

Fig. 6.7 An ectopic pregnancy in the ampulla of the fallopian tube.

previous caesarean section scar or in the abdomen. The incidence of EP is 1% of pregnancies; intraperitoneal bleeding from an EP is an important cause of maternal mortality. Early recognition and appropriate care are the key to effective treatment.

CLINICAL PRESENTATION

Clinical presentations in cases of EP are highly variable, ranging from no symptoms to cardiovascular collapse. Risk factors for the development of EP include:
- Previous ectopic pregnancy
- History of pelvic inflammatory disease
- Pregnancy with an intrauterine contraceptive device in place
- Previous pelvic surgery – for example, tubal surgery, appendicectomy, caesarean section
- History of subfertility, including pregnancies conceived after assisted conception
- Pregnancy whilst taking the progesterone-only contraceptive pill
- Smoking
- Advanced maternal age

CLINICAL PRESENTATION AND DIAGNOSIS

The history should include the date of the last menstrual period, date of positive pregnancy test and presence of risk factors for EP. Symptoms of EP classically include pelvic pain with vaginal bleeding following an interval of amenorrhoea. Other symptoms include breast tenderness, diarrhoea, dizziness, fainting, shoulder tip pain, passage of tissue from the vagina rectal pressure, or pain on defaecation. Women presenting with pain or bleeding in early pregnancy should be referred to an early pregnancy assessment service (or out-of-hours gynaecology service depending upon local service provision) for clinical assessment and an ultrasound scan.

Clinical signs include pelvic tenderness, adnexal tenderness, cervical motion tenderness (cervical excitation), rebound tenderness over the abdomen (peritonism), pallor, abdominal distension, tachycardia and/or hypotension. During clinical assessment of women of reproductive age, a pregnancy test should be undertaken even in the presence of non-specific symptoms since the symptoms and signs of EP can mimic the symptoms and signs of other conditions, such as gastrointestinal infection or urinary tract infection. Nearly a third of women with EP will have no recognised risk factors. The level of serum hCG facilitates both diagnosis and treatment.

A transvaginal ultrasound scan is the investigation of choice to identify the location of the pregnancy and make a diagnosis. Ultrasound signs indicating a tubal EP include an adnexal mass containing a gestational sac with a yolk sac or a fetal pole moving separately to the ovary or a complex, inhomogeneous adnexal mass, again moving separately to the ovary. An empty uterus or a collection of fluid within the uterine cavity (sometimes described as a 'pseudo sac') can indicate a possible EP. 'Free fluid' seen on a scan in this context, is likely to be blood in the peritoneal cavity, due to bleeding from an EP.

A transabdominal ultrasound scan may be more suitable for women with pelvic pathology, such as fibroids or an ovarian cyst, or if a transvaginal ultrasound scan is declined, in which case the limitations of transabdominal scanning should be explained. Concurrent EP and intrauterine pregnancy is rarely encountered (heterotopic pregnancy, 1 in 7000 to 1 in 30,000 pregnancies) but is more common after in vitro fertilization than spontaneous conception.

CARE OF WOMEN WITH AN ECTOPIC PREGNANCY

Options for care depend on the clinical picture, the location and ultrasound scan features of EP, along with the serum hCG level. Tubal EP (the most common location of ectopic pregnancy) can be treated surgically (salpingectomy or salpingotomy), medically (using methotrexate) or, occasionally, expectantly. Care must be tailored to the clinical condition and the woman's future fertility preferences.

Expectant

Expectant management should be considered as an option for women who are asymptomatic and clinically stable with a confirmed diagnosis of tubal EP measuring less than 35 mm with no visible heartbeat, a serum hCG level less than 1500 IU/L and who are able to attend regularly for follow-up.

Medical

Methotrexate is a folic acid antagonist which prevents the growth of rapidly dividing cells by interfering with DNA synthesis. Medical treatment with methotrexate is suitable for women who are haemodynamically stable with serum hCG levels less than 1500 IU/L, who have an unruptured tubal ectopic pregnancy less than 35 mm in diameter with no fetal heart activity, and no significant fluid collection in the peritoneal cavity or pouch of Douglas. Clinically stable women meeting these criteria with a serum hCG level between 1500 IU/L and 5000 IU/L can also be offered the option of medical treatment with methotrexate or surgery.

Women should be informed of the importance of attending regular follow-up appointments to measure the serum hCG and assess their clinical condition, and the need to use reliable contraception for at least 3 months following treatment. Administered as a single intramuscular injection (50 mg/m^2 body surface area), success rates of up to 92% are reported, with subsequent intrauterine pregnancy rates of 58% and rates of a recurrent EP of 9%. Approximately 15% of women require a repeat dose of methotrexate; 7% may require surgery because of intrapertioneal bleeding.

Most women experience abdominal pain with the use of methotrexate and it may be difficult at times to differentiate between tubal miscarriage and tubal rupture. Clinical features and scan findings guide as to what is the most appropriate care in these situations.

Surgical

If the woman is haemodynamically unstable, does not meet criteria for medical or expectant management, or prefers to have surgical treatment, then surgical management should be offered.

Surgery should be considered for women who have an adnexal mass >35 mm, an EP with a fetal heartbeat, significant free fluid in the pouch of Douglas, a serum hCG more than 5000 IU/L, or symptoms and signs consistent with intraperitoneal bleeding from an ectopic pregnancy. If the woman is not haemodynamically stable, the most expedient method of surgical management should be chosen after initial resuscitation. If the woman is haemodynamically stable (the majority), a laparoscopic approach is preferable to laparotomy, as it is associated with less blood loss, lower analgesia requirements, shorter hospital stay and quicker postoperative recovery.

Salpingectomy (removal of the fallopian tube) is preferred to salpingotomy (incision of the tube and removal of the pregnancy tissue) when the contralateral tube appears healthy as it is associated with lower rates of persistent trophoblast and recurrent EP but with similar cumulative subsequent intrauterine pregnancy rates (55%–60%). However, salpingotomy should be considered in suitable cases if the woman has contralateral tubal disease or an absent contralateral fallopian tube and desires future fertility.

RHESUS ISOIMMUNISATION

All non-sensitized rhesus negative women who have undergone a surgical procedure for a miscarriage or EP should be offered anti-D immunoglobulin at a dose of 250 IU. Anti-D prophylaxis is not recommended in the first trimester for women who undergo medical treatment for an ectopic pregnancy or miscarriage, or who have a threatened or complete miscarriage or a pregnancy of unknown location. If there is doubt as to the exact gestation of a pregnancy loss, it is preferable to offer anti-D to avoid the risk of rhesus isoimmunisation on subsequent pregnancies.

After Pregnancy Loss

Pregnancy loss, irrespective of gestation or location of pregnancy, is a bereavement. Whilst the emotional trauma experienced is variable, the potential adverse impact should not be underestimated. Information about support groups, such as the Miscarriage Association and The Ectopic Pregnancy Trust, should be provided to all women experiencing pregnancy loss.

Key Points

- Miscarriage is the loss of a pregnancy before 24 weeks' gestation.
- Management of miscarriage is centred on accurate diagnosis, counselling and minimizing complications.
- Care must be taken to avoid uterine evacuation if there is any possibility of a continuing pregnancy. A 'wait and see' approach must be adopted until the diagnosis is certain.
- There should be a low threshold of suspicion for ectopic pregnancy.
- Care should be provided in a dedicated early pregnancy unit.

Chapter 7

Heavy Menstrual Bleeding, Dysmenorrhoea and Pre-Menstrual Syndrome

Jenifer Sassarini, Kay McAllister

Chapter Outline

Heavy Menstrual Bleeding

Heavy menstrual bleeding (HMB) is defined, for clinical purposes, as bleeding that has an adverse impact on the quality of life of a woman. It may occur alone or with other symptoms. Menstrual blood loss can be measured, but this is usually performed only for research purposes. HMB was often called 'menorrhagia' in the past, but this term is better avoided as it means different things to different people (e.g., the definition in the United States is different from that in the United Kingdom). HMB is the most common cause of iron-deficiency anaemia in women in high-resource settings.

Menstrual problems are becoming more prevalent, as women experience more periods in their lifetime now than their predecessors did 100 years ago (approximately 400 vs. 40 periods). This is because women have fewer children and breastfeed less (leading to lactational amenorrhoea). Only 50% of women who complain of excessive heavy bleeding, however, actually suffer from blood loss that falls out-side the normal range for women not complaining of any menstrual abnormality (>80 mL/month).

The medical and surgical treatments of HMB represent an appreciable burden to health service resources. HMB is a common indication for hysterectomy, although the number of these procedures performed has fallen in the last 3 decades with the introduction of effective alternative treatments. Although a commonly performed operation, hysterectomy is a major surgical procedure. Its use needs to be balanced against the potential associated mortality and morbidity. Satisfaction rates with hysterectomy are very high, however.

CAUSES OF HMB

A classification system for the causes of abnormal uterine bleeding (AUB) has been described by the International Federation of Gynecology and Obstetrics (FIGO), which is called the PALM-COEIN System (Table 7.1). Clinicians should remember that, using this classification, a woman may have more than one entity that could contribute to AUB and that structural entities such as polyps are often asymptomatic.

Uterine Pathology

HMB is associated with both benign pathology (e.g., uterine fibroids, endometrial polyps, adenomyosis, pelvic infection) and, extremely rarely, malignant pathology (e.g., endometrial cancer). Over half of women with an excessively heavy blood loss of >200 mL/period will have fibroids. With the advent of high-quality ultrasound that is readily available in outpatient clinics, pathology is identified in a greater proportion of women.

Endometrial polyps are common benign localized overgrowths of the endometrium. They consist of a fibrous tissue core covered by columnar epithelium, and it is believed that they arise as a result of disordered cycles of endometrial apoptosis and regrowth. Although it is uncertain that they cause HMB, it is likely that intrauterine endometrial polyps do increase the likelihood of irregular bleeding (Fig. 7.1). However, it is unlikely that small endocervical polyps detected at the time of a routine cervical smear have the same effect. Malignant transformation of such polyps is very rare.

Uterine fibroids (leiomyomas) are benign tumours of the myometrium that are present in approximately 20% of women of reproductive age. They are well-circumscribed whorls of smooth muscle cells and collagen, and may be single or multiple (Fig. 7.2).

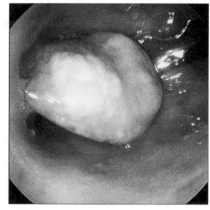

Fig. 7.1 Hysteroscopic view of intrauterine polyp. (© KARL STORZ – Endoskope, Germany)

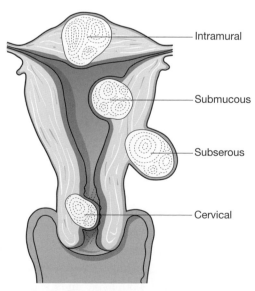

Fig. 7.2 Sites of fibroids throughout the uterus.

TABLE 7.1 **PALM-COEIN Classification System for Abnormal Uterine Bleeding Proposed by the International Federation of Gynecology and Obstetrics (FIGO)**	
Polyp	Coagulopathy
Adenomyosis	Ovulatory dysfunction
Leiomyoma	Endometrial
Malignancy and hyperplasia	Iatrogenic
	Not otherwise classified

Size varies from microscopic growths to tumours that weigh as much as 40 kg, and they are more common in women of Afro-Caribbean origin. Submucous fibroids project into the uterine cavity, intramural fibroids are contained within the wall of the uterus and subserosal fibroids project from the surface of the uterus. Cervical fibroids arise from the cervix.

Many are asymptomatic, but when symptoms do occur, they are often related to the site and/or size of the fibroid. Presenting symptoms include menstrual dysfunction, infertility, miscarriage, dyspareunia and pelvic discomfort. The mechanism by which fibroids adversely affect reproduction is unclear but may be related in part to distortion of the uterine cavity, affecting implantation. Fibroids that do not distort the cavity are unlikely to have an adverse impact. Women with fibroids may also present because of pressure effects on surrounding organs, such as increased frequency of micturition as a result of pressure on the bladder or even hydronephrosis due to ureteric compression. Sex steroids mediate the growth of fibroids; therefore, they grow during pregnancy and shrink after the menopause. Occasionally, necrosis of the fibroid ('red degeneration') leads to acute abdominal pain during pregnancy. The incidence of malignant change (leiomyosarcoma) in fibroids is considered to be extremely low (0.1%).

HMB in the Absence of Pathology

The term 'abnormal uterine bleeding' is commonly used in clinical practice and includes the symptoms of HMB, irregular menstruation and intermenstrual bleeding. HMB in the absence of recognisable pelvic pathology or systemic disease is a diagnosis of exclusion and is probably the most common 'diagnosis' reached after investigating women with HMB. Some HMB with no pathology may be 'anovulatory' or 'ovulatory', although this is not an important distinction clinically, as treatment is the same in both cases. The underlying cause is likely to reside at the level of the endometrium, although the precise nature of the vascular and endocrine abnormality remains elusive.

Medical Disorders and Clotting Defects

Very rarely, HMB is associated with medical problems, such as thyroid disease (both hypo- and hyperthyroidism), hepatic disease and renal disease (although the majority of women with end-stage renal failure are amenorrhoeic). Other symptoms of the underlying medical disorder are likely to be present.

Certain coagulation abnormalities (e.g., von Willebrand disease) and platelet defects (e.g., thrombocytopenia) are associated with an increased incidence of HMB.

ASSESSMENT OF HMB

History

The number of sanitary towels used, duration of bleeding and passage of clots seem to have little correlation with the actual volume of blood lost. However, complaints of 'flooding' (leakage of heavy blood loss onto clothing) and having to use 'double sanitary protection' (pad and tampon) to prevent leakage of blood onto clothes are indicative of HMB, and are likely to have a negative impact upon the woman's quality of life. Therefore, it is important to ask about the degree of inconvenience experienced, such as time lost from work, or becoming housebound during menses owing to fear of social embarrassment from an episode of flooding in public.

A history of irregular bleeding, dyspareunia, pelvic pain or intermenstrual or post-coital bleeding may raise the suspicion of underlying pathology, and often requires additional investigation. These can be termed 'red flag' symptoms.

The woman should also be questioned about symptoms suggestive of anaemia, such as fatigue and lightheadedness. A history suggestive of systemic disease such as a thyroid disorder or a clotting abnormality would signal that further investigation for such causes is required. The woman should also be questioned about risk factors for endometrial cancer, such as unopposed estrogen use, tamoxifen use, polycystic ovary syndrome or family history of endometrial or colon cancer. It is also important to establish whether she has a history of thromboembolism, as many medical treatments for HMB are hormonal; thus, their use may be relatively or absolutely contraindicated.

Examination

The woman should be examined for signs of anaemia. Abdominal, bimanual and speculum examinations should be considered; however, if the history suggests HMB without structural or histological abnormality, pharmaceutical treatment can be started without carrying out a physical examination or other investigations at initial consultation in primary care. An enlarged, 'bulky' uterus suggests uterine fibroids; tenderness suggests endometriosis, pelvic inflammatory disease, or adenomyosis.

Investigations

Laboratory Tests

A full blood count should be carried out in all women with HMB to diagnose/exclude anaemia. Thyroid function tests and coagulation tests should be performed only if there are features in the history. No other endocrine tests are routinely indicated.

Ultrasound

Ultrasound is the first-line diagnostic tool for identifying structural abnormalities, and a pelvic ultrasound scan should be performed if either history or examination suggests structural uterine pathology. Imaging should also be undertaken in women in whom pharmaceutical treatment has failed or if it is not possible to assess the uterus clinically because of obesity. The site and size

of abnormalities such as fibroids can be determined, together with assessment of the ovaries (Fig. 7.3).

Endometrial Assessment

This should be performed in all women aged >45 years as well as in younger women with persistent HMB in spite of medical treatment, red flag symptoms such as irregular bleeding, or risk factors for endometrial cancer. This can take the form of an endometrial biopsy or a hysteroscopy, both of which can be carried out either as an outpatient or inpatient procedure (Fig. 7.4 and p. 151).

Cervical Cytology

This should be performed if it is due, or if the cervix looks suspicious.

CARE OF WOMEN WITH HMB

Polyps

Benign intrauterine polyps will usually be removed by polypectomy using hysteroscopic techniques. If

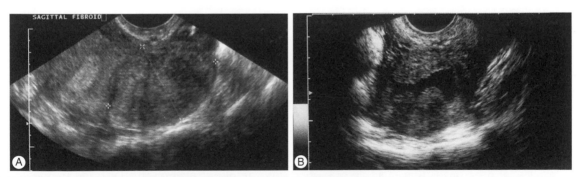

Fig. 7.3 Uterine fibroids. (A) A large intramural fibroid. **(B)** Two submucous fibroids projecting into the cavity of the uterus, which contains a small amount of fluid (saline infusion ultrasound scan).

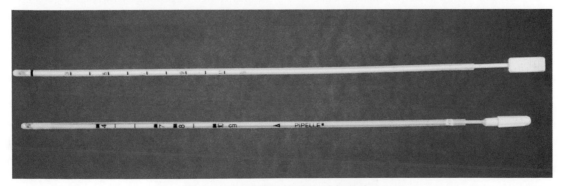

Fig. 7.4 Two varieties of endometrial samplers.

malignant pathology is detected, then this should be treated as appropriate.

Fibroids

Fibroids may be treated medically or surgically.

Medical

Pharmaceutical treatment should be considered when fibroids measure less than 3 cm and cause no distortion of the uterine cavity. If contraceptive and/or hormonal treatments are acceptable, the following treatments can be offered:

- Levonorgestrel-releasing intrauterine system (LNG-IUS);
- Tranexamic acid, non-steroidal anti-inflammatory drugs (NSAIDs), or combined oral contraceptive (COC);
- Norethisterone (15 mg) daily from days 5 to 26 of the menstrual cycle, or;
- Injected long-acting progestogens.

Unfortunately, the symptoms caused by fibroids respond poorly to medical treatments used when there is no pathology. Therefore, in women with fibroids measuring 3 cm or more or with fibroids causing distortion of the uterine cavity, ulipristal acetate should be offered. The drug is started when menstruation has occurred, and should be taken as one 5-mg tablet daily for a treatment course of up to 3 months, up to a maximum of four intermittent courses.

Ulipristal acetate is a selective progesterone receptor modulator, a class of drugs that may have a role in the treatment of fibroid-related HMB. Treatment with this class of drugs leads to a rapid decrease in bleeding in 80% of women without leading to hypo-estrogenism or inhibiting ovarian cyclicity. Concerns have been raised regarding ulipristal acetate in the care of women with fibroids and HMB since they can cause unique changes in the endometrium that are difficult to interpret. Furthermore, cases of severe liver injury requiring transplant associated with its use have been reported. Its use in the United Kingdom is currently restricted to treating uterine fibroids in premenopausal women for whom surgical procedures are not appropriate or have not worked.

Since growth of fibroids is hormone dependent, gonadotrophin-releasing hormone (GnRH) analogues (which result in hypo-estrogenism) may be used to shrink fibroids. GnRH analogues are derivatives of natural GnRH, with modifications that confer greater potency and longer activity. Depot injection of GnRH analogues, however, leads to pituitary downregulation with hypo-estrogenism. Fibroids shrink by approximately 50% over 3 months of treatment, but regrowth occurs upon cessation of treatment. During treatment, hypo-estrogenism can result in symptoms such as hot flushes and may also cause loss of bone density. In view of concerns about osteoporosis, GnRH analogues are limited to short-term use (<6 months). 'Add-back' hormone replacement therapy (HRT) is required to minimize the risk of osteoporosis and other side effects.

Surgical

Hysteroscopic resection of small submucous fibroids is often possible, which can lead to improved fertility and relief of menstrual problems. Endometrial ablation in the presence of small fibroids is possible (see later discussion).

Myomectomy involves incision of the fibroid pseudocapsule, enucleation of the bulk of the tumour and closure of the resulting defect. The operation is usually performed as an open abdominal procedure, although laparoscopic techniques are sometimes employed. Myomectomy is associated with a similar degree of morbidity to hysterectomy. There is a risk of haemorrhage (due to the vascularity of fibroids) and a small possibility that an emergency hysterectomy may need to be performed during surgery to arrest uncontrollable bleeding. Furthermore, there is a risk of adhesion formation, which could compromise fertility (as a result of tubal obstruction), and the possibility that residual seedling fibroids may grow, leading to the recurrence of fibroids. GnRH analogues are often used preoperatively to shrink fibroids, with associated decreased intraoperative blood loss. Women who have undergone myomectomy are often recommended to birth by caesarean in any subsequent pregnancy because of concerns regarding uterine rupture during labour.

Uterine artery embolization (UAE), which is performed by interventional radiologists, is an effective and safe technique. It involves interruption of the blood supply to the fibroid by blocking the uterine arteries with coils or foam delivered through a catheter placed in the femoral artery. The healthy myometrium revascularizes immediately, owing to the development of collateral circulation from vaginal and ovarian vessels. Fibroids, however, do not appear to revascularize, and shrink by about 50%, a reduction which appears to be sustained. Pain following occlusion of the vessels is often severe and usually requires opiate analgesia. Potential complications include infection, fibroid expulsion and adverse effects due to exposure of the ovaries to ionizing radiation. The incidence of these is low and immediate morbidity is less than that following hysterectomy, although pain and fever from post-embolization syndrome is not uncommon and deaths (though rare) have occurred.

UAE, myomectomy, or hysterectomy should be considered in cases of HMB in which large fibroids (greater than 3 cm in diameter) are present and bleeding is having a severe impact on a woman's quality of life. Women should be informed that UAE or myomectomy may potentially allow them to retain their fertility. Studies indicate that fertility outcomes are better in younger women, women with fewer fibroids, and when fibroids that have been distorting the endometrial cavity have been removed. There is evidence that a successful pregnancy is possible following UAE and even after failed myomectomy, although rates of miscarriage may be higher and rates of caesarean section and postpartum haemorrhage may be higher. There are also reports of transient or permanent ovarian failure after UAE in up to 5% of cases. This occurs most often in women over the age of 45 years, but there have been case reports of ovarian dysfunction in younger women.

If childbearing is complete and the woman is experiencing severe symptoms as a result of her fibroids, then hysterectomy may be considered (see later discussion).

Other Causes

In the majority of cases of HMB, no specific cause is found. Sometimes, a woman is seeking reassurance that there is no pathology and does not necessarily wish treatment. Most women, however, request treatment. The following treatments may be considered.

Medical

Intrauterine Progestogens The LNG-IUS delivers progestogen directly to the uterus (Fig. 7.5). It is a first-line treatment for HMB that is particularly suitable for women requiring contraception, as it is a highly

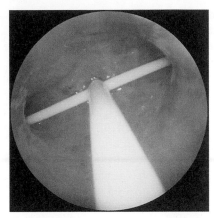

Fig. 7.5 An intrauterine progestogen-releasing system in the uterus. (© KARL STORZ – Endoskope, Germany)

effective reversible method of contraception and can stay in place for up to 5 years. After 12 months, menstrual blood loss is reduced by around 95%, and many women are amenorrhoeic. The main problems with the LNG-IUS are the high incidence of irregular bleeding, particularly within the first 3 to 6 months after insertion, and an expulsion rate of 5%.

Prostaglandin Synthesis Inhibitors NSAIDs taken during menstruation reduce menstrual blood loss by around 25% by reducing endometrial prostaglandin concentrations. The NSAID most commonly used for treatment of HMB is mefenamic acid, although other NSAIDs have similar efficacies. Side effects include gastrointestinal complaints, dizziness and headache. These drugs are also of benefit for treating dysmenorrhoea.

Antifibrinolytics Antifibrinolytics, such as tranexamic acid, work by inhibiting plasminogen activator, thereby reducing the fibrinolytic activity in the endometrium. This increases clot formation in the spiral arterioles and reduces menstrual blood loss. Taking tranexamic acid during menstruation reduces blood loss by around 50%. Gastrointestinal side effects, nausea and tinnitus can occur. The drug should not be taken by women who are predisposed to thromboembolism.

NSAIDs and antifibrinolytics are the best options for women wishing to conceive, as they are taken only during menstruation and do not suppress ovulation.

Combined Oral Contraceptive Pill This reduces blood loss by approximately 50%. Its mechanism for doing so is thought to be due to suppressive effects on the endometrium. There is no age restriction on the use of the COC in women at low risk of cardiovascular complications (see p. 235).

Systemic Progestogens Oral progestogens are widely prescribed for HMB. Studies have shown that taken as a long or short course, they reduce menstrual blood loss compared with baseline. Long course treatment (up to 9 months) is more effective than short courses (up to 2 weeks). Taken in a cyclical fashion, oral progestogens are also useful in regulating otherwise irregular cycles. If the depot injectable progestogen (medroxyprogesterone acetate) is administered for long enough, amenorrhoea frequently results. During the initial months of use, however, bleeding can be unpredictable and heavy. Side effects of progestogens include nausea, bloating, headache, breast tenderness, weight gain and acne.

GnRH Analogues Amenorrhoea occurs as a result of pituitary downregulation, which leads to inhibition of ovarian activity. However, women may experience problems associated with the resultant hypo-estrogenism—particularly, hot flushes and vaginal dryness. GnRH analogues are usually reserved for short-term use only (up to 6 months), and add-back HRT is usually prescribed to relieve symptoms of hypo-estrogenism.

Danazol Danazol is a synthetic androgen with anti-estrogenic and anti-progestogenic activity that reduces menstrual blood loss but is no longer recommended because of its adverse side-effect profile, which includes irreversible virilization.

Surgical

Endometrial Ablation Using a number of different techniques, it is possible to destroy most or all of the endometrium, thereby lessening or stopping menstrual blood loss altogether. Because the endometrium regenerates from the basal layer, it is essential to ablate to the endomyometrial border. Endometrial ablation offers a safer method of symptom control, much shorter hospital stay and shorter recovery period than hysterectomy. Early techniques involved a hysteroscopic procedure under general anaesthesia, during which the endometrium was treated under direct visualization by laser, diathermy, or resection. Newer, non-hysteroscopic procedures included ablation with a heated balloon and bipolar radiofrequency impedance-controlled endometrial ablation (e.g., NovaSure); other

approaches are being developed all the time (Fig. 7.6). These newer procedures carry fewer risks than the hysteroscopic resections, and some can be performed under local anaesthesia.

The success rates of the different ablative techniques are broadly similar. All are associated with a 70% to 80% overall satisfaction rate in addition to an amenorrhoea rate of 20% for balloon treatment and around 50% for impedance-controlled ablation. Complications are rare but include uterine perforation, hyponatraemia and infection. Pregnancy is contraindicated after an ablation procedure. Women are urged to use a reliable, if not permanent, form of contraception after ablation.

Hysterectomy This is the only treatment that guarantees amenorrhoea; as a consequence, it is associated with a high level of satisfaction. Hysterectomy is performed via the abdominal or vaginal route, the latter with or without laparoscopic assistance (laparoscopically assisted vaginal hysterectomy [LAVH]). Abdominal hysterectomy involves a laparotomy incision, which is usually transverse; a vaginal hysterectomy involves an incision through the vaginal wall. The choice between the various procedures depends on the size of the uterus, the degree of uterine descent, whether the ovaries will be removed (which is difficult by the vaginal route) and the skills and preferences of the surgeon (Table 7.2). In current practice, hysterectomy is increasingly carried out entirely laparoscopically (either by LAVH or by total laparoscopic hysterectomy). The decision to proceed with laparoscopic hysterectomy will depend on the experience of the surgeon, the presence of other gynaecological conditions or disease, size of the uterus, presence and size of fibroids and history of previous abdominal surgery (including caesarean section). Robotic-assisted laparoscopic hysterectomy is available in some centres.

Complications of hysterectomy include haemorrhage, bowel trauma, damage to the urinary tract, infection, postoperative thromboembolism and risk of vaginal prolapse in later years. Complications are more common in those with uterine fibroids. Women undergoing a vaginal procedure recover more quickly from the operation than do those undergoing an abdominal hysterectomy, but the incidence of major complications, although low, is slightly higher with the vaginal route.

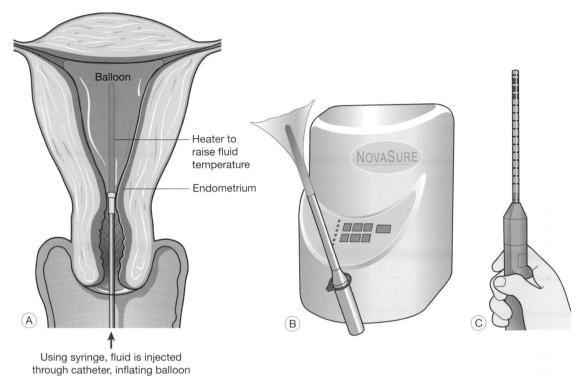

Fig. 7.6 **Conservative surgical treatments for menorrhagia. (A)** A thermal balloon, **(B)** impedance-controlled ablation and **(C)** microwave endometrial ablation.

TABLE 7.2	Pros and Cons of Different Hysterectomy Methods	
	Pros	**Cons**
Total abdominal hysterectomy (TAH)	Cervix is removed; therefore, no further need for smears and no further risk of cervical malignancy (thus, particularly suitable for those with a history of abnormal cytology) Good access to ovaries	Longer recovery compared with vaginal and laparoscopic methods
Subtotal abdominal hysterectomy	Fewer complications than TAH (↓bleeding, ↓infection, ↓bladder injury, ↓ureteric damage) Good access to ovaries	Risk of cervical cancer remains as before Longer recovery compared with vaginal and laparoscopic methods
Vaginal hysterectomy	May be lower incidence of bladder and bowel injury in straightforward cases (compared with abdominal hysterectomy) No painful abdominal wound	Limited ovarian access Contraindicated with: • large uterus • restricted uterine mobility • limited vaginal space • adnexal pathology • cervix flush with vagina
Laparoscopically assisted vaginal hysterectomy and total laparoscopic hysterectomy	Shorter postoperative recovery time Quicker return to work and normal activities Good access to ovaries Smaller scars and better cosmetic results compared with abdominal hysterectomy	Higher postoperative pain scores (compared with vaginal hysterectomy) Longer operating time Increased costs

For women with no pathology who are undergoing an abdominal hysterectomy and who have a history of normal cervical cytology, there is the choice of having a 'subtotal' hysterectomy. This involves removing the body of the uterus but leaving the cervix behind. The advantages of a subtotal hysterectomy compared with a 'total' hysterectomy are that the operation is quicker and entails less risk of damage to structures surrounding the cervix (bowel and urinary tract, Fig. 7.7). It has also been reported (though not proven) that these advantages include less postoperative disruption to bowel, bladder and sexual functioning. If the cervix is left intact, the surgeon must be careful to remove any residual endometrium in the cervical canal at the time of surgery to minimize the small risk that menses would continue from the endometrium in the cervical canal. The disadvantages of a subtotal hysterectomy are that the woman must continue the cervical cytology screening programme. The risk of cervical cancer arising in the stump of the cervix is extremely small (<0.1%) provided that cervical cytology was normal prior to the operation.

Whether the ovaries are removed at the time of abdominal hysterectomy depends on several factors, including the woman's preferences, her age, her family history of breast or ovarian carcinoma and her attitude towards HRT. Removal of healthy ovaries at the time of hysterectomy should not be undertaken routinely. In women under age 45 years considering hysterectomy for HMB with other symptoms that may be related to ovarian dysfunction—for example, pre-menstrual syndrome (PMS)—a trial of pharmaceutical suppression for at least 3 months should be used as a guide to the need for oophorectomy. If removal is being considered, the impact of this procedure on the woman's well-being and need for HRT should be discussed pre-operatively. Women with a significant family history of breast or ovarian cancer should be referred for genetic counselling prior to a decision about oophorectomy. There is no doubt that removal of ovaries at the time of hysterectomy will reduce the risk of later development of ovarian cancer (lifetime risk 1 in 52 in the United Kingdom), but recent data suggest that women aged 35 to 45 years who have a hysterectomy with ovarian conservation are at lower risk of all-cause mortality and have lower death rates from ischaemic heart disease and cancer compared with women whose ovaries are removed at the time of hysterectomy. It has therefore been suggested that removal of this biologically active organ may have harmful effects in the long term. Women should also be informed about the risk of possible loss of ovarian function even if ovaries are retained during hysterectomy. It may therefore be appropriate to discuss 'routine' oophorectomy in women over 45 and ovarian conservation in women under 45 years. The decision must remain a very individualized consideration, however.

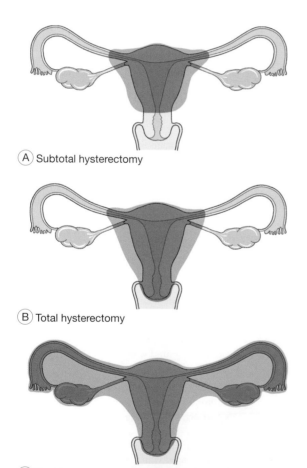

(A) Subtotal hysterectomy

(B) Total hysterectomy

(C) Total hysterectomy with bilateral salpingo-oophorectomy

Fig. 7.7 Types of abdominal hysterectomy. (A) Subtotal abdominal hysterectomy, **(B)** total abdominal hysterectomy and **(C)** total abdominal hysterectomy with bilateral salpingo-oophorectomy.

Medical Disorders and Clotting Defects

Referral should be made to an appropriate physician/haematologist to institute further investigation and treatment of the underlying condition.

Dysmenorrhoea

Excessive menstrual pain (dysmenorrhoea) is a significant clinical problem. It characteristically involves cramping lower abdominal pain that may radiate to the lower back and legs and may be associated with gastrointestinal symptoms or malaise. It has been estimated that dysmenorrhoea affects 30% to 50% of menstruating women. It is also one of the most frequent causes of absenteeism from school and days taken off work. As with HMB, dysmenorrhoea may be idiopathic (primary dysmenorrhoea) or due to pelvic pathology (secondary dysmenorrhoea).

PRIMARY DYSMENORRHOEA

This generally begins with the onset of ovulatory cycles, typically within the first 2 years of menarche. Pain is usually most severe on the day of or the day prior to the start of menstruation. There is good evidence that prostaglandins are involved in the aetiology, as higher concentrations of PGE_2 and $PGF_{2\alpha}$ are found in the menstrual fluid of women who suffer from dysmenorrhoea than those who do not. $PGF_{2\alpha}$ increases the contractility of the myometrium and can lead to the dysmenorrhoea.

Management of Primary Dysmenorrhoea

Pelvic examination may not be helpful in primary dysmenorrhoea and is not appropriate when dealing with an adolescent. A transabdominal ultrasound scan will reveal normal pelvic organs and provide considerable reassurance to a young woman and her family. Discussion and reassurance are an essential part of the management. If dysmenorrhoea is unresponsive to standard medical therapy (see later discussion), then consideration should be given to the possibility of underlying pathology and appropriate investigation instituted.

Care of Women With of Primary Dysmenorrhoea

Prostaglandin Synthesis Inhibitors

NSAIDs reduce the uterine production of $PGF_{2\alpha}$ and, thus, dysmenorrhoea. Most NSAIDs have been shown to be effective treatments, but mefenamic acid and ibuprofen are preferred in view of their favourable efficacy and safety profiles.

Combined Hormonal Contraceptives

Suppression of ovulation with the combined contraceptive pill is highly effective in reducing the severity of dysmenorrhoea.

Depot Progestogens

The injectable progestogen-only contraceptive suppresses ovulation and, thus, may be a useful treatment in alleviating dysmenorrhoea.

Levonorgestrel-Releasing Intrauterine System (LNG-IUS)

In addition to reducing menstrual blood loss, the LNG-IUS is effective at reducing dysmenorrhoea.

SECONDARY DYSMENORRHOEA

This is, by definition, associated with pelvic pathology. Its onset usually occurs many years after menarche. Common associated pathologies are endometriosis, adenomyosis, pelvic infection and fibroids. It may also be associated with the presence of an intrauterine contraceptive device. In contrast, the LNG-IUS is associated with reduced dysmenorrhoea.

Care of Women With Secondary Dysmenorrhoea

Women who have no complaints other than dysmenorrhoea and who have no abnormalities upon abdominal, pelvic, or speculum examination may be safely treated without further investigation. Swabs from the genital tract, however, are helpful in excluding active pelvic infection, particularly *Chlamydia trachomatis*.

If pelvic masses such as fibroids are suspected, a pelvic ultrasound may be helpful. A laparoscopy is indicated if endometriosis or pelvic inflammatory disease is suspected, or in those women for whom standard medical therapy has been ineffective. Treatment is dependent on the underlying pathology (see Chapter 8 for the management of endometriosis).

Pre-Menstrual Syndrome

PMS can usefully be defined as 'a condition manifesting with physical, behavioural and psychological symptoms in the absence of organic or psychiatric disease, which regularly occurs during the luteal phase of each ovarian cycle and which disappears or significantly regresses by the end of menstruation'. PMS is considered severe if it impairs work, relationships, or usual activities. Some observers note that as many as 40% of women suffer mild symptoms and, of these, 5% to 8% have symptoms severe enough to disrupt their lives, principally in the 2 weeks leading up to the start of menstruation. Symptoms will settle during pregnancy.

Over 150 symptoms have been attributed to PMS, but particularly:

- Mood changes/irritability
- Abdominal bloating
- Breast tenderness (cyclical mastalgia)
- Headaches.

Aetiology

The exact aetiology of PMS remains unknown, although ovulatory cycles are generally considered to be a necessary prerequisite. There are suggestions that it is the changing patterns of hormone levels, rather than the absolute levels, that are important. Coupled with this, some women may be sensitive to progesterone and/or progestogens. A second theory involves the neurotransmitters serotonin and gamma-aminobutyric acid (GABA). The levels of both have been associated with the occurrence of PMS symptoms. GABA levels are altered in women with PMS symptoms, whilst selective serotonin reuptake inhibitors (SSRIs) improve PMS symptoms.

Clinical Presentation

As there are no specific biochemical tests for PMS, the diagnosis is dependent on a prospective charting of symptoms over a minimum of two cycles to confirm that there is a true exacerbation in the luteal phase when compared with the follicular phase of the cycle (Fig. 7.8). There are a variety of online symptom trackers, although a simple calendar record of the presence or absence of a woman's principal symptoms and days of menstruation is helpful to make the diagnosis. There are numerous specific criteria, although many of them are research tools that are not necessarily always applied strictly to clinical practice. An example of one of these tools is shown in Box 7.1. A symptom diary should be completed prior to commencing treatment, especially if it involves medication.

Differential Diagnosis

Symptoms that can be worse in the follicular phase are not attributable to PMS. Other conditions—such as endometriosis, migraine headaches, depression and

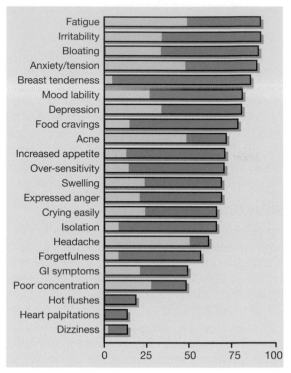

Fig. 7.8 Reported incidence (cycles, %) of individual symptoms in the follicular phase of the cycle (open bars) and the luteal phase of the cycle (filled bars) in 170 women. *GI*, Gastrointestinal.

anxiety disorders—are exacerbated premenstrually. However, again, they should not be confused with the more specific diagnosis of PMS. Perimenopausal mood changes are usually non-cyclical; in these circumstances, a serum follicle-stimulating hormone (FSH) measurement should be considered. A normal FSH level does not exclude menopause, but the investigation may be of particular value in women who have had a hysterectomy with ovarian conservation (since there is no menstruation) or in those who are using a progestogenic method of contraception. The breast pain associated with PMS is usually cyclical, bilateral, poorly localized, and commonly involves 'lumpiness'. By contrast, non-cyclical breast pain is precisely localized and rarely bilateral.

In those with abdominal bloating, it is important to consider intra-abdominal pathology—such as ovarian cysts, ascites, or irritable bowel syndrome. The abdominal bloating associated with PMS is rapidly relieved by the onset of menstruation, perhaps owing

BOX 7.1 EXAMPLE OF A SET OF DIAGNOSTIC CRITERIA FOR PMS

1. The presence, by self-report, of at least one of the following somatic and affective symptoms during the 5 days before menses in each of the three previous cycles

Affective Symptoms	Somatic Symptoms
Depression	Breast tenderness
Angry outbursts	Bloating
Irritability	Headache
Anxiety	Swelling
Confusion	
Social withdrawal	

2. Relief of these symptoms within 4 days of the onset of the menses, without recurrence until day 12 of the cycle
3. Presence of the symptoms in the absence of any pharmacological therapy, hormone ingestion, or drug or alcohol misuse
4. Reproducible occurrence of symptoms during two cycles of prospective recording
5. Identifiable dysfunction in social or economic performance by one of the following criteria:
   • Discord in relationship confirmed by partner
   • Difficulties in parenting
   • Poor work or school performance
   • Increased social isolation
   • Legal difficulties
   • Suicidal ideation
   • Medical attention sought for somatic symptoms

From Mortola, J. F., Girton, L., Beck, L., & Yen, S. S. (1990). Diagnosis of premenstrual syndrome by a simple, prospective, and reliable instrument: the calendar of premenstrual experiences. Obstetrics and Gynecology, 76(2), 302–307.

to the relaxing effect of progesterone on smooth muscle or to the comparative stasis of the gut in response to morphine-like endorphins. Hypothyroidism and anaemia should be considered in those complaining predominantly of fatigue. The characteristics of endogenous depression are different from those of the mood changes and irritability commonly observed in PMS. However, as both conditions are relatively common, it is not unusual to encounter both in the same woman.

Care of Women With Pre-Menstrual Syndrome

Women with mild PMS do not usually need medical treatment and may be helped by reassurance and information. General health measures should be encouraged in all women, such as improved diet with a low glycaemic index, increased exercise, self-relaxation, and reducing smoking and drinking. Some women find self-help groups supportive, while others choose yoga or hypnosis.

SYMPTOMATIC TREATMENT

A number of symptomatic treatments are in use, although the evidence supporting their effectiveness is limited. Women with pre-menstrual bloating can be treated in the same way as those with irritable bowel syndrome, and those with oedema may respond to a diuretic such as spironolactone. Breast tenderness can also be treated with diuretics, evening primrose oil, or low-dose danazol. Women should be counselled regarding the potential irreversible virilising effects of low-dose danazol. Effective contraception must also be used at the same time. Mood changes are considered in more detail later.

TREATMENT AIMED AT THE HYPOTHESIZED UNDERLYING CAUSE

A wide variety of medical treatments for PMS have been considered, many of which are still in current use. Close scrutiny, however, reveals that only a limited number of these are of proven value. These treatment modalities are classified accordingly in Box 7.2. The 'probably effective' group consists of treatments demonstrated to be effective by good-sized trials, usually randomised placebo-controlled trials. The use of a placebo arm is particularly important in PMS research, as most placebo treatments demonstrate symptom

BOX 7.2 POSSIBLE TREATMENTS FOR PMS

Probably effective
• SSRIs
• Psychological approaches, including cognitive behavioural therapy
• Suppression of ovulation
• Oophorectomy

May be effective
• Diet
• Exercise
• Vitamin B_6
• Complementary therapy
• Evening primrose oil

Probably not effective
• Progesterone

improvements of around 30%. Treatments classified as 'probably not effective' have also been examined in well-conducted studies, and no significant benefit has been demonstrated over placebo. The 'may be effective' group includes therapies for which studies have been inconclusive, often because of small patient numbers. These three groups will be considered in more detail in the next section.

Probably Not Effective

Progesterone or Progestogens

The rationale for the use of progesterone or progestogens in the management of PMS is based on the unsubstantiated premise that the condition is due to a progesterone deficiency. Although initial data suggest that women with PMS have low serum concentrations of progesterone metabolites (pregnenolone and allopregnanolone), there is no consistent evidence that these women have low concentrations of progesterone. In addition, systematic reviews of randomised trials do not suggest any useful clinical benefit of treatment with these hormones. However, intramuscular or subcutaneous depot administration of medroxyprogesterone may be helpful due to its anovulatory effect.

May be Effective

Diet

Diet should be altered so that more of the meals consumed have a low glycaemic index. It is suggested that an increased carbohydrate intake increases serotonergic activity, which, in turn, improves symptoms.

Exercise

Aerobic activity leads to increased endorphin levels, which is known to improve mood. Several studies suggest that this may be of some benefit in the treatment of PMS.

Complementary Therapy

Studies have explored the use of homeopathy, relaxation, massage, reflexology, chiropractic therapy and biofeedback. While there were some positive findings, there is no compelling evidence to support the regular use of any of these therapies. Despite the lack of an evidence base, these complementary therapies should be discussed as possible treatment options as part of an integrated holistic treatment plan.

Food Supplements

Similar to complementary therapies, there are mixed results in randomised, placebo-controlled trials.

Vitamin B_6 (Pyridoxine)

Pyridoxine is involved in the metabolism of dopamine and serotonin, low levels of which lead to high levels of prolactin and aldosterone, possibly explaining the fluid retention experienced by women with PMS. It may also account for some of the psychological symptoms attributable to alterations in neurotransmitter levels.

Vitamin B_6 can be taken on a continuous basis or during the second half of the menstrual cycle. Owing to safety concerns (i.e., the peripheral neuropathy that may result from taking high doses), a maximum dose of 10 mg/day is recommended.

Evening Primrose Oil

This contains essential fatty acids, including gamolenic acid. Trials demonstrate some clinical improvement, principally in the relief of mastalgia. Other supplements with mixed reviews include *Vitex agnus castus Ginkgo biloba* and magnesium.

Probably Effective

Psychological Approaches

Techniques aimed at reducing stress may be beneficial. Cognitive behavioural therapy (CBT), which encourages relaxation, and the use of 'coping skills' can be helpful and should be considered as a first-line option for women with severe symptoms.

Selective Serotonin Reuptake Inhibitors

PMS often presents with symptoms similar to those of anxiety and depression. This association has resulted in treatment with a variety of antidepressants. Reduced platelet uptake of serotonin and reduced levels of serotonin in the blood of women with PMS during the luteal phase suggest that there is a role for SSRIs in PMS treatment. Meta-analysis shows that SSRIs are effective, with around 60% of women with severe PMS reporting a reduction in physical and behavioural symptoms compared with around 30% of controls. This effectiveness is often apparent after only one or two cycles. Side effects include insomnia, gastrointestinal disturbances, fatigue and loss of libido, but may be acceptable at the recommended low dose. Intermittent use in the luteal phase is as effective as continuous daily dosing, and may help to limit side effects. A gradual rather than abrupt withdrawal is appropriate if the SSRI has been taken on a continuous basis in order to avoid symptoms of withdrawal. SSRIs can be offered as a first-line treatment option but should be stopped before and during a pregnancy, as there is a possible association with congenital malformations.

Ovarian Suppression

Because the majority of PMS symptoms can be attributed to cyclical ovarian hormone production, the suppression of ovulation is a logical treatment option. The effectiveness of second-generation combined hormonal contraceptives (CHCs) for the treatment of PMS is uncertain. Some research suggests an improvement in symptoms, whereas other research suggests symptom exacerbation. There is now evidence to support the use of CHCs containing drospirenone. This can be attributed to its antimineralocorticoid and antiandrogenic properties. Recent results suggest that more benefit is obtained from continuous rather than cyclical administration. Depot medroxyprogesterone, a long-acting injectable progestogen, may also be helpful.

The synthetic androgen danazol suppresses ovulation, and a relatively low dose of 200 mg twice daily is effective in improving the symptoms of mastalgia. Use of danazol is limited by its potential for irreversible virilisation, and effective contraception should be used to avoid virilisation of a female fetus.

Transdermal estradiol (100–200 µg/day), by way of patches designed for HRT, is associated with an improvement in PMS symptoms. If the woman has not had a hysterectomy, progestogen is required to avoid endometrial stimulation, hyperplasia and possible malignant transformation. The lowest dose of progestogen required for endometrial protection is recommended; micronized progesterone taken orally or vaginally for 10 to 12 days during each cycle should be considered first-line treatment. The LNG-IUS is also particularly suitable since the serum level of progestogen is very low, thus minimizing the risk of progestogenic side effects (which may mimic/exacerbate PMS); it also provides contraceptive cover. Any unscheduled bleeding in women taking high-dose transdermal estradiol should prompt early investigation.

GnRH analogues are a highly effective way of suppressing ovarian function; therefore, they are an effective treatment for severe PMS. As estrogen is suppressed to postmenopausal levels, the PMS symptoms may be replaced by menopausal ones, including hot flushes, and there is an increased risk of osteoporosis. These can be minimized with the use of add-back HRT, either tibilone or a continuous combined preparation. A therapeutic trial of GnRH analogues with add-back HRT is often beneficial in clarifying the diagnosis if the symptom diary is not conclusive. It also helps to establish that the woman can tolerate an HRT preparation should oophorectomy become appropriate. Use of GnRH analogues for more than 6 months must include add-back HRT and regular measurement of bone density—for example, annual dual-energy X-ray absorptiometry scanning. Although generally accepted as a treatment option, GnRH analogues are not specifically licensed for use in women with PMS.

Bilateral Oophorectomy

This is an effective treatment for PMS. However, it is a surgical procedure; therefore, it is not without significant short-term surgical risks. The procedure can usually be undertaken laparoscopically. There are also longer-term risks from premature ovarian insufficiency if HRT is not taken postoperatively. Thus, this surgical option is suitable only for those very likely to benefit from it as suggested by a definite response to a GnRH analogue and only in those who have completed their family. It is reasonable not to opt for this procedure if natural menopause is likely to be occurring in the near future. Some clinicians recommend that bilateral oophorectomy should be combined with hysterectomy since this avoids the need for a progestogen-containing HRT regimen postoperatively. In some women, the use of progestogens can trigger PMS symptoms.

INDIVIDUAL MANAGEMENT STRATEGY

Given the large number of treatments advocated, it can be difficult to determine which is the optimum approach for a specific woman. As PMS is usually a chronic condition, it is important to consider the side-effect profile of treatments that may be used over many years. Once the diagnosis is established by prospective symptom diary-keeping, it seems sensible to try those treatments with fewest significant side effects, which should initially include diet modification, regular aerobic exercise and techniques aimed at stress reduction. A significant proportion of women will benefit from trying these three together. Drug therapy can then be considered for those who do not improve sufficiently.

Appropriate first-line therapy includes CBT, a low-dose SSRI, or a drospirenone-containing CHC. The next stage is a high-dose SSRI, estradiol patches, or ovarian suppression with a GnRH analogue. However, successful symptom improvement can pose a dilemma, as continuous treatment may not be appropriate. Long-term suppression with medroxyprogesterone acetate administered every 3 months intramuscularly or subcutaneously should be considered as an alternative. Bilateral oophorectomy should be reserved for the most severe cases, with a preoperative trial of GnRH analogue essential beforehand.

Key Points

- HMB can be classified as being related to structural uterine pathology (e.g., fibroids) or not. Very rarely, HMB may be secondary to some specific medical disorders, including clotting defects.
- Medical treatment includes prostaglandin synthesis inhibitors, antifibrinolytics, the COC pill, systemic progestogens, intrauterine progestogens, GnRH analogues and danazol.

With the exception of GnRH analogues, these treatments are less successful in the presence of fibroids. Endometrial ablation and hysterectomy are the two surgical options.

- Dysmenorrhoea may be idiopathic (primary dysmenorrhoea) or due to pelvic pathology (secondary dysmenorrhoea). Treatment is with prostaglandin synthesis inhibitors, the combined contraceptive pill, or depot injection of intrauterine progestogens.
- PMS can be defined as a regular pattern of symptoms occurring before menstruation, with a lessening of symptoms soon after the start of bleeding.
- The aetiology of the condition is poorly understood, and diagnosis is dependent on prospectively charting the symptoms to confirm that there is a true cyclical variation.
- Only a limited number of treatments are more effective than placebo, listed in Box 7.2. Initial treatment should include dietary advice, regular aerobic exercise and techniques aimed at stress reduction. An SSRI is an appropriate first-line drug. If unsuccessful, it may be appropriate to institute a trial of ovarian suppression. Long-term suppression with medroxyprogesterone acetate or surgical oophorectomy may be considered.

Chapter 8

Pelvic Pain and Endometriosis

Neelam Potdar

Chapter Outline

Pelvic Pain

Physiological pelvic pain with menstruation or childbirth is almost universal, but many women have pelvic pain for other reasons. Pelvic pain can be acute (associated with miscarriage, ectopic pregnancy, or appendicitis) or it can be chronic, lasting for many months or years.

With acute pain, there is usually a well-defined pathological cause that either resolves spontaneously or can be effectively treated. It is important to recognise that chronic pelvic pain (CPP) is a symptom, not a diagnosis. CPP is as common as migraine or lower back pain. Aiming for accurate diagnosis and effective management from the first presentation may help to improve the woman's quality of life, and may avoid a succession of referrals, investigations and operations.

Pelvic pain is considered under the two headings of 'acute' and 'chronic', and there is often significant overlap. Although there are many gynaecological causes of pelvic pain, the non-gynaecological causes are also important. Therefore, a multidisciplinary approach, particularly for women with CPP, is required.

Pain is a subjective phenomenon, meaning it is a symptom experienced solely by the woman. Many of the factors affecting pain are centrally mediated; hence, pelvic pain is often made worse by psychological, psychiatric, or social distress. The organs within the peritoneal cavity (the viscera) are sensitive to inflammation, chemicals and distortion caused by specific stimuli (e.g., adhesions or gaseous distension). The sensitivity of different organs to stimuli is an important factor influencing the amount of pelvic pain experienced. Compression of the bowel is associated with minimal discomfort, whereas stretching and distension cause severe pain. Unlike painful cutaneous stimuli, it is often very difficult to localize visceral pain.

History

The history is the most important factor in determining how quickly the diagnosis is reached and appropriate treatment is started. Particular attention should be given to the time of onset of the pain; the characteristics, radiation and severity of the pain; exacerbating and relieving factors; cyclicity; and analgesic requirements. Associated symptoms of gastrointestinal, urological or musculoskeletal origin should be ascertained. It is also important to take a detailed menstrual history – in particular, the frequency and character of vaginal bleeding, any intermenstrual bleeding or vaginal discharge, and their relationship to the pain. A sexual history may be of help, particularly superficial or deep dyspareunia, contraception and sexually transmitted infections (STIs). There may be a family history of gynaecological disorders (e.g., endometriosis). A cervical screening history should be recorded.

With chronic pain, there is often value in taking a detailed family and social history, including any relationship problems, pressure at work, financial worries and whether there has been previous sexual abuse. Listening is centrally important to the history taking and may, in itself, be therapeutic for some women. Asking open-ended questions such as 'What do you think the cause of your pain might be?' and 'How is the pain affecting your life?' gives the woman an opportunity to tell you about aspects of the problem that might not be apparent from a more systematic history.

If the history suggests there is a non-gynaecological component to the pain, referral to the relevant health care professional – such as a gastroenterologist, urologist, genitourinary medicine physician, physiotherapist, psychologist, or psychosexual counsellor – should be considered.

Examination

A detailed account of how to undertake a gynaecological history and examination is described in Chapter 2. Clinical examination is most usefully undertaken when there is time to explore the woman's fears and anxieties. The examiner should be prepared for new information to be revealed at this point. Observation of the woman's general demeanour is important when assessing the severity of pain. Collateral accounts from other health professionals and friends or family may

also be helpful. The temperature, pulse and blood pressure should be recorded and a urinary pregnancy test (UPT) performed when appropriate.

Abdominal examination should include inspection for distension or masses, palpation for tenderness, rebound, guarding and abdominal auscultation if gastrointestinal obstruction or ileus is suspected. Inspection of the vulva and vagina at speculum examination may reveal abnormal discharge (suggestive of infection) or bleeding. A bimanual examination may reveal uterine or adnexal enlargement suggestive of a pelvic mass, fibroids, or an ovarian cyst. Cervical excitation (pain associated with digital displacement of the cervix) is associated with ectopic pregnancy and pelvic infection. Tenderness or pain elicited by bimanual palpation of the pelvic organs themselves is suggestive of an ongoing inflammatory process, which may be infective (e.g., *Chlamydia*) or non-infective (e.g., endometriosis). A fixed, immobile uterus suggests multiple adhesions, and nodules felt on the uterosacral ligaments can be a feature of endometriosis.

Acute Pelvic Pain

There are many causes of acute pelvic pain, but the most important gynaecological conditions are ectopic pregnancy, miscarriage, pelvic inflammatory disease and torsion or rupture of ovarian cysts (Box 8.1). If the UPT is negative, a high vaginal swab, endocervical swab and full blood count should be performed to investigate for infection. All sexually active women below the age of 25 years who are being examined can be offered opportunistic screening for *Chlamydia*. An ultrasound scan is helpful in identifying ovarian cysts.

The management of miscarriage, pelvic inflammatory disease and ovarian cysts is discussed in the appropriate chapters. Pain experienced mid-cycle with ovulation, the so-called 'mittelschmerz', is a self-limiting,

---

BOX 8.1 CAUSES OF ACUTE PELVIC PAIN

- *Gynaecological:* Ectopic pregnancy, miscarriage, acute pelvic infection, ovarian cysts
- *Gastrointestinal:* Appendicitis, constipation, diverticular disease, irritable bowel syndrome, inflammatory bowel disease
- *Urinary tract:* Urinary tract infection, renal stones
- *Other causes:* Musculoskeletal

physiological cause of pain. This pain is usually sudden in onset, can be quite severe, and, if persistent in each cycle, will respond to ovulation suppression with hormonal contraception.

Chronic Pelvic Pain (CPP)

The definitions of CPP are numerous, but one suitable definition is 'intermittent or constant pain in the lower abdomen or pelvis of at least 6 months' duration, not occurring exclusively with menstruation or intercourse and not associated with pregnancy'. A comparison between acute pelvic pain and CPP is shown in Table 8.1. CPP can lead to loss of employment and relationship difficulties, including divorce. Health care costs associated with CPP are considerable and do not take into consideration the disability and suffering of the woman and loss of earnings to both the individual and wider society. Among high-quality studies, the rate of dysmenorrhoea was 16.8% to 81%, that of dyspareunia was 8% to 21.8%, and that of non-cyclical pain was 2.1% to 24% worldwide.

The care of women with CPP is particularly challenging, as there are many possible causes and contributory factors (Box 8.2). Association with dysmenorrhoea, dyspareunia, irregular menstruation, abnormal vaginal discharge, cyclical pain and subfertility may all be helpful in suggesting an underlying gynaecological problem. Altered bowel habits, excess flatulence, intermittent abdominal bloating, constipation, or diarrhoea, on the other hand, point to a gastrointestinal problem, particularly irritable bowel syndrome (IBS). However, these bowel symptoms can also be associated with the presence of gynaecological pathology, such as endometriosis. Psychiatric, urological and musculoskeletal causes of chronic pain are further possibilities. Physical and sexual abuse can also predispose women to CPP.

Known gynaecological causes of CPP include endometriosis, adhesions and pelvic varices. Adhesions

BOX 8.2 DIFFERENTIAL DIAGNOSES FOR WOMEN WITH CHRONIC PELVIC PAIN

- *Gynaecological*: Endometriosis, adhesions, adenomyosis, leiomyoma, pelvic congestion syndrome, ovarian cysts
- *Gastrointestinal*: Adhesions, appendicitis, constipation, diverticular disease, irritable bowel syndrome, inflammatory bowel disease
- *Urinary tract*: Urinary tract infection, calculus, interstitial cystitis
- *Skeletal*: Degenerative joint disease, scoliosis, spondylolisthesis, osteitis pubis
- *Myofascial*: Fascitis, nerve entrapment syndrome, hernia
- *Psychological*: Somatization, psychosexual dysfunction, depression
- *Neuropathic*: Pudendal nerve entrapment, spinal cord neuropathies

can cause pain if there is associated organ distension, stretching, or tethering. Division of dense adhesions has been shown to relieve pain. Symptoms suggestive of IBS or interstitial cystitis are often present in women with CPP. These conditions may be the primary cause of or a component of CPP.

Up to 40% of women with CPP, despite extensive investigation, do not have an identifiable cause. It is therefore important to consider, in consultation with the woman, which investigations are worthwhile. In gynaecology, investigation can involve a diagnostic laparoscopy, the findings of which guide the approach to care.

PELVIC INFECTION

Chronic pelvic infection is associated with a high incidence of tubal damage and, consequently, an increased incidence of ectopic pregnancy, subfertility, or CPP. It may occur due to relapse of infection after inadequate treatment, reinfection from an untreated partner, post-infection tubal damage, or further STIs. Each episode of pelvic inflammation is associated with an increase in the incidence of CPP.

OVARIAN CYSTS

The majority of ovarian cysts are benign, particularly those presenting with acute pain. Pain may occur because of cyst torsion, cyst rupture, or bleeding into the cyst. Management depends on the presenting clinical situation, but ovarian torsion requires urgent surgical intervention to relieve the pain and treat the cyst.

TABLE 8.1 Comparison of Acute and Chronic Pelvic Pain	
Acute	**Chronic**
Well-defined onset	Ill-defined onset
Short duration	Unpredictable duration
Rest often helpful	Rest usually not helpful
Variable intensity	Persistent with exacerbations

Other

Endometriosis is discussed in the subsequent section. If investigations do not identify a cause and there remains significant diagnostic uncertainty about gynaecological origin of pain, it may be worth considering a 3-month trial of ovarian suppression with a gonadotrophin-releasing hormone (GnRH) analogue. In around 75% of women who experience a marked reduction of symptoms following suppression and recurrence after treatment stops, a hysterectomy and bilateral salpingo-oophorectomy may lead to long-term improvement in symptoms. Many, however, may not wish to have major fertility-ending surgery, and there is a risk that there will be no improvement in symptoms despite hysterectomy.

NO CAUSE FOR CPP IDENTIFIED

Treating a woman with CPP without a specific diagnosis is particularly difficult because of the problems involved in choosing an appropriate therapeutic intervention. In these cases, CPP can be considered a disease entity in its own right, and strategies are required to relieve the physical, psychological and social distress that it causes.

Options include psychological therapy, pain medication (including use of anticonvulsants such as gabapentin and neuropathic agents such as amitriptyline), hormonal treatments, antidepressants and surgery – including pelvic clearance. Communication with the woman should include sharing of information and an honest discussion of the treatment options with a realistic assessment of the likely outcomes.

Encouragement to lead as full a life as possible whilst investigation and treatment are ongoing is acknowledged to be very important. This includes encouraging the woman to return to work, exercise, maintain a healthy diet, avoid the inappropriate use of analgesia and look for alternatives to analgesia where possible. Complementary approaches, such as acupuncture and cognitive behavioural therapy, may be helpful.

The risks of inappropriate medical interventions and treatments associated with CPP can be minimized by adopting a sympathetic and caring multidisciplinary approach or by referral to health care professionals with a special interest and expertise in managing this condition. A multidisciplinary team approach should ideally include expertise in pain management, gastroenterology, gynaecology, neurology, psychiatry and psychology. Specific psychological approaches to the management of CPP, with input from psychologists and liaison psychiatrists, may be helpful to many women. These approaches include behavioural therapy, cognitive behavioural therapy, group therapy and pharmacological therapy. Pharmacological therapy (e.g., antidepressants and anxiolytics) may be valuable for those individuals with concurrent depression.

Endometriosis

Endometriosis is the presence of endometrial-like tissue outside the uterus, which induces a chronic inflammatory reaction. This tissue usually lies within the peritoneal cavity, predominantly in the pelvis and commonly on the uterosacral ligaments behind the uterus (Fig. 8.1). Rarely, it can also be found in distant sites such as the umbilicus, abdominal scars, perineal scars, pleural cavity and nasal mucosa. Like the true endometrium, it responds to cyclical hormonal changes and bleeds at menstruation.

Adenomyosis occurs when there is endometrial tissue within the myometrium of the uterus. The uterus is enlarged and feels 'boggy'. There is painful and heavy menstruation. Previously, adenomyosis could only be diagnosed from histology after a hysterectomy was performed. With advances in imaging technology, adenomyosis can be identified on ultrasound scan or by magnetic resonance imaging (MRI) of the pelvis. It is considered to be a separate entity from endometriosis, occurring in a different population and having a different aetiology.

Incidence

The reported incidence of endometriosis varies widely. For example, in asymptomatic women undergoing laparoscopy for other reasons, the presence of endometriosis has been reported in up to 43% of cases. Endometriosis is more commonly identified in subfertile women. Most cases of endometriosis are diagnosed in women aged 25 to 35 years, although the symptoms of endometriosis can present as early as the onset of puberty. It is rarely diagnosed postmenopausally, but recurrence has been associated with the use of hormone replacement therapy.

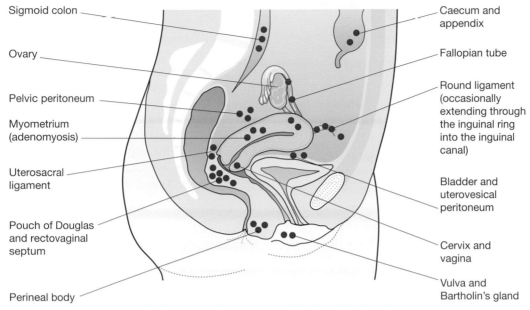

Fig. 8.1 Recognised sites for endometriotic deposits in the pelvis.

Aetiology

The precise aetiology of endometriosis remains unclear, with no single explanation reliably explaining all of its features. Sampson's 'implantation' theory postulates that endometrial fragments flow in a retrograde manner along the fallopian tube during menstruation, 'seeding' themselves on the pelvic peritoneum. Retrograde menstruation occurs in 90% of ovulating women. Seeding onto scars (such as after caesarean section or on perineal scars after childbirth) has been observed. In animal studies that involved artificial retrograde menstruation, endometriosis developed in 50% of cases.

This theory, however, cannot be the only mechanism of endometriosis formation, as endometriosis has been reported in women with congenitally obstructed fallopian tubes. Meyer's 'coelomic metaplasia' theory proposes that cells of the original coelomic membrane transform to endometrial cells by metaplasia, possibly as a result of hormonal stimulation or inflammatory irritation. This could explain the presence of endometriosis in nearly all distant sites, although it is also possible that spread from the uterus to these distant sites occurs by venous or lymphatic channels.

Questions remain as to why endometriosis becomes established in some, but not all, women – why the extent of endometriosis does not always correlate well with the extent of the symptoms experienced. It is possible that there is some genetic or immunological predisposition that accounts for such wide variation. Endometriosis is significantly more common in first-degree relatives of women with the disease; twin studies also support a genetic basis.

Clinical Presentation

Endometriosis is the most common cause of secondary dysmenorrhoea. There is usually continuous non-spasmodic pain that is worse immediately before and throughout menstruation. Colicky dysmenorrhoea may also occur in association with heavy menstrual loss and the passage of clots. In addition, there may be dyspareunia, which may relate to endometriotic deposits in the pouch of Douglas or to ovarian endometriomas. Typically, this pain settles when the period ends, but some women also describe continuous lower abdominal pain that is not specifically related to their cycle or to sexual activity. The common presenting symptoms of endometriosis are outlined in Box 8.3.

BOX 8.3 THE COMMON PRESENTING SYMPTOMS OF ENDOMETRIOSIS

- Severe dysmenorrhoea
- Chronic pelvic pain
- Deep dyspareunia
- Pain during ovulation
- Cyclical or perimenstrual symptoms (e.g., bladder or bowel), with or without abnormal bleeding or pain
- Chronic fatigue
- Pain on defaecation (dyschezia)
- Subfertility (especially with dysmenorrhoea)

Extensive deposits leading to the scarring of the pouch of Douglas and involving the ovaries, fallopian tubes, and other pelvic organs may be completely asymptomatic. Conversely, women with peritoneal lesions only a few millimetres across may be debilitated by pain.

Menstrual disturbances may be associated with endometriosis and, in particular, with adenomyosis. Where there is also significant ovarian involvement, the menstrual cycle may become erratic. Rarely, postcoital bleeding is experienced in the presence of endometriosis involving the cervix or where deposits in the pouch of Douglas penetrate into the posterior fornix.

Endometriosis at distant sites is rare but may generate local symptoms, such as cyclical nose bleeding with nasal deposits and pneumothorax or menstrual haemoptysis with pleural deposits. Rectal bleeding at the time of menstruation may occur if the bowel is affected, or haematuria with bladder involvement.

Examination

The clinical diagnosis of endometriosis is aided by the following findings:

1. Blue nodules seen in the posterior vaginal fornix on speculum examination
2. A fixed (immobile) retroverted uterus
3. Thickened uterosacral ligaments, which may be nodular
4. Tenderness in the lateral and posterior fornices with applied pressure on the uterosacral ligaments
5. Adnexal mass if there is an endometrioma.

Nodules are most reliably detected when clinical examination is performed during menstruation.

Attempts to gently palpate the uterus may also provoke pain. This pain often resembles the presenting symptom, particularly when it was dyspareunia.

With the exception of visualizing endometriotic nodules, none of these features is diagnostic of endometriosis; and conversely, their absence does not exclude the disease. There are many other causes of pelvic pain, such as IBS and recurrent urinary tract infection, which can confuse the differential diagnosis. In particular, chronic conditions such as pelvic inflammatory disease and adhesions mimic many features of endometriosis. Laparoscopy may be needed to make the diagnosis.

Endometriosis and Fertility

Endometriosis is commonly diagnosed in women who are undergoing laparoscopic investigations for subfertility but who do not have specific endometriosis-related symptoms. Although endometriosis and subfertility are associated more frequently than can be explained by chance, the exact mechanism of their relationship is uncertain (Table 8.2).

Severe disease can cause subfertility by forming adhesions around the fallopian tubes and ovaries and by affecting ovarian tissue directly (due to the formation of ovarian cysts called endometrioma or 'chocolate cysts'). However, the association between mild endometriosis and subfertility is less clear. Theoretically,

TABLE 8.2 Possible Mechanisms by Which Endometriosis May Reduce Fertility

System	Mechanism
Sexual function	Dyspareunia, leading to reduced frequency of intercourse
Sperm function	Inactivation and phagocytosis of spermatozoa by macrophages in inflammatory peritoneal fluid caused by endometriosis
Tubal function	Fimbrial damage
	Reduced tubal motility with prostaglandins
Ovarian function	Anovulation
	Luteinized unruptured follicle syndrome

high prostaglandin production from endometriotic tissue could impede tubal motility or the spermatozoa may be affected by adverse immunological factors. Another possibility is that subfertility caused by some unrelated factor may predispose women to endometriosis because in the absence of pregnancy the affected women will have more periods. An association with luteinized unruptured follicle (LUF) syndrome, in which follicular development proceeds along apparently normal lines but oocyte release does not occur, provides another explanation. As endometriosis is more common in women with this condition, it has been proposed that failure to release follicular fluid mid-cycle may result in an environment that promotes the establishment of endometriosis.

Investigation

Transvaginal ultrasound can detect endometriosis involving the ovaries (endometriomas/chocolate cysts), and MRI can delineate the extent of active endometriotic lesions greater than 1 cm in diameter in deep tissues, for example, the rectovaginal septum. Laparoscopy remains the standard diagnostic method (Fig. 8.2). Active endometriotic lesions are classically described as red, puckered and inflamed, or as 'burnt match heads' (cigarette burns). Inactive lesions look like scars. The endometriotic lesions can be superficial or deep and infiltrating. However, the degree to which laparoscopic visualization alone may be adequate has been questioned (Box 8.4). It has been proposed that clinicians should confirm a positive laparoscopy with a biopsy of the lesion so that the diagnosis can be confirmed with histology.

The natural course of endometriosis is unknown, with an assumption that mild disease can progress to more severe disease. The prompt return of symptoms after treatment, seen in many patients, may represent re-extension of uneradicated residual disease.

It is impossible to guarantee a cure after treatment. Therefore, routine repeat laparoscopy after completion of treatment has limited prognostic value and is probably best reserved for those patients with recurrent symptoms.

While the tumour marker CA125 may be elevated in endometriosis, measuring serum CA125 levels has no value as a diagnostic tool.

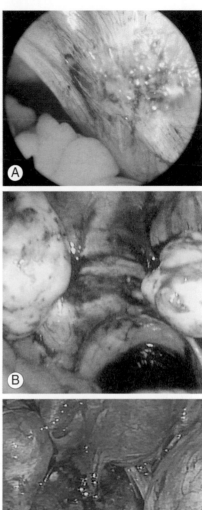

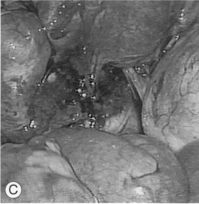

Fig. 8.2 Peritoneal appearances of endometriosis. Laparoscopic views show **(A)** clear blisters ('sago' granules), 'blood blisters', yellow-brown patches, 'powder burns', atypical vascularity and telangiectasia; **(B)** bilateral endometriomas; and **(C)** severe endometriosis with adhesions. (Parts [B] and [C] © KARL STORZ – Endoskope, Germany)

Care of Women With Endometriosis

Medical treatment with non-steroidal anti-inflammatory drugs and/or simple analgesics is widely employed, and many women will be taking these prior to

BOX 8.4 LAPAROSCOPIC AND HISTOLOGICAL APPEARANCE OF ENDOMETRIOTIC LESIONS

- Haemosiderin deposits covered with peritoneum resemble the classical appearance of endometriosis but may arise from local haemorrhage of any origin. Most often, the typical chocolate cysts that are seen in the ovary are endometriomas. However, the histological examination occasionally shows that these have arisen from haemorrhage into a follicular or corpus luteum cyst.
- A wide range of subtle peritoneal changes, such as clear 'sago' blisters, glandular papillae, white opacified patches, red flame-like lesions and peritoneal defects, may prove on biopsy to be a result of endometriosis.

diagnosis. Medical treatment with ovulation suppression is most useful for symptomatic relief but is of no value for the treatment of endometriosis in patients wishing to conceive. Treatment duration is usually limited to between 3 and 6 months. Surgical treatment may be conservative, with laser or diathermy ablation/excision of lesions, or radical, involving hysterectomy and oophorectomy.

MEDICAL TREATMENT

Medical treatment is founded upon the observation that endometriosis improves during both pregnancy and menopause. Thus, creating a 'pseudo-pregnancy' with progestogens or combined oral contraceptives or a 'pseudo-menopause' with GnRH analogues is appropriate and frequently effective.

For symptomatic endometriosis, continuous progestogen therapy (e.g., medroxyprogesterone acetate 10 mg twice daily for 90 days or a progesterone-only contraceptive pill) is most cost-effective, has fewer side effects and is more suitable for long-term use compared with more expensive alternatives. Progestogens act directly on endometrial tissue, both in the uterus and in the endometriosis lesions, by binding to progestogen receptors. This produces decidualization and thinning of the endometrial tissue. The combined oral contraceptive pill is an appropriate alternative; it is usually taken continuously or in a tricycle regimen in order to reduce the frequency of menstrual periods. The combined contraceptive pill can be used in the long term by women who find it effective and are not at additional risk of adverse events from the pill, such as venous thrombosis or

stroke. The levonorgestrel-releasing intrauterine system (such as Mirena) is an effective option used to reduce endometriosis-associated pain.

Second-line drugs are the GnRH analogues, which can be administered by nasal spray, implants, or injection. GnRH analogues bind to GnRH receptors in the pituitary gland. They initially stimulate gonadotrophin release, but the pituitary gland becomes rapidly desensitized to GnRH stimulation, thereby suppressing gonadotrophin release and, in turn, ovarian production of estrogen and progesterone. The profound hypo-estrogenic state that is produced not only affects endometrial tissue but also causes side effects mimicking menopause. Therapy is limited to 3 to 6 months, and it is routine to prescribe 'add-back' hormone replacement therapy (e.g., tibolone) to alleviate the predictable vasomotor side effects (flushing and sweating) and reduction in bone mineral density. The use of add-back therapy does not reverse the effect of treatment on pain relief. Danazol, an oral steroid-like drug with anti-estrogen action, although effective, is now seldom used due to irreversible androgenic side effects.

Medical treatment can also be used as an aid to reaching a diagnosis. If amenorrhoea and symptom relief are achieved with a trial of medical management, then it is more likely that the symptoms were due to endometriosis. If symptoms persist, a review of the diagnosis is necessary, as the endometriosis may be present incidentally, and alternative causes of pelvic pain must be considered again.

SURGICAL TREATMENT

When continued fertility is required, conservative surgery is appropriate. This is usually carried out laparoscopically and includes ablation (destruction of lesions using energy from diathermy, plasma, or laser devices), and excision of endometriosis deposits. It may bring about symptom relief and has a role in women with subfertility. Cystectomy, rather than drainage and coagulation, should be performed for an ovarian endometrioma more than 3 cm in diameter to reduce the risk of endometrioma recurrence.

Hysterectomy with bilateral oophorectomy for women who have completed their childbearing can be helpful. Hormone replacement may be needed depending on the woman's age at the time of surgery.

A combined (estrogen and progesterone) hormone replacement approach is usually recommended to avoid inadvertent stimulation of any residual endometriosis.

The surgical management of deep infiltrating endometriosis is complex and should be undertaken in a centre with the appropriate multidisciplinary expertise. In the United Kingdom, specialist endometriosis centres have been established.

Fertility Treatment

Surgical ablation or excision of minimal and mild endometriosis does improve fertility, but whether surgery has a role in moderate and severe endometriosis is less clear. Surgical treatment of large ovarian endometriotic cysts (measuring 5 cm or greater) probably enhances spontaneous pregnancy rates and will improve transvaginal access to the ovaries for oocyte retrieval (see Chapter 5) if in vitro fertilization is needed. In cases of moderate and severe endometriosis, assisted reproduction techniques should be considered as an alternative to surgery or following unsuccessful surgery.

Complications, Prognosis and Long-Term Sequelae

Depending upon the severity of the disease, adhesions and fibrosis may distort the bowel, bladder, ureters and other adjacent structures, leading to chronic problems with these systems. The physical and psychological morbidity from long-term pain can be considerable.

Key Points

- Acute pelvic pain and CPP have numerous, occasionally overlapping, causes (see Boxes 8.1 and 8.2).
- Many women already have a theory or a concern about the origin of the pain. These ideas should ideally be addressed in the initial consultation.
- The multifactorial nature of CPP should be discussed and explored from the start. The aim should be to develop a partnership between women and clinicians to formulate a care plan.
- Transvaginal ultrasound and MRI are useful tests for diagnosing adenomyosis.
- Women with cyclical pain should be offered a therapeutic trial using the combined oral contraceptive pill, progesterone-only pill, or a GnRH analogue for a period of 3 to 6 months before having a diagnostic laparoscopy.
- Women with symptoms suggestive of IBS should be offered a trial of antispasmodic medication alongside dietary advice.
- While the most common causes of CPP are endometriosis and chronic pelvic infection, over one-third of women with CPP will have no identifiable cause. It is important to avoid unnecessary investigations by accepting the 'CPP syndrome' as a disease entity in its own right.
- Endometriosis is caused by the presence of endometrium-like tissue outside the uterine cavity. Endometrium-like tissue growing within the uterine wall is referred to as adenomyosis.
- Endometriosis is a common gynaecological problem; the incidence is higher among women with subfertility. Symptoms include dysmenorrhoea, dyspareunia, lower abdominal pain and heavy menstrual bleeding.
- Medical management of endometriosis is achieved by the administration of progestogens, the combined oral contraceptive pill, GnRH analogues, or the use of a levonorgestrel-releasing intrauterine system. Surgery may involve laparoscopic ablation or excision of deposits, ovarian cystectomy, or hysterectomy with bilateral oophorectomy.

Chapter 9

Menopause and Hormone Replacement Therapy

Nick Panay

Chapter Outline

Introduction

'Menopause' is derived from the Greek term for cessation of the last monthly period. The definition is 12 months of absent periods in a woman with a uterus who is not pregnant or not taking hormones that might affect the menstrual cycle. Due to the increase in life expectancy in the last century, menopause has now become merely a midlife point for many women.

This is contrary to the rest of the animal kingdom, in which the reproductive lifespan is closely aligned with maximum lifespan. From an anthropological perspective, a prolonged non-reproductive stage allows for the long-term quality care of pre-existing offspring (The Grandmother Hypothesis).

The years leading up to and the year beyond menopause are known as 'perimenopause'. This

TABLE 9.1	The Possible Consequences of Estrogen Deficiency	
Short-term problems	Vasomotor symptoms (80% of women)	Hot flushes
		Night sweats
		Headaches
		Palpitations
	Psychological	Insomnia
		Irritability
		Poor concentration
		Poor short-term memory
		Depression/ low mood
		Lethargy
		Decreased self confidence
	Sexual problems	Decreased libido
		Dyspareunia
	Musculoskeletal	Joint aches
Intermediate-term problems	Urogenital	Atrophic vaginitis
		Vaginal dryness
		Urethral symptoms
		Urge incontinence/ frequency
Long-term problems	Circulation	Cardiovascular disease
		Cerebrovascular disease
	Skeletal	Osteoporosis
		Hip fracture
		Vertebral fracture

stage is associated with fluctuating and eventually low levels of estrogen that result from declining ovarian reserve. Although physiological, menopause has important adverse short- and long-term effects on health (Table 9.1), which can be offset in part by the use of hormone replacement therapy (HRT). The pros and cons of HRT will be discussed in detail in this chapter and will need to be carefully considered on an individual basis before treatment is started. Lifestyle, exercise and dietary approaches should underpin any medical interventions. Complementary and non-hormonal approaches will also be considered for women who do not require or wish to use HRT or for those in whom HRT is contraindicated.

Physiology

Perimenopause (or climacteric) may begin months or years (average 4 years) before the last menstrual period, and symptoms may continue for years afterwards. The median age at menopause in the United Kingdom is 50.8 years and occurs when the supply of oocytes becomes exhausted. A newborn girl has over half a million oocytes in her ovaries; one-third of these disappear before puberty and most of the remainder is lost during reproductive life. In each menstrual cycle, some 20 or 30 primordial follicles begin to develop and most become atretic. As only about 400 cycles occur during an average woman's lifetime, most oocytes are lost spontaneously through ageing rather than through ovulation.

Menopause before the age of 45 years is referred to as early and before the age of 40 years is premature; the latter is now referred to as premature ovarian insufficiency (POI). The following factors are all causes of POI: genetic, for example, Turner syndrome and Fragile X; autoimmune, for example, adrenal; infective, for example, mumps and TB; environmental toxins, for example, smoking; and iatrogenic, for example, chemo/radiotherapy or surgery. However, the idiopathic category (unknown) is still the largest. Genome-wide associated studies and other genetic studies are now uncovering other causative genes which are likely to make up the remainder of the 'unknown' category.

In premenopausal women, estradiol is produced by the granulosa cells of the developing follicle. However, as menopause approaches, this production becomes very variable. The proportion of anovulatory menstrual cycles increases and progesterone production declines. Pituitary production of follicle-stimulating hormone (FSH) and luteinizing hormone (LH) rises because of diminishing negative feedback from estrogen and other ovarian hormones, such as inhibin, but other pituitary hormones are not affected. Serum levels of FSH over 40 IU/L, when associated with irregular or absent periods, can be used clinically to clarify the diagnosis of menopause (see later discussion), although levels begin to rise significantly around the age of 38 years in normally cycling women. Anti-Müllerian hormone (AMH) is a better marker of follicular reserve than FSH and is used particularly to assess the response to ovarian stimulation during assisted conception. Recent research has shown that AMH can be used to predict the age of menopause, although it is still not sufficiently reliable to detect POI. AMH is independent of the day of cycle and its predictive value of ovarian reserve is claimed to last for up to 2 years from when the sample is taken.

Circulating androstenedione and dehydroepiandrosterone sulphate, mainly of adrenal origin, are converted by fat cells mainly into estrone, a less potent form of estrogen than estradiol. After menopause, estrone is the predominant type of circulating estrogen rather than ovarian estradiol.

Signs and Symptoms

See Table 9.1 and Figs 9.1 and 9.2.

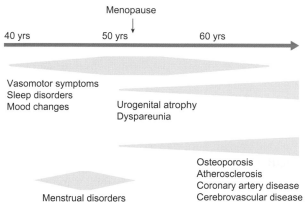

Fig. 9.1 The impact of estrogen deficiency on quality of life and longer-term health.

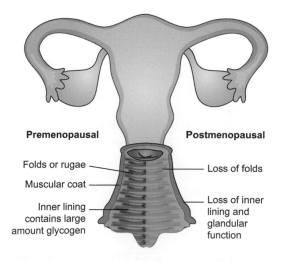

Fig. 9.2 Postmenopausal changes in the vaginal epithelium.

VAGINAL BLEEDING

Irregular periods before menopause are often due to anovulatory menstrual cycles as ovarian reserve drops, which results in inadequate progesterone production in the luteal phase of the cycle and, therefore, unpredictable shedding of the endometrium. However, if erratic bleeding persists, a pelvic ultrasound scan should be performed to assess the endometrial thickness and to look for other pathological features, such as endometrial polyps or fibroids. Further endometrial assessment may be required through hysteroscopic assessment of the endometrial cavity and biopsy of the endometrium to exclude the possibility of endometrial hyperplasia or carcinoma.

Diagnosis of menopause is made retrospectively, one year after the final menstrual period. Further vaginal bleeding after this time frame is 'postmenopausal' and is usually investigated urgently, ideally within 2 weeks of the episode being reported. Approximately 10% of those with postmenopausal bleeding are eventually diagnosed with a gynaecological malignancy.

HOT FLUSHES

A 'hot flush' is an uncomfortable subjective feeling of warmth in the upper part of the body, usually lasting around 3 minutes. Approximately 50% to 85% of menopausal women experience such vasomotor symptoms, although only 10% to 20% seek medical advice. Flushes are often accompanied by sweating; there may also be other symptoms, such as nausea and palpitations. Night sweats may be particularly troublesome, leading to severe insomnia and chronic tiredness. These vasomotor symptoms are now known to originate in the arcuate nucleus of the hypothalamus, which has been identified as the control centre for thermoregulation and which is responsive to both estrogen and ambient temperature. Studies have shown that, in this centre, there is a group of sex steroid–responsive neurons that co-express kisspeptin, neurokinin B and dynorphin, referred to as the KNDy neurons. In the menopausal state, it is thought that these neurons are in a state of hypertrophied hyperactivation due to estrogen withdrawal, which disrupts baseline thermoregulation and triggers hot flushes. Modulation of these neurons with neurokinin-receptor antagonists in recent clinical trials has demonstrated that these could be a viable therapeutic alternative to estrogen for controlling hot flushes.

About 20% of women begin experiencing flushes while still menstruating regularly. Flushes usually subside as the body adjusts to the new lower estrogen concentrations, but recent data suggest that these symptoms continue for 7 to 8 years in many women and in some (5%–10%), they continue indefinitely. These symptoms can be extremely distressing, impairing personal, social and professional quality of life. Exogenous estrogen administration, in the form of HRT, is effective in relieving these symptoms in about 90% of cases.

GENITOURINARY/VULVOVAGINAL ATROPHY (GU/VVA)

The genital system, urethra and bladder trigone are estrogen dependent and undergo gradual atrophy after menopause (see Fig. 9.2). Thinning of the vulval and vaginal skin (vulvovaginal atrophy [VVA]) can cause vulval irritation, vaginal dryness, pain during intercourse and bleeding problems. Loss of vaginal glycogen causes a rise in pH, which can predispose to local infection. Urgency of micturition and recurrent urinary tract infections may result from atrophic change in the bladder trigone and urethral mucosa. A new classification system which encompasses VVA and urinary tract problems has recently been proposed in North America called Genitourinary Syndrome of Menopause (GSM) and could be adopted universally in due course.

Unlike flushes, these atrophic symptoms may appear years after menopause and do not improve spontaneously. It is estimated that approximately 50% of women will eventually suffer genitourinary atrophy symptoms if left untreated. The symptoms respond extremely well to topically applied ultra-low-dose estrogen, but this usually needs to be continued indefinitely to prevent recurrence.

OTHER SYMPTOMS

There are many other symptoms which are thought to be related to menopause although not diagnostic of it. The most distressing include low mood and cognitive problems, musculoskeletal aches and pains, tiredness, loss of libido and weight gain.

Studies have suggested that many of these symptoms can be improved by HRT more effectively than by placebo. However, although low mood may be associated with menopause and can be relieved by HRT, the same may not be true for clinical depression, which is not usually caused directly by estrogen withdrawal. The response to estrogen in this situation is therefore uncertain and may also depend on the presence of other symptoms such as hot flushes, night sweats or insomnia.

Long-Term Effects

It is thought that menopause alters a woman's susceptibility to breast cancer, cardiovascular disease (CVD), osteoporosis and dementia.

BREAST CANCER

Breast cancer increases with increasing age. However, the rate of increase slows after menopause. The risk of breast cancer is decreased if menopause occurs prematurely and is increased if it occurs late. A woman who has had menopause in her late 50s has double the risk of breast cancer when compared with a woman who has had menopause in her early 40s.

CARDIOVASCULAR DISEASE

CVD is the principle cause of morbidity and mortality in women. Women are protected against cardiovascular disease before menopause; this protective effect is thought to be mediated by the favourable effect of estrogen on lipids/lipoproteins, insulin sensitivity and arterial vasodilation. A premenopausal woman's risk of developing coronary artery disease is less than one-fifth of that of a man of the same age, a sex difference that disappears with increasing age. The incidence of CVD rises exponentially in both sexes, but the risk factors for CVD differ between the sexes, as does the impact of preventative measures. Data from epidemiological studies and the known physiological effects of estrogen support a protective effect against cardiovascular disease, although the difference in risk factors referred to previously may also be contributory.

Studies looking at the effect of postmenopausal estrogen therapy suggest that long-term estrogen treatment may reduce the risk of CVD. Meta-analyses of randomised controlled trials have shown a significant reduction in cardiovascular morbidity and mortality.

However, this effect appears to rely on HRT having been started before the age of 60 years, now referred to as the 'window of opportunity'. HRT started later than this may have an initial harmful effect through the prothrombotic effect of oral estrogen and some progestogens on blood vessels which already have significant atherosclerosis. It is possible that this effect can be mitigated through the use of lower doses of metabolically favourable progestogens and transdermal estradiol. This area requires further research before HRT can be recommended routinely for primary prevention of CVD.

OSTEOPOROSIS

Osteoporosis is a skeletal disorder of the bone matrix resulting in a reduction of bone strength such that there is an increased risk of fracture when falling from one's own height. It is predominantly a disease of women, who achieve a lower peak bone mass than men and are also subjected to accelerated loss of bone density due to low estrogen after menopause. Women lose 50% of their skeleton by the age of 70 years; men only lose 25% by 90 years. Loss of height occurs due to loss of collagen in the intervertebral discs as well as due to vertebral fractures.

Bone resorption by osteoclasts is accelerated by menopause (Fig. 9.3). Estrogen receptors have been demonstrated on bone cells, and estrogens stimulate osteoblasts directly. Calcitonin and prostaglandins may also be involved as intermediate factors in the link between estrogen and bone metabolism. In the first 4 years after menopause, there is an annual loss of 1% to 3% of bone mass, falling to 0.6% per year thereafter. This leads to an increased rate of fractures, particularly of the distal radius, vertebral body and upper femur. One or more of these fractures will affect 40% of women over 65 years old. Wedge compression fractures of the spine leading to the so-called 'dowager's hump' affect 25% of white women over 60 years of age (Fig. 9.4), and fractures of the hip have occurred in 20% of women by the age of 90 years. Women who are underweight have a higher risk of osteoporosis, which may be caused in part by reduced peripheral conversion of androgens to estrogen. Women of Afro-Caribbean origin have a smaller risk of osteoporosis than white or Asian women, as they have a greater initial bone mass.

Normal trabecular bone	Trabecular bone with resorption areas

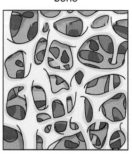 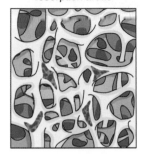

Trabecular bone with microcracks	Osteoporotic trabecular bone

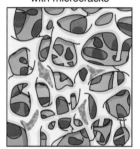 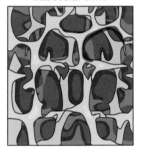

Fig. 9.3 Various stages of bone resorption due to estrogen deficiency of menopause.

Osteoporosis has important consequences for women and for health services. In the United Kingdom, over 35,000 postmenopausal women suffer femoral fractures every year and 17% of them die in hospital. HRT has a very significant benefit in reducing the incidence of osteoporosis and osteoporotic fractures. Although it is proven that estrogen decreases fracture risk, it is not currently recommended as a first-line treatment by the regulatory authorities, as the long-term risks are considered to outweigh the benefits. However, the view of the menopause societies in the United Kingdom and globally is that HRT should be one of the first-line options for osteoporosis in women starting treatment before the age of 60 years.

DEMENTIA

During menopause transition, cognitive problems are common. Although these symptoms do not usually persist, the incidence of Alzheimer dementia is higher in women compared with men. Estrogen has been

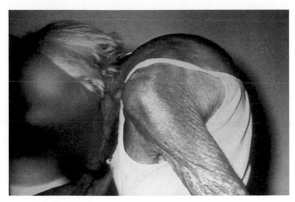

Fig. 9.4 Severe osteoporosis of the spine. (Reproduced with permission from *A woman's guide to osteoporosis*, Wyeth Laboratories.)

shown to improve cerebral perfusion and cognition in women under 60 years and promotes neuronal growth and neurotransmission. Therefore, HRT may prevent diseases such as vascular dementia and Alzheimer dementia if started early (earlier than 60 years old) but long-term randomised data are required to confirm this. The failure of estrogen to show benefit for dementia in women commencing HRT over 60 years of age probably reflects the predominance of the thrombotic effects of estrogen in this age group.

Diagnosis

Menopause may be confused with pre-menstrual syndrome, depression, thyroid dysfunction, pregnancy and, rarely, phaeochromocytoma or carcinoid syndrome. Vasomotor symptoms may be caused by calcium antagonists and by anti-depressive therapy, especially tricyclics.

The diagnosis of postmenopause is primarily clinical and can only be made in retrospect after 12 months of amenorrhoea (possibly 4 months in women under 40 years of age). If there is clinical confusion, such as in a younger woman, the serum FSH level should be measured, which should be >40 IU/L postmenopausally. In younger women (<40 years) two FSH levels should be measured 6 weeks apart, as levels of FSH often fluctuate considerably during perimenopause. In the United Kingdom, guidance from the National Institute for Health and Care Excellence (NICE) states clearly that a blood test is not required in women

45 years or older with vasomotor symptoms before treating them with HRT. If there is diagnostic doubt about whether a woman is perimenopausal, especially over 45 years of age, a therapeutic trial of HRT can be considered. Absence of a satisfactory response suggests that symptoms are unrelated to low levels of estrogen. Perimenopausally, FSH levels may be in the premenopausal range; it should be noted that FSH levels peak physiologically in mid-cycle, making it worth re-checking unexpected levels a second time. Ideally, FSH levels should be checked on days 2 to 3 in women who are still menstruating.

Hormone Replacement Therapy

Estrogen supplementation is the basis of replacement therapy. Although progesterone and progestogens (synthetic progesterone) may have a small role in relieving vasomotor symptoms, they are added to estrogen to protect the endometrium. Estrogens may be systemically administered as daily oral tablets, twice-weekly or weekly transdermal patches, daily transdermal estradiol gel or spray, or subcutaneous implants administered every 6 to 8 months. Whatever the route of administration, women who have not undergone hysterectomy should be prescribed a regimen which includes progesterone or progestogen to minimize the risk of endometrial hyperplasia and cancer associated with unopposed estrogen therapy. This advice also applies to women who have undergone endometrial resection. Women who have had a hysterectomy do not require a progestogen unless they are thought to have a significant risk of recurrence of endometriosis.

ORAL PREPARATIONS

The oral route of administration may have a more beneficial effect than parenteral therapy on lipid profiles, leading to higher high-density lipoprotein (HDL) levels, which is non-atherogenic, and lower low-density lipoprotein (LDL) levels, which is atherogenic. However, the trade-off is that it is potentially thrombogenic because of an increase in clotting factors from first-pass liver metabolism. Tablets may be given as an estrogen-only preparation for those who have had a hysterectomy or as a combined estrogen–progesterone/progestogen preparation for those who have not. The combined form may be administered cyclically or continuously. Cyclic preparations, which usually lead to monthly withdrawal bleeds, are used perimenopausally. Continuous combined preparations, so-called 'no-period' HRT, are an option from more than 2 years after the final menstrual period in women less than 50 years old or more than 1 year in women more than 50 years of age. This continuous combined therapy is more convenient for the vast majority who do not suffer unscheduled bleeding, but breakthrough bleeding beyond the first 6 months of treatment warrants further investigation.

Alternatives to the estrogen–progesterone/progestogen preparations are tibolone, raloxifene and estrogen/bazedozifene. Tibolone is a synthetic steroid with weak estrogenic, progestogenic and androgenic effects, which may be started 1 to 2 years after periods have ceased in a similar way to the continuous combined preparations. Raloxifene, a synthetic selective estrogen receptor modulator (SERM), has estrogenic effects on bone and lipid metabolism, but has a minimal effect on uterine and breast tissue. It is ineffective for controlling perimenopausal symptoms but can be used for osteoporosis of the spine and it does not cause vaginal bleeding. The combination of estrogen with the SERM bazedoxifene has recently provided a useful option for women who are intolerant of the 'premenstrual syndrome-type' side effects of progesterone/progestogens. Bazedoxifene provides protection of the endometrium instead of progesterone/progestogens. In the pipeline is another type of estrogen usually produced in the fetal liver (estetrol rather than estradiol), which is thought to avoid breast tissue stimulation and may even protect against breast cancer.

TRANSCUTANEOUS ADMINISTRATION

Transdermal patches are available as an unopposed estrogen form in various doses or as cyclical or continuous estrogen–progestogen combinations. Skin reactions, ranging from hyperaemia to blisters, affect a small percentage of users but the modern small "dot matrix" patches minimize these side effects. The clinical advantage of transcutaneous administration is that it does not increase the risk of thrombosis since it minimizes the effect on hepatic production of coagulation factors. It may also avoid gastrointestinal side effects and changes in lipoprotein levels. Patches are usually applied to the buttock and each patch lasts for between 3 and 7 days depending on the formulation.

This method appears to be as effective as oral preparations in treating symptomatic women and for the prevention of osteoporosis.

Percutaneous estrogen gels and sprays are also available. A measured dose is applied to the skin on a daily basis and avoids the prolonged skin contact of patches. They can reduce skin reactions and provide an 'invisible' transdermal treatment but do require daily application. They do not contain progesterone or progestogen; therefore, women with a uterus require additional endometrial protection when being treated with these products.

SUBCUTANEOUS IMPLANTS

Estradiol pellets may be implanted in the subcutaneous fat, usually in the lower abdomen, at intervals of no less than 5 or 6 months. The estradiol level does not always fall away to baseline before symptoms recur and there is a risk of tachyphylaxis (persistent symptoms despite ever-increasing estradiol levels) unless strict dose control is observed. However, provided that pre-implant estradiol levels are monitored and high doses avoided, the risk of tachyphylaxis is minimized. Testosterone implants can also be used to treat distressing low libido. For commercial reasons, the licenced implants were withdrawn but unlicenced implants can still be obtained by specialist centres.

HRT in Women With Premature Ovarian Insufficiency

Women with POI (less than 40 years old) usually require higher doses of HRT in order to fully control their symptoms and because these are physiological for them. It is also important to remember that HRT in this age group is recommended not only to control symptoms but also to protect against long-term risks of osteoporosis, cardiovascular disease and dementia. Therefore, treatment should be continued at least until the average age of menopause (51 years). If pregnancy is not desired, then treatment can start with the oral contraceptive pill, but data suggest that HRT is more favourable from a bone and metabolic perspective.

TREATMENT OF GENITOURINARY/VULVOVAGINAL GU/VVA SYMPTOMS

Treatment includes estradiol vaginal tablets, low-dose estradiol-releasing silastic ring pessaries and estriol vaginal pessaries and vaginal cream. A newer option is vaginal dehydroepiandrosterone (DHEA, prasterone) pessaries; the DHEA is converted locally by aromatase enzymes to estradiol and testosterone. Low-dose vaginal preparations are safe as well as effective in the treatment of atrophic symptoms since the systemic absorption is very small after the first few weeks of administration. However, these treatments should be continued indefinitely for benefits to be maintained. Other options for GU/VVA symptoms include orally administered ospemifene, which is a SERM, and carbon dioxide or erbium laser treatments. The latter require further data for effectiveness and safety, but initial data are promising.

Testosterone

In women with distressingly low libido, it is possible that treatment with female physiological doses of testosterone could be of benefit. There are particularly good data for women who have had surgical menopause but benefit is seen even in women with natural menopause. Treatment should be driven by symptoms, not by low testosterone levels, although baseline and regular tests should be done to avoid high levels. Due to the lack of licenced female testosterone options, it is usually necessary to prescribe one-tenth of the male dose of 1% gels. Licenced testosterone patches and implants for female use were withdrawn for commercial reasons, but a 1% testosterone cream has recently been licenced in Australia. A minimum trial of 3 months is required and serious androgenic adverse effects, such as deep voice/clitoromegaly are rare with physiological doses, although some localized hair growth and acne can occur in a small percentage of women.

Risks and Side Effects of HRT

General

Nausea and breast tenderness occur in about 5% to 10% of patients. Uterine bleeding is common, particularly with high-dose regimens. In general, the lowest dose that controls symptoms should be used. Irregular bleeding should be investigated as appropriate. There is a slight risk of cholelithiasis with oral preparations. Diabetes control is improved and the incidence is lower in those taking HRT.

Endometrial Carcinoma

Unopposed therapy (i.e., estrogen only) increases the incidence of endometrial cancer four-fold. Therefore, it should be used only for those who have had a hysterectomy. The incidence is reduced to a relative risk of <1.0 with opposed therapy. Typically, the addition of progesterone/progestogen for 10 to 12 days per cycle is required to give adequate protection. The levonorgestrel-releasing intrauterine system protects the endometrium effectively when used in conjunction with estrogen-only HRT in postmenopausal women. This is particularly useful in women who are still menstruating when starting HRT and also provides very effective contraception.

Breast Cancer

A link between sex hormone treatment and breast cancer is biologically plausible because of the connection between late menopause and breast cancer. There is a small increase in likelihood of being diagnosed with breast cancer with combined HRT although estrogen alone in hysterectomized women is associated with little or no excess risk. Recent data suggest that the excess risk is largely promotional on pre-existing undetected breast cancers and becomes apparent 3 to 5 years after HRT is started. In the US Women's Health Initiative randomised trial, the excess risk of breast cancer with combined HRT was approximately 1 extra case per 1000 women per year. Eventually, the excess risk subsides when HRT is stopped but may remain elevated for up to 10 years. The progestogen type has a significant influence on this risk. In general, the more androgenic the progestogen the greater the risk; natural progesterone and the most similar progestogen, dydrogesterone, appear to confer the smallest risk.

Other Cancers

The evidence of any adverse effect of HRT on ovarian cancer is controversial and no more than one extra case per 5000 women per year. The risk of cervical and vulval cancer does not appear to be increased. The incidence of colon cancer is decreased by up to one-third in women taking HRT.

Venous Thromboembolic Disease

There is an increased risk of venous thromboembolic disease in the first year of oral HRT treatment, with a relative risk of approximately 4 in the first 6 months and 3 in the second 6 months (baseline risk, 1.3/1000 per year). This increased risk is largely confined to the first year of use. There is no increased risk in those taking transdermal HRT according to many studies. Routine pre-treatment screening for thrombophilia is not recommended, but it should be discussed with a haematologist in those with a personal or family history of venous thromboembolic disease. It is not known whether transcutaneous administration of estrogen is associated with an increased risk of secondary venous thromboembolism (VTE) and it would usually be avoided in those who have had a prior thrombotic episode. If all other treatment options had been tried, then it is possible for prophylactic anticoagulation to be used in combination with HRT in the highest-risk patients. The care of these patients should be in collaboration with a haematologist.

Stroke

There is a significant increase in the risk of stroke in all age groups with oral HRT, although the impact is small in younger menopausal women, as the baseline risk of stroke is so low. The dose and route of administration of HRT is important in this context. Low-dose oral and transdermal HRT appear to confer little or no excess risk in younger menopausal women (50–59 years old).

CONTRAINDICATIONS TO HORMONE TREATMENT

Venous thromboembolic disease that was associated with pregnancy and a history of recurrent VTE are recognised contraindications to HRT, as are liver disease and undiagnosed vaginal bleeding. Treated hypertension and other cardiovascular risk factors are not contraindications if effectively managed.

HRT is also contraindicated following breast cancer (including intraductal cancer). However, in women with intractable symptoms who have tried all other options, HRT may occasionally be prescribed in specialist centres, particularly if the tumour was hormone receptor negative. HRT may also be prescribed for women with *BRCA* genes undergoing risk-reducing bilateral salpingo-oophorectomy, especially in the younger age group (<45 years old). This does not appear to attenuate the benefit of the surgery for breast/ovarian cancer risk reduction.

HRT is also contraindicated in women with endometrial carcinoma although those who have had surgery for early-stage disease (I and II) are occasionally treated with HRT depending on age, severity of symptoms and failure to respond to non-hormonal alternatives.

DURATION OF HORMONE REPLACEMENT THERAPY

When HRT is prescribed for vasomotor symptoms, it is generally continued for a few years to provide relief of these symptoms. Then, discontinuation is attempted through dose reduction to see whether the symptoms are continuing. The decision to continue therapy beyond this time depends on whether symptoms recur and on a weighing up of the risks of osteoporosis against the potential side effects, including breast cancer, for that particular individual. Most menopause societies advise that arbitrary limits not be placed on treatment duration but that there should be at least an annual re-evaluation of the pros and cons of continuing with therapy.

Non-Hormonal Treatment

DRUGS

Vasomotor symptoms may be reduced by clonidine, which acts directly on the hypothalamus. However, in practice, it is of limited value as it is no more effective than placebo in randomised controlled trials. The selective serotonin reuptake inhibitors have also been shown to be effective. However, some types should be avoided in women on tamoxifen – for example, fluoxetine and paroxetine – as they reduce its effectiveness. Venlafaxine, which is a serotonin and noradrenaline reuptake inhibitor, is one of the most commonly used alternatives to HRT in breast cancer patients. Gabapentin and oxybutynin have also been shown to reduce vasomotor symptoms but are not without side effects, such as drowsiness. Palpitations and tachycardia may be improved by beta-blockers. Sedatives, hypnotics and antidepressants may be helpful in the treatment of non-vasomotor symptoms. Recent research has focused on the role of neurokinin receptor antagonists, which appear to be as effective as HRT for alleviation of vasomotor symptoms. However, at the time of this writing, they were still at phase 3 clinical trial stage.

Herbal preparations are taken by many women, but conclusive evidence of their benefit is lacking. Recent meta-analyses have shown some benefit for St John's Wort and soy/red clover isoflavones. However, there are drug interactions with the former and caution should be exercised in using the latter in patients with hormone-dependent malignancies.

The first-line treatment for osteoporosis in women over 60 years old is currently bisphosphonates; estrogen is used only for those for whom this is inappropriate. In younger women, treatment with bisphosphonates is not recommended due to risk of adverse effects and long-term reduction in bone turnover unless there is a history of fracture. In elderly women, supplementation with calcium, calcitonin and vitamin D reduces the risk of hip fractures. Moderate weight-bearing exercise may slow the rate of bone loss, though compliance with exercise programmes is often poor.

PSYCHOLOGICAL SUPPORT

Since menopausal symptoms often resolve with time, some women with these symptoms need only reassurance. Others may have particular stresses at this time of life, such as children leaving home, which may accentuate their perimenopausal symptoms and can severely compromise quality of life. The marked placebo benefits in various studies show the importance of psychological support and a sympathetic ear. However, there is now good evidence that cognitive behavioral therapy can also be of significant benefit for menopause-related symptoms.

Key Points

- The average age of women experiencing spontaneous menopause in the United Kingdom is 51 years.
- Menopause is defined as 1 year of amenorrhoea in the presence of a uterus and in the absence of another cause, such as low body mass or excess exercise.
- Menopause is caused by ovarian insufficiency, as the supply of oocytes is depleted. FSH rises as estrogen production falls; an FSH of >40 IU/L is indicative of menopausal status.

- Cessation of periods is often preceded by irregular bleeding. A vaginal bleed more than a year after menopause warrants urgent investigation.
- Vasomotor symptoms, such as hot flushes, affect more than two-thirds of women and may continue for more than 5 to 10 years after menopause. They can severely affect quality of life and should not be dismissed. Other symptoms include genitourinary atrophy, musculoskeletal and possibly psychological and cognitive symptoms.
- Long-term health risks of the postmenopause include CVD, osteoporosis and dementia. Fractures of the radius, vertebral body, or femoral neck affect 40% of women over the age of 65 years.
- HRT is offered to treat menopausal symptoms and to reduce long-term hypo-estrogenic side effects.
- If the woman still has a uterus, opposed HRT (estrogen and progesterone/progestogen) is necessary to avoid the risk of endometrial carcinoma. Oral, transcutaneous and vaginal preparations are available in addition to subcutaneous implants.
- Vaginal hormonal preparations are usually the most effective for GU/VVA symptoms although physiological moisturisers can be helpful in women who wish to avoid HRT altogether.
- Oral selective estrogen receptor modulators can now be used for GU/VVA symptoms and for vasomotor symptoms when combined with estrogen.
- Women should be offered the option of testosterone supplementation if they are suffering with distressingly low libido and psychosexual causes have been excluded.
- Women with early menopause or premature ovarian insufficiency should be advised to use hormone replacement at least until the average age of menopause.
- Side effects of HRT include an increased incidence of breast cancer with combined HRT and venous thromboembolic disease with oral preparations.

Chapter 10

Pelvic Organ Prolapse

Karen Guerrero

Chapter Outline

Introduction

Pelvic organ prolapse (POP) is described as the descent of one or more of the pelvic organs into the vagina. It can affect any of the compartments of the vagina: anterior (bladder), posterior (bowel) or apical (uterus/cervix or vault if the woman has previously had a hysterectomy). Although prolapse in a single compartment can happen, typically more than one compartment will be involved (e.g., bladder and uterine prolapse co-existing).

These organs are supported in the pelvis by the muscles, ligaments and fascia of the pelvic floor. If the pelvic floor is damaged or weakened – for example, as a result of childbirth – the organs descend into the vagina, causing prolapse. One-third of women who have had children will develop a symptomatic prolapse; the lifetime risk of requiring surgery for prolapse is around 11% for women. Stress urinary incontinence (SUI) has the same aetiology and can co-exist with prolapse in any compartment.

Aetiology

POP is caused by injury to the pelvic floor. The injury can be to the muscles (levator ani) or the fascial supports, including many important ligaments (e.g., the uterosacral and cardinal ligaments). The most likely time to injure the pelvic floor is during childbirth. However, chronic constipation and other factors, which lead to an increase in intra-abdominal pressure, can contribute.

CHILDBIRTH

Childbirth results in trauma to the pelvic floor and loss of support to the female pelvic organs. Direct trauma, such as avulsion of the levator ani or ligaments, can happen at the time of vaginal delivery, especially with forceps deliveries. Pelvic nerve damage also plays a part. The pudendal nerve may be compressed against the bony pelvis during labour; the longer the woman is in labour, the worse the damage is likely to be. Forceps deliveries also increase the risk of levator ani damage. A prolonged labour – in particular, a prolonged second stage with a large baby and subsequent instrumental delivery – increases the risk of prolapse even further.

MENOPAUSE

The menopausal state, characterised by estrogen deficiency and loss of connective tissue strength, has been implicated as a contributing factor in the development of prolapse. However, prolapse can also occur in young women before menopause. Thus, simply being menopausal is not always implicated.

CONGENITAL

Congenital weaknesses, or neurological deficiency of the tissues, account for prolapse in a very small proportion of women, as can connective tissue disorders (e.g., Ehlers-Danlos syndrome). Very rarely, children may be born with congenital cloacal abnormalities, which result in abnormal genitalia.

GYNAECOLOGICAL SURGERY

Although surgery is often used to treat prolapse, it can be responsible for some types of prolapse. A colposuspension, an operation done for SUI (see Chapter 11), alters the anatomy of the vagina. The bladder neck is lifted up behind the symphysis pubis to support the bladder, but this results in gravitational effects on the posterior vaginal wall which can then lead to posterior wall prolapse in up to 25% of women who undergo this operation. Vaginal vault prolapse is a recognised sequelae of hysterectomy.

GENETIC

Genetic factors have been implicated in the development of prolapse. It is uncommon, for example, in the women of African origin, possibly related in some way to the different collagen content of tissues.

Types of Prolapse

The main types of prolapse, and the main symptoms, are summarized in Table 10.1. It is important to remember that a single prolapse is very rare, with most women having 'multicompartment' prolapse, that is, more than one of these listed next.

URETHROCELE

The term 'urethrocele' is occasionally used to describe descent of the part of the anterior vaginal wall over which the urethra sits. This is approximately the lower 3 to 4 cm of the anterior wall. Descent here leads to urethral hypermobility, which can disrupt the urethral continence mechanism, predisposing to SUI. This is not treated by prolapse surgery; rather, it is treated by SUI surgery (see Chapter 11).

CYSTOCELE

The bladder rests on the anterior vaginal wall and its supporting mechanisms. A cystocele occurs when

TABLE 10.1	Types of Pelvic Organ Prolapse	
Compartment	Prolapse	Symptoms[a]

Anterior	Urethrocele
	Cystocele
		Stress urinary
		  incontinence
		Poor bladder
		  emptying, residual
		  urine, frequency
		  and urinary
		  infection

Apical	Uterine
	  (procidentia)
	Vault
	  (enterocele)
		Bleeding and/or
		  discharge from
		  ulceration in
		  association with
		  procidentia
		
		Backache

Posterior	Enterocele	Pressure, backache
	Rectocele	Difficulty in bowel emptying

[a]In addition to the general symptoms of discomfort, dragging, the feeling of a 'lump' and, rarely, coital problems.

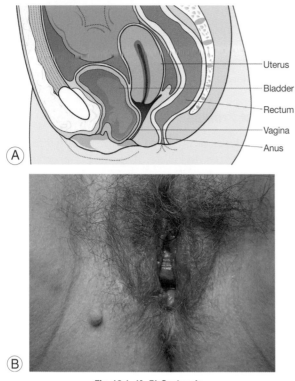

Fig. 10.1 (A, B) Cystocele.

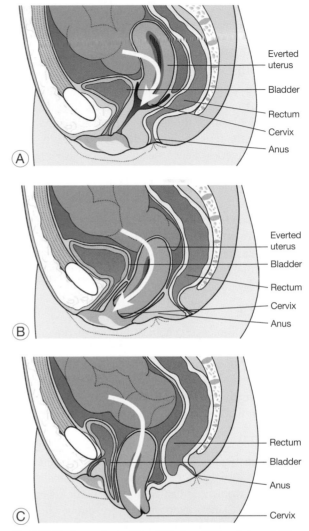

Fig. 10.2 Uterine prolapse. Stage I (A), stage II (B) and stage III (C).

there is descent in the anterior compartment and the bladder prolapses into the vagina (Fig. 10.1).

UTERINE PROLAPSE

The cervix, with the uterus on top, normally sits in the upper third of the vagina. When apical supports are lost, it descends and is called a uterine prolapse (Fig. 10.2).

RECTOCELE

Weakening of the tissue that lies between the vagina and rectum (rectovaginal fascia) allows the rectum to protrude into the lower posterior vaginal wall, causing a rectocele (Fig. 10.3). Laxity of the perineum may also be present, which gives a gaping appearance to the fourchette (the posterior margin of the introitus).

ENTEROCELE

An enterocele occurs in the upper vagina (Fig. 10.4). Weakness in the support mechanism here leads to descent of the vagina and a peritoneal sac, potentially containing small bowel or omentum. Enteroceles are

apical prolapses, that is, the top of the vagina. Therefore, they are commonly found with uterine prolapses or, if the woman has had a hysterectomy, the top of the vagina descends with an enterocele in it. This is called a 'vault prolapse'.

Prolapse Staging

Many different classification systems have been described to attempt to stage (size) POP, and these are shown in Fig. 10.5. The universally recommended tool is the pelvic organ prolapse quantification

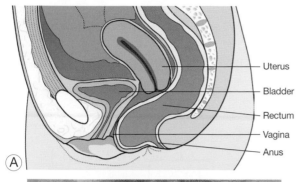

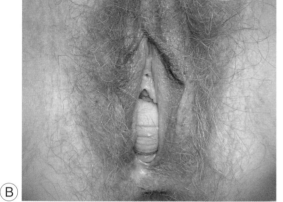

Fig. 10.3 (A, B) Rectocele.

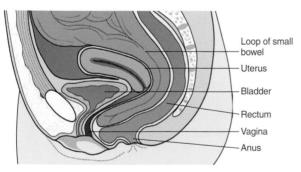

Fig. 10.4 Enterocele.

system (POP-Q). This system describes location in addition to the size of prolapse. The simplified staging system shown in Table 10.2 is the one commonly used in clinical practice. 'Procidentia' is a term used when the cervix, uterus and vaginal wall have completely prolapsed through the introitus, that is, stage IV prolapse.

Symptoms

Prolapse is often asymptomatic and may be detected only when women attend for a cervical smear test. The only real symptom of POP is that of feeling a lump or swelling coming from the vagina. Women will describe it in different ways. The most common description used by women is of 'something coming down', usually accompanied by discomfort and a dragging sensation. Some will describe a lump that they can see or feel, others will describe a swelling that 'hangs out', 'pops in/out', or that they need to push in themselves. The feeling of things coming down will sometimes cause a sensation of pulling.

Women sometimes describe backache, which improves when lying down, although this can often be for other reasons – for example, arthritis and not the prolapse. If the POP is protruding outside the vagina, it may rub on the woman's clothes. This may lead to ulceration of the cervix and thickening of the vaginal mucosa, which can bleed and be sore. Prolapse itself, however, 'does not' cause pain. Women who are in a lot of pain may have a prolapse, but it is not the cause of their pain.

POP may lead to difficulties with sexual intercourse. Although sexual intercourse is usually possible with a POP, women are worried they should not have intercourse because of concern that they may make things worse or because they often feel embarrassed by their perceived appearance of their vagina.

Although a very large POP that protrudes outside the vagina can lead to urethral kinking, which may lead to voiding difficulties or problems emptying their bowels, it is very rare for this to occur. However, functional bladder and bowel symptoms (i.e., urinary or faecal incontinence, constipation, difficulty passing urine or urine infections) will co-exist in most women with POP. This is not because they are necessarily caused by the POP but because they have the same aetiology. Taking a history must include asking for these symptoms so that these problems can be addressed, but managing the prolapse alone will not improve these symptoms in most women.

Signs

Examination for prolapse forms part of the general gynaecological examination. Abdominal examination, although historically done to detect a pelvic mass that

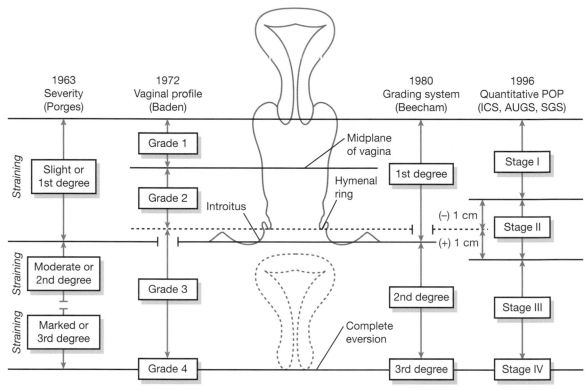

Fig. 10.5 Classification systems that have been used to stage (size) POP.

TABLE 10.2	The Simplified Staging System Commonly Used to Stage Pelvic Organ Prolapse

Pelvic Organ Prolapse Quantification System (POP-Q)	
Stage 0	No prolapse demonstrated
Stage I	The most distal portion of the prolapse is more than 1 cm above the level of the hymen
Stage II	The most distal portion of the prolapse is 1 cm or less proximal or distal to the plane of the hymen
Stage III	The most distal portion of the prolapse is more than 1 cm below the plane of the hymen but protrudes no further than 2 cm less than the total vaginal length in cm
Stage IV	Essentially complete eversion of the total length of the lower genital tract is demonstrated

may be pushing the pelvic organs downwards, is more likely to detect a palpable bladder, which, if found after voiding, is a sign of urinary retention.

Pelvic examination is then performed, initially with the woman supine. The woman is asked to abduct her legs. On inspection of the vulva, one may note atrophic changes (scanty hair, thinning of the labia). Vaginal atrophy may be seen, suggesting the need for estrogen treatment. Urinary leakage should be looked for on coughing, and an assessment of the perineum is made. By gently parting the labia majora with the thumb and index finger of the left hand, prolapse may be seen appearing at the introitus. The woman should be asked to strain or cough to push down any prolapse, making it easier to identify. A bimanual examination may then be performed which may give a useful indication of uterine size and, possibly, descent.

Examination in the left lateral position can also be helpful (see Fig. 2.6). This allows a systematic examination of the entire vagina, exerting gentle traction with the speculum on the posterior vaginal wall. Sponge forceps are occasionally used during this examination to reduce a large prolapse or to enable the examiner to distinguish the anatomy. The speculum can then be slowly withdrawn along the posterior wall of the vagina and the full extent of any rectocele will come into view. If a prolapse is not apparent with the woman lying down, it may sometimes be necessary to examine her in the standing position.

Care of Women With Pelvic Organ Prolapse

As with many conditions, POP can be managed surgically or non-surgically. Non-surgical management is termed 'conservative management'. In the case of POP, it should be tried before resorting to surgery.

CONSERVATIVE MANAGEMENT

No Treatment

If a POP is not causing symptoms and the woman is unaware of it, then she does not require any treatment. Simply because a doctor notices a prolapse within the vagina does not mean that it requires management.

Many women are aware of the presence of a POP; however, it may not be troubling them or interfering with their quality of life or daily activities. It is perfectly reasonable to reassure these women that they do not have serious pathology and that no intervention is required.

Lifestyle Advice

Women should be advised about weight reduction and smoking cessation. Fluid and dietary advice will also be helpful for concomitant bladder and bowel symptoms.

Pelvic Floor Exercises

Supervised pelvic floor muscle exercises by trained physiotherapists have been proven to improve symptoms in stage I–II prolapse, reducing the need for surgery. The key word here is 'supervised'. Simply giving the woman a leaflet about pelvic floor exercises and telling her to go and do them, although unlikely to

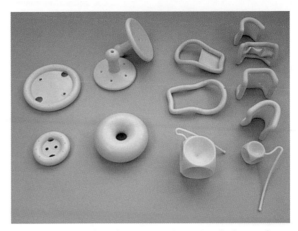

Fig. 10.6 A selection of the commonly used vaginal pessaries.

do any harm, is also unlikely to produce any benefit. Sending an enthusiastic woman to an enthusiastic physiotherapist, however, can produce cure/improvement rates of 60% to 70%.

Pelvic floor physiotherapy is of less proven benefit in women with stage III–IV POP, but it still has a role in the treatment of associated urinary and bowel symptoms.

Vaginal Pessaries

These are devices specifically made for women to wear in their vagina. A pessary does not cure prolapse but provides support while the woman is wearing it, thereby relieving POP symptoms. Pessaries are commonly used. They come in various shapes and sizes, some of which are shown in Fig. 10.6.

The most commonly used pessary is called a 'ring' pessary. It is an inert plastic ring, which is placed in the vagina so that one edge of the ring is behind the symphysis pubis and the other is in the posterior fornix (Figs 10.7 and 10.8). The ring stretches the vault of the vagina and, thus, supports the uterus. Traditionally, once a pessary is fitted, arrangements are usually made to change it every 4 to 6 months by a health care professional. At this examination, the vagina is inspected thoroughly for atrophic changes and ulceration due to pressure necrosis. The pessary is either washed and reused or replaced depending on the type. Many of the newer pessaries are amenable to self-management and women remove it themselves, choosing when to wear it. Therefore, sexual activity is

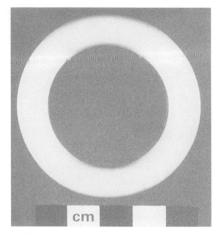

Fig. 10.7 Ring pessary (50 mm diameter).

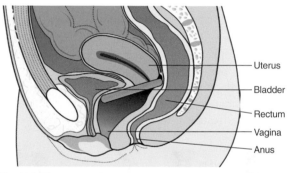

Uterus
Bladder
Rectum
Vagina
Anus

Fig. 10.8 Ring pessary in situ. Note that the anterior vaginal wall is elevated to reduce the cystocele and the uterine prolapse has been corrected.

possible with pessary use and sexually active women should not be excluded from this treatment option.

Complications from pessaries may include urinary symptoms (frequency, infection), vaginal discharge, bleeding, or, very rarely, fistula formation (if the pessary is neglected).

Vaginal Estrogen Therapy

If atrophy of the lower genital tract is noted, with or without association with POP, topical estrogen therapy (commonly administered topically as a cream) may help. Systemic absorption of estrogen is negligible and is safe to use in most women. It improves vaginal tissue thickness, quality and sensitivity. Therefore, it may improve many symptoms the woman may be experiencing that are not necessarily caused by the POP. It can also help decrease the incidence of vaginal pessary

complications in postmenopausal women. In some women, it may also be sensible to use preoperatively to help improve vaginal skin.

SURGICAL MANAGEMENT

The choice of surgical procedure will depend on the woman's age; type and stage of prolapse; whether she is sexually active; any comorbidities, including high body mass index (BMI); and, ultimately, the woman's wishes.

Complications can occur with all type of surgery, not just prolapse surgery. These include infection, bleeding and organ injury, which could be life-threatening. Chronic pain can also occur with all surgery, including prolapse surgery. Prolapse surgery can result in vaginal scarring and narrowing, making sexual intercourse difficult and sometimes impossible.

Recurrence of prolapse after surgical correction is common, with up to 30% of women having vaginal prolapse repairs requiring a second operation within 5 years. Careful counselling of women must therefore not only be about what operation to have but also about complications and risk of recurrence and, thus, the importance of trying conservative treatments first.

Operations can be performed via the vaginal route, abdominally or laparoscopically. The following procedures can be considered, either in isolation or performed in combination. It may also be appropriate in some women to combine them with surgery for SUI (see Chapter 11).

Anterior Repair (Colporrhaphy)

This is a vaginal operation performed to treat a cystocele. The principle of an anterior repair is to make a midline incision through the vaginal skin and to reflect the underlying bladder off the vaginal mucosa. Once this is achieved, supporting sutures are placed into the fascia in order to elevate the bladder. The remaining redundant vaginal skin that has been 'ballooning' down is excised, and the vaginal skin is sutured closed.

Posterior Repair (Colporrhaphy)

This is a vaginal operation performed to treat rectoceles. The principles of a posterior repair are similar to those of an anterior repair. An incision is made in the posterior vaginal wall and the rectum is separated from

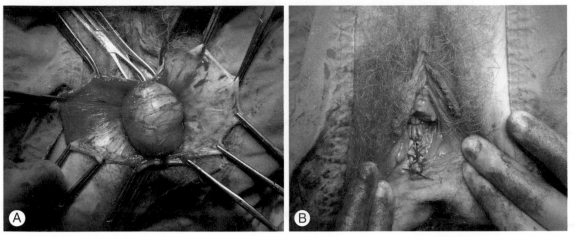

Fig. 10.9 Posterior colporrhaphy. (A) The posterior wall is opened in the midline to expose the rectum. **(B)** The posterior wall is closed after reducing the prolapse.

the vagina (Fig. 10.9). Supporting sutures are placed in the disrupted rectovaginal fascia to reduce the prolapse. The lax vaginal skin is then excised and the incision closed. This operation can be combined with a repair of the perineal body to support the perineum (perineoplasty). Again, particular care must be taken not to narrow the vagina and cause dyspareunia.

Vaginal Hysterectomy

Vaginal hysterectomy is performed for uterine prolapse. The aim is not simply to remove the uterus, that is, the prolapsing organ, as the vaginal vault will descend instead. Once the uterus is removed, the supporting uterosacral ligaments are shortened and reattached to the vaginal vault to support the upper vagina.

Manchester Repair

Manchester repair (also called 'Fothergill repair') has a role in treating a woman with cystocele and a uterine prolapse, but is not commonly performed. A vaginal approach is used. The skin around the cervix is incised. The uterosacral and transverse cervical (cardinal) ligaments are divided and shortened, the cervix is amputated, and the shortened ligaments are approximated anterior to the cervical stump. The anterior repair is performed and completed as before.

Sacrospinous Ligament Fixation

This is a vaginal operation performed for apical prolapse, typically post-hysterectomy vault prolapse

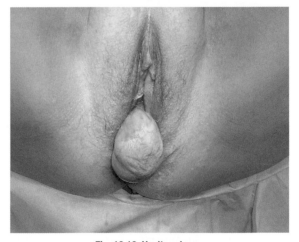

Fig. 10.10 Vault prolapse.

(Fig. 10.10), but it can also be performed for a uterine prolapse. The procedure requires the surgeon to suture the top of the vaginal vault, or uterus (hysteropexy), to the sacrospinous ligament, a ligament that runs from the base of the sacrum to the ischial spine in the lower back/buttocks (Fig. 10.11).

Vaginal Implant Repairs

Colporrhaphy procedures can be supported with the use of an implant. These were thought to add to the strength of the repair and potentially decrease recurrence. Implants can be biological (e.g., porcine dermis) or synthetic (e.g., polypropylene mesh similar to

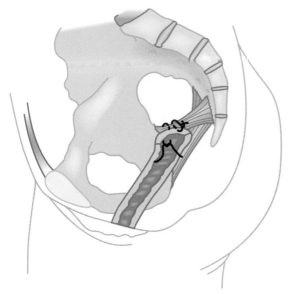

Fig. 10.11 Sacrospinous ligament fixation (for post-hysterectomy vault prolapse).

those used in abdominal hernia repairs), absorbable or non-absorbable.

Implants and synthetic meshes in particular have been associated with an increased risk of complications (e.g., vaginal exposure, organ perforation and chronic pain), however, without much proven benefit. Therefore, they are currently not recommended for use in vaginal prolapse surgery.

Sacrocolpopexy (Sacrohysteropexy)

This operation for prolapse is done abdominally, either open via an incision or laparoscopically. It is performed for apical or multicompartment prolapse involving the vaginal apex (vault or uterus) and has a higher success rate with lower recurrence rates than vaginal apical procedures.

Sacrocolpopexy involves suturing the vaginal vault to the body of the sacrum indirectly by using a poly-propylene mesh interposed between the two structures. If the uterus is still in place, a hysterectomy may be required first to be able to attach the mesh

to the anterior vagina. In women wishing to conserve their uterus (e.g., preference, family not complete) the mesh can be wrapped around the cervix instead. This is called a 'sacrohysteropexy'.

While concerns have been raised about the use of these mesh implants and their potential complications, guidelines in the United Kingdom recommend that this procedure is one of the choices that should be offered to women for correction of an apical prolapse. However, it is advised that outcomes and complications resulting from this type of operation should be closely scrutinized.

Key Points

- **POP is the descent of the pelvic organs (urethra, bladder, uterus and bowel) into the vagina.**
- **The biggest risk factor is childbirth. Other contributing factors include obesity, menopause, gynaecological surgery, age and conditions that increase intra-abdominal pressure.**
- **Prolapse can be the following: anterior compartment (urethrocele or cystocele – urethra or bladder prolapse, respectively); apical (uterus or vaginal vault post-hysterectomy); or posterior (rectocele and enterocele – prolapse of the rectum or small bowel, respectively). Prolapse is rarely found in isolation and most women have a combination of the above.**
- **Women with prolapse tend to present with a 'something coming down' discomfort, but may also have urinary or bowel symptoms.**
- **Asymptomatic prolapse does not need to be treated.**
- **Treatment should first be conservative (i.e., pessaries, pelvic floor exercises) before resorting to surgical repair.**
- **Surgical options can be either vaginal or abdominal and may often need to be combined.**

Chapter 11

Urinary Incontinence

Veenu Tyagi

Chapter Outline

Introduction

Urinary incontinence (UI) is defined as any involuntary loss of urine, which is a social or hygienic problem. UI is common – it is reported by 46% of women attending primary care clinics in the United Kingdom but is often underdiagnosed and undertreated. The incidence of UI increases with age. Overactive bladder (OAB) symptoms are present in up to half of elderly women in care homes. UI is a major quality of life (QOL) issue because it causes distress and can have negative physical and psychological impacts.

Types of Urinary Incontinence

The most common types of UI in women are:
- Stress urinary incontinence (SUI)
- Overactive bladder (OAB)
- Mixed incontinence (SUI and OAB)
- Urinary retention with overflow
- Genitourinary fistula

SUI is the most common cause of UI, accounting for 40% of cases. It is defined as involuntary leakage of urine on effort or physical exertion, including sporting activities, or on sneezing or coughing, in the absence of any detrusor contraction. 'Activity-related incontinence' might be the preferred term in some languages to avoid confusion with psychological stress.

OAB accounts for about 30% of cases of UI in women. Women complain of a sudden, compelling desire to pass urine which is difficult to postpone (urgency). This is usually associated with daytime urinary frequency (more than previously deemed normal for the woman). As the problem tends to be both day and night, however, women can have nocturia (interruption of sleep one or more times because of need to micturate) and, in severe cases, enuresis (bed wetting). Urge urinary incontinence (UUI) is a severe form of OAB.

In **mixed urinary incontinence (MUI)**, women experience incontinence associated with both urgency and physical exertion. This accounts for around 30% of cases.

Urinary retention with overflow is common in elderly women with an underactive bladder or in those with certain neurological problems. The bladder fills, the woman no longer has a sensation to pass urine, and urine leaks once the bladder reaches maximum capacity and no further filling is possible.

A **fistula** is an abnormal communication between two epithelial surfaces. Any such communication between the lower urinary tract (ureter, bladder or urethra) and the genital tract (uterus or vagina) will result in continuous dribbling UI. When it occurs, it is usually a complication of surgery. Fistulae can also occur following obstructed labour, particularly when there is a prolonged delay until birth occurs. Rates of obstetric fistula are low in countries where women have prompt access to maternity care, including safe caesarean section. Fistula accounts for only 1 in 1000 cases of incontinence in women in the United Kingdom.

The Mechanism of Urinary Continence

Urinary continence is maintained at the bladder neck.
1. **Proximal urethral sphincter mechanism** is present in the region of the bladder neck: the proximal urethra is a water-tight seal, which maintains the pressure in the urethra at greater levels than the pressure in the bladder. The

anatomical basis of that seal is considered to be a series of arteriovenous anastomoses within the wall of the proximal urethra. They allow some degree of turgor pressure to be exerted circumferentially around the urethra, which results in keeping the urethra occluded.

2. **Distal urethral sphincter mechanism.** The distal urethra is surrounded by striated muscle within the wall of the urethra and is innervated by sacral nerve roots S2–4 via the pudendal nerve.

3. **Supporting tissues around the urethra** include the pubourethral ligaments, derived from the fascia of the pelvic floor and, to a lesser degree, the pelvic floor musculature – namely, the levator ani muscle. They maintain the proximal urethra in an intra-abdominal position. Any rise in intra-abdominal pressure is transmitted equally to the bladder and the proximal urethra. The pressure difference between urethra and bladder will not change; therefore, continence will be maintained. Weakness or damage to the supporting tissues can make the urethra hypermobile, and any rise in intra-abdominal pressure makes it move below the pelvic floor leading to unequal distribution of pressure, which may predispose to SUI (Fig. 11.1).

Bladder stability refers to the concept that the bladder muscle (detrusor) should relax during bladder filling and contract during micturition. This involves a complex interaction between the anatomical parts of the urinary tract and the nervous system. Women with OAB have involuntary detrusor contraction. If the contraction is modest, then the woman will feel the contraction as urinary urgency. If the contraction is strong enough to elevate the pressure in the bladder above that in the urethra, then there will be associated leakage in addition (UUI).

Aetiology of Incontinence
STRESS URINARY INCONTINENCE

SUI requires some degree of weakness of one or both of the proximal and distal urethral sphincter mechanisms or supporting tissues around the urethra. While

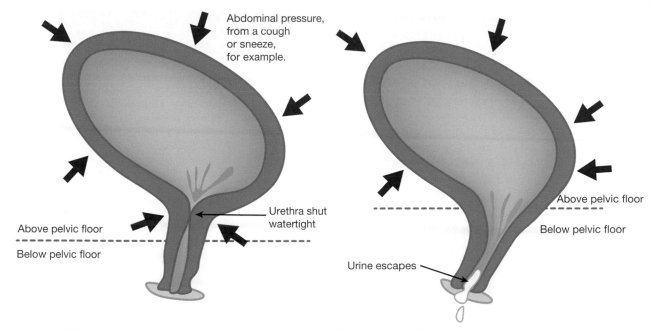

Abdominal pressure, from a cough or sneeze, for example.

Urethra shut watertight

Above pelvic floor

Below pelvic floor

Above pelvic floor

Below pelvic floor

Urine escapes

1) Normal
The bladder neck is well supported and the muscle sphincter squeezed tight shut. A rise in abdominal pressure acts evenly on squeezing the bladder and sealing the urethra – no leakage of urine

2) Stress incontinence
The bladder neck has fallen and the muscle sphincter is strained. So a rise in abdominal pressure acts more by squeezing the bladder than sealing the urethra – urine escapes

Fig. 11.1 Aetiology of stress urinary incontinence.

no single aetiological factor exists in all women with SUI, there are a series of predisposing factors that often explain the condition. These include:

- Pregnancy
- Pelvic organ prolapse
- Menopause
- Collagen disorder
- Obesity

Pregnancy

SUI is more common in women who have had previous pregnancies. The risk seems to be present regardless of how the baby is born, as the additional abdominal pressure from the gravid uterus and the smooth muscle relaxation caused by progesterone seem to have an effect. There is more risk of subsequently developing SUI when a baby has been born vaginally, either due to muscle injury to the pelvic floor or some loss of pudendal nerve function.

Prolapse

Prolapse and SUI co-exist in over 50% of cases. While these conditions are often concurrent and have overlapping predisposing factors, the prolapse may be mild or asymptomatic. Prolapse can worsen SUI in some cases, as the anatomical change can compromise continence mechanisms further.

Menopause

Many women date the onset of their symptoms from menopause. There is evidence that lack of estrogen weakens the urethral sphincter complex and reduces maximal urethral closure pressure (intrinsic sphincter deficiency), leading to SUI. The effect of this pressure reduction in the urethra is that a smaller rise in intra-abdominal pressure can result in SUI.

Collagen Disorder

Collagen is a major component of the pubourethral ligaments. There is evidence that there are different types of collagen in the pubourethral ligaments of women who have incontinence compared with those who do not.

OVERACTIVE BLADDER

In most women, the aetiology of an OAB is unknown (idiopathic). Neurological conditions – typically, multiple sclerosis, stroke or spinal cord injury – are known to be a cause of OAB. There is a link between psychological diagnoses and OAB, with a higher incidence of anxiety in women with this condition.

VOIDING DIFFICULTY

Voiding difficulties in women are mainly due to an underactive detrusor (hypotonia in 90% of cases) and, less commonly (10%), due to anatomical obstruction (due to previous surgery or increased urethral sphincter activity). The aetiology of the detrusor hypotonia is either due to ageing, with the natural reduction in muscle fibres and muscle strength, or pregnancy and childbirth, due to nerve damage (pudendal neuropathy). There is some evidence that women who postpone voiding despite the urge to do so and void infrequently are more prone to this problem. Women with neurological disease may have voiding difficulty due to either detrusor hypotonia or obstruction – in the latter case, secondary to inappropriate contraction of the urethral sphincter or incoordination (dyssynergia) between bladder and urethral sphincter complex.

Clinical Presentation

This will depend on the underlying cause for UI. Women may complain of symptoms related to OAB – for example, frequency, urgency, nocturia with or without associated UUI and enuresis, or UI associated with physical activity or constant leakage. It is important to enquire about voiding symptoms, for example, hesitancy, straining to void, poor or intermittent urinary stream and post-micturition symptoms, such as sensation of incomplete emptying and post-micturition dribbling. Accompanying 'red flag' symptoms, such as haematuria, persistent bladder or urethral pain, or recurrent urinary tract infection (UTI), warrant urological assessment of the lower and upper urinary tracts to exclude malignancy or other serious pathology.

TABLE 11.1	Effect of Urinary Incontinence Upon Quality of Life
Emotions	Feelings of stigma and humiliation. Social and recreational withdrawal. Fear and anxiety related to being incontinent in public.
Relationships	Reduced intimacy, affection and physical proximity. Relationship breakdown.
Employment	Absence from work. Loss of concentration. Interruption of work for toilet breaks.
Sleep	Nocturia is common and quality and amount of sleep is affected. Tiredness the next day. Risk of falls, especially in the elderly.
Exercise and sport	A barrier to exercise.
Travel	Reluctance to travel for work or leisure.

Nearly half of women with SUI have co-existing pelvic organ prolapse. Therefore, an enquiry about symptoms and impact on QOL is essential. Bowel dysfunction can be associated with UI and must be explored.

UI is a major QOL issue that can prevent a woman from socializing and restrict her physical activities (Table 11.1). Severe UI can have a significant psychological impact, leading to depression, loss of self-esteem and anxiety. It can also have a significant negative impact upon a woman's sex life; incontinence during intercourse can lead to avoidance of sexual activity. Nocturia can affect concentration and work performance. Nocturia in the elderly also carries the risk of falls, with a fractured neck of the femur a common outcome. It should be noted that in the elderly, UI is the second most common reason for a person being unable to return to independent living.

Clinical Assessment

CLINICAL EXAMINATION

All women should undergo an abdominal and pelvic examination. Abdominal examination may reveal a palpable bladder, suggesting urinary retention, and, infrequently, an otherwise unsuspected pelvic mass as the cause for the symptoms. Pelvic examination may reveal pelvic organ prolapse or vaginal atrophy. Useful observations during your assessment include:

- **SUI (clinical stress leakage):** Observation of involuntary urine leakage from the urethra synchronous with straining or coughing with no associated urgency.
- **Extra-urethral incontinence:** Observation of urine leakage through channels other than the urethral meatus – for example, a fistula or ectopic ureter (a congenital abnormality in which the ureter is joined to a site other than the trigone of the bladder).
- **Focused neurological examination,** if appropriate. This may include assessment of cognitive function, ambulation and mobility, hand function and lumbar and sacral spinal segment function.
- **Rectal examination:** If symptoms of anal incontinence are present, the anal sphincter tone should be determined by digital examination, with low or absent tone suggestive of abnormal pelvic innervation.

INVESTIGATIONS

Urinalysis

Every woman presenting with lower urinary tract symptoms should have a urinalysis performed. The presence of leucocytes and nitrites suggests a UTI, which may be causing or worsening the woman's symptoms. If the woman is symptomatic of a UTI, treatment with a broad-spectrum antibiotic is started and a midstream specimen of urine sent. Recurrent UTIs and/or presence of persistent haematuria should prompt cystoscopy and ultrasound of the upper renal tracts. The presence of glycosuria may suggest diabetes, which can predispose to recurrent UTIs and urinary frequency.

Frequency-Volume Chart (Bladder Diary)

Bladder diaries should be used in the initial assessment. Women should be encouraged to complete a minimum of 3 days of the diary, covering variations in their usual activities, such as both working and leisure days. The amount, type and timing of fluid intake should be recorded along with the timing and amount of voiding and episodes of UI. It is a simple, non-invasive way to assess urinary frequency, urgency, diurnal and nocturnal cycles, functional bladder capacity and total urine output. Fluid intake and pad changes can give an indication of the severity of wetness. This may also be used for monitoring the effects of treatment and act as feedback. Table 11.2 shows an example from four women.

- Woman A has normal frequency but is incontinent when not needing the toilet. This is likely to represent SUI.
- Woman B has a normal bladder capacity (400 mL) but is emptying her bladder with as little as 50 mL in it, which is typical of an OAB. In addition, she has leaked urine before going to the toilet – further evidence of OAB.

TABLE 11.2 Frequency-Volume Chart (Bladder Diary)								
	Woman A		Woman B		Woman C		Woman D	
Time	Intake	Urine	Intake	Urine	Intake	Urine	Intake	Urine
0800	250	500	50	400*	500	450	200	100
1000	200	*	300	200*	500	400		150
1200		300	400	50*	500	350	150	100
1400	300			50*	500	400	400	150
1600		200	200		500	500		150
1800	450			250	500	350	250	100
2000		350		75*	500	400	200	150
2200	500	*	250			400		150
0000				200				150
0200				100				100
0400		250		50				150
Total	1700	1600	1200	1375	3500	3250	1200	1450

*Intake and Urine volumes in ml. * indicates an episode of incontinence*

- Woman C is drinking large volumes, which is giving her urinary frequency and high urinary output.
- Woman D has a small-capacity bladder, which may be as a result of chronic bladder inflammation.

Cystoscopy

This is not required in the initial investigation of UI. Cystoscopy is indicated if women have haematuria or recurrent UTIs or refractory OAB with previous vaginal mesh surgery.

Ultrasound Measurement of Post-Void Residual (Bladder Scan)

This is a non-invasive test that should be performed if incomplete emptying, voiding dysfunction or recurrent UTIs are suspected to check for post-void residual volume.

Pelvic ultrasound (to assess the pelvic organs) has a limited role in evaluation of women with UI other than if pelvic masses are suspected.

Quality-of-Life Questionnaires

There are several disease-specific validated QOL questionnaires for subjective assessment of lower urinary tract symptoms in women, including sexual dysfunction. This should be a part of the assessment of every woman both before and after treatment, along with an impression of what she expects from treatment. Shared goals with shared decision-making will improve satisfaction.

Urodynamic Studies

These tests are a dynamic assessment of the lower urinary tract that offer objective information about bladder and urethral function. However, they are invasive, time-consuming and expensive, and some women find them embarrassing. Furthermore, they are not certain to always provide a confident diagnosis. The indications for urodynamic studies are listed in Box 11.1.

BOX 11.1 INDICATIONS FOR URODYNAMIC STUDIES

Women wishing surgery for stress urinary incontinence who have any of the following:
1. Symptoms of predominant overactive bladder or urinary incontinence in which the type is unclear
2. Symptoms suggestive of voiding dysfunction
3. Anterior or apical compartment prolapse
4. Previous surgery for stress urinary incontinence

Care of Women With Urinary Incontinence

Initial assessment is aimed at identifying 'red flag' symptoms that warrant further investigations and trying to categorise predominant symptoms – for example, SUI predominant (Table 11.3). If a woman is thought to have MUI, treatment should be directed towards the predominant symptom.

Ongoing care depends on the type of incontinence and should start with conservative treatment, which usually includes two distinct approaches: lifestyle interventions and bladder retraining by a continence advisor or clinical nurse specialist.

Conservative

LIFESTYLE INTERVENTIONS

Lifestyle changes are an essential component which forms the foundation of all other treatments. These are outlined in Box 11.2.

TABLE 11.3 Difference in Women's Symptoms With OAB, SUI and MUI

Symptoms	OAB	SUI	MUI
Urgency (strong, sudden desire to void)	Yes	No	Yes
Frequency with urgency (>8 times/24 h)	Yes	No	Yes
Leaking during physical activity, e.g., coughing, sneezing, lifting, etc.	No	Yes	Yes
Amount of urinary leakage with each episode of incontinence	Large	Small	Variable
Ability to reach the toilet in time following urge to void	Often no	Yes	Variable
Waking to pass urine at night	Usually	Seldom	Variable

MUI, Mixed urinary incontinence; *OAB,* overactive bladder; *SUI,* stress urinary incontinence.

BOX 11.2 LIFESTYLE INTERVENTIONS

- Aim for fluid intake of around 1.5 L/day. Excessive fluid intake may worsen frequency and incontinence; some women with overactive bladder over-restrict the amount of fluid they drink, increasing the risk of bladder irritation.
- Restrict alcohol and caffeine. These drinks should constitute no more than a third of the total daily fluid intake.
- Aim for a body mass index under 30.
- Stop smoking.
- Avoid carbonated drinks.
- Treat chronic constipation and chronic cough.

BLADDER RETRAINING

This involves analysis and alteration of the woman's behaviour and her environment to alter a maladaptive voiding pattern, and should be offered for a minimum of 6 weeks. The objective is to re-establish voluntary control over voiding. The woman's bladder diary is reviewed and based on this; the time interval between voids is gradually increased to achieve a less problematic micturition pattern.

PHYSIOTHERAPY

Supervised pelvic floor muscle training by a physiotherapist for at least 3 months is the first-line treatment for women with SUI and MUI. Treatment involves muscle training using pelvic floor exercises (Kegel exercises), which are repetitive voluntary contractions and relaxations of the pelvic floor muscles. The aim is to increase the strength of the voluntary pelvic floor muscle contraction and teach voluntary contraction of the muscles before increases in abdominal pressure (counter brace). Guidance in the United Kingdom advises against the use of perineometry or pelvic floor electromyography for biofeedback as a routine part of pelvic floor muscle training.

Cones can be inserted vaginally for short periods to produce contractions to retain them. Women exercise daily with increasing weights, retaining the cone for 10 to 20 minutes each time. There is no evidence that biofeedback or the use of vaginal cones is better than supervised pelvic floor exercises. However, in women who cannot actively contract their pelvic floor muscles, they may aid motivation to continue with the exercises and with treatment.

DRUG THERAPY

Overactive Bladder

There are several pharmacological treatments for UI, and antimuscarinic (also known as anticholinergic) medication remains the mainstay of medical treatment for OAB. There are several preparations available with comparable effectiveness but they vary in their dosage, frequency, side effects, tolerability and cost. Some of the available anticholinergics include oxybutynin, solifenacin and tolterodine. When offering anticholinergic medicines for OAB, clinicians should take into account other medicines that could affect the woman's total 'anticholinergic load', as there is a risk of worsening cognitive impairment.

Antimuscarinic medications reduce bladder contractility by competitively inhibiting postganglionic acetylcholine receptors (M2, M3), meaning that the problematic bladder contractions which occur with OAB are reduced. Antimuscarinics have their effect during bladder filling. They are effective in about 50% of women who will have up to 50% improvement. The main side effects include dry mouth, dizziness, nausea and constipation. While the presence of dry mouth and constipation may indicate that the medicine is starting to have an effect, these effects may result in the woman discontinuing treatment. Medications need to be tried for at least 4 weeks before any substantial benefit is seen, and further improvement in symptoms may occur over time. If treatment is not effective or not well tolerated, then either the dose can be changed, an alternative antimuscarinic drug can be offered or a drug can be administered by a different route (e.g. transdermally).

Mirabegron is a beta-3 adrenoreceptor agonist that works by actively relaxing the bladder, helping the bladder to fill and store more urine. It is indicated in women in whom antimuscarinics are contraindicated, have been ineffective or have unacceptable side effects.

Stress Urinary Incontinence

Medical therapy for SUI comprises vaginal topical estrogen and duloxetine. Vaginal estrogen can be offered to all women with UI who have signs of vaginal atrophy even if they are on systemic hormone replacement therapy.

Duloxetine is a combined serotonin and noradrenaline reuptake inhibitor licensed for use in moderate to severe SUI. It is recommended that duloxetine is offered to women only if they prefer pharmacological over surgical treatment or are not suitable for surgical treatment. Blockade of serotonin and noradrenaline reuptake in the spinal cord stimulates pudendal motor neurons, increasing stimulation of urethral striated muscles in the sphincter and enhancing contraction. Duloxetine improves SUI by increasing urethral closure pressure and electrical activity of the sphincter. Adverse effects are related to increases in noradrenaline and serotonin and include gastrointestinal disturbances, dry mouth, headache and – very rarely – suicidal ideation.

SURGERY

Surgical treatment of SUI and OAB are very different, and treating one does not usually improve the other. OAB infrequently requires major surgery, which has significant risk of complications. Hence, surgery solely for OAB is rarely performed.

Surgery for SUI

There are various surgical procedures for SUI. When surgery is indicated, women should be provided with appropriate information to make an informed choice between all options (including mesh surgeries). The use of patient decision aids may be helpful.

Discussion with the woman considering surgery for SUI should include:

- The benefits and risks of all surgical options
- The uncertainties about the long-term adverse effects for all procedures, particularly those involving the implantation of mesh materials
- Differences between procedures in the type of anaesthesia, expected length of hospital stay, surgical incisions and expected recovery period
- Any social or psychological factors that may affect the woman's decision

The following procedures, discussed next, are offered in the United Kingdom at the time of writing:

1. Retropubic mid-urethral mesh sling
2. Autologous rectus fascial sling
3. Colposuspension
4. Urethral bulking agents

Mid-Urethral Sling (MUS)

This involves the placement of a strip of non-absorbable tape (sometimes referred to as a mesh;

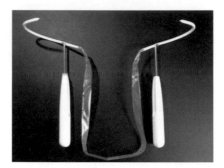

Fig. 11.2 Polypropylene mesh (tape).

Fig. 11.2) from the vagina at mid-urethral level through either the retropubic or obturator space, with entry or exit points at the lower abdomen or groin, respectively. The tape is an artificial, non-absorbable, synthetic material made of type 1 polypropylene. The tape is placed under the mid-urethra (between the urethra and vagina) without tension, being held in place by its serrated edges in the surrounding tissue. Although the tape is effective immediately after insertion, it can take several weeks before it is invaded by fibroblasts which reinforce and fix the tape in place. This forms a hammock which then prevents urethral hypermobility with an increase in abdominal pressure, thus preventing leakage.

The success with tape procedures for SUI is 85% to 90%. Complications differ for different types of tape (Table 11.4). Public concern was raised about uncommon but severe complications related to use

TABLE 11.4	Complications With MUS
Failure to cure SUI	10%–15% (short term)
New OAB	5%–15%
Voiding difficulty	5%–10% short term (higher with TVT)
	1%–3% long term
Urinary infection	10%
Mesh exposure in the vagina	2%–4%
Thigh pain	5%–10% (higher with TOT)
Operative blood loss	Higher with retropubic tapes
Bladder injury	5%–8% (highest with retropubic tapes)
Urethral trauma	1%

MUI, Mixed urinary incontinence; *MUS,* mid-urethral sling; *OAB,* overactive bladder; *SUI,* stress urinary incontinence; *TOT,* transobturator tape; *TVT,* tension-free vaginal tape.

of tapes and mesh for SUI and vaginal pelvic organ prolapse surgery. In 2018, the UK Government temporarily halted the use of transvaginal mesh surgery altogether in the management of both pelvic organ prolapse and SUI. These restrictions have since been lifted, and new processes are in place to ensure that this type of surgery is used only after additional measures regarding assessment of suitability and fully informed consent.

There are three types of procedure for SUI which use tape:

a) *Retropubic tape (tension-free vaginal tape TVT).* This was the first tape to be developed and used clinically. It was introduced to UK practice in 1998. The tape is inserted vaginally, bypasses the bladder neck and bladder in the retropubic space, and exits suprapubically (Fig. 11.3).

b) *Transobturator tape (TVTO or TOT).* This procedure was first described in 2002. Here, after the same insertion point in the vagina, the tape is passed through the obturator membrane on either side and laterally towards the adipose tissue of the thigh (Fig. 11.4). TOT has the advantage over TVT of less risk of damage to the abdominal organs and urinary retention but has significantly higher incidence of thigh

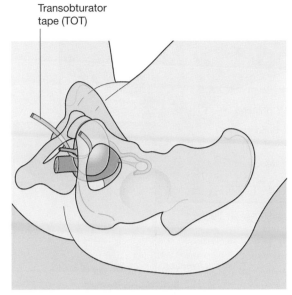

Fig. 11.4 Transobturator tape.

pain (see Table 11.4). It is recommended that a transobturator approach is avoided unless there are specific clinical circumstances in which the retropubic approach should be avoided, such as previous pelvic surgery and scarring.

c) *Single incision tapes – 'mini tapes'.* The first 'mini tape' was introduced with the proposed benefit of less likelihood of damage to vessels, nerves and pelvic organs, as there was no need to tunnel the tape through the retropubic space or obturator membrane. The tape is inserted through a similar vaginal incision but then anchored into the woman's tissues without exiting through the skin.

Rectus fascial sling. Sling procedures can be performed using either autologous (meaning from the same person), allograft or xenograft material. Autologous rectus fascial slings are currently the only biological material in SUI surgery that is recommended for use in the United Kingdom. To make the sling, a strip of rectus fascia is excised from the abdominal wall and is placed in a similar fashion as a retropubic MUS. The same hammock-shaped support is formed, causing urethral closure when the sling is stretched with increasing intra-abdominal pressure. This reduces many of the complications associated with mesh, because there is no synthetic material involved.

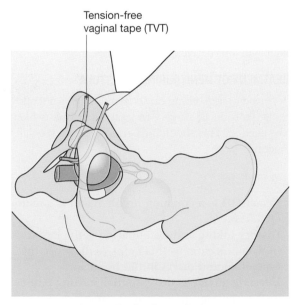

Fig. 11.3 Tension-free vaginal tape.

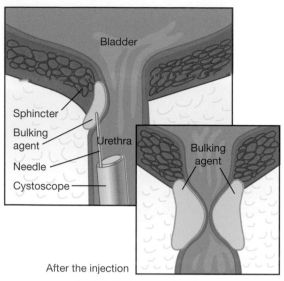

Bladder

Sphincter

Bulking
agent

Needle

Cystoscope

Urethra

Bulking
agent

After the injection

Fig. 11.5 Bladder neck injection.

Colposuspension. This is an operation in which the bladder neck and proximal urethra are elevated by suturing the paravaginal fascia at the level of the bladder neck to the iliopectineal ligament (Cooper ligament). The success rate is similar to MUS (85%–90%) and, even when performed laparoscopically rather than at open surgery, it has higher short-term morbidity with a longer hospital stay and longer recovery, higher rates of voiding difficulties (10%–15%), detrusor overactivity, and posterior vaginal wall prolapse. This procedure was commonly performed for SUI before the MUS was introduced. However, with the recent controversies regarding the use of tapes for surgery for SUI, more women are now opting to have this procedure.

Intramural bulking agents. The procedure involves injecting bulking agents composed of synthetic materials, bovine collagen or autologous substances to augment the urethral wall at the level of proximal or mid-urethra. This achieves better function of the urethral mucosa to increase urethral pressure (Fig. 11.5). This is a minimally invasive procedure and can be performed under local anaesthesia as a day case procedure. These are less effective than the other definitive procedures (66% success) and provide temporary improvement in the symptoms. Hence, injections need to be repeated after a few months. They are a good treatment choice for young

women who have not completed their family, women not keen for definitive surgery, or older women with comorbidities for whom anaesthesia required for a more invasive procedure would carry additional risk.

Invasive Treatment for an Overactive Bladder

If medical treatment fails (refractory OAB), then the woman can be offered either intravesical botulinum toxin type A (Botox) injections or sacral nerve root stimulation. These are specialized procedures performed by a urologist or a specialist urogynaecologist. The botulinum toxin injections, performed during cystoscopy, temporarily paralyse the detrusor muscle, which allows for an increase in bladder capacity alongside reduced OAB symptoms. A sacral nerve stimulator is an implanted electronic device, connected by wire to the sacral nerve, in order to override the sensation of the urge to urinate.

Rarely, women with OAB with a small-capacity or neurogenic bladder may require extensive urological surgery, such as urinary diversion, detrusor myomectomy or augmentation cystoplasty.

TREATMENT OF VOIDING DISORDERS

The treatment of voiding difficulty due to underactive detrusor is clean intermittent self-catheterization (CISC). Women with botox treatment for OAB can sometimes be affected by this and be prepared to perform CISC. An indwelling catheter (urethral or suprapubic) in women who are unable to perform CISC may be an alternative.

TREATMENT OF GENITOURINARY FISTULA

If a period of indwelling catheterization does not allow the fistula to heal, surgery to treat the fistula is likely to be needed. This should be performed by a specialist surgeon.

Key Points

- **Female UI is a common problem and is a major QOL issue.**
- **History taking and examination is the key step in women's care, as this helps to diagnose the type of UI and direct initial treatment.**
- **Lifestyle advice is the essential starting point in the treatments for incontinence.**

Chapter 12

Ovarian Neoplasms

Claire Thompson

Chapter Outline

Introduction

Ovarian neoplasms, or tumours, encompass a wide range of conditions: benign, malignant and indeterminate lesions, known as borderline. Pathologically, these are distinct, as shown in Fig. 12.1. They pose challenges for both early detection and correct diagnosis.

Ovarian cancer is the second most common gynaecological malignancy in high-income countries (endometrial cancer being the most common). There are many histological subtypes of ovarian cancer; epithelial ovarian cancer (EOC) represents 90% of cases. In the United Kingdom, there are approximately 7400 cases diagnosed each year, and approximately 4300 women die from the disease annually. The continuing challenge with ovarian cancer is that 70% of women present at an advanced stage of disease (Stage III or IV). Consequently, the overall 5-year survival remains around 40% despite many advances in treatment. EOC is the leading cause of death from gynaecological cancer in the United Kingdom. The most common and most lethal subtype of EOC is high-grade serous carcinoma (HGSC).

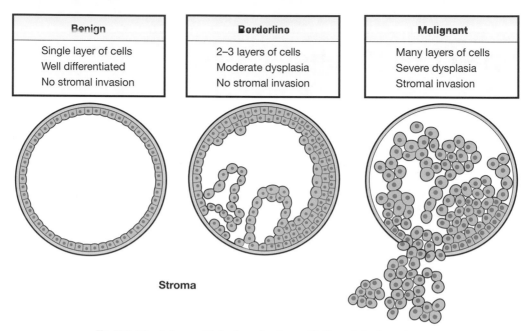

Benign	Borderline	Malignant
Single layer of cells	2–3 layers of cells	Many layers of cells
Well differentiated	Moderate dysplasia	Severe dysplasia
No stromal invasion	No stromal invasion	Stromal invasion

Stroma

Fig. 12.1 Morphology and behaviour of surface epithelium–derived neoplasms.

Risk Factors

Ovarian cancer is predominantly a disease of older, postmenopausal women with the majority (>80%) of cases being diagnosed in women over 50 years. The lifetime risk of developing ovarian cancer is 1 in 54 and there are a number of risk factors identified associated with its development. A woman's reproductive history appears to contribute to her lifetime risk – women who have had pregnancies have a lower risk than those with no pregnancies. Early menarche, late menopause and obesity also seem to contribute to a greater risk of ovarian cancer. Family history plays a very important role in the development of ovarian cancer – direct genetic risk is discussed on page 141.

Conversely, the use of the oral contraceptive pill, tubal ligation, breastfeeding and suppression of ovulation appear to offer protection against ovarian cancer. These factors support the theory that a higher number of ovulations correlate with the risk of developing ovarian cancer. However, our knowledge of how EOC develops has advanced significantly and it is now considered that some of these cancers arise not from the ovary itself but from the fallopian tube.

Natural History

There are 3 broad categories of ovarian tumour based on their cell of origin: epithelial, sex cord/stromal and germ cell. These are divided into different histological subtypes, as shown in Fig. 12.2.

EOCs were believed to only arise from the surface epithelium of the ovary and include the subtypes of serous (high and low grade), endometrioid, clear cell and mucinous. However, recently it has been discovered that the majority of ovarian and peritoneal HGSC tumours may originate not from the ovary but from the fimbria of the fallopian tube via the development of a serous tubal intraepithelial carcinoma (STIC) lesion. The STIC lesion forms and sheds onto the ovary surface and progresses to form HGSC (Fig. 12.3). This method of development is particularly relevant for women who carry a *BRCA* gene mutation and has led to the development of risk reduction strategies in which *BRCA* mutation carriers are offered prophylactic bilateral salpingo-ophorectomy (BSO). The theory that some of these cancers arise other than from the ovary itself is also supported by the fact that ovarian-like tumours can arise in the peritoneum of women who have previously

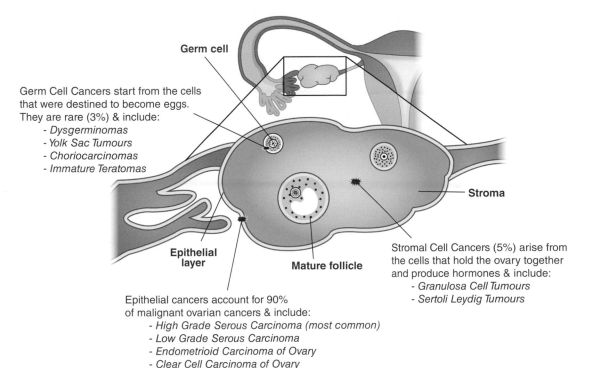

Germ cell

Germ Cell Cancers start from the cells that were destined to become eggs. They are rare (3%) & include:
- *Dysgerminomas*
- *Yolk Sac Tumours*
- *Choriocarcinomas*
- *Immature Teratomas*

Stroma

Epithelial layer

Mature follicle

Stromal Cell Cancers (5%) arise from the cells that hold the ovary together and produce hormones & include:
- *Granulosa Cell Tumours*
- *Sertoli Leydig Tumours*

Epithelial cancers account for 90% of malignant ovarian cancers & include:
- *High Grade Serous Carcinoma (most common)*
- *Low Grade Serous Carcinoma*
- *Endometrioid Carcinoma of Ovary*
- *Clear Cell Carcinoma of Ovary*
- *Mucinous Carcinoma of Ovary (rare)*

Fig. 12.2 **Ovarian neoplasms principally arise from three tissue components.**

had both ovaries and fallopian tubes removed. Cancer in this case is called 'primary peritoneal cancer'.

Endometriosis is associated with the development of clear cell and endometrioid carcinomas. Borderline tumours, which have malignant potential, can evolve, as evidenced by cases of serous borderline tumours being the precursor to a proportion of low-grade serous carcinomas.

Genetics

The development of cancer (oncogenesis) results from mutations in one or more of the vast array of genes that regulate cell growth and programmed cell death. When cancer occurs as part of a hereditary cancer syndrome, the initial cancer-causing mutation is inherited through the germline and, therefore, is present in every cell of the body. Up to 10% to 15% of cases of ovarian cancer are believed to be familial. The majority of these are *BRCA1* and *BRCA2* mutations, and Lynch syndrome.

BRCA genes function as tumour suppressor genes by helping to repair DNA breaks which could

otherwise lead to cancer and the uncontrolled growth associated with tumours. However, when these genes are mutated (*BRCA* positive), it results in an inability

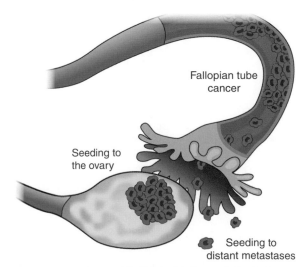

Fallopian tube cancer

Seeding to the ovary

Seeding to distant metastases

Fig. 12.3 **Source of serous tubal intraepithelial carcinoma lesions as a cause of ovarian cancer.**

to repair DNA in damaged cells and, therefore, stop cancer cells from proliferating.

Women with *BRCA* mutation positive ovarian cancer have better outcomes than women with non-hereditary ovarian cancer. Reasons for this include that they develop serous histology and have high response rates to first and second lines of platinum-based chemotherapy. Newer therapies, including poly (ADP-ribose) polymerase (PARP) inhibitors, take advantage of the fact that *BRCA* mutation carriers cannot repair deoxyribonucleic acid (DNA) effectively, as PARP inhibitors block an enzyme that makes it harder for cancer cells to repair, leading to cell death. Focused family history taking and referral to genetic clinics can lead to identification of carriers and testing of their family members. These genes are inherited in an autosomal-dominant manner.

Although there is still no effective screening method for ovarian cancer, prophylactic surgery will reduce the risk of developing cancer in these higher-risk women.

Lynch syndrome, also known as 'hereditary non-polyposis colorectal cancer' (HNPCC), predisposes to the development of several cancers – most notably, colorectal ovarian and endometrial cancer. This is a mismatch repair mutation involving a number of genes, such as *MLH1*, *MSH2*, *MSH6*, *PMS2* and *EPCAM*. The lifetime risk for the development of *BRCA* and Lynch syndrome–associated cancer in presented in Table 12.1.

Pathology

Table 12.2 summarizes the pathological classification of ovarian tumours.

TABLE 12.1   Lifetime Risk (Up to Age 70 Years) of Cancer With *BRCA* and Lynch Syndrome

BRCA

Type of Cancer	General Population	BRCA1	BRCA2
Ovarian cancer	2%	40%–60%	10%–20%
Breast cancer in women	11%	60%–85%	45%–60%

Lynch Syndrome

Type of Cancer	General Population	Lynch Syndrome	
Ovarian cancer	2%	9%–12%	
Colorectal cancer	5.5%	Up to 80%	
Gastric cancer	<1%	11%–19%	
Endometrial cancer	2.4%	30%–60%	

TABLE 12.2   Pathology of Ovarian Tumours

Type	Subtype		
Epithelial	Serous	Common	Benign or malignant
	Mucinous	Common	Benign or malignant; associated with pseudomyxoma peritonei
	Endometrioid	Uncommon	Usually malignant
	Clear cell	Uncommon	Usually malignant
	Urothelial-like (Brenner)	Uncommon	Rarely malignant
	Borderline	Common	Separate clinical entity; do not invade
Sex cord/stromal	Granulosa cell	Rare	Low grade; often secrete sex hormones
	Thecoma/fibroma	Uncommon	Rarely malignant; may secrete sex hormones; Meigs syndrome
	Sertoli/Leydig	Rare	May secrete sex hormones
Germ cell tumours	No differentiation	Rare	Dysgerminoma; may secrete hCG
	Extra-embryonic differentiation	Rare	Yolk sac tumours (endodermal sinus tumours), malignant ovarian choriocarcinoma
	Embryonic differentiation (teratoma)	Common	Mature teratomas (benign) may contain epithelium, hair, teeth and greasy white sebum; immature (malignant) are rare
Metastases		Common	Especially endometrial, gastrointestinal tract and breast

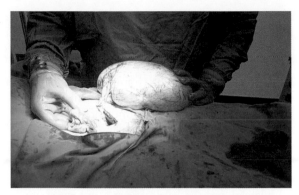

Fig. 12.4 A unilateral benign cystadenoma.

BORDERLINE TUMOURS

Borderline ovarian tumours are a distinct pathological group of neoplasms that demonstrate higher proliferative activity when compared with benign neoplasms, but which do not show stromal invasion. They are often called tumours of low malignant potential and constitute 10% to 15% of all epithelial ovarian neoplasms. They affect younger age groups and carry an excellent prognosis, with a 5-year survival of 90% across all stages. The two most common histological subtypes of borderline tumours are serous and mucinous. Extra-ovarian tumour implants are found in 20% to 40% of cases. Despite their excellent prognosis, long-term follow-up is required as late recurrences (>10 years) can occur.

EPITHELIAL TUMOURS

Serous Tumours

Serous tumours are the most common ovarian neoplasm, accounting for almost 70% of ovarian cancers. Serous cystadenocarcinomas involve both ovaries in over 50% of cases and may have both cystic and solid components. They also account for 20% of all benign ovarian tumours (serous cystadenomas), occurring primarily in women of reproductive age. Serous cystadenomas are usually unilateral, unilocular cysts, filled with serous (straw-coloured) fluid, and are of variable size (Fig. 12.4).

Mucinous Tumours

These comprise 20% of all ovarian tumours and less than 5% are malignant. Benign tumours are usually unilateral. Mucinous tumours are usually multiloculated and contain mucinous fluid of variable viscosity. They are generally the largest in size of the common epithelial tumours. Uncommonly, pseudomyxoma peritonei may also be present, which is characterised by a gelatinous tumour within the peritoneal cavity. These pose histological challenges in determining the primary origin, which may be ovarian or a primary mucinous tumour of the appendix.

Endometrioid Tumours

Endometrioid tumours are usually malignant and closely mimic endometrial cancer in histological appearance. In around 30% of cases, there is a co-existent second primary tumour of the endometrium.

Clear Cell Tumours

These are virtually all malignant and may be a variant of endometrioid tumours. They are the most frequent epithelial tumour found in association with ovarian endometriosis. It must be emphasized, that ovarian cancer developing from endometriosis is uncommon.

Urothelial-Like Tumours

Urothelial-like, or Brenner, tumours are uncommon—usually unilateral and rarely malignant. They in part comprise epithelium of urothelial type, but their main component is ovarian stroma. A rare aggressive variant is urothelial or transitional cell carcinoma.

SEX CORD/STROMAL TUMOURS

This is a group of rare neoplasms that comprise around 5% of all ovarian tumours.

Granulosa Cell Tumours

These are functional, low-grade cancers that account for around 3% to 5% of ovarian malignancies. Three-quarters secrete sex hormones, most commonly estrogen which, depending upon the age of the woman, may lead to precocious pseudopuberty, irregular menstrual bleeding or postmenopausal bleeding. They tend to recur late but can be monitored with serum inhibin B and anti-Müllerian hormone (AMH) measurements, as these are produced by granulosa cells. These tumour markers have largely replaced monitoring estradiol levels, as up to 30% of granulosa cell tumours may not produce estradiol. Characteristically, granulosa cell tumours contain cells with 'coffee bean' nuclei and 'gland-like' spaces, called 'Call–Exner bodies', which are pathognomonic of the condition.

Thecoma/Fibroma

These tumours are usually unilateral and rarely malignant. They contain cells ranging from theca cells to fibroblastic-type cells. Tumours containing the former are estrogenic, although they are less common than granulosa cell tumours. Rarely, ovarian fibromas may present with non-malignant ascites and pleural effusion, which resolve after removal of the tumour (Meigs syndrome).

Sertoli/Leydig Cell Tumours

These are rare, accounting for <1% of ovarian tumours. They occur in young women, typically in their mid-20s. They are unilateral and commonly produce male sex hormones, which can be androgenic, resulting in virilisation in nearly 85% of women. Only a few are estrogenic. They contain either Sertoli cells or Leydig cells; in the case of the latter, they may be accompanied by stroma-derived fibroblasts.

GERM CELL TUMOURS

This heterogeneous group of tumours affects mainly children and young women and comprises 20% to 25% of all ovarian tumours. Overall, around 3% are malignant. However, they represent the majority of ovarian tumours in children, in whom around one-third are malignant.

Teratoma

Teratomas are often referred to as 'dermoid cysts', are common, and are almost always benign. They characteristically contain elements from all three embryonic germ cell layers and are thought to occur via parthenogenesis, a form of reproduction in which the ovum develops without fertilization. Mature teratomas may contain epithelium, hair, teeth and greasy white sebum, and constitute 20% of all ovarian neoplasms. They are the most common in women in their 20s but account for 50% of ovarian neoplasms in females under 20 years. Malignant change, usually squamous cell, is rare (<1%) and usually occurs in postmenopausal women.

Immature teratomas are rare, characteristically occurring in children under 15 years of age. Specialised tissue derivatives from a single germ layer are found in 3% of teratomas, notably among those with predominantly thyroid tissue (struma ovarii) and carcinoid tumours.

Dysgerminoma

Dysgerminoma is the most common malignant germ cell tumour, comprising at least 50% of this group. Nevertheless, it is relatively uncommon and represents only 3% of all ovarian cancers. Some 75% occur in females aged 10 to 30 years, the median age being 22 years, and it is the most frequently encountered ovarian malignancy in pregnancy. Approximately 10% are bilateral and the level of serum human chorionic gonadotrophin (hCG) is often raised.

Endodermal Sinus or Yolk Sac Tumour

This is the second most common malignant germ cell tumour of the ovary, but comprises only 1% of all ovarian cancers. It rarely affects women over 40 years, the median age being 19 years. Presentation is commonly with a sudden onset of pelvic symptoms and a pelvic mass. Elevated serum levels of alpha-fetoprotein (AFP) are found along with normal hCG levels. Co-existent teratomas are found in 20% of cases.

Choriocarcinoma

These secrete hCG and may present with precocious pseudopuberty. They have a poor prognosis and do not respond well to chemotherapy (unlike uterine trophoblastic disease; see p. 169.

METASTATIC TUMOURS

Secondary tumours in the ovaries are relatively common. Cervical cancer only rarely metastasizes to the ovaries but spread from endometrial cancer is more frequent. Breast cancer may also metastasize to the ovaries; women presenting with single or bilateral ovarian masses should be examined carefully to exclude a breast lesion.

Cancers of the gastrointestinal tract also metastasize to the ovary and, in the case of gastric cancer, give rise to the so-called Krukenberg tumour. This contains mucin-producing 'signet ring' adenocarcinoma cells. Such tumours may elicit a stromal response in the ovary, which may cause hormone production; as a result, virilisation may be a presenting feature. In such cases, confusion with sex cord/stromal tumours may arise, although these, unlike Krukenberg tumours, are usually unilateral.

Spread

Ovarian cancer spreads trans-coelomically, whereby a tumour is 'seeded' directly within the peritoneal cavity onto the surfaces of the intraperitoneal structures and organs. Death from these tumours is usually a result of intestinal obstruction and cachexia as a consequence of widespread intraperitoneal disease. Malignant pleural effusions are encountered. Para-aortic lymph node metastases are found in up to 18% of cases where the disease appears to be confined to the ovary.

Presentation

Presence of a pelvic mass is a common clinical problem affecting women of all ages. Although many will be benign, the primary goal of clinical and diagnostic evaluation is to assess for malignancy.

Rarely, ovarian cancers are diagnosed incidentally during pelvic or abdominal palpation for another reason. In general, the symptoms are diverse and non-specific and women often do not recognise the sinister nature of these symptoms.

Symptoms associated with ovarian cancer (particularly when present for more than 1 year and/or occurring more than 12 times per month) are persistent abdominal distension, abdominal bloating, early satiety and/or loss of appetite, pelvic or abdominal pain and increased urinary urgency and/or frequency. Other symptoms may include postmenopausal bleeding, unexplained weight loss, fatigue or changes to bowel habit.

The disease may progress insidiously until abdominal distension develops due either to ascites or masses. This can evolve into gastrointestinal complications with bowel obstruction secondary to widespread intraperitoneal malignancy. UK guidance from the National Institute for Health and Care Excellence (NICE) emphasises the importance of investigating persistent, non-specific symptoms.

Investigation

Clinical examination and serum CA125 measurement should be considered in women with symptoms suggestive of ovarian cancer. If the CA125 is ≥35 IU/mL or if a pelvic mass or other abnormality is identified on examination, an ultrasound scan of the abdomen and pelvis should be undertaken. For women with a normal CA125 (<35 IU/mL), or a CA125 ≥35 IU/mL associated with a normal ultrasound, careful clinical assessment for other causes of their symptoms is required.

The risk of malignancy index (RMI) aids in the differentiation of benign from malignant lesions and may be estimated as follows: RMI = ultrasound score × menopausal score × CA125. An ultrasound score of 1 is assigned if one concerning feature is seen and a score of 3 if more than one feature is seen. These include multilocular cysts, solid areas, metastases, ascites and bilateral lesions. A score of 1 is assigned to pre-menopausal women, whereas postmenopausal women are assigned a score of 3. An RMI score of greater than 200 indicates a risk of malignancy of 70%; women with that high a score should be further investigated and treated in a gynaecological oncology centre.

Women below 40 years of age with suspected ovarian cancer serum AFP and hCG should be assayed in addition to CA125 in an effort to identify women with non-epithelial ovarian lesions. Inhibin B and AMH should be measured if a granulosa cell tumour is suspected.

If there is clinical concern regarding ovarian cancer or if the RMI is high (>200), then computed tomography (CT) of the chest, abdomen and pelvis (or magnetic resonance imaging) should be undertaken in addition to the tumour markers mentioned earlier. A CT scan of the chest is important to look for pleural effusions or chest metastases. Clinicians should keep an open mind, as a proportion of these women will have cancers other than ovarian, such as bowel or pancreatic. Until a mass has been assessed histopathologically, it is not possible to be certain of its exact nature.

In the United Kingdom, gynaecological cancer services are organised into cancer networks consisting of cancer units and cancer centres. Women with features suggestive of ovarian cancer should be referred to a centre with a gynaecological oncology multidisciplinary team (MDT) of gynaecological oncologists, medical oncologists, pathologists, radiologists and nurses. Evidence suggests that this is associated with an improved prognosis.

Tumour Markers

Around 80% of EOCs are associated with elevated levels of a tumour marker called CA125. This marker is of value in the assessment of women presenting with pelvic masses as well as in sequentially monitoring the response to treatment and to help identify pre-symptomatic relapse during follow-up. However, CA125 may also be elevated in benign conditions such as endometriosis or where peritoneal irritation has taken place, such as appendicitis or pancreatitis. It can also be elevated in cardiac failure (particularly right-sided), hepatic failure and some systemic inflammatory conditions. Therefore, a positive result of >35 U/mL, while suggestive of possible ovarian cancer, is far from diagnostic. Conversely, a negative result does not exclude a diagnosis of ovarian cancer, since 50% of Stage I (confined to the ovary) ovarian cancers will have a normal CA125. About 65% of ovarian germ cell tumours produce elevated serum levels of hCG, AFP or both. When elevated, these markers can be very useful in monitoring response to therapy and in detecting tumour recurrence.

There is no current routine screening for ovarian cancer. Large trials, including the UK Collaborative Trial of Ovarian Cancer Screening (UKCTOCS) trial, showed that CA125 and/or ultrasound were not effective in screening for ovarian cancer.

FIGO Staging

Ovarian cancer is staged according to the International Federation of Gynaecology and Obstetrics (FIGO) System. (Table 12.3).

Care of Women With Benign Tumours

Where possible, benign tumours require excision rather than drainage in order to allow full histological assessment and to prevent recurrence. This can usually be performed laparoscopically. There may often be difficulties in deciding whether a cyst is benign or malignant prior to removal. Although unilateral cysts in young women with no concerning ultrasound features tend to be benign, it is good practice to remove the cyst intact and, if achieved by laparoscopy, to place into a waterproof retrieval bag prior to drainage in order to ensure no intra-abdominal spillage. Dermoid cysts are typically solid and contain elements such as hair and teeth. Again, avoiding spillage is advised, as this can result in peritonitis due to irritation.

Surgery for Early Ovarian Cancer

The aim of surgery for early-stage ovarian cancer (Stages I and II) is complete macroscopic tumour resection and adequate surgical staging. Early-stage disease may be an unexpected postoperative histological

TABLE 12.3 **Staging of Ovarian and Fallopian Tube Cancer**
Stage I. Tumour confined to ovaries or fallopian tube(s).
1A: Tumour limited to 1 ovary (capsule intact) or fallopian tube surface.
1B: Tumour limited to both ovaries (capsules intact) or fallopian tubes; no tumour on ovarian or fallopian tube surface.
1C: Tumour limited to 1 or both ovaries or fallopian tubes, with any of the following:
Surgical spill, capsule ruptured before surgery, or malignant cells in the ascites or peritoneal washings
Stage II. Tumour involves 1 or both ovaries or fallopian tubes with pelvic extension (below pelvic brim) or primary peritoneal cancer.
IIA: Extension and/or implants on uterus and/or fallopian tubes and/or ovaries.
IIB: Extension to other pelvic intraperitoneal tissues.
Stage III. Tumour involves 1 or both ovaries or fallopian tubes, or peritoneal cancer, with cytologically or histologically confirmed spread to the peritoneum outside the pelvis and/or metastasis to the retroperitoneal lymph nodes.
IIIA: Microscopic peritoneal spread.
IIIB: Macroscopic peritoneal metastasis beyond the pelvis up to 2 cm in greatest dimension.
IIIC: Macroscopic peritoneal metastasis beyond the pelvis more than 2 cm in greatest dimension.
Stage IV. Distant metastasis.

Modified from FIGO 2018 (Int J Gynecol Obstet 2018; 143 (Suppl. 2): 59–78).

finding in cases that have been managed as a benign condition. A re-staging procedure by a gynaecological oncologist should be recommended to establish stage and whether adjuvant treatment is required.

Young women who are suitable for fertility-sparing surgery should be identified by the MDT and the risks and benefits of this approach discussed with the woman so that she can make an informed choice. The affected ovary and tube will be removed alongside peritoneal washings, omentectomy and assessment/biopsy of lymph nodes and peritoneum. The uterus and contra-lateral ovary can be retained as long as there is no visible residual malignancy.

Adequate (non-fertility-sparing) primary surgery for apparent early-stage ovarian cancer consists of peritoneal washings/ascitic sampling taken prior to manipulation of the tumour, BSO, total hysterectomy, multiple peritoneal biopsies, which can include the para-colic spaces or sub-diaphragmatic spaces, omentectomy, pelvic and para-aortic lymph node assessment.

If the tumour is suspected to be mucinous, lymph node dissection can be avoided as the rate of positive nodes is very low. However, in addition an appendicectomy should be performed.

Surgery for Advanced Ovarian Cancer

The aim of surgery in the management of advanced-stage ovarian cancer is to achieve resection of all visible disease in women fit enough to undergo this procedure, as this has been shown to be associated with an improved overall survival. This is often referred to as 'cytoreductive surgery'. Primary cytoreductive surgery followed by 6 cycles of adjuvant chemotherapy remains the preferred pathway of care, where optimal (no visible disease remaining) cytoreduction can be achieved. However, the clinical outcomes of primary surgery versus neoadjuvant chemotherapy with interval cytoreduction (surgery following 3 cycles and then further chemotherapy) has been the subject of many studies.

Neoadjuvant chemotherapy with interval cytoreductive surgery after 3 cycles of platinum-based chemotherapy is not inferior to primary surgery and adjuvant chemotherapy. Therefore, in situations in which there is uncertainty about the possibility of optimal removal of tumour (Fig. 12.5), it should be preferred; this includes cases with Stage IV disease.

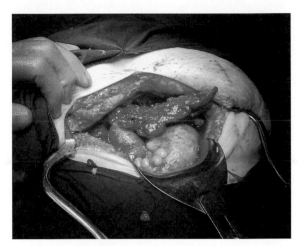

Fig. 12.5 The omentum in Stage IIIC cystadenocarcinoma is almost completely replaced with tumour, and in this case optimal debulking was not achieved.

Women with advanced disease (Stage III/IV) should have their treatment planned by a specialist MDT at a cancer centre in order to ensure the availability of experienced surgical teams who can perform all surgical procedures required, with the aim of having no residual macroscopic disease. This can often involve additional procedures such as bowel resections, splenectomy, urological procedures and removal of large amounts of the peritoneum.

Chemotherapy and Targeted Therapies

In cases of EOCs, the conventional chemotherapy agents are carboplatin and paclitaxel. Following primary surgery, the conventional approach has been to use 6 cycles of carboplatin and paclitaxel, at 3-weekly intervals. Alternative agents include topotecan, liposomal doxorubicin and gemcitabine.

In germ cell tumours the combination used most often is called BEP, and includes the chemotherapy drugs bleomycin, etoposide and cisplatin. If the cancer is a dysgerminoma, these are usually very sensitive to chemotherapy and can sometimes be treated with the less toxic combination of carboplatin and etoposide.

For EOCs, there are new developments in agents to be administered along with chemotherapy. Bevacizumab (BEV) is a monoclonal antibody that targets the vascular endothelial growth factor (VEGF) receptor. In the last decade, interest has been focused on the addition of BEV to conventional chemotherapy. Studies have demonstrated an improvement in progression-free survival, although not overall survival. Nevertheless, this is an important finding in the development of a maintenance strategy for treatment of ovarian cancer.

The latest developments are PARP inhibitors. PARP proteins are used by cells in several DNA repair processes. PARP inhibition can result in preferential death of cancer cells when another mechanism for repairing DNA is defective, such as in *BRCA* gene mutations. Three PARP inhibitors, olaparib, niraparib and rucaparib, have been approved as maintenance therapy for platinum-sensitive EOC. As evaluation of these PARP inhibitors continues, the indications for their use are broadening.

Recurrence

Unfortunately, the majority of women with advanced ovarian cancer will have recurrence of disease. Further chemotherapy will likely be considered in these cases but the use of secondary surgery is frequently an option.

The choice of chemotherapy agent will depend on the woman's response to platinum-based chemotherapy or what is called their 'platinum sensitivity status'. 'Platinum-refractory' describes women whose disease progresses during therapy or within 4 weeks after the last dose. 'Platinum-resistant' describes women whose disease progresses within 6 months, and 'partially platinum-sensitive' when there is disease progression between 6 and 12 months. Platinum-sensitive women are those with an interval of more than 12 months free of disease after treatment.

Many women will have several lines of chemotherapy over a number of years before eventually dying of their disease. As most women will eventually die of their disease progression, it is important to consider palliative care when appropriate.

Survival

The 5 year overall survival of ovarian cancer is 40%. This improvement over the last 2 decades is due to new treatments, better surgery and continuing research. Certain subtypes of ovarian cancer do have better outcomes, such as germ cell tumours, which have a 5-year overall survival of 75%. Many women may require repeated treatments over a series of years.

Key Points

- Ovarian cancer is the second most common gynaecological cancer and the most lethal. There are around 7000 newly diagnosed cases each year in the United Kingdom.
- The overall 5-year survival is about 40%, as most new cases present with advanced disease (Stage III or IV).
- Genetic factors have been identified, for example, *BRCA1* and *BRCA2* mutations of tumour suppressor genes, which identify a small proportion of women at risk.
- Presentation is usually with vague abdominal symptoms, pelvic mass and malaise.
- Treatment is primarily surgical, although advances in chemotherapy and targeted therapies—particularly with platinum-based drugs, taxanes, bevacizumab and PARP inhibitors—provide new treatment avenues.
- Research strategies are directed towards earlier diagnosis and improved chemotherapies.
- Currently available tests do not fulfil the criteria for a screening programme aimed at low-risk women.

Chapter 13

Uterine Neoplasms

Malcolm Farquharson, Kevin Burton

Chapter Outline

Introduction

The uterus consists of both the cervix and the body (or 'corpus') of the uterus. For many reasons, including their causative factors and their treatment, tumours arising from the corpus and the cervix are usually regarded as originating from two separate organs. This chapter will consider cancers arising from the uterine body; cancers arising from the cervix are discussed in Chapter 14.

The majority of malignancies arising from the uterine body arise from the endometrium. The endometrium consists of both glandular and supporting (or 'stromal') elements; it is possible for either to undergo malignant change. The majority of uterine malignancies are adenocarcinomas arising from the endometrial glands (Figs 13.1 and 13.2A). Sarcomas of the muscle of the uterus, the myometrium or the stromal tissues of the endometrium are rare (see Fig. 13.2B).

Incidence

In the United Kingdom, the incidence of endometrial cancer has been increasing. It is now the fourth most common cancer in women after breast, bowel and lung cancers. Each year, there are around 9000 cases diagnosed annually in the United Kingdom.

Approximately 90% of cases will be diagnosed after menopause whereas only around 1% of endometrial carcinomas will develop in women under the age of 40 years. The incidence is rising in high-resource settings.

Aetiology

The majority of endometrial cancers are associated with conditions in which there are prolonged, high levels of estrogen. Therefore, it is postulated that estrogen has a role in the development of the disease (Box 13.1).

High levels of estrogen may be physiological, as observed in the presence of obesity (due to the

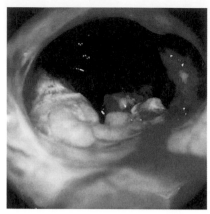

Fig. 13.1 A hysteroscopic view of an endometrial carcinoma arising from the posterior uterine wall. (© KARL STORZ - Endoskope, Germany)

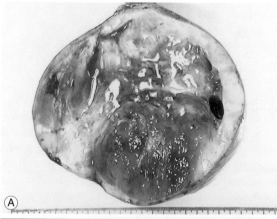

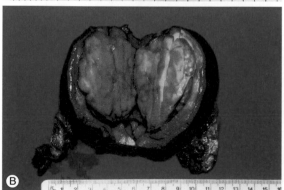

Fig. 13.2 Macroscopic picture of endometrial carcinoma (A) and endometrial sarcoma (B). (Courtesy of Dr N. Wilkinson, Department of Pathology, Leeds.)

BOX 13.1 RISK FACTORS FOR ENDOMETRIAL CARCINOMA

Increase Risk
- Obesity
- Nulliparity
- Late menopause
- Unopposed estrogen therapy, tamoxifen
- Estrogen-secreting tumours (granulosa/theca cell ovarian tumours)
- Personal history of breast or colon cancer
- Family history of breast, colon or endometrial cancer

Decrease Risk
- The combined oral contraceptive pill
- Progestogens

aromatisation in body fat of peripheral androgens to estrogens), or with conditions such as polycystic ovary syndrome (due to chronic anovulation) and late menopause. Around one-third of cases are related to obesity.

Non-physiological causes of increased estrogen include unopposed (without progesterone to protect the endometrium) estrogen hormone replacement therapy (HRT), which increases the risk four-fold. This risk is reduced to a relative risk of <1.0 with opposed HRT (i.e., with the addition of progestogen for at least 10 days per cycle). Tamoxifen, which is commonly used in the treatment of breast cancer, increases the risk of endometrial cancer. Rarely occurring estrogen-secreting tumours also increase the risk of endometrial carcinoma.

Endometrial cancer is diagnosed less frequently in women who have used the combined oral contraceptive pill, probably because it induces regular withdrawal bleeding. Women who smoke, and are thereby likely to reach an earlier menopause, also have a lower than expected incidence of the disease.

The more common estrogen-dependent type of endometrial cancer is called 'type I cancer' and is diagnosed in women around the time of menopause. It is generally diagnosed at an earlier stage and, as a result, can have a better prognosis. There may be a premalignant phase (see Endometrial Hyperplasia section, later in this chapter) and the tumour cells of type I disease usually have estrogen and progesterone receptors.

Type II endometrial cancers are not generally related to estrogen production. They are diagnosed in older women, can progress more rapidly, and are not associated with a premalignant phase. The likelihood of surviving 5 years after being diagnosed with this type of cancer are lower than for type I disease.

Endometrial cancer is inherited in 2% to 5% of cases. Lynch syndrome is caused by an autosomal-dominant inherited mutation in DNA mismatch repair genes. In addition to colorectal cancer, Lynch syndrome is associated with an increased risk of endometrial cancer (both types I and II) with a 30% to 60% lifetime risk of developing the disease.

Clinical Features and Diagnosis

CLINICAL FEATURES

Abnormal uterine bleeding is the cardinal symptom of endometrial carcinoma. The bleeding is most commonly postmenopausal. Postmenopausal bleeding is defined as spontaneous bleeding occurring more than 12 months after the final menstrual period. Around 5% of women with postmenopausal bleeding will have a primary or secondary malignancy, most commonly endometrial cancer (80%), cervical cancer, or, rarely, an ovarian tumour. As the condition can occur in premenopausal women, any irregular uterine bleeding in those over 40 years of age should also be investigated, especially if the woman is obese or has other risk factors for endometrial carcinoma.

A less common mode of presentation in postmenopausal women is that of vaginal discharge – either blood stained, watery or purulent (a pyometrium). Pain is rarely associated with early disease and usually indicates metastatic spread. Endometrial carcinoma can be detected with cancerous endometrial cells found on a cervical smear test.

The mode of spread is principally direct and will usually involve the myometrium to a greater or lesser degree. The cervix, fallopian tubes and the local supporting tissues (parametrium) can also become involved with more locally advanced cases. Lymphatic and haematogenous spread may occur.

DIAGNOSIS

There are three methods of investigation. The method chosen depends on the woman's risk factors and the local facilities. In current practice, most women will be investigated through dedicated clinics. In many cases, these clinics will be 'one stop', where all investigations are performed during a single attendance.

Ultrasound

Transvaginal scanning, often a first-line investigation, is used to measure the endometrial thickness and appearance in postmenopausal women (Fig. 13.3). If the thickness is less than 4 mm and the endometrium is smooth and regular, endometrial cancer is very unlikely. If the endometrium measures over 4 mm and the woman is not on HRT, then a hysteroscopy is recommended. A threshold of 5 mm is employed when a woman is taking HRT.

Endometrial Biopsy

An outpatient biopsy can be obtained using one of a number of samplers, for example, the Pipelle® (Fig. 13.4). This Pipelle is a thin (3 mm diameter) plastic tube with a plunger. It is passed through the cervix to obtain a sample of endometrium for histological analysis.

Hysteroscopy

The inside of the uterine cavity can be visualized directly using a hysteroscope (narrow telescope), which can be introduced with or without anaesthesia depending on the instrument, the local facilities and the woman's preference (see Fig. 13.1). Biopsy or curettage can also be performed during the same procedure. Hysteroscopy with biopsy is considered to be

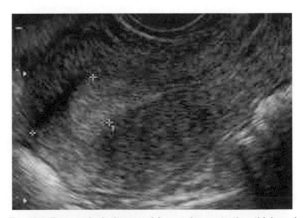

Fig. 13.3 Transvaginal ultrasound image demonstrating thickened endometrium. (Courtesy of Dr C. Hardwick, Glasgow.)

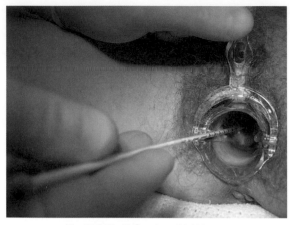

Fig. 13.4 Pipelle® endometrial biopsy.

the 'gold standard' investigation of women presenting with postmenopausal bleeding.

Pathology

Endometrial pathology can be divided into hyperplasia, carcinoma or sarcoma.

ENDOMETRIAL HYPERPLASIA

Endometrial hyperplasia is a risk factor for the development of cancer, believed to result from persistent and prolonged estrogenic stimulation of the endometrium. Hyperplasia is characterised by an increased number of endometrial cells due to proliferation, which results in a thicker endometrium. The nomenclature of this condition can be confusing: the terms 'simple hyperplasia', 'glandular hyperplasia', 'cystic glandular hyperplasia' and 'endometrial hyperplasia' are synonymous. Classification has been simplified to a binary classification on the basis of the presence or absence of cellular atypia, that is, hyperplasia without atypia, and hyperplasia with atypia. The atypia may be severe enough to create difficulty in distinguishing the hyperplastic state from a well-differentiated carcinoma.

Cytological atypia includes a loss of polarity of cells within the glands, an increase in the nuclear–cytoplasmic ratio, and nuclear irregularity with hyperchromatic changes, chromatin clumping and prominent nucleoli. This atypia is the only feature distinguishing benign endometrial lesions from those with invasive potential.

In 30% to 50% of cases of atypical hyperplasia, there is co-existing endometrial carcinoma. In the absence of endometrial carcinoma, it is believed that 10% to 20% of untreated cases of atypical hyperplasia will develop carcinoma within 10 years.

Hyperplasia is usually discovered by endometrial biopsy as part of the investigation of abnormal uterine bleeding. Hyperplasia without atypia ('simple') often occurs in anovulatory teenagers and in the perimenopausal years. It is common to treat hyperplasia with progestogens in young women. The levonorgestrel intrauterine system, which delivers progesterone to the endometrium, is often used to treat abnormal uterine bleeding in pre-menopausal women and is likely to have a protective effect in those with endometrial hyperplasia. Hysterectomy is the usual recommended treatment for those with atypical hyperplasia, or regular repeat biopsy to detect progression or regression, in those who decline hysterectomy.

ENDOMETRIAL CARCINOMA

Endometrial adenocarcinoma can have a variety of histological appearances depending upon whether it is purely glandular, has areas of squamous differentiation, or whether it demonstrates a serous or clear cell pattern. The latter two forms are associated with a poorer prognosis and are considered to be type II cancers.

ENDOMETRIAL SARCOMA

Endometrial sarcomas are rare but tend to be aggressive tumours that metastasize early and are generally associated with a poor prognosis.

GENETICS

Advances in genetics and molecular biology have improved our knowledge of cancer. The Cancer Genome Atlas Research Network (TCGA) has divided endometrial cancer into four distinct subtypes according to various genetic and epigenetic features: an ultramutator phenotype caused by DNA polymerase epsilon (POLE) mutations, a hypermutator phenotype caused by DNA mismatch repair deficiency, a copy number low phenotype and a copy number high phenotype.

POLE, the catalytic subunit of DNA polymerase, is implicated in nuclear DNA replication and repair. Women with POLE mutations have a more favourable prognosis; however, treatment based on molecular subtyping rather than clinical-pathological staging is yet to be established.

Prognostic Factors

Endometrial cancer is often – but falsely – regarded as a less aggressive tumour than other gynaecological malignancies. This is because it more commonly presents at an earlier stage (Table 13.1). Stage for stage, endometrial cancer has a prognosis similar to that of cancer of the cervix. There are many factors that affect the prognosis, the most significant being the stage of disease. This is an indication of how far the cancer has spread, as well as how aggressive the tumour is. The histological type of endometrial cancer is also important. Papillary serous cancer, which is more common in older women, spreads in a manner similar to cancer of the ovary and is associated with a poorer prognosis. Other factors that affect the prognosis are outlined in Box 13.2.

TABLE 13.1	FIGO Staging of Endometrial Carcinoma
IA	Tumour confined to the uterus, no or <½ myometrial invasion
IB	Tumour confined to the uterus, >½ myometrial invasion
II	Cervical stromal invasion, but not beyond uterus
IIIA	Tumour invades serosa or adnexa
IIIB	Vaginal and/or parametrial involvement
IIIC1	Pelvic node involvement
IIIC2	Para-aortic involvement
IVA	Tumour invasion of bladder and/or bowel mucosa
IVB	Distant metastases, including abdominal metastases and/or inguinal lymph nodes

Uterine sarcomas were staged previously as endometrial cancers, which did not reflect clinical behaviour. Therefore, a new corpus sarcoma staging system was developed based on the criteria used in other soft-tissue sarcomas. *FIGO,* International Federation of Gynecology and Obstetrics.

BOX 13.2 PROGNOSTIC FACTORS IN ENDOMETRIAL CANCER

- Histological type
- Histological differentiation
- Stage of disease
- Myometrial invasion
- Peritoneal cytology
- Lymph node metastasis
- Adnexal metastasis

Care of Women With Endometrial Carcinoma

Endometrial carcinoma is staged using the International Federation of Gynecology and Obstetrics (FIGO) scheme (see Table 13.1). This is a surgico–pathological system based on histology results from the excised uterus, tubes, ovaries and lymph nodes. Before surgery, most women will be investigated with cross-sectional imaging, usually in the form of an MRI scan. This is to determine the degree of involvement of the tissues near the tumour as well as to allow an assessment of the lymph nodes. Sometimes CT scanning is used, but MRI gives a better indication of infiltration into the myometrium (Fig. 13.5).

The mainstay of treatment is surgical, in the form of hysterectomy and bilateral salpingo-oophorectomy. This procedure is often performed laparoscopically, which reduces length of hospital stay and time to recovery. Peritoneal cytology is usually obtained, although this is not currently part of the FIGO staging. There is

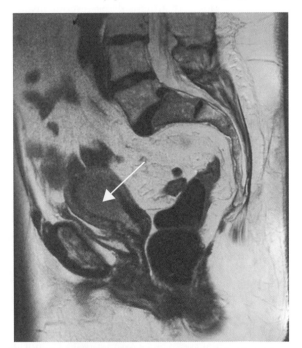

Fig. 13.5 A sagittal image through the uterus, showing the endometrial cavity distended by tumour. The tumour extends into the endocervical canal and is invasive posteriorly at the fundus. (Courtesy of Dr S. Swift, Department of Radiology, St James's Hospital, Leeds.)

debate as to whether the pelvic lymph nodes should be removed, sampled or left undisturbed. The balance is the trade-off between potential complications of lymph node removal and the additional information (positive or negative) that will be obtained. Having certainty of a negative lymph node status can reduce or limit the extent of adjuvant radiotherapy. A sentinel lymph node (the first lymph node that cancer cells are most likely to spread to) biopsy may provide a balance between achieving adequate staging whilst minimizing morbidity. More evidence is required before this procedure becomes routine practice. If, during the preoperative investigations or at the time of surgery, the disease is discovered to have spread beyond the uterus, treatment should be individualized. Treatment of disease in the fallopian tubes or ovaries is with surgery, followed by adjuvant treatment. More widespread tumour, however, should be treated depending on the degree and location of spread and the overall best interests of the woman.

Treatment after surgery is related to the stage of the disease. Radiotherapy may be used as an adjuvant (postoperative) treatment if the tumour invades the myometrium deeply, as there is a higher risk of extrauterine disease. Radiotherapy limited to the vault of the vagina (brachytherapy) is aimed at preventing a recurrence developing in this area. Radiotherapy to the whole pelvis (external beam radiotherapy) will also prevent local disease recurring in this area but does not improve overall survival. An argument for performing a lymphadenectomy or sentinel node biopsy is that if the nodes are free of tumour, then radiotherapy can be avoided in cases where it might otherwise have been recommended.

Radiotherapy may be used for treatment of local disease if the woman is medically unfit for major surgery. However, this is becoming less common, as most women's comorbidities can be optimised sufficiently to proceed with surgery.

If disease is widespread, or in Stage III, chemotherapy may be considered. The most useful drugs are cisplatinum and doxorubicin; the addition of chemotherapy to standard radiotherapy is associated with improved survival. In a woman who is unfit or unable to undergo surgery, high-dose progestogens can be used to slow the progression of the disease, as these tumours are often hormone sensitive. Their use is not as effective as standard treatment options but in selected cases can be of benefit.

Recurrence

Most women treated for endometrial cancer will not experience a recurrence and the prognosis will be good. Most relapses occur within 2 years of primary treatment. Recurrence is most common in the vault of the vagina and, less commonly, in the lymph node chains, lungs, bone and liver. Unfortunately, 80% of those with distant recurrent disease will die within 2 years. Care should be taken to maximize quality of life over this time rather than subject the woman to treatments with high morbidity and a slim chance of success.

Those women with a recurrence, especially an isolated vault recurrence, who have not received radiotherapy should be considered for this treatment. For the remainder, the choice is between hormonal therapy and chemotherapy. The main hormonal option is high-dose progestogens, with the aim of slowing progression of the disease. Chemotherapy can produce tumour shrinkage in some cases. However, its use needs to be balanced with the associated potential toxicity.

Summary

Endometrial cancer is often considered to be easily treatable and usually is. However, stage for stage, its survival approximates that of other gynaecological cancers. It is in many ways fortunate that most women with endometrial cancer present with postmenopausal bleeding in the early stages of the disease.

To ensure the optimal outcome, women who present with bleeding 12 months or more after their last menstrual period should be referred urgently for a gynaecological opinion. Once a diagnosis is made, referral to a cancer centre specializing in the treatment of gynaecological cancer is likely to give the woman the best chance of cure and long term survival.

Key Points

- Endometrial cancer is the most common gynaecological cancer in the United Kingdom and is generally a postmenopausal disease.
- Exposure to estrogen without progesterone is known to increase the risk of developing the disease.
- Endometrial cancer typically presents with postmenopausal bleeding or abnormal uterine bleeding. Less commonly, the presentation can be with vaginal discharge.

- Diagnosis is made by biopsy of the endometrium. The cavity can be directly visualized with a hysteroscope, and the tissue sampled by curettage or using an outpatient sampling device. In postmenopausal women, endometrial carcinoma is very unlikely if the endometrial thickness is <4 mm.
- In early stage disease treatment is generally surgical (hysterectomy and removal of the ovaries and fallopian tubes). In some cases, lymphadenectomy may be advisable.

Chapter 14

Cervical Neoplasms

Claire Thompson

Chapter Outline

Introduction

Approximately 1 in 10 female cancers diagnosed worldwide are cancers of the cervix; in countries without effective screening programmes, little is changing. Cervical cancer remains the most common cancer among women in many countries without accessible effective screening programmes, with over 450,000 cases each year worldwide. In the United Kingdom, there are 3100 cases of cervical cancer diagnosed each year and 1300 women die from the disease annually.

The discovery of a precursor or premalignant lesion, which can be detected by cytology, has revolutionised the prevention of this cancer. The 'cervical smear' fulfils many of the criteria for a suitable screening programme. Both the incidence and mortality associated with cervical cancer have fallen considerably since the introduction of this screening programme, and the introduction of the human papillomavirus (HPV) vaccine aims to reduce this further still.

The Transformation Zone

Understanding the transformation zone is key to understanding cervical cancer screening. The endocervix is lined by columnar epithelium and the ectocervix by squamous epithelium. Under the influence of estrogen, part of the endocervix everts, thereby exposing the columnar epithelium to the chemical environment of the upper vagina (Fig. 14.1). The change in pH, along with other factors, causes the delicate columnar epithelium cells to transform into squamous epithelium through the process of metaplasia. This area is called the 'transformation zone' and is relatively unstable. As a consequence, premalignant changes can develop in the transformation zone; it is this area that is sampled by the cervical smear test.

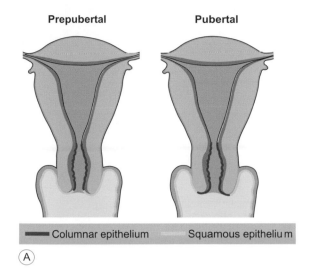

Prepubertal   **Pubertal**

━━ Columnar epithelium   Squamous epithelium

Ⓐ

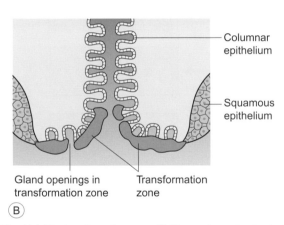

Columnar epithelium

Squamous epithelium

Gland openings in transformation zone

Transformation zone

Ⓑ

Fig. 14.1 The transformation zone. (A) The cervix everts at puberty, exposing the columnar epithelium of the endocervical canal. **(B)** This epithelium, referred to as the 'transformation zone', gradually undergoes metaplasia to squamous epithelium.

In addition to examining the cervical cells from the transformation zone, cervical smear reports may also identify infections such as candida, trichomoniasis, or wart (HPV) virus. Rarely, they may identify cells from other parts of the genital tract, such as malignant cells from the endometrium.

The Cervical Screening Programme (UK)

The aim of the NHS Cervical Screening Programme (NHSCSP) is to reduce the incidence of and mortality from cervical cancer through a systematic, quality-assured population-based screening programme for women aged 25 to 65 years.

Historically, cytology was assessed microscopically, first for evidence of cellular abnormalities, termed 'dyskaryosis', which were graded as negative (normal), borderline, mild, moderate, and severe. Moderate and severe dyskaryosis cases were referred for further assessment by colposcopy. There was debate regarding the value of referral of the low-grade lesions (borderline and mild dyskaryosis), which led to the implementation of HPV triage. With the knowledge that the vast majority of cervical cancer is caused by HPV, these low-grade abnormalities were tested for high-risk HPV. If positive, they were referred for colposcopy; if negative, they were returned to normal screening.

This strategy has evolved into primary HPV screening, which has been demonstrated within randomised controlled trials to be more sensitive than cytology in the detection of premalignant disease of the cervix. Improved sensitivity leads to a reduction in the incidence of both adenocarcinomas and squamous carcinomas of the cervix when compared with screening by cytology alone.

As a result, a national programme of primary HPV screening with triage by cytology is now in operation (Fig. 14.2). The NHSCSP sends the first invitation for cervical screening when a woman reaches 24.5 years of age. Individuals are then recalled every 3 years until they turn 50 years of age, when the recall interval changes to every 5 years. The smear test can diagnose dyskaryosis and/or HPV, whereas colposcopy facilitates assessment of the cervix and biopsy or treatment to be performed. Histology of colposcopically directed biopsies identifies the presence of the premalignant conditions of cervical intraepithelial neoplasia (CIN) or cervical glandular neoplasia (cGIN) or whether there is evidence of cancer. CIN arises from the squamous cells of the ectocervix, whereas cGIN arises from the glandular cells of the endocervical canal and is less common. The degree of dyskaryosis (cytology) tends to correlate with the degree of CIN (histology; Figs. 14.3–14.5). Both precancerous lesions tend to be asymptomatic; therefore, screening is the best method of detection. Not every woman with one of these precancerous changes will develop cervical cancer. However, if left untreated, they may evolve into cancer over time. This time can vary significantly but is estimated to be an average of 10 years.

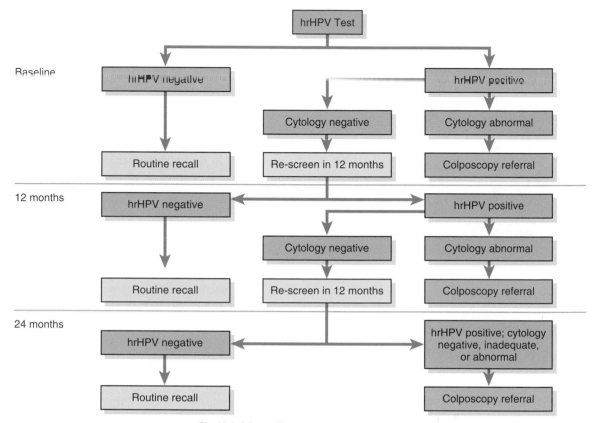

Fig. 14.2 Primary HPV screening pathway (UK).

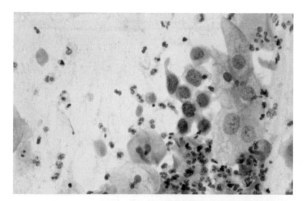

Fig. 14.3 Slide prepared from a cervical smear. There is moderate dysplasia with hyperchromasia, irregular nuclei, and multinucleation. This slide also shows *Trichomonas vaginalis*, leucocytosis, and a spermatozoon.

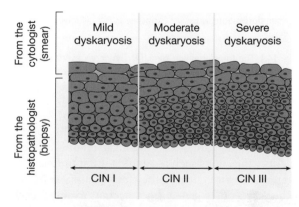

Fig. 14.4 The CIN grading system.

COLPOSCOPY

This is a procedure by which the cervix is visualized using a type of binocular microscope referred to as a

'colposcope' (Fig. 14.6). The woman lies in the lithotomy position and a bivalve speculum is inserted to allow visualization of the cervix. It is important to identify the squamocolumnar junction. Abnormal epithelium, such as CIN, contains an increased amount of protein

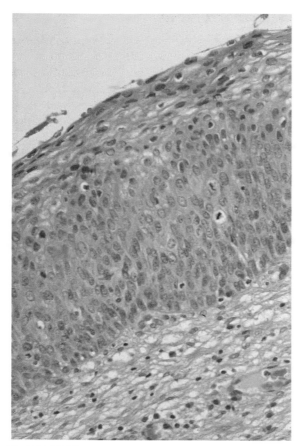

Fig. 14.5 CIN II in a biopsy specimen. There are abnormal cells arising from the basal layer but not extending to the full thickness of the epithelium.

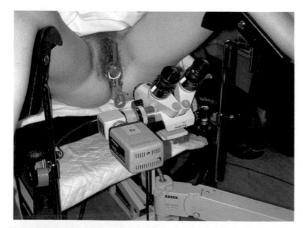

Fig. 14.6 Colposcopy, using a high-powered microscope, allows detailed examination of the cervix.

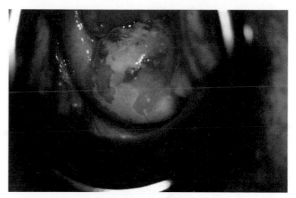

Fig. 14.7 Acetic acid coagulates protein and the abnormal cells, which have more protein, appear 'aceto-white'.

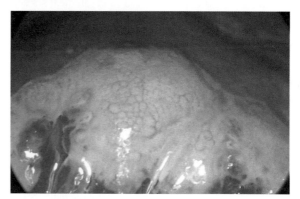

Fig. 14.8 Patches of aceto-white may be separated by areas of blood vessels, creating a mosaic pattern.

and lower levels of glycogen than normal epithelium. If acetic acid is applied to the cervix, the protein coagulates, and the abnormal cells appear white: 'aceto-white' (Fig. 14.7). There may also be a 'mosaic' pattern with patches of aceto-white separated by areas of red vessels (Fig. 14.8). Some of the vascular patterns may appear 'punctated' if the vessels are viewed end on. The inter-vessel distance increases with more severe lesions, and bizarre branching with coarse punctation and atypical vessels suggests invasive disease (cancer). Lugol iodine (Schiller iodine) stains glycogen mahogany brown – the abnormal cells, which have less glycogen and therefore take up less iodine, can be viewed in this way also.

These features of dense aceto-white uptake, punctuation, and mosaicism are suggestive of premalignant or malignant change. These alert the colposcopist to what may be a 'high-grade lesion'. A biopsy should be performed to make a histological diagnosis.

The premalignant stages are classified as:

- Mild or cervical intraepithelial carcinoma I (CIN I; also called low-grade squamous intraepithelial lesion [LSIL])
- Moderate or CIN II or high-grade squamous intraepithelial lesion (HSIL)
- Severe or CIN III (HSIL)
- cGIN.

TREATMENT OF CERVICAL INTRAEPITHELIAL NEOPLASIA

High-grade CIN (CIN II and CIN III) and cGIN require treatment (Table 14.1). With CIN I, there is more controversy and, generally, a period of cytological surveillance will be employed, as many of these lesions will spontaneously resolve. If high-grade CIN is suspected colposcopically, the options are to treat immediately (termed 'see-and-treat') using an excisional method, for example, large loop excision of the transformation zone (LLETZ), or to biopsy to confirm high-grade CIN and treat thereafter. This choice depends on the certainty of the colposcopic findings, the woman's fertility wishes, and other factors, such as the likelihood that the woman will attend for follow-up.

If undertaking LLETZ, the cervix is infiltrated with local anaesthetic and a loop diathermy excision is performed. The alternative treatment of ablating the area has the disadvantage that the histological assessment is less complete.

Smoking is an aetiological factor in the development of CIN; thus, smoking cessation should be discussed with the woman.

FOLLOW-UP

This is defined by the national screening guidelines. Any woman who has had CIN, whether treated or not, continues to be at risk of developing cervical cancer due to either incomplete treatment of her CIN or the development of new disease. Follow-up is usually carried out by repeating cervical smears. Colposcopy can also be used. Protocols vary but, in the UK, a smear with HPV testing ('test of cure') is performed 6 months following treatment. If this is negative with no evidence of high-risk HPV type, then the woman is returned to routine screening. If not, the woman is invited to return for further assessment by colposcopy.

RESULTS OF THE UK CERVICAL SCREENING PROGRAMME

The aim of screening is to identify women at high risk of cervical cancer to enable intervention at a time that allows treatment to substantially reduce this risk. The NHSCSP in England is believed to save 4500 lives per year. Although successful, it will not be able to prevent all cervical cancers. It is estimated that the NHSCSP, when undertaken in women aged between 25 and 49 years, 3-yearly screening prevents 84 cervical cancers out of every 100 that would otherwise develop without screening.

Cervical Cancer

AETIOLOGY

As noted earlier, cervical cancer arises from areas of CIN or cGIN. At least 30% of women with CIN III, if left untreated, will probably go on to develop invasive disease over a period of 5 to 20 years. All cases of cervical

TABLE 14.1	Treatment Modalities for Cervical Intraepithelial Neoplasia		
Method	**Summary of Method**	**Pros**	**Cons**
Loop excision of the transitional zone	Wire loop with high-frequency current	Easy outpatient procedure. Tissue is available for pathology.	Small association with cervical insufficiency and stenosis.
Laser vaporization	Destruction with CO_2 laser	Easy outpatient procedure. Known depth of tissue destruction.	No tissue available for pathology.
'Cold' coagulation	Heating to approximately 120°C	Easy outpatient procedure.	No tissue available for pathology. Depth of tissue destruction not known.
Cone biopsy	Surgical excision, often under anaesthesia	Large specimen obtained. Tissue is available for pathology.	Often needs general anaesthesia. Associated with cervical insufficiency and stenosis.

cancer should be referred and managed by a gynaecological oncology multidisciplinary team in specialist centres.

Sexual Behaviour

Cervical cancer is typically a disease of sexually active women and is associated with HPV. Compared with unaffected women, women with cervical cancer are likely to have had more sexual partners, to have started intercourse at a younger age, and are less likely to have used barrier methods of contraception.

Human Papillomavirus (HPV)

More than 99% of cervical cancers are caused by infections with certain subtypes of HPV. At least 13 subtypes of HPV are known to cause cervical cancer; of these, serotypes 16 and 18 alone or together are responsible for 70% of cervical cancer cases.

Certain serotypes of HPV may act by producing proteins (E6/7) that affect the action of the *p53* gene product. The *p53* gene is important in repairing DNA and, if damaged, may predispose to malignant change. HPV is very common, present in around one-third of all women in their 20s in the United Kingdom. The central role of HPV is the basis for both HPV triage in the CSP as well as for the HPV vaccination programme.

The Combined Oral Contraceptive Pill

Prolonged use (over 10 years) of the combined oral contraceptive pill (COCP) increases the risk of cervical cancer up to four-fold, but only in women who carry HPV. The increased risk is diminished once women stop taking the COCP. However, for many women, this increased risk does not outweigh the benefits for them of taking the COCP. There is no definitive evidence that the progesterone-only pill increases the risk of cervical cancer.

Smoking

Women who smoke are at an increased risk of developing cervical cancer. This may be due to alterations in immune function in the cervical epithelium or due to chemical carcinogenesis.

PREVENTION

As certain subtypes of HPV are known to be the main aetiological factors responsible for the development of cervical cancer, vaccines have been developed with the aim of protection from the common oncogenic HPV subtypes. Cervarix®, Gardasil® and Gardasil®9 are available in many countries. For these vaccines to be most effective, girls should be inoculated before they become sexually active. HPV immunisation was added to the UK vaccination programme for girls in 2008, and extended to boys in 2019. HPV vaccination is now recommended for all children aged 12 to 13 years, currently with Gardasil®, which contains HPV 6, and HPV 11 (causing genital warts) and HPV 16 and HPV 18 (common oncogenic subtypes). This is expected to change to Gardasil®9 (which covers an additional 5 oncogenic subtypes) from 2022. This vaccine will also reduce the incidence of vulval, anal and some head and neck cancers, as well as genital warts. Not every cervical cancer will be prevented; thus, it remains important to participate in the cervical screening programme.

PRESENTATION

Women with cervical cancer may present with abnormal vaginal bleeding, post-coital bleeding, intermenstrual bleeding, or an offensive vaginal discharge. These symptoms are relatively common in young women and are more frequently related to a physiological cervical ectropion, unexplained menstrual irregularity, breakthrough bleeding associated with hormonal contraception, and chlamydia infection. However, malignancy should always be considered. In early-stage cases, there may be no symptoms, and the diagnosis is made as an incidental finding after abnormal cervical cytology is reported. Other symptoms – such as backache, referred leg pain, leg oedema, haematuria, or alteration in bowel habit – are typically associated with advanced-stage disease, when the cancer has begun to infiltrate adjacent anatomical structures. General malaise, weight loss, and anaemia are also features of advanced disease.

Women should undergo history and examination, including a pelvic and speculum examination with the cervix clearly visualized. Any suspicion of a cancerous lesion should be referred urgently to a colposcopy clinic and seen within 2 weeks.

Three categories of clinical appearance are described:

1. The most common is an exophytic lesion (Fig. 14.9). It usually arises on the ectocervix, often producing a large, friable polypoid mass, which bleeds easily. It can also arise from within

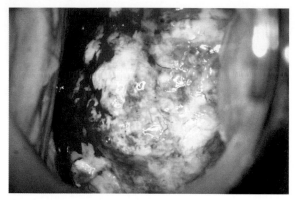

Fig. 14.9 Squamous carcinoma of cervix.

the endocervical canal so that the canal becomes distended and 'barrel shaped'.
2. An infiltrating tumour shows little ulceration or exophytic growth but tends to produce a hard, indurated cervix.
3. An ulcerative tumour erodes a portion of the cervix and vaginal vault, producing a crater with local infection and a seropurulent discharge.

PATHOLOGY

There are two main types of cervical cancer: squamous (80%) and adenocarcinoma (15%–20%). Squamous cancers may be of keratinizing (the most common), large-cell, non-keratinizing, and small-cell subtypes. Adenocarcinomas develop from the glandular cells of the cervix. Rare types of cancer of the cervix include sarcomas, lymphomas, clear cell, and neuroendocrine, none of which are associated with HPV.

SPREAD

Cervical cancer spreads by direct extension into adjacent structures and via the draining lymphatics. Blood-borne metastases are rare. Direct invasion beyond the cervix is usually into the parametrium, upper vagina, and pelvic sidewall, where a tumour may lead to ureteric obstruction. There may also be invasion of the bladder and rectum. There is no predictable pattern of lymphatic spread, with paracervical, parametrial, and both internal and external iliac nodes potentially involved. There may also be a spread to the common iliac, para-aortic, and left supraclavicular nodes.

The risk of lymph node metastases correlates with both stage and tumour volume. Approximately 5% to 10% of women with apparent Stage I disease have pelvic node involvement. The incidence of para-aortic node involvement is less, involving around 5% of women with Stage I disease, but this increases to 25% with Stage III disease.

STAGING, INVESTIGATION, AND PROGNOSTIC FACTORS

Cervical cancer staging is according to the FIGO staging system, updated in 2019 (Table 14.2). Prior to this, FIGO staging was based on clinical examination in order to maintain consistency in countries where radiological imaging may have been difficult to obtain. However, now, like all other gynaecological staging systems, it takes lymph node status into account. All women should still undergo a formal pelvic examination, including a rectovaginal examination to assess parametrial involvement. Examination under anaesthetic (EUA) may still be required in certain cases and to assist in obtaining a biopsy. However, EUA, along with cystoscopy, have largely been superseded by radiological imaging. The most sensitive modality for assessment of local invasion by the tumour is MRI. Systemic assessment can be via CT or, where available, positron emission tomography (PET) CT, which provides increased sensitivity for determining lymph node involvement. If nodes are radiologically suspicious of tumour involvement, it is likely to be more appropriate to avoid surgery and treat with chemotherapy and radiotherapy. Determining the extent of involvement, that is, whether the pelvic and/or para-aortic lymph nodes are positive, allows improved decision-making regarding the extent of the radiation field for treatment.

In countries where effective screening is accessible, a greater proportion of cases present with Stage I disease. Globally, the majority (>75%) of women with cervical cancer present with advanced-stage disease (Stage III/IV). The prognosis for women with early-stage disease is relatively good. Five-year survival is 95% for Stage I disease and 75% for Stage II. However, this falls to 40% for Stage III and 15% for Stage IV disease.

CARE OF WOMEN WITH CERVICAL CANCER
Stage IA1–IA2

Stage IA1 can be cured by simple excision. If preservation of fertility is required, a cone biopsy (in which a cone-shaped wedge of cervical tissue is removed,

TABLE 14.2   Staging of Cervical Cancer[a]

Stage	Description
IA1	Invasive carcinoma confined to the cervix. Stromal invasion < 3 mm.
IA2	Invasive carcinoma confined to the cervix. Stromal invasion ≥ 3 mm and < 5 mm in depth.
IB1	Invasive carcinoma confined to the cervix, ≥ 5 mm depth of stromal invasion and < 2 cm in greatest dimension.
IB2	Invasive carcinoma confined to the cervix ≥ 2 cm and < 4 cm in greatest dimension.
IB3	Invasive carcinoma ≥ 4 cm in greatest dimension.
II	The carcinoma invades beyond the uterus but has not extended onto the lower 1/3 of the vagina or to the pelvic wall.
IIA	Involvement limited to the upper 2/3 of the vagina without parametrial involvement.
IIA1	Invasive carcinoma < 4 cm in greatest dimension.
IIA2	Invasive carcinoma ≥ 4 cm in greatest dimension.
IIB	With parametrial involvement but not onto the pelvic wall.
III	The carcinoma involves the lower 1/3 of the vagina and/or extends to the pelvic wall and/or causes hydro-nephrosis or non-functioning kidney and/or involves pelvic and/or para-aortic lymph nodes.
IIIA	The carcinoma involves the lower 1/3 of the vagina but no extension onto pelvic wall.
IIIB	Extension onto the pelvic wall and/or hydronephrosis/non-functioning kidney (unless known to be due to another cause).
IIIC	Involvement of pelvic and/or para-aortic lymph nodes, irrespective of tumour size and extent (with r and p notations).
IVA	Spread to adjacent pelvic organs.
IVB	Spread to distant organs.

[a]Modified from FIGO Committee Report: Revised FIGO staging for carcinoma of the cervix uteri. Bhatla et al. 2019..

including high into the cervical canal) may be adequate treatment. Clear margins of invasive disease and CIN are required. Close cytological follow-up at 6 and 12 months after treatment, then on a yearly basis for 9 years, is required. Where preservation of fertility is not important, simple hysterectomy may be preferable. With Stage IA2, there is an approximately 5% chance of nodal involvement. In these women, local excision, as discussed earlier, should be combined with pelvic lymphadenectomy. If these nodes are positive, adjuvant radiotherapy will be required. Sentinel lymph node biopsy (SLNB) can be considered, where available. SLNB is a technique in which the first draining lymph nodes (known as 'sentinel lymph nodes') are removed and examined. It has a high sensitivity for detection of metastases in tumours <2 cm but is less accurate for larger tumours. Combined use of technetium-99m colloid (99mTc) lymphoscintigraphy and blue dye is a reliable method of detection. Near infrared (NIR) fluorescence imaging is a more recent technique, which uses medical dyes that show fluorescence in the NIR spectrum when a specialised camera is used. Indocyanine green is the most common dye used. This technique reduces the risk of lymphadenectomy-related morbidity, most notably, the development of lymphoedema.

Stage IB–IIA

The choice between radical hysterectomy and radical radiotherapy is determined by the size and distribution of the cancer, as well as the clinical condition of the woman. There is no difference in survival between the two methods, but there are significant differences in morbidity.

Radical hysterectomy and pelvic lymphadenectomy involve total hysterectomy, excision of the parametria and upper vagina, as well as dissection and removal of the pelvic lymph nodes. The key surgical principle is to obtain a satisfactory surgical margin and to be able to histologically assess the draining lymphatics. Salpingectomy is performed and oophorectomy may be performed, if appropriate. The ovaries are rarely the site of metastatic spread in squamous cancer and usually can be safely conserved in young women. The operative mortality is <1%, although potential morbidity includes infection, thromboembolic disease, haemorrhage, and ureteric fistulae. There are also medium-term problems with reduced bladder sensation and voiding difficulties, together with long-term problems of high residual urinary volumes, recurrent urinary infections, stress incontinence, and lymphocyst formation. The laparoscopic approach has many potential advantages. However, in this situation, laparoscopic or robotic surgery carries a significantly higher risk of recurrence and death from the disease. Thus, many centres have reverted to open procedures.

Radical radiotherapy usually consists of external beam therapy to the pelvis and local vaginal therapy (brachytherapy). Combining this with cisplatin chemotherapy increases the survival rate; such combined chemo-radiotherapy has become the standard of care. External beam radiotherapy is delivered in fractions over a number of weeks to treat the pelvic lymphatics, whereas with brachytherapy, a vaginal delivery system to irradiate central disease is used. In the United Kingdom, brachytherapy, is now in the form of high-dose radiotherapy, which results in much shorter treatment times. The radiation dose that can be given is limited by the size of the lesion and the proximity of the bladder and bowel, both of which are particularly susceptible to radiation damage. Radiation side effects are described as early and late. Initially, there is often radiation cystitis and radiation proctitis. Late effects include fibrosis, causing vaginal stenosis, sexual dysfunction, and fistula formation. In those found to have positive pelvic nodes postoperatively, it is usual to offer adjuvant chemo-radiotherapy.

Women with Stage IB1 disease will usually be offered surgery. For women with small Stage IB1 lesions (<2 cm) that have been assessed in detail with MRI/CT, and in whom future fertility is important, there is the possibility of radical local treatment. This is called 'radical trachelectomy and lymphadenectomy'. The cervix is removed along with the paracervical tissues, but the uterus is conserved along with insertion of a suture to maintain 'cervical competence'. The lymph nodes are also removed. Although it offers the woman the potential of future pregnancy, it is not without significant problems, and there remains the risk of premature birth in a subsequent pregnancy.

As the tumour grows larger in Stages 1B2 and 1B3 disease, the decision becomes more challenging.

Women will be offered either surgery or chemo-radiotherapy. If there is extension beyond the cervix or involvement of the deep cervical stroma, then chemo-radiotherapy would be advised rather than surgery. The main reason for this is that the morbidity associated with radical surgery plus chemo-radiotherapy is significantly greater than either alone. Also, if the cervix has been removed, it is technically more difficult to give the high doses of brachytherapy that are required to achieve local control. Similarly, for women with Stage IB3 and IIA, chemo-radiotherapy would now normally be advised. The reason for this is that even if radical surgery were to be successful, the likelihood of an unsatisfactory margin or positive nodes is sufficiently great to make adjuvant treatment likely.

Stage IIB–IV

The treatment of advanced-stage disease usually involves radical radiotherapy in combination with cisplatin chemotherapy. Failure to cure inoperable cervical cancer may result from suboptimal treatment of the central disease or the existence of lymph node metastases. With large lesions, the sensitivity of adjacent structures to radiation may prevent the use of curative radiation doses at the tumour periphery and, furthermore, some tumours may be radio-resistant. However, as with many other cancers, there have been many improvements in care, including the use of targeted treatments such as bevacizumab and immunotherapy.

RECURRENT DISEASE

Those women with recurrence have a 1-year survival of only 10% to 15%. If the woman has not been previously treated with radiotherapy, this may be a treatment option. However, the majority of women will have already had radical radiotherapy. Women with a central pelvic recurrence may be cured by pelvic exenteration. A total pelvic exenteration involves removal of the uterus, cervix, vagina, bladder, urethra, rectum, and possibly levator ani muscles with urinary reconstruction by an ileal conduit, an end colostomy, and plastic surgery techniques, where required. With careful selection, up to 60% of these cases may survive 5 years, but the operation is associated with major morbidity.

The remaining women may benefit from chemotherapy to palliate symptomatic recurrence or radiotherapy to palliate recurrence involving bone or nerve roots. The most commonly used second-line agents are platinum/paclitaxel, mitomycin/5FU, gemcitabine and topotecan, and combinations based on these drugs, which may cause tumour shrinkage. The main benefit from chemotherapy is the relief of disease-related symptoms, such as pelvic pain, but chemotherapy itself can cause considerable toxicity and does not improve survival for these women.

SUPPORT FOR WOMEN WITH CERVICAL CANCER

Over 49,000 women are living with or beyond cervical cancer in the United Kingdom today, and it is currently the most common cancer in women under 35 years of age. Survival is improving, but the impact of many of the treatments can lead to long-term quality of life issues. Physical implications, such as loss of fertility, pain, urinary or bowel dysfunction, lymphoedema, fistula formation, and loss of sexual function are common and understandably have a huge impact on the lives of women and their families. The psychological impact should not be underestimated. Providing support – including survivorship clinics, psycho-oncology service, and multidisciplinary team involvement for gastrointestinal and urology complications – is vital to reduce long-term morbidity.

Key Points

- Cervical cancer is the most common cancer among women in many developing countries. There are over 450,000 cases worldwide each year.
- The risk of cervical cancer is related to HPV exposure. Early age of first intercourse and a high number of sexual partners are risk factors. Smoking also increases the risk.
- The most important causative agent is HPV, particularly serotypes 16 and 18. In the United Kingdom and many other countries, children receive vaccination to protect against these HPV serotypes.
- Screening is possible because of a relatively long precancerous phase and involves a programme of regular cervical smears. HPV primary screening has been introduced across the United Kingdom.
- When cervical smears demonstrate HPV and/or dyskaryosis, colposcopy allows identification of abnormal epithelium suggestive of CIN to be located, biopsied, and treated.
- Although 80% of cervical cancers are of mainly squamous type, around 10% to 25% are adenocarcinomas.
- FIGO staging of cancer is from Stages I to IV. Stage I can be treated by surgery or radiotherapy. More advanced cancer can be treated by radiotherapy ± chemotherapy.

Chapter 15

Gestational Trophoblastic Disease

John Tidy

Chapter Outline

Introduction

Gestational trophoblastic disease (GTD) comprises a group of diagnoses, each characterised by the abnormal proliferation of trophoblast cells with constitutive human chorionic gonadotropin (hCG) production. GTD can be divided into premalignant and malignant forms, with the premalignant diagnoses of complete and partial molar pregnancies and the malignant forms including invasive moles, choriocarcinoma, placental site trophoblastic tumour (PSTT), and epithelioid trophoblastic tumour (ETT; Table 15.1). The malignant forms of GTD have a number of important differences from other more common types of cancer in terms of aetiology, genetic structure, pathophysiology, and responsiveness to treatment. Malignant forms of trophoblastic disease, such as invasive mole and choriocarcinoma, are extremely sensitive to chemotherapy, which routinely results in cure, even in women presenting with advanced metastatic disease. PSTT and ETT are less sensitive to chemotherapy; thus, surgery plays a more important role in the management of such cases.

Overall, GTD is rare; molar pregnancies, which are the most common form of GTD, have an estimated incidence of around 1 to 3 cases for every 1000 live births. The incidence has previously been thought to vary significantly across different geographical regions and racial groups, with historical estimates showing a near 10-fold higher incidence in Korea, the Philippines, and China compared with Europe and the United States. However, more recent data indicate that similar rates of 1 to 3 cases per 1000 are reported in nearly every modern series worldwide.

The incidence of molar pregnancies is significantly higher at the extremes of reproductive age, at approximately 1 in 30 in those aged under 15 years and as high as 1 in 5 for women in their late 40s or early 50s. As these extremes of the reproductive age group make up only a very small proportion of the women who become pregnant, over 90% of molar pregnancies occur in women aged 18 to 40 years.

Choriocarcinoma, PSTT, and ETT are even rarer, occurring in approximately 1 in 50,000 and 1 in 200,000 pregnancies, respectively. In view of the rarity of the diagnoses and the complexity of care, the management of all trophoblast disease after the initial uterine evacuation is best provided by a specialist centre.

TABLE 15.1   Classification of Gestational Trophoblastic Disease

Classification	Pathology	Usual Karyotype	Clinical Features
Premalignant			
Partial hydatidiform mole	Focal hyperplasia of villi Benign	69,XXY: two paternal haploid sets and one maternal haploid set.	Difficult to diagnose on ultrasound, as a fetus can be present during the first 8–10 weeks. Most present as failed pregnancies. Less than 1% require additional treatment after evacuation.
Complete hydatidiform mole	Generalized hyperplasia Benign	46,XX: two haploid sets, both paternal ('andro-genically diploid').	Uterine cavity filled with vesicular mole tissue on ultrasound without an embryo. Approximately 15%–20% become malignant and require additional therapy.
Malignant			
Invasive mole	Features of invasion	Virtually all are androgeni-cally diploid.	Molar tissue invading the myometrium that may cause uterine rupture if not treated.
Choriocarcinoma	Columns and sheets of malignant trophoblast cells containing syncytiotrophoblast and cytotrophoblast cells, frequent haemorrhage and an absence of villi.	Contains maternal and paternal chromosomes (unlike choriocarcinoma of ovarian origin).	Most follow a live birth, stillbirth, miscarriage, or ectopic pregnancy but can arise from a hydatidiform mole. There is frequently metastatic spread. Highly curable with chemotherapy.
Placental site trophoblastic tumour	Malignant intermediate trophoblast cells infiltrating muscle. No cytotrophoblast cells, and no villi. Positive stain for human placental lactogen (hPL).	May contain maternal and paternal chromosomes.	Slow-growing malignancy invading the myometrium and potentially metastasizing to the lung. Human chorionic gonadotropin (hCG) levels are less elevated than in choriocarcinoma. Usually treated with surgery and chemotherapy.
Epithelioid trophoblastic tumour	Malignant chorionic type intermediate trophoblas-tic cells that form nest or solid masses with a nodular pattern. Can be confused with cervical carcinoma.	May contain maternal and paternal chromosomes.	Slow-growing malignancy invading the myometrium and potentially metastasizing to the lung. hCG levels are less elevated than in choriocarcinoma. Usually treated with surgery and chemotherapy.

Trophoblast Cells in Health and Disease

In a healthy pregnancy, the trophoblast cells make up a key component of the placental tissue. Their role is to promote invasion of the conceptus into the lining of the uterus, promote angiogenesis, and produce hCG.

The malignant forms of GTD, both those arising from molar pregnancies and those arising from malig-nant transformation of cells in healthy placentae, share many of these characteristics. In addition to the abil-ity to invade the lining of the uterus and stimulate new blood vessels, the malignant cells are also able to spread to other organs of the body and grow at a very fast rate, without any control on their division. Fortunately, despite these changes, the production of hCG is always retained. This is extremely helpful in establishing a diagnosis and in monitoring the response to treatment.

Premalignant Gestational Trophoblastic Disease

Premalignant GTD (see Table 15.1) is divided into partial and complete molar pregnancies. The original derivation of the historical term 'hydatidiform mole' – from the Greek *hydatis*, meaning a watery vesicle, and the Latin *mola*, meaning a shapeless mass – is an accurate description of the appearance of a complete molar pregnancy evacuated after the first trimester. With the near-universal use of first-trimester ultrasound, however, this florid appearance is now rarely seen in high-resource settings.

PARTIAL MOLAR PREGNANCY

Molar pregnancies occur as the result of an error, either in the production of the oocyte or at the time of fertilization. Normally, fertilization combines a 23,X set of haploid chromosomes from the ovum with either a 23,X or 23,Y haploid set from the sperm, the result being a diploid 46,XX or 46,XY zygote, which has the correct balance of maternal and paternal genes. In contrast, a partial molar pregnancy has 69 chromosomes, 23 from the mother, and the other 46 paternally derived, usually from the entry of two separate sperm into the ovum (Fig. 15.1).

In a partial molar pregnancy, there is usually an embryo, which may be seen on an early ultrasound. The ultrasound may have been 'routine' or have been carried out because of vaginal bleeding, vaginal discharge, abdominal pain, or excessive morning sickness. Partial molar pregnancies can be associated with an enlarged placenta or cystic changes within the decidual reaction in association with either an empty sac or a delayed miscarriage. However, many only become apparent after histological tissue examination is carried out following a failed pregnancy. The features are of focal hyperplasia and swelling of the villi, though many areas do not exhibit these obvious changes, and pathologically distinguishing a partial mole from a hydropic miscarriage can be difficult. Fortunately, the risk of malignant change after a partial molar pregnancy is less than 1%. Thus, very few women with partial moles require chemotherapy.

COMPLETE MOLAR PREGNANCIES

In contrast to partial molar pregnancies, complete molar pregnancies have the correct number of chromosomes, with the majority having a 46,XX karyotype. In complete molar pregnancies, however, all of the genetic material is from the father. Therefore, they are termed 'androgenetic' in origin.

There appear to be two mechanisms by which this genetic combination arises:

- The maternal 23,X haploid set of chromosomes in the ovum may be lost at the time of fertilization, and the 23,X haploid paternal chromosomes from the fertilizing sperm may duplicate themselves, giving rise to the 46,XX cell.
- Alternatively, an 'empty' ovum may be fertilized by two separate spermatozoa (dispermy), which also leads to a paternally derived karyotype.

In a complete molar pregnancy, there is no fetal material and the placental tissue has marked hyperplasia and gross vesicular swelling of the villi. Ultrasound features, which suggest a complete molar pregnancy, include a polypoid mass between 5 and 7 weeks or thickened cystic appearance of the villous tissue after 8 weeks' gestation with no identifiable gestational sac. The classical macroscopic 'bunch of small grapes' appearance of a complete molar pregnancy generally occurs later in the second trimester. Thus, as most molar pregnancies are now diagnosed in the first trimester, this appearance is seen less often (Fig. 15.2). In areas without routine ultrasound, the presentation may be later with abnormal clinical findings, including a large-for-dates uterus (from the bulk of the tumour), hyperemesis, or, more rarely, thyrotoxicosis, resulting from the supra-physiological levels of hCG, which mimics the action of thyroid-stimulating hormone on the thyroid gland.

Approximately 15% to 20% of complete molar pregnancies become malignant and will require chemotherapy after their surgical evacuation.

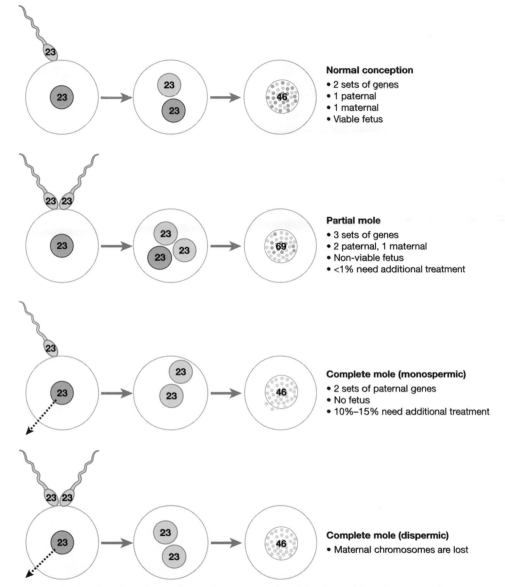

Fig. 15.1 Genetic make-up of normal pregnancy and partial and complete molar pregnancies.

Malignant Gestational Trophoblastic Disease

INVASIVE MOLE

Invasive molar pregnancy is rare in areas with routine first-trimester ultrasound but occurs when the molar tissue invades predominantly into the myometrium. The clinical presentation is with a uterine mass and an elevated hCG level. As a result of the myometrial invasion,

the tumour can lead to uterine rupture and present with abdominal pain and bleeding. Histologically, invasive mole has a similar appearance to a complete molar pregnancy and is routinely curable with chemotherapy.

CHORIOCARCINOMA

Choriocarcinoma is a highly malignant tumour arising from malignant transformation of the placental

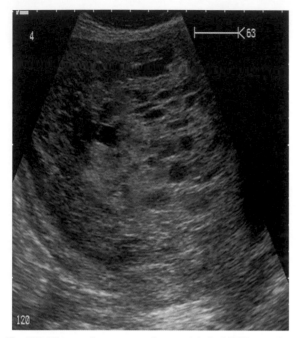

Fig. 15.2 Ultrasound appearance of a complete hydatidiform mole.

trophoblast cells. Histologically, it is characterised by haemorrhage, necrosis, and intravascular growth, and can occur after any pregnancy event. Choriocarcinoma lacks the villous structure of the normal trophoblast or molar pregnancy and is very rare; post-partum choriocarcinoma occurs in approximately 1 case per 50,000 live births. Choriocarcinoma may become apparent shortly after a pregnancy or can present after an interval of up to 20 years after the causative pregnancy.

Presentation of postpartum choriocarcinoma is usually with persistent vaginal bleeding and a markedly raised hCG (the serum hCG level, which is usually <100,000 IU/L at the time of delivery, should fall to normal within 3 weeks postpartum). Diagnosis can also follow presentation of a metastasis in:

- The lung, causing haemoptysis or dyspnoea
- The brain, leading to neurological abnormalities
- The gastrointestinal tract, causing chronic blood loss or melaena
- The liver, leading to jaundice
- The kidney, causing haematuria

The finding of an elevated hCG level in a woman with advanced cancer is highly suggestive of choriocarcinoma.

In contrast to molar pregnancies, there do not appear to be any specific risk factors or higher-risk groups for the development of choriocarcinoma.

PLACENTAL SITE TROPHOBLASTIC TUMOUR

PSTT is a rare type of gestational tumour, with approximately 1 case for every 200,000 live births. In contrast to choriocarcinoma, PSTT is believed to arise from the intermediate trophoblastic cells that develop slightly later in pregnancy. These cells have a lower capacity to invade and make relatively less hCG than the syncytiotrophoblast cells that give rise to choriocarcinoma.

The presentation of PSTT is similar to that of choriocarcinoma. Interestingly, though, it occurs predominantly after the delivery of a female infant and is more likely to be associated with hCG-induced amenorrhoea. PSTT usually presents rather later than choriocarcinoma, tends to grow more slowly, and is less chemosensitive.

Epithelioid Trophoblastic Tumour

ETT has only been described as a separate trophoblastic tumour over the past 20 years. It develops from the chorionic-type intermediate trophoblastic cells and forms nest or solid masses with a nodular pattern. ETT can be mistaken for cervical cancer. Its management is similar to PSTT.

Care of Women With Molar Pregnancies

Following an ultrasound scan suggestive of a molar pregnancy, the first step is to arrange a uterine evacuation. In a complete molar pregnancy, in which there are no fetal parts, the evacuation should be performed by a suction procedure. The risks of bleeding and perforation during surgical evacuation are significant. The procedure should be performed by a senior surgeon and with cross-matched blood available. Medical evacuation may be appropriate for a partial mole, particularly if larger fetal parts are present, but this should be followed with a surgical evacuation of any retained products of conception. It is recommended that oxytocin is avoided until after the uterine evacuation is completed to minimize the risk of distant spread by uterine contractions.

Following the evacuation, the diagnosis is confirmed on histological examination and supported, if needed, by cytogenetic studies of the trophoblast cells.

Follow-Up After a Molar Pregnancy

Following the evacuation of a complete molar pregnancy, there is an approximately 15% to 20% chance of persistent disease and the development of malignancy, while after a partial molar pregnancy, the risk is only 1%. There is no effective prospective method of determining which women will develop persistent disease and will therefore require further treatment. However, hCG follow-up after the evacuation allows this group to be identified.

To ensure that this is meticulously carried out, in the United Kingdom, follow-up of molar pregnancies is organized through three central trophoblast centres (in London, Sheffield, and Dundee). Each case of molar pregnancy is registered with the nearest laboratory, which will then organize the hCG follow-up directly. This system has been a major factor in producing the extremely high cure rates now seen for the disease, and the clinical experience in these centres has led to most of the major therapeutic developments in these rare tumours.

For the majority of women with molar pregnancies, the hCG values fall to normal levels within 2 months, and relapse after this point is very rare. The standard advice is that follow-up is needed for only 6 months from the time of the evacuation or for 6 months from the first normal hCG level in those in whom the rate of fall is slower. It is also recommended that women postpone a further pregnancy during the follow-up period, as the hCG from the new pregnancy could mask the hCG from relapsed disease, which would delay diagnosis and treatment.

There is an increased risk of a further molar pregnancy in subsequent pregnancies, with the risk estimated at approximately 1:70. For women unfortunate enough to have had two molar pregnancies, the risk of a third in a later pregnancy is in the order of 1:10.

Care of Women With Malignant Gestational Trophoblastic Disease

Following evacuation of a molar pregnancy, there are a number of indications for further treatment (Box 15.1). The most frequent of these is a rise or a plateau in the hCG levels after the evacuation. The majority of women receive treatment with simple single-agent chemotherapy, which has a high cure rate and is generally well tolerated (Fig. 15.3). A few women who have completed their families and have no evidence of disease spread may opt instead for a hysterectomy. However, they still require careful follow-up, as occult extrauterine disease may exist and chemotherapy could still be required.

Most, but not all, women with choriocarcinoma occurring after a pregnancy require chemotherapy. However, some cases, even with metastatic disease to the chest, will spontaneously resolve. Surgery in this group is rarely useful.

Women who develop persistent disease, referred to as 'gestational trophoblastic neoplasia' (GTN), require treatment, usually with chemotherapy. To help determine which type of treatment is required, the International Federation of Gynaecology and Obstetrics (FIGO) scoring system can be used (Table 15.2). This system calculates a score based on eight variables.

BOX 15.1 INDICATIONS FOR TREATMENT AFTER A MOLAR PREGNANCY IN UK TROPHOBLASTIC CENTRE

- hCG levels ≥ 20,000 IU/L after one or two uterine evacuations
- hCG plateau of four values ± 10% over a 3-week period
- hCG increase of >10% of three values over a 2-week period
- Persistence of hCG for more than 6 months after molar evacuation
- Histological diagnosis of choriocarcinoma, PSTT, or ETT
- Heavy vaginal bleeding, evidence of gastrointestinal or intraperitoneal haemorrhage in the presence of raised hCG levels
- Metastases in the liver, gastrointestinal tract, or brain
- Pulmonary metastases with static or rising hCG levels

ETT, Epithelioid trophoblastic tumour; *hCG,* human chorionic gonadotrophin; *PSTT,* placental site trophoblastic tumour.

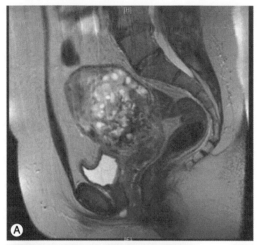

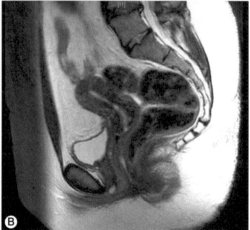

Fig. 15.3 Invasive complete molar pregnancy. (A) Magnetic resonance imaging appearance prior to chemotherapy treatment. **(B)** Follow-up scan performed 3 months after chemotherapy completion.

Women scoring ≤6 points (low risk) initially receive single-agent chemotherapy, while those scoring ≥7 (high risk) are treated with multi-agent chemotherapy. In the United Kingdom, low-risk treatment is with intramuscular methotrexate. High-risk women are treated with intravenous etoposide, methotrexate, actinomycin D, cyclophosphamide, and vincristine (EMA-CO).

Women who present with PSTT or ETT localized to the uterus are offered hysterectomy and bilateral salpingectomy, as both types of tumour are less responsive to chemotherapy. Women with metastatic PSTT or ETT require platinum-based multi-agent chemotherapy.

In the United Kingdom, overall cure rates of 100% for those in the low-risk treatment group and approximately 94% for those in the high-risk group, including those women presenting with advanced disease (Fig. 15.4), can be expected. The small number of women who are difficult to cure usually present unwell with multi-organ involvement or metastatic PSTT and ETT with a long interval (>4 years) from their causative pregnancy.

After the completion of chemotherapy, most women recover fairly rapidly, and fertility is retained in nearly all cases. An interval of 12 months from the completion of chemotherapy to the next pregnancy is usually recommended, and the majority of women are able to have more children. There is thought to be little or no excess risk of fetal abnormalities in this post-chemotherapy group.

TABLE 15.2	FIGO Prognostic Score System for Gestational Trophoblastic Disease (2000)			
	Score			
	0	**1**	**2**	**4**
Age	<40 y	≥40 y	–	–
Antecedent pregnancy	Mole	Miscarriage	Term	–
Interval	<4 mo	4–6 mo	7–13 mo	≥14 mo
Pre-treatment hCG (IU/L)	<1000	1000–10,000	10,000–100,000	>100,000
Largest tumour size	<3 cm	3–5 cm	>5 cm	–
Site of metastases	Lung	Spleen, kidney	Gastrointestinal tract	Brain, liver
Number of metastases	0	1–4	5–8	>8
Previous chemotherapy	–	–	Single agent	Two or more drugs

FIGO, International Federation of Gynaecology and Obstetrics; *hCG,* human chorionic gonadotropin.

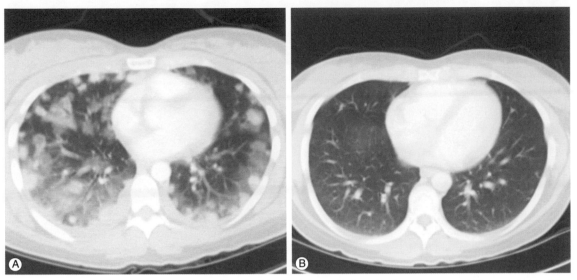

Fig. 15.4 Choriocarcinoma. (A) Computed tomography (CT) scan of the chest, demonstrating extensive pulmonary metastases and haemorrhage, in a woman with choriocarcinoma presenting 1 month after a normal delivery. **(B)** A CT scan performed 6 months later shows the complete resolution of the disease in response to chemotherapy.

Key Points

- Gestational trophoblastic disorders represent an abnormal proliferation of trophoblastic tissue and may be benign (molar pregnancy) or malignant (invasive mole, choriocarcinoma, PSTT, or ETT).
- Trophoblastic tumours always produce hCG, which acts as an excellent marker for diagnosis, assessing response to treatment, and for follow-up.
- A hydatidiform mole may be complete or partial. A complete mole is diploid (however, all the chromosomes are paternally derived), and there is no fetal tissue (only trophoblast). A partial mole is usually triploid (with 46 of the 69 chromosomes being paternally derived), and there may be a fetus.
- The diagnosis of a molar pregnancy is often suggested by ultrasound, in which there is homogeneous solid tissue with a vesicular appearance. The diagnosis is confirmed by histopathological examination of tissue.

- The initial management of a molar pregnancy is to carry out an evacuation of the uterus, and follow-up is required to ensure that the hCG level is falling. Further treatment, usually chemotherapy, is required if the hCG rises progressively following the uterine evacuation or if the pathology is reported as choriocarcinoma.
- Choriocarcinoma is rare but can occur after any type of conception, including a normal pregnancy, miscarriage, or hydatidiform mole.
- Most types of GTN, including choriocarcinoma, are exquisitely sensitive to chemotherapy, and the cure rate is high. Women with PSTT or ETT localized to the uterus are treated with surgery. Women with metastatic PSTT or ETT and more than a 4-year interval between the antecedent pregnancy and presentation have a very high mortality, >75%.
- Following a molar pregnancy, there is a modest increase in risk of molar pregnancy in any subsequent pregnancies.

Chapter 16

Disorders of the Vulva

Michelle Kent, Kevin Burton, Kate Darlow

Chapter Outline

Introduction

The vulva consists of the mons pubis, labia majora (singular: labium majus), labia minora (singular: labium minus), clitoris, and the vestibule (see Fig. 2.1). It is covered with keratinizing squamous epithelium, unlike the vaginal mucosa, which is covered with non-keratinizing squamous epithelium. The labia majora are hair-bearing and contain sweat and sebaceous glands: from an embryological viewpoint, they are analogous to the scrotum. Bartholin glands are situated in the posterior part of the labia, one on each side of the vestibule. The lymphatics of the vulva drain to the inguinal nodes, and then to the external iliac nodes. The area is richly supplied with blood vessels.

Points to Note in the History

The presenting symptoms may include pain, burning, itching, bleeding, presence of an ulcer, or swelling. Ask about general skin complaints, such as eczema or psoriasis, which can also affect the vulval skin. Some skin care products, such as strongly perfumed soaps, may be an irritant to the vulva. Enquiring about any changes to products the woman is using, as well as any topical treatments she has already tried, is important. Note any medical history that could be related, such as poorly controlled diabetes, Crohn disease, or immunosuppression. Finding out how vulval complaints are affecting a woman's quality of life is important. A multidisciplinary approach to management – including gynaecology, dermatology, clinical psychology, and pain management – may be valuable.

Examination of the Vulva

Before direct examination of the vulva, a general dermatological examination is often useful, particularly:

- The nail beds for signs of pitting – found in psoriasis
- The extensor surfaces (elbows and knees), also for features of psoriasis
- The flexor surfaces for lichen planus and dermatitis
- The mouth for other features of lichen planus.

The vulva may then be inspected under a good light, as described on page 21. If necessary, closer inspection is possible using a colposcope. Clinical photography can aid the monitoring of chronic conditions.

Simple Vulval Conditions

URETHRAL CARUNCLE

A urethral caruncle is a polypoidal outgrowth from the edge of the urethra, which is most commonly seen after menopause. The tissue is soft, red, and smooth, appearing as an eversion of the urethral mucosa. Most women are asymptomatic, but others experience dysuria, frequency, urgency, and focal tenderness. If there are any suspicious features, an excision and biopsy may be required to exclude the rare diagnosis of a urethral carcinoma.

BARTHOLIN GLAND CYSTS

The greater vestibular, or Bartholin, glands lie in the subcutaneous tissue below the lower third of the labium majus and open via ducts to the vestibule between the hymenal orifice and the labia minora. They secrete mucus, particularly at the time of intercourse. When the duct becomes blocked, a tense retention cyst forms. If there is super-added infection, a painful abscess develops. The abscess can be incised and drained, usually under general anaesthesia. To prevent the cyst reforming,

the fistula is kept open by suturing its edges to the surrounding skin, a procedure known as marsupialization (Fig. 16.1). Insertion of a balloon catheter (Word catheter) under local anaesthesia is an alternative to incision, drainage, or marsupialization. The aim of this procedure is to allow a sinus tract to develop after 3 to 4 weeks. Carcinoma of the Bartholin gland is very rare.

SMALL CYSTS

The most common small vulval cysts are usually either inclusion cysts or sebaceous cysts. Inclusion cysts form because epithelium is trapped in the epidermis, usually following perineal trauma at the time of childbirth. They

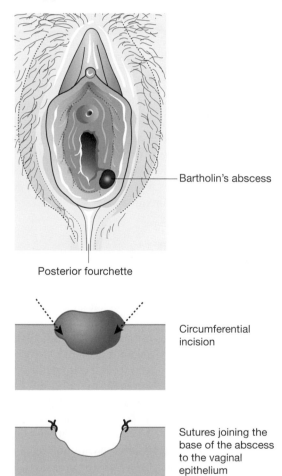

Bartholin's abscess

Posterior fourchette

Circumferential incision

Sutures joining the base of the abscess to the vaginal epithelium

Fig. 16.1 Marsupialization of a Bartholin abscess. The lower part of the abscess cavity granulates and heals during subsequent weeks. (From Pitkin J, Peattie A, Magowan BA. *Obstetrics and Gynaecology. An Illustrated Colour Text.* Edinburgh: Churchill Livingstone; 2003.)

are usually asymptomatic and need no treatment. Sebaceous cysts are usually multiple, mobile, non-tender white or yellow, and filled with a 'cottage cheese-like' substance. Excision may be requested by the woman.

NAEVI

Vulval naevi (moles) are usually asymptomatic but become more pigmented at puberty. Any other change in a vulval naevus is an indication for removal. Of malignant melanomas in women, 2% arise from the vulva.

FIBROMA, LIPOMA, HIDRADENOMA

Fibromas and lipomas are benign, mobile tumours of fibrous tissue and fat, respectively. Hidradenomas are rare tumours of sweat glands near the surface of the labia. All are benign, but the diagnosis is usually only made once they have been excised.

HAEMATOMA

The most common cause of a vulval haematoma is vaginal delivery. It may also occur following surgery to the vulva, or by 'falling astride' accidents (particularly in children, where the possibility of sexual assault should be borne in mind). Vulval haematomas usually present with pain, and surgical evacuation under general anaesthesia is often required.

SIMPLE ATROPHY

Older women develop vaginal, vulval, and clitoral atrophy as part of the normal ageing process of skin. In severe cases, the thin vulval skin, terminal urethra, and fourchette can cause dysuria and superficial dyspareunia, and the labia minora may fuse and 'bury' the clitoris. Introital stenoses can make coitus difficult and sometimes impossible. A simple moisturizer rubbed into the vulva is effective and topical estrogen is often appropriate. There may be a small amount of systemic absorption with topical estrogen therapy. If this route is chosen, treatment should be for no more than 2 or 3 months without either a break or a short course of progesterone to prevent endometrial stimulation.

ULCERS

These may be:
- Aphthous (yellow base)
- Herpetic (exquisitely painful multiple ulceration, pp. 202)
- Syphilitic (indurated and painless, pp. 204)
- Associated with Crohn disease
- A feature of Behçet syndrome (a rare, chronic, painful condition with aphthous genital, oral, and ocular ulceration)
- Malignant (see later discussion)
- Associated with lichen planus (see later discussion) or Stevens-Johnson syndrome
- Tropical (lymphogranuloma venereum, chancroid, granuloma inguinale).

Treatment depends on the cause. The management of Behçet syndrome is challenging and multidisciplinary, but the combined oral contraceptive and topical and oral steroids may be effective.

Infection

Candida, vulval warts, herpes, lymphogranuloma venereum, scabies, granuloma inguinale, tinea, chancroid, and syphilis are discussed in Chapter 18.

Hidradenitis suppurativa is a chronic, unrelenting infection of the sweat glands. The aetiology is uncertain. The glands become obstructed, and chronic inflammation follows. Long-term antibiotics reduce further attacks, but the only potential cure is surgical excision of the affected area.

Dermatoses

Vulval 'dystrophy' is an abnormality of vulval epithelium. Epithelial growth may be hypoplastic, hyperplastic, or abnormal in some other way.

LICHEN SCLEROSUS

This chronic and recurrent condition can present at any age but is more common in the older woman and usually presents with pruritus. Less commonly, presentation is with dyspareunia or pain. It is an autoimmune condition, and there is an association with other autoimmune disorders, including pernicious anaemia, thyroid disease, diabetes mellitus, systemic lupus erythematosus (SLE), primary biliary cirrhosis, and bullous pemphigoid. Histologically, the epidermis appears thin, with loss of rete ridges (epithelial projections into the underlying connective tissue). The superficial dermis is hyalinized, and a band of chronic inflammatory cells is seen beneath it.

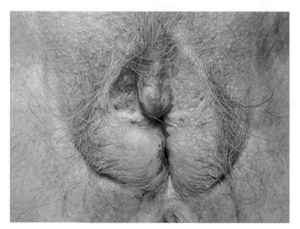

Fig. 16.2 Lichen sclerosus. The skin is white, with some reddened areas, and adhesions have narrowed the introitus.

On examination, the skin appears white, thin, and crinkly but may be thickened and keratotic if there is co-existent squamous cell hyperplasia (Fig. 16.2). There may also be clitoral or labial atrophy, with loss of the normal vulval features, such as recession of the clitoral hood and shrinkage of the labia minora. Diagnosis is usually made on clinical examination but can be confirmed by biopsy. Lichen sclerosus is non-neoplastic but may co-exist with vulval intraepithelial neoplasia (VIN), and there is an association with subsequent development of vulval squamous cell carcinoma in 2% to 5% of cases. Initial follow-up is required to ensure that the woman is managing her symptoms and there are no suspicious skin changes. Once symptoms are controlled, then clinical review should be prompted by a change in symptom, a failure of routine management to control symptoms, or a concern regarding the skin features.

Treatment is required if the condition is symptomatic. Initially, treatment is usually with a potent topical corticosteroid cream (e.g., clobetasol propionate 0.05%), reducing gradually over a few months to a milder preparation (e.g., 1% hydrocortisone). An emollient such as Oilatum or Diprobase is symptomatically beneficial. Avoidance of soaps, perfumed products, and 'baby wipes' is recommended. A non-fragranced, non-biological washing powder should be recommended. Vulvectomy is not appropriate since the recurrence rate after surgery is around 50%.

SQUAMOUS CELL HYPERPLASIA

Squamous epithelial hyperplasia is characterised by thickened hyperkeratotic skin with white, itchy plaques. Pruritus is usually severe. Diagnosis is by skin biopsy, and treatment is as for lichen sclerosus.

OTHER DERMATOSES

Allergic/Irritant Dermatosis

The vulval skin, especially the introitus, is not uncommonly affected by dermatitis. The dermatitis is either due to an irritant (non-immunological) or a true allergy (immunological aetiology). Chemicals causing hypersensitivity of the vulval skin include cosmetics, perfumes, contraceptive lubricants, sprays, and douches. Detergents, dyes, fabric softeners, bleaches, soaps, and chlorine used to clean undergarments can also cause irritation. In severe cases, hypersensitivity to local anaesthetic creams and even corticosteroid preparations may develop.

Women with contact dermatitis have a red, inflamed vulva with features of eczema, and patch-testing may identify local irritants. Temporary relief may be obtained with vulval moisturizers (e.g., Dermol 500 in a daily bath), emollients (e.g., Epaderm), and topical corticosteroids (e.g., a month's course of topical clobetasol). Lesions that do not respond should be biopsied to confirm the diagnosis and exclude sinister changes.

Psoriasis

Psoriasis manifests as a well-circumscribed, erythematous eruption with superficial scaling and may often have a plaque that may extend to the thigh. The diagnosis is easier to make if there is co-existing extragenital psoriasis or nail changes. Because the vulva is often moist, it is often difficult to distinguish psoriasis from candidal infection or dermatitis. *Candida* should be excluded. The lesions may be treated with topical preparations, ultraviolet light, corticosteroid creams, or other suitable formulations.

Intertrigo With *Candida*

Intertrigo refers to a moist inflammatory dermatitis, which can occur in any body fold because of apposition and chafing of skin surfaces. Skin folds are more likely to rub together in those who are overweight.

The skin is sore, macerated, and often red, inflamed, and cracked. Weight loss (where appropriate), local hygiene, and improved ventilation should be encouraged – for example, the use of stockings and cotton underclothes rather than tights and nylon pants.

Candida often complicates intertrigo and should be treated as on page 198. In the absence of candidal infection, steroid creams may be used to relieve inflammation.

Lichen Planus

Lichen planus is a chronic pruritic, purple, papular rash involving the vulva and flexor surfaces. It can affect other flexor surfaces and oral mucous membranes, and the diagnosis may be supported by the finding of other lesions, such as Wickham striae (whitish lines) in the buccal mucosa. It is usually idiopathic but can be drug related. Treatment is with potent topical steroids or ultraviolet light, and it tends to resolve within 2 years. Surgical excision should be avoided.

Pruritus

Pruritus describes an intense itching with a desire to scratch. It is more common in those aged over 40 years, and symptoms are often most severe under times of emotional stress or depression. There are numerous aetiologies (Box 16.1).

A biopsy may be necessary to establish the diagnosis, and patch testing may achieve a diagnosis. It is important to break the 'itch – scratch – itch' cycle; the short-term application of a potent topical corticosteroid will reduce the local inflammation caused by scratching. Application of a strong steroid cream twice daily for 3 weeks, followed by hydrocortisone cream

BOX 16.1 CAUSES OF PRURITUS VULVAE

- Infection (*Candida*, pediculosis, thread worms)
- Eczema
- Dermatitis (consider patch testing)
- Irritation from a vaginal discharge
- Lichen sclerosus
- Lichen planus
- Vulval intraepithelial neoplasia
- Vulval carcinoma
- Medical problems, for example, diabetes mellitus, renal or liver failure
- Psychogenic

1% daily as maintenance, is useful, as is the use of soap substitutes (e.g., Oilatum). Irritants and bath-water additives should be avoided, soap substitutes used, the area dried gently (e.g., with a hairdryer), loose cotton clothing worn, and nylon tights avoided. Antihistamines may also be of help. Co-existing depression may require treatment.

Vulvodynia

This is chronic vulvar discomfort characterised by the complaints of burning, stinging, irritation, or rawness with no other specific diagnosis having been identified. There may also be pruritus. The condition may be localized (vestibulodynia) with associated erythema, severe pain on penetration or to vestibular touch, and tenderness elicited by applying pressure to the vestibule. The condition may also be generalized (dysaesthetic vulvodynia). No single factor can be identified as the specific cause. It may be associated with previous sexual abuse or female genital mutilation (FGM): the World Health Organization (WHO) defines FGM as the partial or total removal of external female genitalia or other injury to the female genital organs for non-medical reasons (see later discussion).

There may be a response to low-dose tricyclic antidepressants (e.g., amitriptyline) or neuromodulators (e.g., gabapentin, pregabalin). Symptomatic relief can also be achieved by the use of topical local anaesthetic. Occasionally, nerve blocks or botulinum toxin is used to treat refractory cases. Due to the complex nature of this symptom, management can be challenging, and refractory cases should be reviewed in specialist multidisciplinary clinics, where physiotherapy, psychological counselling, pain management, and behavioural modification can be explored.

Vulval Intraepithelial Neoplasia

VIN refers to the presence of neoplastic cells within the confines of the vulval epithelium. VIN is categorized by histological appearance. 'Usual type' VIN (uVIN) is often related to exposure to human papillomavirus (HPV). 'Differentiated' VIN (dVIN) is found in association with lichen sclerosus or lichen planus. Both uVIN and dVIN should be considered as a 'high-grade' disorder. In contrast, 'low-grade' is no longer a commonly used term and is generally used to refer to genital warts.

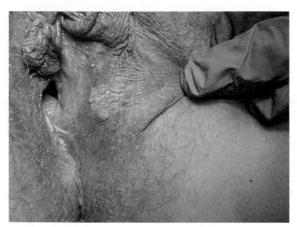

Fig. 16.3 Vulval intraepithelial neoplasia of the left labium majus. In this case, the lesion is rough surfaced, not unlike the appearance of wart virus infection, but lesions are also commonly macular with indistinct borders.

Many cases of VIN are asymptomatic, although pruritus is present in up to two-thirds of cases and pain is an occasional feature. Lesions may be papular and rough surfaced, resembling warts (Fig. 16.3), or macular with indistinct borders. White lesions represent hyperkeratosis, and pigmentation can also be seen. The lesions can be multifocal or unifocal. In HPV-related cases (uVIN), there is an association with intraepithelial neoplasia of the cervix, vagina, and perianal areas.

Diagnosis is by biopsy, which may be taken at the time of vulvoscopy, under either local or general anaesthesia. The opportunity should be taken to examine the cervix at the same time, as there is an association with cervical intraepithelial neoplasia (CIN). As the natural history of VIN is uncertain, treatment is controversial. Spontaneous regression has been observed, but progression of VIN to invasive carcinoma occurs in approximately 5% of cases, and up to 15% of those with VIN may have superficial invading vulval cancer.

Treatment of VIN includes surgical excision to obtain clear margins, with plastic surgical reconstruction for extensive areas; immunomodulators, such as imiquimod cream; or laser ablation where there is no concern regarding malignancy. Close follow-up is required, as the disease can recur. Smoking is a potent co-factor for the development of VIN, and smoking cessation should be encouraged.

PAGET DISEASE (EXTRA-MAMMARY PAGET DISEASE)

In this uncommon condition, there is a poorly demarcated, often multifocal, eczema-like lesion. In 10% of cases, there is a co-existing adenocarcinoma either in the pelvis or at a distant site. The development of symptoms may precede the development of cancer by 10 to15 years. Treatment is by wide local excision. However, due to the indistinct nature of the margins, it can be difficult to obtain clearance. Recurrences are common.

Vulval Carcinoma

Vulval cancer is relatively uncommon. Squamous cell carcinoma accounts for 90% of vulval cancers. Approximately 5% of vulval malignancies are malignant melanomas. The others include Bartholin gland cancer, basal cell carcinomas, and sarcomas. It is usually a disease of older women (60+ years) and, like cervical cancer, is more common in cigarette smokers and women who are immunocompromised. Many squamous vulval cancers also share a common aetiology with cervical cancer in that high-risk HPV is a common cause. HPV vaccination is likely to reduce the future incidence of VIN and HPV-related vulval squamous cell carcinoma.

CLINICAL PRESENTATION

Most women will present with a history of long-standing vulval irritation or pruritus, and some will have had a previous history of lichen sclerosus. A lump or ulcer is common (Fig. 16.4). As the disease advances, the tumour grows, and focal necrosis may cause discharge and pain. The diagnosis is confirmed by histological examination of a biopsy.

PATHOPHYSIOLOGY

Squamous cell carcinoma spreads to the inguinal nodes and, from there, to the external iliac nodes in the pelvis (Table 16.1). Unless the lesion has only penetrated the basement membrane by <1 mm, node involvement can occur and may include both the superficial and deep inguinal lymph node systems.

SURGICAL MANAGEMENT

Vulval cancer should be managed by a gynaecological cancer multidisciplinary team. The treatment of vulval

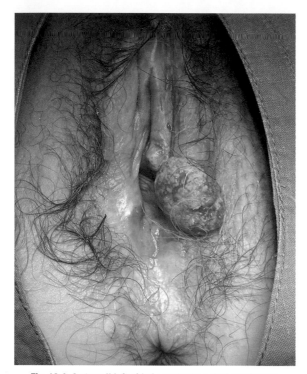

Fig. 16.4 A stage II left-sided squamous vulval carcinoma.

TABLE 16.1	International Federation of Gynaecology and Obstetrics (FIGO) Staging of Vulval Carcinoma	
Stage	**Definition**	
I$_A$	Tumour <2.0 cm in dimension and <1 mm of stromal invasion. No lymphovascular space invasion, and no nodal disease	
I$_B$	Tumour <2.0 cm in dimension but with >1 mm of stromal invasion	
II	Tumour of any dimension invading the lower one-third urethra/vagina or lower one-third anus with negative nodes	
III	Tumour of any size with or without extension to adjacent perineal structures (lower one-third urethra, lower one-third vagina, anus) with positive inguinofemoral lymph nodes	
III$_A$	(i)	With 1 lymph node metastasis (≥5 mm) or
	(ii)	1 – 2 lymph node metastasis(es) (<5 mm)
III$_B$	(i)	With ≥2 lymph node metastases (≥5 mm) or
	(ii)	≥3 lymph node metastases (<5 mm)
III$_C$		With positive nodes with extracapsular spread
IV$_A$	(i)	Upper urethral and/or vaginal mucosa, bladder mucosa, rectal mucosa, or fixed to pelvic bone or
	(ii)	Fixed or ulcerated inguinofemoral lymph node
IV$_B$	Any distant metastases, including pelvic nodes	

carcinoma is surgical excision, either a wide local excision or vulvectomy, where this can be achieved without compromising bladder or bowel function. The addition of groin node lymphadenectomy should be performed where the depth of invasion is >1 mm. It is appropriate to carry out only a unilateral exploration if the lesion is well lateralized, >1 cm from a midline structure such as the clitoris or posterior fourchette. In all other cases, a bilateral groin node dissection is required. Distant metastases are not a contraindication to radical vulval surgery, as death from a large fungating genital neoplasm or erosion of the femoral artery or vein by metastatic groin nodes is very distressing.

The groin explorations are carried out through separate incisions, and the wound will typically be drained for 7 to 10 days under suction, as lymph fluid accumulates and wound breakdown is common. To reduce the associated morbidity from groin node dissection, the technique of sentinel lymph node biopsy (SLNB) has been explored as an acceptable technique, with reduced morbidity and false-negative rates of 1% for women with no suspicious nodes on imaging. SLNB involves injecting dye or a radioactive isotope at the site of the vulval tumour; the first node that the dye or isotope reaches, the sentinel node, is then surgically removed. If there are no malignant cells in the sentinel node, then formal groin node dissection may not be required. If there is significant groin node involvement, it may be necessary to give adjuvant pelvic node radiotherapy.

The most common complication of a radical vulvectomy is breakdown of the wound, which may take weeks to heal. To reduce the morbidity, plastic surgical reconstruction can be offered. In addition, women undergoing this surgery are often elderly, immobile, and are at a high risk of venous thromboembolic disease. Long-term sequelae of surgery include vulval mutilation, if plastic surgical reconstruction is not offered, and lymphoedema. The 5-year survival following treatment is around 80% if groin nodes are negative and 40% if positive.

RECURRENCE

The likelihood of a recurrence of the excised tumour at the primary site is reduced when a 10-mm margin of excision has been achieved. However, the epithelium is likely to be unstable, and there may be multifocal pre-invasive lesions from which new vulval tumours may arise. Treatment of recurrence is surgical, although interstitial radiotherapy may be appropriate.

Female Genital Mutilation

FGM (formerly known as 'female circumcision' or 'cutting') involves partial or complete removal of the female external genitalia for non-medical reasons. The practice is usually carried out by members of the local community on young girls between infancy and 15 years of age. The WHO estimates that more than 200 million girls and women have had FGM carried out, largely concentrated in 30 countries in Africa, the Middle East, and Asia, as well as migrants from these areas. FGM is criminalised (illegal) in many countries worldwide, including most of the countries where it is most prevalent, but reporting of FGM and enforcement of these laws remains variable. It is illegal in the United Kingdom under specific anti-FGM legislation. FGM is internationally recognised as a violation of the human rights of girls and women; one of the United Nations Sustainable Development Goals (SDGs) is to eliminate FGM worldwide by 2030.

TYPES OF FGM

FGM is broadly classified into four types based on examination of the vulva.

Type 1

Partial or total removal of the clitoris and/or the clitoral hood (Fig 16.5).

Type 2

Partial or total removal of clitoris and labia minora with or without removal of the labia majora (Fig. 16.6).

Type 3

Complete removal of labia minora and/or labia majora (with or without removal of the clitoris) with the labia sutured together to create a narrow introitus (Fig 16.7).

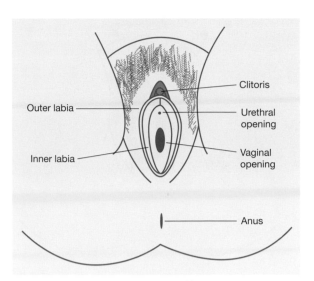

Fig. 16.5 Type 1 FGM.

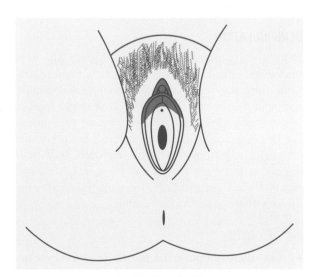

Fig. 16.6 Type 2 FGM.

Type 4

This encompasses all other harmful procedures, including pricking, piercing, incising, and burning the female genitalia.

COMPLICATIONS

Immediate complications of FGM include severe pain, haemorrhage, infection, urinary retention, and death. Long-term complications can include keloid scars,

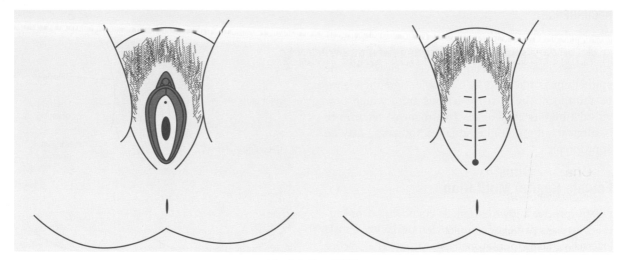

Fig. 16.7 Type 3 FGM.

sexual dysfunction/pain, psychological trauma, and increased risk of complications at delivery.

DEINFIBULATION

Deinfibulation may be required for women who have undergone type 3 FGM in order to allow them to pass urine normally, have sexual intercourse, and/or have a vaginal delivery. It can be carried out under local or regional anaesthetic. For women who are pregnant, it can be carried out antenatally or during labour. When caring for any woman who has endured FGM, it is important to ensure the safety of her daughters and sisters. If she is pregnant, this includes considering the future welfare of the fetus, if female.

Key Points

- A swollen symptomatic Bartholin gland cyst or abscess is usually marsupialized or managed with a balloon catheter.

- Squamous carcinoma of the vulva develops in around 2% to 5% of women diagnosed with lichen sclerosus.
- VIN is analogous to CIN. Treatment of VIN is local excision of severely dysplastic lesions with careful follow-up.
- Vulval carcinoma is usually of squamous cell type and tends to occur in the more elderly population. The treatment is excision ± unilateral or bilateral inguinal lymphadenectomy. Pelvic radiotherapy may also be indicated if there is a significant chance of nodal spread.
- FGM is usually carried out against female infants and young girls, has major immediate and long-term complications, and is internationally recognised as a human rights violation.

Chapter 17

Gynaecological Surgery

Mayank Madhra

Chapter Outline

Introduction

Surgery has a central aim of helping people to live a longer or better life. Translated into medical terminology, this means improved survival and enhanced quality of life (QOL). QOL is a subjective measure, reported by the patient, and multiple factors affect how QOL would be rated at any point in time. An operation is in the middle of a much longer process of selecting the patients in whom surgery is most likely to bring short- or long-term benefit. A surprisingly small part of the process involves what are thought of as traditional surgical skills, such as incising, dissecting, and knot tying.

Preoperative Care

One of the assumptions underlying this framework is that people wishing to have surgery want to improve their survival and QOL. This can transpire in many person-specific forms. From a surgical perspective, it can mean performing surgery in an attempt to alleviate the underlying cause of a symptom which had been negatively affecting QOL, such as removal of an infected and inflamed appendix, with an immediate physical benefit. It could also mean performing surgery to remove both ovaries and fallopian tubes to improve something more intangible, such as 'raised risk of developing cancer

in the future'. In this situation, the benefit in QOL is psychological in the short term and, if successful, in the long term will avoid a future reduction in QOL by preventing the development of cancer.

The baseline, or preoperative, QOL represents what is at risk to the patient if the operation results in complications. A myomectomy (removal of a fibroid), intended to improve fertility, can rarely result in hysterectomy to control bleeding during the operation. This would mean a risk of a permanent, opposite effect on fertility and QOL to that hoped for preoperatively.

Knowing what patients hope to gain from an operation, how any complications would impact their overall QOL, and what they would consider an acceptable compromise are important when the decision to operate is made. An important question to ask is what would happen if no action was taken instead of performing an operation. In the case of myomectomy discussed earlier, the woman is likely to continue to have suboptimal fertility but would avoid the risk of a surgical complication which might remove fertility completely.

Unexpected findings or complications, by definition, occur during the operation. One of the options facing the surgeon is to continue with the operation in the knowledge that the discussion prior to surgery means that they know how to act in the best interests of the patient. Alternatively, the operation can be

183

curtailed, with a subsequent explanation and further discussion with the patient of the implications of the new findings. This leads to an updated decision of whether to proceed with the surgery or not.

All of these factors are input into the consent process. The culmination of this process is represented by the consent form, completed by the patient and the surgeon. This process is ongoing—either party can veto the decision to proceed - even if the doctor thinks the patient is choosing the 'worse' option by declining surgery. This issue is sometimes raised in patients who would decline a blood transfusion. In the United Kingdom, any medical procedure, including transfusion, performed without the consent of the person may be considered assault from a legal standpoint. There are multiple forms of consent—implied, verbal, and written—and, typically, there are exceptions for emergency situations, for instance, when an unconscious patient is given lifesaving treatment. Legal definitions of an adult, a person able to give or withhold consent, and capacity for decision-making vary from country to country.

Preoperative optimisation improves the odds of a good outcome from the operation for the patient. The factors, which can be modified, depend on how much time there is available to do so before the operation. An unwell patient with hypovolaemic shock secondary to bleeding might need a blood transfusion while simultaneously being prepared for anaesthesia. In contrast, a patient who mentions a symptom such as angina incidentally could have a less urgent operation postponed to allow for further investigations. The 'optimisation' might take the form of other major surgery, such as a coronary artery bypass graft. Proceeding to surgery without optimisation can still be preferable if the risks of delaying surgery for preoperative optimisation are thought to be worse. Reducing or stopping smoking is almost always helpful, as is having a body mass index in the normal range. Medications to reduce blood loss and replace iron stores are frequently used for preoperative optimisation prior to gynaecological surgery in women who have heavy menstrual bleeding and anaemia.

The preoperative review of the patient on the day of planned surgery is the final chance to confirm or change the plan. Is the operation still required? Could it be that the heavy menstrual bleeding has stopped or the ovarian cyst has resolved spontaneously? This would mean that physiology has removed the potential gains in QOL hoped for from the operation and would greatly change the balance of benefit and harm to the patient from going ahead. A change in heart from a woman about wishing to try for a pregnancy in the future can mean that a previously planned operation could have the opposite effect to what is now desired.

Safer Surgery Principles

Despite improvements in care, avoidable surgical complications account for a substantial number of preventable injuries and deaths worldwide.

Two key factors making surgery safer are teamwork and communication, which are utterly dependent on each other. When an operation is performed on a patient, it depends on a combination of personnel from the ward, theatres, support staff, anaesthetic, and surgical teams. The exact combination of people working together to help a patient on any particular day is rarely the same. Communicating all relevant information to the whole team assembled can seem like a greater task than the operation itself but can be made much easier by completing a 'Surgical Checklist'.

The World Health Organization produces surgical safety guidance which identifies a core set of safety checks for improving performance at critical time points within the patient's care pathway. The checklist provides structure and guidance for surgical teams, allowing them to work together in a safer and more effective manner. This guidance has been widely adopted in many countries, including the United Kingdom. One of the key features is the introduction of safety checks (briefing, sign in, time out, surgical pause, sign out, and debriefing) for all surgical procedures (Fig. 17.1).

A briefing, which all key members of the team attend, is performed at the start of the operating theatre session. For each patient, the discussion includes the planned procedure, expected duration, any allergies, relevant comorbidities, patient positioning, equipment requirements, any prophylaxis required such as antibiotics, and measures to prevent venous thromboembolism. Further patient-specific checks also take place prior to anaesthesia, prior to skin incision, and at the completion of the procedure. The 'sign out' at

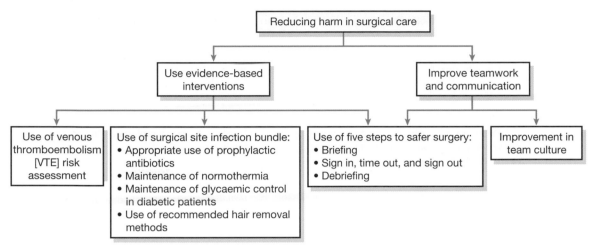

Fig. 17.1 Safer surgery principles.

the end of the operation also includes a check that all surgical equipment—such as instruments, swabs, or needles—are accounted for to guard against anything being unintentionally left inside the patient.

At the end of the surgical session, a review of any problems encountered is needed to ensure that steps are taken to avoid these in the future and promote further improvements in safety and care.

Gynaecological Operations

Gynaecological surgery generally involves removal or repair of the tissues of the female genital tract. In gynaecology cancer surgery, this will also include removal of sites to which gynaecological cancers may have spread, for example, lymph nodes or omentum. Many of these procedures will be discussed in other chapters. Therefore, only an overview will be given here. Common gynaecological operations are listed in Table 17.1.

Hysterectomy is a common operation and can be performed by an abdominal (open), laparoscopic (keyhole), or vaginal approach. Once under anaesthesia, the woman is positioned for surgery, the surgical site disinfected, surgical drapes applied, and a urinary catheter placed.

ABDOMINAL (OPEN) HYSTERECTOMY

Options for the position of the skin incision are shown in Fig. 17.2. The choice between a low transverse incision (Pfannenstiel), a midline incision, or a paramedian incision will depend on the indication for the hysterectomy. A midline approach will allow access to the pelvis and upper abdomen and is usually required for gynaecology cancer surgery. The omentum and lymph nodes can be removed, and the incision can be extended as needed to complete the surgery. This is also required for larger non-cancerous pelvic masses, such as fibroids or large ovarian cysts, especially as it is preferable to remove some types of large cysts intact (e.g., where there is a suspicion of malignancy). Paramedian incisions can help avoid adhesions and reduce risk of bowel or bladder injuries in women with previous midline incisions. The Pfannenstiel incision allows access to the pelvis for most other types of surgery. It is quicker and less painful to recover from and has a lower risk of developing a hernia at the incision site compared with a midline incision.

The skin, subcutaneous layer of adipose tissue, rectus sheath (with rectus muscles separated and pushed aside) and the peritoneum are encountered in turn to reach the peritoneal cavity (Fig. 17.3).

The specific findings in the pelvis will determine the steps to follow. Large cysts may have to be removed first so that the rest of the pelvis can be accessed to perform a hysterectomy. There are steps common to most hysterectomies. The division and suturing of the round ligament on each side will detach the uterus from two of its supporting structures. This allows access to the broad ligament, where the uterine artery

TABLE 17.1 Common Gynaecological Operations

Site	Procedure	Indication
Vulva	Radical vulvectomy	Advanced vulval cancer
	Wide local excision	Early vulval cancer
	Excision biopsy	Vulval intraepithelial neoplasia (VIN)/suspicious vulval lesion
Vagina	Anterior colporrhaphy (anterior vaginal repair)	Cystocele—bladder prolapse into vagina
	Posterior colporrhaphy (posterior vaginal repair)	Rectocele—rectal prolapse into vagina
	Manchester repair (removal of cervix and anterior colporrhaphy)	Vaginal prolapse
	Sacrospinous fixation	Prolapse of the vaginal vault (after hysterectomy or with the uterus preserved)
Cervix	Radical trachelectomy (removal of cervix with preservation of uterus)	Early-stage cervical cancer and wish for fertility preservation
Endometrium	Endometrial ablation (destruction of the endometrium without hysterectomy)	Some causes of abnormal uterine bleeding (AUB), most commonly heavy menstrual bleeding (HMB)
	Endometrial resection (removal of the endometrium without hysterectomy)	Symptomatic fibroids, symptomatic endometrial polyps
Uterus	Total abdominal hysterectomy (removal of uterus and cervix via laparotomy)	HMB
		Symptomatic uterine fibroids
	Subtotal abdominal hysterectomy (removal of the uterus only, without removal of the cervix)	As above, where there is an anticipated low future risk of cervical abnormality
	Total laparoscopic hysterectomy	Early-stage endometrial and cervical cancer
		Some causes of AUB or HMB in which the uterus is not significantly enlarged
	Radical hysterectomy (Wertheim hysterectomy)	Stage 1B1 cervical cancer
	Vaginal hysterectomy	Uterine prolapse
		HMB in which the uterus is not significantly enlarged
	Myomectomy (removal of uterine fibroid without hysterectomy)	Symptomatic fibroids and wish for fertility preservation
		Fibroids contributing to subfertility
Fallopian tube	Salpingectomy (removal of fallopian tube)	Ectopic pregnancy or hydrosalpinx (fluid filled, blocked and presumed non-functional fallopian tube)
	Salpingotomy (removal of pregnancy tissue from the fallopian tube without removal of the tube)	Ectopic pregnancy with previously removed, scarred, or absent fallopian tube on the opposite side to the ectopic pregnancy, and wish to preserve fertility
	Laparoscopic sterilization	Permanent non-hormonal contraception
Ovary	Oophorectomy (removal of ovary; the fallopian tube next to the ovary is often removed at the same time: salpingo-oophorectomy)	Ovarian mass suspicious for malignancy
		Risk-reducing surgery to prevent other disease (ovarian cancer or breast cancer recurrence)
		Severe symptoms of pre-menstrual syndrome
	Ovarian cystectomy (removal of ovarian cyst without removal of ovary)	Ovarian cyst at lower risk of malignancy, with wish to preserve maximal healthy ovarian tissue
Pelvis and upper abdomen	Total abdominal hysterectomy plus bilateral salpingo-oophorectomy plus omentectomy (removal of the omentum) and lymphadenectomy (removal of pelvic or aortic lymph nodes)	Ovarian cancer
		More advanced grade or stage endometrial cancer

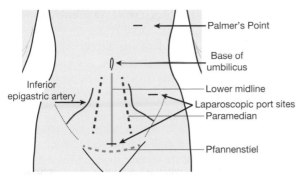

Fig. 17.2 Skin incisions for open and laparoscopic gynaecological surgery.

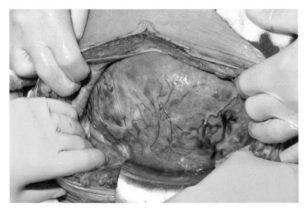

Fig. 17.3 The pelvis at the start of an abdominal hysterectomy. The peritoneal cavity has been opened using a midline incision. This shows placenta accreta invading the lower uterine segment and grossly distorting anatomy. A baby boy was born with a classical uterine incision, the placenta left in place, and then hysterectomy performed.

and ureter pass, and can sometimes allow these structures to be more easily identified. For cases in which the fallopian tubes and ovaries are being removed with a hysterectomy, the infundibulo-pelvic ligaments are cut and sutured on each side. The ovarian ligaments are a continuation of the infundibulo-pelvic ligaments. They run between the ovary and uterus and are cut and sutured if the ovaries are being left in place. The loose peritoneum (utero-vesical fold) between the front of the uterus and the bladder is opened to create space between the cervix and the bladder; this increases the distance between the ureter and the uterine vessels. The uterine artery and vein are cut and sutured on each side of the uterus at the junction between the

uterus and the cervix. The uterus is separated from the cervix at this point in a subtotal hysterectomy (STAH). For a total hysterectomy (TAH), the tissue alongside the cervix (to the point where it joins the vagina) is cut and sutured. The uterus and cervix can now be removed. The circular hole left at the upper part of the vagina, where the cervix was previously attached, is sutured closed. Before closing the abdominal wall, the pelvis is checked for any ongoing bleeding. The peritoneum is usually not sutured; most of the strength of the abdominal wall closure is given by the suture used to close the rectus sheath. Using dissolving sutures to help oppose the subcutaneous layers of fat can be helpful for skin healing. The skin edges are sutured or stapled so that the edges touch, ideally without tension or overlap.

Laparoscopic Hysterectomy

Laparoscopic operations are usually performed, where possible, in preference to an open operation. The benefits of minimally invasive surgery are quicker recovery, less pain, and less thrombo-embolism, amongst others (Box 17.1).

The woman is positioned flat with the hips flexed at 45 degrees, and a urinary catheter placed to empty the bladder. A uterine manipulator instrument is placed into the uterus to help position and reposition it to make certain steps easier during surgery.

Next, the peritoneal cavity has to be filled with carbon dioxide gas to create a pneumoperitoneum. Carbon dioxide is used because it is low cost, not flammable, and any residual gas is readily absorbed and excreted by the body after the procedure. The pneumoperitoneum can be created at the umbilicus with a specially designed device (Veress needle) or by performing a small 1- to 2-cm incision (Hasson technique) to allow the laparoscopic instrument port to be placed into the abdomen. This will be used to

BOX 17.1 ADVANTAGES OF LAPAROSCOPIC SURGERY

- Reduced risk of wound infection
- Shorter hospital stay
- Less postoperative pain
- Reduced blood loss
- Quicker return to normal activities

introduce the gas. Alternatively, transparent laparoscopic ports can be used to first enter the peritoneal cavity under direct vision, and then to introduce the gas. Where adhesions are anticipated underneath the umbilicus, Palmer's point (3 cm below the left costal margin in the left upper quadrant) can be used instead (see Fig. 17.2).

Once the pneumoperitoneum has been created, the laparoscopic camera is used to guide the insertion of other instrument ports. The woman is tilted in a head-down position to move the small bowel out of the pelvis (Fig. 17.4). Laparoscopic devices, which use electrical or ultrasonic energy, are used to cut and seal (rather than suture) the ligaments around the uterus in a similar approach to open hysterectomy. The uterus can be moved in relation to the instruments to facilitate this and guide the surgeon where to divide between the cervix and the vagina. The uterus is removed through the vagina, and then the hole at the top of the vagina is sutured closed. After checking for bleeding, the ports and the carbon dioxide are removed, and the skin incisions infiltrated with local anaesthetic and sutured closed.

VAGINAL HYSTERECTOMY

Vaginal surgery has perhaps the best outcomes for women with less pain and better postoperative mobility. Although the size of the incision used to perform a vaginal hysterectomy, or vaginal prolapse repair, might be larger than laparoscopic surgery, the amount of pain caused appears to be much less, leading to a comparatively faster recovery. It can also be performed

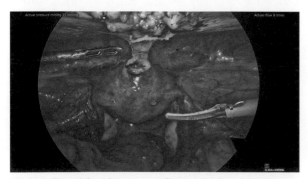

Fig. 17.4 The pelvis at laparoscopy. Dense adhesions following caesarean section between the uterus, bladder, and anterior abdominal wall are being divided with an ultrasonic energy device. Following this, laparoscopic hysterectomy could proceed.

under regional anaesthetics (spinal) in women who are not suitable for a general anaesthetic.

The woman is placed in the lithotomy position, with the legs abducted to almost 90 degrees in order to give as much access for the surgery as possible. The bladder is typically not emptied and left partly filled to make it easier to identify. The first step is to separate the cervix from the vagina using diathermy or a scalpel. Each step in a vaginal hysterectomy allows for further movement of the cervix towards the surgeon. The bladder is pushed upwards away from the cervix and uterus, and the uterine arteries and veins on each side are clamped, cut, and sutured. This allows further movement of the uterus towards the surgeon to cut and suture the ovarian and round ligaments. The uterus can be removed from the vagina, and the incision at the top of the vagina is sutured. Limits on the length of surgical instruments mean that the ovaries are usually retained during vaginal hysterectomy. A urinary catheter is sometimes placed at the end of the procedure to check for haematuria and for postoperative monitoring of urine output.

Postoperative Care

After an operation, the patient usually initially feels worse than preoperatively. This is the point from which the postoperative recovery starts. The rule to follow is that the patient should get better every day. This is true of all patients, particularly younger patients undergoing laparoscopic surgery. A failure to improve could be the first sign of any developing complication, ranging from very minor and self-limiting to serious and warranting urgent subsequent lifesaving surgery. The time frame over which someone gets better every day depends on how much of an impact the operation has had on that individual's baseline health. It will vary greatly from person to person. The more informative comparison is between the patient's condition today and how the patient felt yesterday and the day before that.

Damage to the ureter is one of the more high-profile complications of gynaecological surgery. This is perhaps because the damage can be undetected at the time of surgery, requires the input of another surgical specialty to repair, and, most importantly, can mean multiple subsequent procedures for the woman. The risk of medico-legal action tends to follow the complications, which creates the most negative lasting impact to the patient. Bowel damage is another serious complication that may require a greatly extended stay after the initial operation or a further laparotomy for control of postoperative peritonitis with emergency stoma formation.

In contrast, bleeding and infection are almost ubiquitous risks with surgery. Thus, measures such as having the correct blood type available in case an urgent transfusion is needed or giving prophylactic antibiotics before the first incision can reduce these risks. Gynaecological surgery particularly predisposes to venous thromboembolism. Calf compression and low molecular weight heparin for all but the shortest operations will reduce the risk of harm for the woman.

Voiding of urine can be affected by many gynaecological procedures, particularly when there has been surgery near the bladder. Following removal of a urinary catheter, complete emptying of the bladder should be demonstrated, as residual urine can predispose to urinary tract infection and longer-term voiding difficulties.

Most women will be discharged from the hospital to complete their recovery at home. It can be more useful and realistic to give a range for this. For example, the patient could be informed that "most people have recovered enough to go back to work after 6 to 8 weeks from the operation, with some taking longer even if the operation goes well." This is much more informative than simply predicting a "6-week recovery."

An awareness of what might be signs of complications which present later after surgery is essential. A clear plan as to how the woman can access advice or help after returning home is also needed.

There is typically a follow-up plan. A letter with the results of specimens biopsied, a phone call a few weeks later, a clinic visit, further surgery, or no follow-up at all may be entirely appropriate.

Key Points

- **The decision to have surgery is best made jointly between the woman and the surgeon after a discussion of the advantages, disadvantages, harms, benefits, and all alternative treatment options, including having no treatment.**
- **Consent is a process which runs in parallel to the decision for surgery.**
- **Communication and teamwork are essential to a well-performing surgical team.**
- **The consistent use of surgical checklists improves patient safety.**

Reproductive Health

Section Outline

Chapter 18

Sexually Transmitted Infections

Dan Clutterbuck

Chapter Outline

Introduction

Sexually transmitted infections (STIs) – including syphilis, gonorrhoea, genital herpes, genital warts, chlamydia, trichomoniasis and *Mycoplasma genitalium* – are transmitted via the moist mucous membranes of the vulva, vagina, cervix, anus, rectum and oropharynx during sexual activity. Untreated STIs in women can lead to chronic pain or infertility and may lead to genital cancers, including cervical, vulval and anal carcinoma. Ulcerative STIs increase the risk of transmission of untreated human immunodeficiency virus (HIV) about threefold.

STIs in pregnant women can cause serious complications, including stillbirth, neonatal death, prematurity, neonatal sepsis, low birth weight and congenital abnormalities. Other infections, including bacterial vaginosis (BV) and *Candida albicans*, are a very common cause of symptoms but are not sexually transmitted and do not have serious sequelae. Pelvic inflammatory disease (PID) is associated with STI in a minority of cases.

In 2020, the World Health Organization estimated that there were 374 million new cases of the four major curable STIs (syphilis, gonorrhoea, chlamydia, and trichomoniasis) in adults aged 15 to 49 years throughout the world each year, with 90% in low and middle income countries.

Sexually transmissible blood-borne viruses (BBVs), including hepatitis B and HIV, are transmitted horizontally (through sex) and vertically (from mother to child). Hepatitis B is a highly infectious virus affecting 257 million people worldwide (2015), with the main route of acquisition being by neonates at birth or in the first year of life. Of these, 90% will develop chronic infection, with a 15% to 40% chance of cirrhosis and hepatocellular carcinoma. A total of 38 million people worldwide were living with HIV

at the end of 2019, of whom 25 million were taking antiretroviral therapy (ART); 85% of pregnant women had access to antiretrovirals to prevent mother-to-child transmission, with a 50% reduction in new HIV infections in children since 2010. The worldwide fall in new infections observed since 2010 has been greater in women and girls (27%) than in men and boys (18%), but the global ambition to achieve 'three zeros' by 2030 – zero new HIV infections, zero AIDS-related deaths and zero discrimination – has stalled significantly since 2017.

Rates of all STIs can vary dramatically geographically and over time, affected by social disruption such as war, economic decline or mass migration; the availability of tests and services; treatment and vaccination programmes; and social mores and sexual behaviour. For example, rates of gonorrhoea and syphilis fell dramatically in the United Kingdom and elsewhere with the widespread availability of effective antibiotics following the end of the Second World War, whereas infections increased substantially in much of Eastern Europe in the 1990s following the collapse of the former Soviet Union. In countries including Australia and the United Kingdom, diagnoses of genital warts have fallen dramatically in cohorts vaccinated against human papillomavirus (HPV). However, the prevailing trend for most STIs in the United Kingdom in this century has been upwards, with sustained rises in gonorrhoea, chlamydia, and herpes infections in women since 2006. Contributory factors include changes in sexual behaviour, new ways of sexual mixing (such as the use of mobile phone apps), early sexual debut, increased geographical mobility within and between countries, the emergence of drug-resistant strains, asymptomatic infections and barriers to accessing testing and treatment services, often affecting those most at risk of infection. The longer-term overall effect of multiple and potentially opposing impacts of the global COVID-19 pandemic, in reducing opportunities for social interaction but also limiting access to testing and treatment, are not yet clear.

The risk of STI acquisition is increased with younger age (under 25 years), prior STI diagnosis, frequent partner change or concurrent partners, non-use of condoms and high rates of condom errors. However, for many women, particularly in low-resource settings, it is the social and demographic risk factors affecting the community from which she chooses a regular partner, rather than her own individual risk factors, that determine her STI risk.

Principles of Sexually Transmitted Infection Management

To minimize the harms from STIs in women, the aim is to ensure early diagnosis, appropriate testing, early treatment and partner notification to break the chain of infection. Symptoms of genital infection in women include vaginal discharge, abnormal vaginal bleeding, pelvic pain, genital lumps and ulceration. However, in the majority of cases, women presenting with these symptoms do not have STI. Conversely, most STIs are asymptomatic: about 70% of women with chlamydia, 50% with gonorrhoea, 30% with HPV and 50% with genital herpes have no symptoms. Consequently, performing STI testing solely in all women who present with genital symptoms will result in large numbers of tests being performed on women at very low risk of STI but will miss or delay a diagnosis in women at risk both of serious complications and of onward horizontal and vertical transmission of infection. The use of a recognisable set of signs and symptoms to identify the likely infective cause and guide antimicrobial treatment without diagnostic testing is termed 'syndromic management'. It is increasingly supported by improvements in availability, reliability and speed of diagnostic testing technologies, in particular, nucleic acid amplification tests (NAATs). However, diagnosis on the basis of observed syndromes (e.g., vaginal discharge) remains valuable even in resource-rich settings where sophisticated tests are widely available. Syndromic management is part of a public health approach which includes the following components:

- Syndromic management *without diagnostic testing* in women at low risk of STI or where access to testing technology is limited: women presenting with vaginal discharge may be treated empirically following a clinical diagnosis
- Syndromic management *with diagnostic testing* and treatment before test results are available in women at higher risk of STI: women clinically diagnosed with clinical genital herpes or PID are treated immediately
- Diagnostic testing for STI according to individual or population-based risk assessment, clinical setting and local and national resources
- Partner notification (identifying, tracing, treating and/or testing the partners of women diagnosed with possible STI) to prevent reinfection and/or onward transmission
- Routine population-based screening for infections which are common and/or have serious sequelae in particular subpopulations (e.g., antenatal syphilis, HIV and hepatitis B testing, chlamydia screening in those under 25 years of age)
- Prophylactic treatment in women undergoing procedures associated with the risk of ascending infection (e.g., termination of pregnancy)
- Vaccination – highly effective vaccines against hepatitis B and HPV are widely available; vaccines against HIV, herpes simplex virus (HSV) and other STIs are in development.

In routine clinical practice, the risk of missing a serious STI diagnosis is reduced by maintaining a low threshold for testing in both symptomatic and asymptomatic women, a high level of awareness of the genital and non-genital manifestations of STI and, above all, routinely including an STI risk assessment in clinical history taking.

Once an STI has been diagnosed, partner notification (contact tracing) is essential in the management of bacterial STIs, HIV and hepatitis B, both to prevent reinfection in those who are curable and to avoid further onward transmission. Partner notification strategies include patient referral, in which the patient informs recent partner(s); provider referral, in which details are passed to a health care professional who then contacts the partners; and conditional referral, in which provider referral is initiated if patient referral has not occurred after an agreed period has elapsed. In provider referral, it is usual to protect the identity of the index patient. The use of enhanced partner notification strategies is increasing, which includes providing the patient with antibiotic treatment for the partner or with a pharmacy voucher for treatment and the use of innovative web applications or mobile apps to allow patients to inform partners while preserving anonymity. Patients are advised to abstain from sex until they and their partner(s) have completed treatment.

Sexual History

STI diagnosis and management in individual women depends on an accurate assessment of risk factors for particular STIs. This makes a comprehensive understanding of symptoms, current and past sexual partners, and other risk activities a crucial part of STI management.

A woman presenting with genital symptoms may or may not have considered the possibility of an STI and women attending for other reasons, such as termination of pregnancy, may be unaware of STI risk. Time, sensitivity and privacy must be ensured: interviews should take place in a soundproof setting. Accurate answers to a risk assessment may not be possible with a partner or relative present. Questioning should be sensitive, inclusive and appropriate but direct, avoiding euphemisms. As with all history taking, choice of words and appropriate facial expressions and body language in the questioner are important. Use open language to avoid conveying any impression of being judgmental; examples are the use of inclusive words, such as 'partner' rather than 'boyfriend'.

After eliciting a history of any presenting symptoms, medication, contraception and a gynaecological history, the sexual history should be taken. An introduction such as 'Do you have a (sexual) partner?' may sometimes be used if she is not expecting questions about sexual contacts, followed by the key question 'When did you last have sex?' whether the answer is positive or negative. For recent contact(s), the important factors affecting the risk and site of infection include the partner status (one-off, regular or other), partner gender, the types of sex that took place, use of condoms, the partner's place of origin and consent to sex. The same questions should be asked about other partners in the last 3 months. See Box 18.1 for further suggestions on sexual history taking for STIs. An assessment of lifetime risk may be useful in deciding

BOX 18.1 SEXUAL HISTORY TAKING FOR SEXUALLY TRANSMITTED INFECTIONS (STIs)

A model for sexual history taking for STIs with examples.

1. One simple framing statement before taking the sexual history avoids any sense of apology or embarrassment. 'So, thinking about your sex life …, Some questions about your sex life …'.
2. Open questions should be used at the start. 'Tell me…, Tell me about that …, So tell me the story …'.
3. More open questions are employed to establish detail. 'Tell me more about how this pain developed …, What is the discharge like …?'
4. Straightforward anatomical terms should be used as much as possible ('vagina' is OK, 'vulva' often is not). 'So, you mean on the lips of your vagina?'
5. Focussing on events helps to avoid labels and generalizations. 'When did you last have sex, any sort of sex …?'
6. Permission giving can be included in the question (explicit permission for a range of answers). 'Was that a one-off thing, with a regular partner, or something else? Have your partners been men, women or both? Was that oral sex, vaginal sex, anal sex … or all of them?'
7. The 'non-acceptable' or non-sanctioned answer should be invited. 'So that was without a condom …? Do you ever use condoms? When did you last have sober sex?'
8. Remember that partners' place of origin is a major determinant of STI risk. 'So, was he/she from (this town/city) … or elsewhere? Any partners from outside the UK?'.
9. Gentleness should be balanced with directness. 'So, did everything happen with your consent or perhaps not?'
10. Display innocent inquisitiveness to understand social issues. 'I really don't know much about which dating apps people use to meet up … can you tell me more?'
11. Make every question permissive of a full range of possible answers. 'When did you last have sex with anyone else/any other partner?'
12. Understand and mitigate the ways in which your own values might affect your questioning. 'When was your last previous partner?' (which assumes serial monogamy – so avoid).

on whether testing for BBVs is indicated, although universal testing at antenatal booking and when testing for STI is recommended in most national guidelines and avoids the need for detailed risk assessment:

- When, if ever was she last tested for HIV or hepatitis?
- In young women from areas with higher HIV or hepatitis prevalence (e.g., sub-Saharan Africa), is there any risk of undiagnosed vertical infection?

- Since her last test:
  - Has she been sexually active in an area with higher HIV or hepatitis prevalence?
  - Has she had any male partners she knows to have been bisexual?
  - Has she or any partner used intravenous recreational drugs?

Examination for Genital Infections

Examination should be performed in all women with symptoms. Informed consent is required, following a full description of the examination and any samples taken and the offer of a chaperone regardless of the practitioner's gender. Male clinicians must have a chaperone when examining a woman's genital tract.

Genital examination is directed by the presenting symptoms and the clinician should:

- Inspect the pubic hair and surrounding skin for pubic lice and any skin rashes.
- Palpate the inguinal region for lymphadenopathy.
- Inspect the labia majora and minora, clitoris, introitus, perineum and perianal area for warts, ulcers, erythema or excoriation.
- Inspect the urethral meatus and Skene and Bartholin glands for any discharge or swelling.
- Insert a bivalve speculum into the vagina.
- Inspect the vaginal walls for erythema, discharge, warts and ulcers.
- Inspect the cervix for discharge, erythema, contact bleeding, ulcers or raised lesions. Mucopurulent discharge from the cervix should be noted but is not a reliable indicator of infection.
- Perform a bimanual pelvic examination to assess size and any tenderness of the uterus, cervical motion tenderness and adnexal tenderness or masses.

Taking Samples for Genital Infections

Syndromic management alone is appropriate for women at low risk of STI who present with genital warts or a first episode of uncomplicated vaginal discharge. In most other situations, samples for microbiological testing are indicated. NAATs are widely available for the diagnosis of chlamydia, gonorrhoea, and herpes simplex, and increasingly commonly for trichomoniasis and symptomatic early syphilis (ulcers). The following tests are routinely offered to symptomatic and asymptomatic women at risk of STI in non-specialist settings:

- A lower vaginal swab (obtained by the clinician or by the woman) for NAATs for both chlamydia and gonorrhoea
- A blood sample for syphilis and HIV serology
- Hepatitis B testing* of the same sample if the woman or any of her sexual partners are from areas of high hepatitis B prevalence (e.g., sub-Saharan Africa or Asia)
- Hepatitis B* and C testing, if the woman or any of her sexual partners have ever injected drugs or are men who have sex with men (MSM)
- Additional samples may be indicated depending on presentation:
  - Samples for NAATs for herpes simplex and syphilis may be taken if ulcers or fissures are seen
  - Additional samples for NAATs for chlamydia and gonorrhoea may be taken from other sites of potential exposure (throat and/or rectum)
  - Samples of vaginal discharge may be taken for microscopy in cases of recurrent, complicated or atypical discharge. NAATs and enzyme tests to detect the organisms of BV are available but not widely used.
  - If a woman is to be treated for suspected gonorrhoea, in addition to NAATs as described earlier, swabs for culture for gonorrhoea placed in Amies, Stuart or similar transport media, or directly inoculating a culture plate, may be taken from the urethra and endocervix for antibiotic sensitivity testing.
  - NAAT technology continues to develop in the speed with which results are available, the availability of clinic-based machines, the development of NAAT-based sensitivity testing, and the range of organisms tested. In addition to *Chlamydia trachomatis* and *Neisseria gonorrhoeae*, tests for *Trichomonas vaginalis* (TV), *M. genitalium* and other organisms are increasingly available.

---

*Hepatitis B immunization should be offered if the hepatitis B test is negative and she is at continued risk.

Syndromes Associated With Genital Infections

ASYMPTOMATIC

Many infections are completely asymptomatic; thus, testing should be considered on the basis of risk factors. In many areas, all women attending for health care will be offered HIV testing or those under the age of 25 years will be routinely offered testing for chlamydial infection.

VAGINAL DISCHARGE

An increase in vaginal discharge may be due to a number of infective and non-infective conditions (Table 18.1). Even in areas of high STI prevalence, most women presenting with vaginal discharge alone will not have an STI. Thus, syndromic management of first presentation of vaginal discharge without microbiological testing is often appropriate in women with no recent change of sexual partner.

Symptoms can help to distinguish the causes and anatomical origin of a vaginal discharge, as follows:

- An increase in vaginal discharge without any itch or irritation accompanied by an unpleasant or fishy odour, which may be worse after sexual intercourse and during menstruation, indicates the possibility of BV.
- Vulval itching accompanied by a thick, white vaginal discharge, vulval burning, external dysuria and superficial dyspareunia may indicate candidiasis.
- A purulent or mucopurulent discharge, with blood staining and/or post-coital or intermenstrual bleeding indicates the possibility of a discharge originating from an inflamed cervix, more

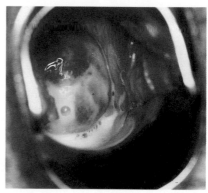

Fig. 18.1 Bacterial vaginosis (BV). BV is due to an overgrowth of anaerobic bacteria, genital mycoplasmas, and *Gardnerella vaginalis*. The discharge is milky white, adherent to the vaginal walls and may be frothy.

commonly associated with STI, including chlamydia and gonorrhoea.

- Abdominal, pelvic or back pain, deep dyspareunia, or systemic symptoms may suggest infection that has ascended to the uterus, ovaries and/or fallopian tubes, or is systemic.
- Signs elicited on examination may assist with the diagnosis:
- An absence of any inflammation of the vulva or vagina and a discharge with a homogeneous, white appearance which is adherent to the vaginal walls and may be malodourous is typical of BV (Fig. 18.1).
- Vulval erythema – sometimes with satellite lesions, fissuring, excoriation and oedema – may indicate vulvovaginal candidiasis. Discharge may be thick or curdy, occasionally with typical white candidal plaques on the vaginal walls (Fig. 18.2).
- A purulent malodourous yellow or grey vaginal discharge with vulval erythema and excoriation and inflammation of the vaginal walls in a sexually active woman raises the possibility of trichomoniasis.
- A purulent or blood-stained cervical discharge may increase the suspicion of chlamydial or gonococcal infection, indicating that tests for these infections should be undertaken.

Additional tests can be performed:

- Narrow-range pH paper can be used to test the pH of the vaginal discharge, avoiding

TABLE 18.1	Causes of Vaginal Discharge
Vaginal infections	Bacterial vaginosis
	Candida albicans
	Trichomonas vaginalis
Cervical infections	*Chlamydia trachomatis*
	Neisseria gonorrhoeae
Physiological discharge	Cervical ectopy
Other causes	Retained tampon
	Retained products of conception

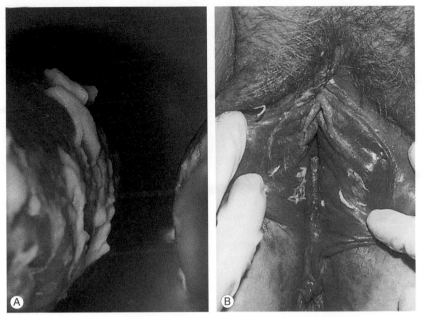

Fig. 18.2 Candidal infection. (A, B) Although *Candida* may present with these 'typical' white plaques, the discharge is sometimes minimal. (**A**, From McMillan A, Young H, Ogilvie MM, Scott GR, eds. *Clinical Practice in Sexually Transmissible Infections*. WB Saunders; 2003. **B**, From Clutterbuck D. *Specialist Training in Sexually Transmitted Infections and HIV*. Mosby; 2005.)

contamination with cervical mucus, which has a pH of 7 and will give a falsely high reading. A pH of >4.9 suggests the presence of anaerobic organisms (which metabolize nitrogen into amine compounds) and supports a diagnosis of BV or, less commonly, trichomoniasis. The pH of the vagina with normal flora or with candidal infection is below 4.5.

- A swab of vaginal secretions is taken from the lateral vaginal walls and the posterior fornix. Samples are inoculated onto glass slides for immediate Gram staining and wet-mount direct microscopy in the specialist sexual health clinic or the swab is sent to the laboratory in a transport medium (e.g., Amies) for examination.
  - Microscopy of a Gram-stained sample may reveal depletion of normal lactobacilli and mixed organisms diagnostic of BV, or the Pseudohyphae and spores of candidal infection.
  - Examination of a wet mount (suspending the discharge in a drop of saline) may reveal Clue cells (epithelial cells covered with bacteria that are 'clues' to the diagnosis of BV) or the motile flagellate trichomonads of TV.
- Culture of vaginal samples is not routinely indicated and is rarely helpful.

Infections of the Vagina

BACTERIAL VAGINOSIS

Background Information

BV is the most common cause of vaginal discharge in women of reproductive age, found in around 9% of women in general practice, 12% of pregnant women, and 30% of women undergoing termination of pregnancy. BV is due to an overgrowth of anaerobic bacteria, genital mycoplasmas and *Gardnerella vaginalis* (all of which can normally be present in small numbers in the vagina). Risk of BV is clearly linked to sexual activity and is associated with multiple male or female partners, having a new sexual partner, and non-use of condoms. However, treating male partners of women with BV does not affect recurrence. Thus, it is not regarded as an STI. Partner notification and treatment is not recommended.

About 50% of women with BV are asymptomatic. A total of 30% to 50% of women are colonized with *G. vaginalis*, anaerobes and mycoplasmas as part of their normal vaginal flora; thus, culture is not helpful in the diagnosis of BV.

Treatment

Asymptomatic non-pregnant women do not need treatment. Treatment is recommended in all women with symptoms and those undergoing gynaecological surgery (including surgical termination of pregnancy).

Treatments include:
- metronidazole 400 mg twice daily for 7 days
- intravaginal clindamycin cream 2% once daily for 7 days.

Complications

BV increases vaginal vault infection following hysterectomy, postpartum endometritis following caesarean section and post-abortal PID after surgical termination of pregnancy.

It increases a woman's risk of acquiring HIV infection two- to threefold, and may also increase the risk of transmission of HIV to a male partner.

CANDIDAL INFECTIONS
Background Information

Some 75% of all women experience at least one episode of symptomatic *Candida* in their lifetime. About 20% of asymptomatic women have vaginal colonization with *Candida*. Increased rates of colonization (30%–40%) are found in pregnancy and uncontrolled diabetes. Factors associated with symptomatic *Candida* are pregnancy, diabetes, immunosuppression, antimicrobial therapy and vulval irritation/trauma. It is not sexually acquired; thus, sexual partners do not need to be treated.

Diagnosis

Microscopy and culture is the most sensitive method of diagnosis. However, in many cases, syndromic management without testing is appropriate. The sensitivity of clinical diagnosis increases with the number of symptoms and signs present. Up to half of women who self-diagnose candidal infection have another condition.

Treatment

Azole antifungals are widely used for treatment:
- oral fluconazole 150 mg single dose (oral azoles are contraindicated in pregnancy)
- clotrimazole pessaries for 1, 3 or 6 nights.

Complications

There are no known long-term complications from candidal infections.

TRICHOMONAS VAGINALIS
Background Information

TV is uncommon in the United Kingdom. However, in other parts of the world – for example, Africa and Asia – it remains a major cause of vaginal discharge. It is sexually transmitted and infects only the urogenital tract. It may be asymptomatic in 10% to 50% of women but can cause significant vulval and vaginal inflammation.

Treatment

The recommended treatment is:
- metronidazole 2 g single oral dose, or
- metronidazole 400 mg orally twice daily for 5 to 7 days.

Of women with TV, up to 30% have gonorrhoea and/or chlamydia. Thus, they should be tested for other STIs. Women should abstain from sex until they and their partner(s) have completed treatment.

Complications

TV increases a woman's risk of acquiring HIV infection and in pregnancy is associated with low birth weight and pre-term delivery.

Infections of the Cervix
CHLAMYDIA TRACHOMATIS
Background Information

C. trachomatis is the most frequently seen bacterial STI, affecting 3% of all women aged 16 to 24 years who have ever had a sexual partner in the United Kingdom and around 14% of those aged 20 to 24 years attending sexual health clinics. The prevalence of chlamydial infection falls steeply with age. The natural history of infection is not fully understood; in more than 50%

of cases, the infection resolves spontaneously without complications. However, it can cause PID, chronic pain and tubal infertility. Screening for, and treating, asymptomatic chlamydia may reduce the rate of PID. England has a chlamydia screening programme.

Symptoms and Signs

- The cervix is the primary site of infection, but the urethra is also infected in about 50% of cases. Chlamydia can also infect the pharynx and rectum.
- Approximately 70% of women with chlamydia are asymptomatic.
- If symptoms are present, they are usually non-specific, such as post-coital bleeding, increased vaginal discharge and dysuria.
- Lower abdominal pain, dyspareunia and inter-menstrual bleeding may be present if the infection has spread beyond the cervix.
- On examination, there may be mucopurulent cervicitis (Fig. 18.3) and/or contact bleeding (Fig. 18.4) but the cervix may also look normal.

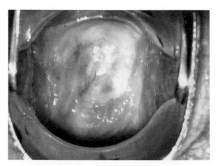

Fig. 18.3 Mucopurulent cervicitis. This may be a feature of infection with *Chlamydia trachomatis* or *Neisseria gonorrhoeae*. The cervix, however, can look normal.

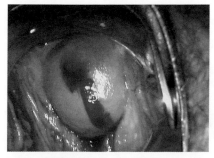

Fig. 18.4 Contact bleeding. This can occur for a number of reasons, one of which is *Chlamydia trachomatis* infection.

Diagnosis

NAATs such as polymerase chain reaction (PCR) have a sensitivity of over 90% for chlamydia and can be performed on vulvovaginal, cervical, pharyngeal, rectal or urine samples. Self-taken vulvovaginal swabs are at least as sensitive as physician-taken cervical swabs and may be used for home-based testing or in the clinic if examination is not otherwise indicated.

Treatment

Uncomplicated chlamydial infection can be treated with:

- doxycycline 100 mg twice daily for 1 week
- azithromycin 1 g single dose, followed by 500 mg daily for 2 days.

Azithromycin is extensively used for the treatment of chlamydia in pregnancy, although this is an unlicenced indication. Women should abstain from sex until they and their partner(s) have completed treatment. A test of cure is not necessary except after treatment in pregnancy. However, reinfection rates are 10% to 30%; thus, re-testing after 6 to 12 months is often advised.

Complications

C. trachomatis can spread beyond the lower genital tract, causing Skene and Bartholin gland abscesses, endometritis, salpingitis and perihepatitis. Around 3% to 10% of women with untreated chlamydia develop symptomatic ascending infection (PID), which may lead to tubal damage, predisposing to tubal pregnancies and tubal infertility, as well as causing chronic pain. Although asymptomatic upper genital tract infection also leads to tubal damage, the proportion of women who develop infertility following asymptomatic chlamydial infection is thought to be low (<1%). Chlamydial infection during pregnancy can cause miscarriage, pre-term birth, postpartum infection, and neonatal ocular and respiratory infection. In genetically susceptible people, sexually acquired reactive arthritis can occur (Reiter syndrome).

NEISSERIA GONORRHOEAE

Background Information

Gonococcal infection rates are around fivefold lower than those of chlamydia in the United Kingdom but have increased dramatically in recent years. In 2019, gonorrhoea rates in England were the highest since records began in 1918 (i.e., long before the antibiotic era). *N. gonorrhoeae* is a highly adaptive organism and gonococcal antibiotic resistance is an increasing global health concern.

Symptoms and Signs

- The cervix is the primary site of infection, but the urethra is also infected in 70% to 90% of cases. Gonorrhoea also commonly affects the pharynx and rectum.
- About 50% of women with gonorrhoea have no symptoms.
- The most common symptoms are increased vaginal discharge, dysuria and post-coital bleeding.
- Lower abdominal pain and intermenstrual bleeding may also be present if the infection has spread beyond the cervix.
- On examination, there may be purulent (Fig. 18.5) or mucopurulent cervicitis and/or contact bleeding – but, again, the cervix may look normal.

Diagnosis

NAATs for *N. gonorrhoeae* are widely used and offer increased sensitivity and convenience over culture. Confirmation of NAAT-positive results by culture allows antibiotic sensitivity testing, although NAAT-based tests for mutations conferring antibiotic resistance are now available. If gonorrhoea is detected in a genital site (e.g., cervix or vulvovaginal swab), non-genital sites (throat, rectum) should also be tested and a test of cure from these sites performed. Treatment

failure, leading to the emergence of resistance, is more likely in non-genital sites.

Treatment

Uncomplicated gonorrhoea in all women, including pregnant and breastfeeding women, can be treated with ceftriaxone 1 g intramuscular (IM) single dose.

Oral cephalosporins are no longer recommended for treatment of gonorrhoea due to worldwide concerns about the emergence of resistance. About 40% of females with gonorrhoea also have *C. trachomatis* infection; thus, they should be tested and treated for chlamydia. Women should abstain from sex until they and their partner(s) have completed treatment.

Complications

N. gonorrhoeae can spread locally beyond the lower genital tract, causing Skene and Bartholin gland abscesses, endometritis, salpingitis, and perihepatitis. About 10% to 20% of women with acute gonococcal infection will develop ascending infection (PID), the resulting damage predisposing to tubal pregnancies and tubal infertility. Infection in pregnancy can cause miscarriage, pre-term birth, postpartum infection, and neonatal infection. Rarely, gonococcal septicaemia can occur and present as an acute arthritis/dermatitis syndrome (disseminated gonococcal infection).

LOWER ABDOMINAL AND PELVIC PAIN

Lower abdominal and pelvic pain can be caused by a number of differing conditions (Table 18.2). PID is particularly common in young (under 25 years) sexually active women.

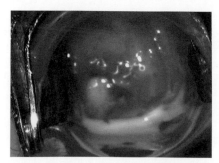

Fig. 18.5 Purulent cervicitis. The cervix is the primary site of infection in 90% of cases of gonococcal infection; a purulent discharge may be seen.

TABLE 18.2	Causes of Lower Abdominal Pain
Uterus	Endometritis (PID)
	Endometriosis
Fallopian tubes	Salpingitis (PID)
	Ectopic pregnancy
Ovary	Torsion of, or haemorrhage into, an ovarian cyst
Urinary tract	Cystitis
Bowel	Acute appendicitis
	Irritable bowel syndrome

PID, Pelvic inflammatory disease.

PELVIC INFLAMMATORY DISEASE

PID results when infections ascend from the cervix or vagina into the upper genital tract. It includes endometritis, salpingitis, tubo-ovarian abscess and pelvic peritonitis. No specific symptoms, signs or laboratory tests are diagnostic of PID. The diagnosis is often made on clinical findings (presence of lower abdominal pain, increased vaginal discharge, cervical motion tenderness and adnexal tenderness on bimanual examination), which together have a positive predictive value (PPV) of 65% to 90% compared with laparoscopy.

The history can help to distinguish PID from lower abdominal and pelvic pain of other cause and anatomical origin:

- Clinical symptoms of PID vary from none to very severe.
- The onset of symptoms often occurs in the first part of the menstrual cycle.
- Lower abdominal pain (usually bilateral) is the most common symptom. Pain affecting the pelvis with deep dyspareunia suggests involvement of the reproductive tract.
- Increased vaginal discharge, irregular or intermenstrual bleeding and post-coital bleeding may indicate cervical or vaginal infection.
- Consider differential diagnoses, including urinary tract infection, appendicitis and ectopic pregnancy.
  - When was her last menstrual period? What contraception has she been using and is there any possibility of her being pregnant?
  - Has she any dysuria, urinary frequency, nocturia or haematuria?
  - Has she any nausea, vomiting, diarrhoea or constipation?

Examination findings support the diagnosis:

- The cervix may have a mucopurulent discharge with contact bleeding, indicative of cervicitis.
- Uterine tenderness, adnexal tenderness or cervical motion tenderness on bimanual examination along with lower abdominal or pelvic pain is sufficient for a diagnosis of PID. Pyrexia and a palpable adnexal mass may also be present.

Diagnosis

- Tests for STIs, including chlamydia and gonorrhoea, should always be performed. Positive results are supportive evidence. Negative results do not exclude the diagnosis.
- Non-specific tests of inflammation such C-reactive protein may be raised, along with the neutrophil count. The absence of pus cells on a slide taken from the cervix or vaginal wall is a sensitive marker of the absence of PID. Laparoscopy, with microbiological specimens from the upper and lower genital tract, is considered the 'gold standard' for diagnosis, but this is not usually appropriate, particularly for those with mild symptoms. Clinical symptoms and signs do not accurately predict the extent of tubal disease found at laparoscopy.

Background Information

C. trachomatis and *N. gonorrhoeae* are important sexually transmitted causes of PID, but *G. vaginalis* and anaerobes associated with BV are also implicated. *M. genitalium* may be associated with PID, but testing for this organism is not routine. PID is commonly and increasingly seen in women without STI. Sometimes, in women with laparoscopically proven PID, no bacterial cause is found. The true incidence of PID is unknown because about two-thirds of cases are asymptomatic.

Treatment

Treatment should not be delayed while waiting for bacteriological test results, as early antibiotic therapy improves outcomes. Outpatient therapy with oral antibiotics is appropriate for clinically mild-to-moderate disease. However, hospitalization is required if there is diagnostic uncertainty, severe symptoms or signs, or failure to respond to oral therapy. Intravenous therapy for the first few days is recommended in women with severe clinical disease. Therapy requires broad-spectrum antibiotics, including cover for gonorrhoea and anaerobes.

Recommended regimens for outpatient therapy include ceftriaxone 1 g IM single dose plus doxycycline 100 mg (oral) twice daily plus metronidazole 400 mg (oral) twice daily for 14 days. For parenteral therapy, second-generation cephalosporins, including cefotetan or cefoxitin plus doxycycline, are preferred.

Appropriate analgesia should be given. Women should abstain from sex until they and their partner(s) have completed treatment. Women with moderate or severe clinical findings should be reviewed after 2 to 3 days to ensure that they are improving. Lack of response to treatment requires further investigation, intravenous therapy and/or surgical intervention. All women should be seen after treatment to check their clinical response and that medication has been completed.

Complications

The main complications from PID are due to tubal damage, with the risk of all complications increasing with severity of infection. Tubal infertility occurs in 10% to 12% of women after one episode of symptomatic PID, 20% to 30% after two episodes and 50% to 60% after three or more episodes. The risk of ectopic pregnancy is increased 6- to 10-fold, with higher rates in women with several episodes. Abdominal or pelvic pain for longer than 6 months occurs in 18% of women. Women with a past history of PID are 5 to 10 times more likely to need hospital admission and undergo hysterectomy.

About one-third of women have repeated infections. This may be due to relapse of infection because of inadequate treatment, reinfection from an untreated partner, post-infection tubal damage, or further acquisition of STIs. In 5% to 15% of women with salpingitis, the infection spreads from the pelvis to the liver capsule, causing perihepatitis (Fitz-Hugh–Curtis syndrome).

DYSURIA

Dysuria is usually due to acute bacterial cystitis, urethritis or vulvitis (Table 18.3). STIs affecting the distal urethra (such as chlamydia and gonorrhoea) occasionally present with dysuria. External dysuria in the absence of frequency or abdominal pain may indicate irritation at the urethral meatus due to candida or genital herpes.

Questions that help distinguish between the causes are:

*   Is the dysuria external, that is, is it as the urine comes into contact with the vulval mucosa?
*   Is there any urinary frequency, nocturia or haematuria?
*   Is there any vaginal discharge, post-coital or intermenstrual bleeding or abdominal pain?

VULVAL ULCERS

Infective lesions are the most common cause of vulval ulcers, with genital herpes the most common cause of genital ulcers in the United Kingdom (Table 18.4).

GENITAL HERPES

Genital herpes can be caused by HSV type 1 or 2. The two viral types are clinically similar: symptoms range from none (asymptomatic); mild irritation and soreness; multiple painful ulcers; or a severe systemic illness with extensive, confluent anogenital ulceration. After an initial episode (often the most severe), HSV ascends the peripheral sensory nerves into the dorsal root ganglion, where latent infection develops. This can reactivate, resulting in recurrent episodes which may or may not be symptomatic but are potentially infectious. Around 75% of first-episode infections are acquired from an asymptomatic partner. Some 90% of people with HSV-2 infection and 60% with HSV-1 will develop recurrences within the first year. The median number of recurrences in year 1 is one in HSV-1 infection and four in HSV-2. Long-term studies show that symptomatic recurrences gradually decrease with time.

Initial Episode

This may be primary infection – the first-ever exposure to either HSV-1 or HSV-2. Over 50% of first-episode genital herpes in the United Kingdom is due to HSV-1:

TABLE 18.3	Causes of Dysuria
Acute bacterial cystitis	Coliform bacteria
	Staphylococcus saprophyticus
Urethritis	*Chlamydia trachomatis*
	Neisseria gonorrhoeae
Vulvitis	Genital herpes
	Candidal infection
	Trichomonas vaginalis
	Vulval dermatological conditions

TABLE 18.4	Types of Vulval Ulcers
Infective	Genital herpes
	Syphilis
Non-infective	Aphthous ulcers
	Behçet syndrome

oral-to-genital transmission is common. Non-primary, initial-episode genital herpes occurs in people with previous orolabial HSV-1 who then acquire genital HSV-2 infection. There is some cross-protection from this prior infection, resulting in a milder illness than in primary infection. These non-primary infections are more likely to be asymptomatic than are primary infections.

Recurrent Herpes

These episodes may be asymptomatic (subclinical shedding). If symptoms are present, they are usually milder than in first infections.

The history can help to determine whether genital ulcers are caused by HSV and establish the stage of infection:

- Multiple painful herpetic ulcers may be preceded by a prodrome of tingling, itching or pain in the area.
- Soreness, itch and external dysuria may initially be mistaken for (and treated as) candidiasis.
- One or more previous similar episodes may be reported in those presenting with recurrence.
- The presence of orolabial or genital sores in a partner supports the diagnosis.
- A history of sex with bisexual males or non-UK partners increases the likelihood of other causes of ulceration, including infectious early syphilis.

On examination:

- Multiple painful superficial ulcers with evidence of lesions at the recognised erythematous, vesicular, ulcerative and resolving stages (Fig. 18.6) confirms the syndromic diagnosis. Tender inguinal lymphadenopathy is present in about 30% of cases.
- In recurrences, there are usually just a few ulcers confined to a small area or the lesions may appear or as fissures or splits.
- Single and/or painless ulcers raise the possibility of other infections (e.g., syphilis) or non-infective ulcers.

Diagnosis

NAATs of swabs from the lesions for HSV-1 and HSV-2 should be performed routinely. In atypical or painless ulcers, syphilis must be excluded by serological testing and NAATs for syphilis on the ulcer swab should be requested if available. Type-specific

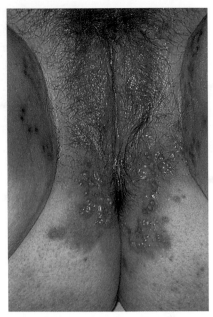

Fig. 18.6 Primary herpes. Multiple painful superficial ulcers are present. (From Clutterbuck D. *Specialist Training in Sexually Transmitted Infections and HIV.* Mosby; 2005.)

serological tests for HSV-1 and HSV-2 are not routinely used for diagnosis but may be useful in assessing the susceptibility of a partner to primary infection (e.g., during pregnancy).

Treatment

Primary and First-Episode Genital Herpes

Antiviral drugs reduce the severity and duration of the symptoms. They do not prevent latency; thus, they have no effect on future recurrences.

Recommended regimens include:

- Aciclovir 400 mg three times daily for 5 days
- Valaciclovir 500 mg twice daily for 5 days.

Aciclovir can be used in pregnancy and breastfeeding.

Analgesia and saline bathing are recommended. Women can be advised to pass urine in a bath or under a shower spray of warm water to ease external dysuria. Topical analgesia (such as lidocaine ointment) may be helpful. The natural history of HSV infection should be explained, covering recurrences, subclinical viral shedding, the potential for sexual transmission and treatments that are available.

Recurrent Genital Herpes

Recurrences are self-limiting and can often be managed with supportive therapy. Infrequent but severe recurrences can be treated with episodic antiviral therapy. If started early, therapy will reduce the severity and sometimes the duration of an attack but will not reduce the number of recurrences. The woman should initiate treatment at home as soon as a recurrence is noticed.

Episodic treatment regimens include:
- Aciclovir 800 mg three times a day for 2 days
- Valaciclovir 500 mg twice daily for 3 days.

For frequent recurrences (more than six recurrences in a year) suppressive therapy may be considered. In around 80% of cases, recurrences are stopped altogether. Therapy does not modify the natural history of infection; however, after 12 months of treatment, about 20% of women will have fewer recurrences due to the natural decay in episode frequency. It may be restarted if frequent recurrences persist.

Suppressive treatment regimens include:
- Aciclovir 400 mg twice daily
- Valaciclovir 500 mg once daily.

Women should be advised to avoid sexual contact with uninfected partners during the prodrome and recurrence, as this is when the risk of transmission is highest. It should be explained that a low risk of transmission remains, even when they have no obvious recurrence, because of subclinical viral shedding. Condoms reduce this risk and suppressive therapy has an additional effect.

Complications

Women who acquire primary genital herpes during pregnancy, particularly in the third trimester, may transmit the infection to the baby at the time of delivery. Herpes neonatorum, though rare in the United Kingdom, carries a risk of death or serious disability. The risk of perinatal transmission with recurrent HSV is low. Genital herpes increases the acquisition and transmission of HIV two- to threefold, although providing suppressive antiviral treatment to women with herpes who are at risk of HIV has not been successful in preventing infection.

Many people with recurrent HSV infection fear rejection by sexual partners and a minority develop psychological problems. Aseptic meningitis and autonomic neuropathy can occasionally occur with primary infection, even leading to urinary retention. Rarely, the infection can disseminate, causing a life-threatening condition. This is more likely in the immunocompromised and in pregnancy.

SYPHILIS

Background Information

Syphilis is caused by the spirochaete *Treponema pallidum*. Infectious syphilis in women in the United Kingdom was almost eradicated by the mid-1990s, but has returned to significant levels in this century. Between 20 and 30 cases of congenital syphilis are diagnosed annually in the United Kingdom. Over 1 million pregnant women had active syphilis infection in 2016, syphilis being the second leading cause of stillbirth worldwide.

Symptoms and Signs

Syphilis can be asymptomatic and identified on screening serology, such as in antenatal testing.

There are several stages of symptomatic syphilis infection:
- *Primary syphilis*: About 3 weeks after exposure, a chancre appears. This is usually a single, painless ulcer with rolled indurated edges, which usually goes unnoticed in women. Even without treatment, it heals spontaneously. Syphilis serology may still be negative at this stage of infection.
- *Secondary syphilis*: After several weeks, a generalized illness develops, with fever, malaise and skin and mucosal rashes. The rash is present on the trunk, limbs, palms and soles. Wart-like, moist papules occur on the vulva (condylomata lata). Even if untreated, these symptoms and signs resolve after 3 to 12 weeks. Syphilis serology is strongly positive at this stage of infection.
- *Late syphilis:* Up to 40% of untreated individuals will develop symptomatic late syphilis, with neurosyphilis, cardiovascular syphilis or gummata.

Diagnosis

Syphilis can be diagnosed by serological testing, commonly using an enzyme immunoassay for syphilis antibodies. NAATs for syphilis ulcers are increasingly available.

Treatment

Long-acting penicillins remain the treatment of choice. Care, including treatment and follow-up, should be undertaken by a specialist sexual health service.

Complications

Without adequate treatment, complications of late syphilis can occur. Syphilis in pregnancy can cause miscarriage and stillbirth, and can be transmitted to the infant, causing congenital syphilis.

VULVAL LUMPS

Raised lesions on the vulva can be due to infections or anatomical variants. Genital warts are by far the most common cause of vulval lumps (Table 18.5).

GENITAL WARTS

Background Information

Genital warts are painless, benign epithelial tumours caused by HPV types 6 and 11. The prevalence of infection with HPV types 6 and 11 in women aged 19 to 23 years was 23% in a study performed prior to the introduction of a national vaccination programme against oncogenic HPV types (16 and 18) for girls aged 13 years in the United Kingdom from 2008. From 2012, this was replaced by a quadrivalent vaccine, also protecting against HPV 6 and 11, and was expanded to include boys from 2020. Between 2009 and 2017 in the United Kingdom, diagnoses of genital warts declined by 90% in 15- to 17-year-old girls and 70% in 15- to 17-year-old boys.

For those who are unvaccinated, HPV is highly infectious: two-thirds of sexual partners will develop warts. HPV infection is also seen in adolescents who have had only non-penetrative sexual contact. The incubation period of months to years means that warts may appear some time into an exclusively monogamous relationship. The immunosuppression of pregnancy may cause warts to appear or recur.

Symptoms and Signs

- Genital warts are painless; thus, in women, they may be asymptomatic.
- If symptomatic, it is usual that the woman has felt the vulval lumps.
- There may be a slight itch and discomfort as the warts develop. However, pain, bleeding, or other symptoms suggest an alternative or co-existing diagnosis.
- On examination, the flesh-coloured papules can be seen around the introital opening. They can spread onto the labia, perineum and perianal area. They may be single but are usually multiple (Fig. 18.7).
- On the mucous membranes, they are usually soft and cauliflower-like (condylomata acuminata).
- On the drier surfaces, they are harder and keratinized.

Diagnosis

They are diagnosed by their clinical appearances. Atypical lesions should be biopsied, particularly in older women, as premalignant and malignant lesions can look similar.

TABLE 18.5	Causes of Vulval Lumps
Viral infections	Genital warts
	Molluscum contagiosum
	Vulval intraepithelial neoplasia and vulval cancer
Bacterial infections	Syphilitic condylomata lata
	Skene or Bartholin gland abscesses owing to *Chlamydia trachomatis* or *Neisseria gonorrhoeae*
Anatomical variants	Sebaceous glands
	Vulval papillae
Other	Sebaceous cysts

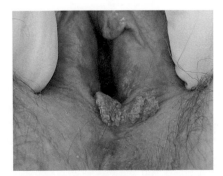

Fig. 18.7 Flesh-coloured papules characteristic of warts. (From Clutterbuck D. *Specialist Training in Sexually Transmitted Infections and HIV*. Mosby; 2005.)

Treatment

Warts may resolve spontaneously. No one treatment modality has been shown to be effective in all cases. Fewer (<5) or keratinized warts can be treated with ablative therapy, such as cryotherapy, trichloroacetic acid, curettage or electrocautery. All of these can be used in pregnancy and a single treatment may be effective. Multiple soft warts (condylomata acuminata) can be treated with topical self-applied treatments, including podophyllotoxin solution or cream, Catephen ointment (a green tea extract) or imiquimod cream, which stimulates local cell-mediated immunity. All topical treatments are contraindicated in pregnancy and can have recurrence rates of up to 25% because of residual subclinical viral infection. Treatment failure should be followed by change of treatment, and management algorithms improve outcomes. Women with genital warts should be offered testing for other STIs. There is evidence that condoms reduce the spread of HPV; thus, women should be advised to use condoms with new partners.

Complications

Genital warts are mainly a cosmetic problem. Psychological morbidity may arise because of their appearance, fears about cervical cancer, or concerns about fidelity if they appear in a regular relationship. Physical complications are rare; HPV 6 and 11 are not associated with cervical cancer and vertical transmission is rare.

Systemic Presentations of Sexually Transmitted Infections

STIs do not always present with genital symptoms or signs. Syphilis becomes a systemic infection following the primary phase, and herpes, gonorrhoea and chlamydia can all cause disseminated infections, producing symptoms and signs in other systems. HIV is a systemic viral infection which may present with direct effects of viral infection or opportunistic infections and malignancies in any body system.

HIV INFECTION

Background Information

HIV infection can be transmitted by contact with body fluids (either sexually or through needles or blood transfusion) and by vertical transmission from mother to baby. It was estimated that 28,000 women were living with HIV in the United Kingdom in 2018. The rate of undiagnosed infection in women is significantly lower than in men in the United Kingdom, partly due to the effective antenatal screening programme introduced in the 1990s. ART allows a near-normal life expectancy for people diagnosed with HIV at an early stage, but deaths from acquired immunodeficiency syndrome (AIDS) still occur in people diagnosed too late for therapy to allow immune recovery. Rates of infection have fallen in all groups since a peak in 2014 and prevention efforts in the United Kingdom have moved to the aim of eliminating HIV transmissions by 2030 through early testing, the universal provision of ART, and the use of oral pre-exposure prophylaxis (PrEP).

Symptoms and Signs

- Most people with HIV have no symptoms in the first few years of infection.
- There may be a systemic illness with fever, malaise and rash at the time of seroconversion, 6 to 12 weeks after infection. This is rarely recognised as being HIV related.
- As immune function is starting to deteriorate, infections such as oral candidiasis and herpes zoster may occur.
- Women with HIV infection get more frequent episodes of vaginal candidiasis and recurrent HSV. They are also subject to higher rates of HPV-related abnormalities, such as cervical intraepithelial neoplasia.
- Opportunistic infections and HIV-related malignancies can present in many different ways. Common early presentations are shown in Fig. 18.8.

Diagnosis

A fourth-generation serological test for antibodies to HIV and HIV antigen is the preferred method of diagnosis. Point-of-care tests for HIV are widely available and used for routine testing, providing a result in as little as 1 minute. They can be particularly helpful in the obstetric setting, for example, when a woman from an area of high HIV prevalence presents in labour. HIV testing should always be a routine part of antenatal care and STI screening, and should be recommended when a woman presents with any HIV clinical indicator

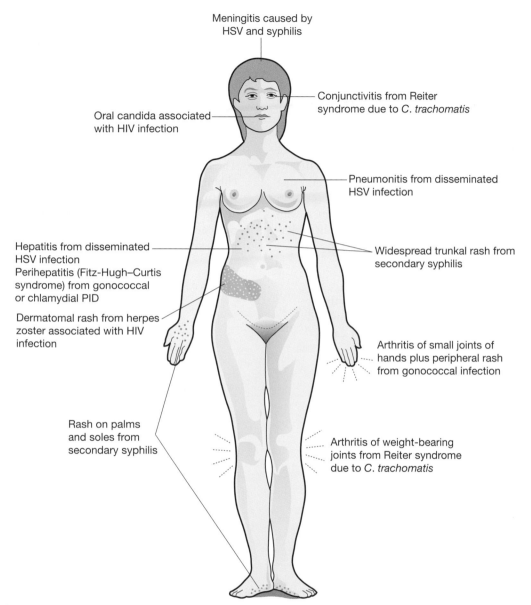

Fig. 18.8 Systemic presentations of sexually transmitted infections (STIs). *C. trachomatis, Chlamydia trachomatis; HIV,* human immunodeficiency virus; *HSV,* herpes simplex virus; *PID,* pelvic inflammatory disease.

condition. Clinical indicator conditions seen in gynae-cology include cervical cancer, cervical intraepithelial neoplasia (grade II and above) and vulval and vaginal intraepithelial neoplasia. Testing requires informed consent but not specialist counselling, which can be performed by any clinician.

Treatment

Women should have their CD4 count (this measures cell-mediated immune function) and HIV viral load (this measures the level of viral replication) performed about every 6 months. ART, usually with two or three drugs in combination, is recommended for all

HIV-infected individuals at any stage of infection and eradicates the risk of horizontal transmission through sex (Undetectable = Untransmittable: U = U).

Complications

Without treatment, there is increasing damage to cell-mediated immunity. This leads to susceptibility to opportunistic infections and, eventually, death a median of 9 to 12 years after infection. Treating the pregnant woman with triple ART and avoiding breast-feeding reduces vertical transmission. Rates of transmission are now as low as 1%. Delivery by caesarean section reduces vertical transmission in women who are not taking ART, but is not thought to offer additional benefit in those on effective treatment.

Key Points

- STIs in females are often asymptomatic. Detection depends on risk assessment and testing in all women presenting for care.

- High rates of STIs are found in sexually active women aged less than 25 years.
- Testing for HIV infection is routine in women attending for antenatal care and termination of pregnancy, and should also be done in any woman presenting with an indicator condition.
- Syndromic management, with or without the support of diagnostic testing for STIs, can help to ensure early treatment.
- The management of STIs – particularly chlamydia, gonorrhoea and PID – includes treatment of the sexual partner(s) and advice about abstinence from sex until the woman and partner(s) have completed treatment in order to prevent reinfection.

Chapter 19

Sexual Problems

David Gerber

Chapter Outline

Introduction

It is important for any doctor to be able to take a sexual history and to have some idea of how sexual problems are managed. Understanding the physiology of the normal sexual response will allow the doctor to better understand many of the uncomplicated sexual problems.

This chapter is divided in its discussion into issues affecting anatomical males and anatomical females. People with gender incongruence may have sexual problems which may or may not be related to their surgical or hormonal treatment. For simplicity, the issues described in this chapter relate to genital anatomy regardless of a person's gender identity.

Scientific investigation of the normal sexual response is necessary to our understanding. However, because of conservative attitudes, few scientists have chosen to work in this area until fairly recently. Early researchers were:

- Sigmund Freud (1856–1939), an Austrian doctor, was the founder of psychoanalysis and the first to recognise the importance of childhood influences on sexuality. His studies were on patients rather than normal subjects.
- Havelock Ellis (1859–1939) studied medicine at St Thomas Hospital, London. His seven-volume *Studies in the Psychology of Sex* (1897–1928) caused controversy but was the first detached treatment of the subject.
- Alfred Kinsey (1894–1956), an American zoologist, became director of Indiana University's

Institute for Sex Research in 1942. To investigate 'normal' sexual experience, 18,500 Americans were interviewed. *Sexual Behavior in the Human Male* was published in 1940 and *Sexual Behavior in the Human Female* in 1953.

- Masters and Johnson: William Masters (1915–2001), a doctor, and Virginia Johnson (1925–2013), a psychologist, working at Washington University, St Louis, carried out the first direct observations on sexual activity under laboratory conditions. *Human Sexual Response* appeared in 1966, and *Human Sexual Inadequacy* in 1970.
- The field of sexual medicine, or sexology, has developed significantly since the early work of these pioneers and is now a flourishing specialty in itself. There are numerous societies, conferences and journals devoted to the field. Despite this, it is still a niche specialism and not everyone has access to services for sexual problems.

Normal Sexual Response

The normal human sexual response can be regarded as having five phases: desire, arousal, orgasm, resolution and the refractory phase (Fig. 19.1). This is the most widely accepted model, first published by Masters and Johnson. There are criticisms of this model and others have developed slightly different models, but this version serves as a useful introduction to the topic.

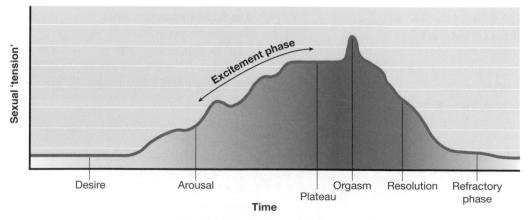

Fig. 19.1 The normal sexual response.

DESIRE

Sexual desire refers to the general level of interest in sexual pleasure. It is modulated by hormones – hence, the change in sexual interest at puberty. The main hormonal modulator is testosterone. Desire is also dependant on contextual factors, such as mood, environment and levels of sexual attraction.

AROUSAL

This phase has three components: central arousal, genital response and peripheral arousal.

Central Arousal

This refers to the response to sexual stimuli, which may be visual or tactile or may result from internal imagery or from a relationship. These stimuli act through the cerebral cortex (Fig. 19.2). The areas of the brain involved in sexual arousal are thought to be in the limbic system. There are thought to be excitatory centres with endorphins as the neurotransmitter and inhibitory centres linked to the centres for pain and fear.

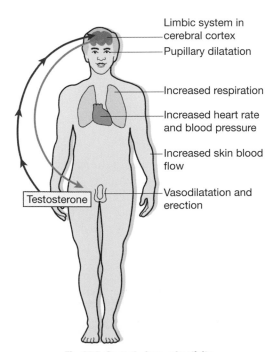

Limbic system in cerebral cortex
Pupillary dilatation
Increased respiration
Increased heart rate and blood pressure
Increased skin blood flow
Testosterone
Vasodilatation and erection

Fig. 19.2 Control of sexual activity.

Genital Response

The spinal pathways leading to the genitalia are not precisely known but appear to be near the spinothalamic pathways for pain and temperature. Genital responses are due to vasocongestion and neuromuscular changes. Arteriolar dilatation is probably controlled by the parasympathetic sacral outflow at S2, 3 and 4 via the nervi erigentes. Thoracic sympathetic outflow also plays a part. The local neurotransmitters involved include vasoactive intestinal polypeptide, a potent vasodilator found in the penis and vagina.

For male anatomy, engorgement of the corpora cavernosa is due mainly to arteriolar dilatation and probably a reduction in the venous outflow, which results in penile erection (Fig. 19.3). The scrotum tightens due to contraction of the dartos muscle and the testes are elevated due to contraction of the cremaster muscle.

For female anatomy, there is engorgement of the venous plexus surrounding the lower part of the vagina and of the erectile bulbs of the vestibule on either side of the introitus (Fig. 19.4). There is reddening and pouting of the labia minora. The clitoris becomes erect and later is said to retract against the symphysis pubis.

The vagina becomes lubricated by a transudate as the blood supply to the vaginal wall increases. This fluid is not the product of mucous glands. Mucous secretion from the cervix makes relatively little contribution to vaginal lubrication (which is, therefore, usually unaffected by hysterectomy). Secretion from the Bartholin glands, formerly thought to be mainly responsible for lubrication, is only moderate in amount and occurs relatively late during arousal.

Relaxation of the anatomic female's pelvic floor muscles occurs after vaginal lubrication has started. In the later stages of arousal, the uterus becomes engorged, increases in size and rises in the pelvis. The upper part of the vagina 'balloons' and there may be slow, irregular contractions of the lower third of the vagina.

In all sexes, but particularly in those with male anatomy, the genital response interacts with the central response so that arousal becomes self-amplifying, that is, having an erection leads to a desire for sexual pleasure.

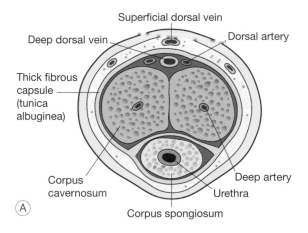

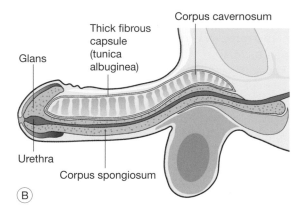

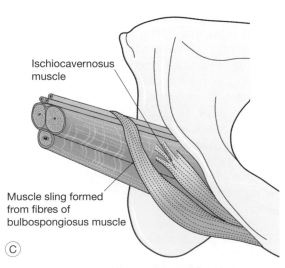

Fig. 19.3 The penis. (A) Cross-section showing erectile spaces and principal blood vessels. **(B)** Erectile tissues. Each crus of the corpora cavernosa is inserted into the pubic bone. **(C)** Muscles.

Peripheral Arousal

Sexual arousal causes:

- A rise in systolic and diastolic blood pressure (which may only be transient)
- General flushing of the skin
- Change in heart rate (either an increase or decrease)
- Respiratory changes
- Pupillary dilatation

Plateau Phase

When arousal is heightened, there may be a 'plateau' phase during which the couple prolongs the pleasure of intercourse before orgasm.

ORGASM

Orgasm involves genital, muscular and sensory changes, as well as cardiovascular and respiratory responses.

In the Male

First, there is smooth muscle contraction of the epididymis, vas deferens, seminal vesicle, prostate and ampulla, propelling seminal and prostatic fluid into the urethral bulb. Then, the person becomes aware that orgasm is imminent and ejaculation usually follows within a few seconds. The internal bladder sphincter remains shut but the external sphincter relaxes and semen is propelled along the urethra by rhythmic contractions of the bulbospongiosus and ischiocavernosus muscles.

In the Female

A few seconds after the onset of the subjective experience of orgasm, there is a spasm of the muscles surrounding the lower third of the vagina (the 'orgasmic platform') followed by a series of rhythmic contractions. Uterine contractions may also occur.

In All Sexes

There is contraction of rectus abdominis, pelvic thrusting, contraction of the anal sphincter and sometimes carpopedal spasm. Systolic and diastolic blood pressure rises by at least 25 mmHg, and hyperventilation occurs. There is a feeling of intense pleasure and an alteration of consciousness to a variable degree.

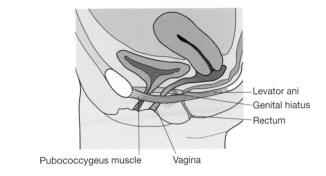

Levator ani
Genital hiatus
Rectum

(A)   Pubococcygeus muscle   Vagina

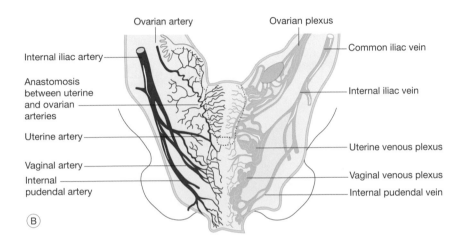

Ovarian artery   Ovarian plexus

Internal iliac artery

Common iliac vein

Anastomosis
between uterine
and ovarian
arteries

Internal iliac vein

Uterine artery

Vaginal artery

Uterine venous plexus

Internal
pudendal artery

Vaginal venous plexus

Internal pudendal vein

(B)

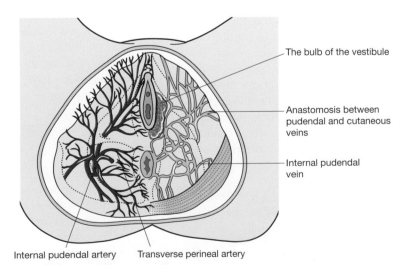

The bulb of the vestibule

Anastomosis between
pudendal and cutaneous
veins

Internal pudendal
vein

(C)   Internal pudendal artery   Transverse perineal artery

Fig. 19.4 Female reproductive organs. (A) The muscular supports of the vagina. This shows the sling of muscle fibres that surround the urethra, vagina and rectum, running from the pubic bone to the coccyx. The levator plate formed by these fibres supports the rectum and vagina in its non-aroused horizontal position. **(B)** Arteries and veins supplying the female reproductive organs. **(C)** Blood vessels of the pelvic floor, showing the rich arterial and venous networks surrounding the vaginal opening.

RESOLUTION

The events of arousal are gradually reversed. In those with male anatomy, there is a moderate immediate loss of erection, followed by a slower complete reversal. In those with female anatomy, if no orgasm has occurred, pelvic congestion may take hours to resolve and can be uncomfortable. In all sexes, there is a subjective feeling of relaxation, though its duration may differ between individuals.

REFRACTORY PHASE

There follows an interval during which further stimulation does not produce a response. In males, this varies from minutes in young males to many hours in older males. Some females do not experience a refractory period; only a minority of females (14% according to Kinsey) can have multiple orgasms.

The Effect of Age

Normal sexual behaviour differs from couple to couple. It also alters with age and with the evolution of a sexual relationship. Couples may present with problems due to difficulties in adjusting to the change from one phase to the next of a relationship.

ADOLESCENCE

Adolescents usually have a higher capacity for sexual arousal and a need to explore the bounds of their sexuality. However, coupled with the need to learn about sexual behaviour, adolescents are subject to emotional vulnerability. This can lead to high-risk sexual behaviour. Unsatisfactory sexual experience at this time can result in sexual problems in later life. Young women in their teens are at a higher risk of unwanted pregnancy due to uncertainty about contraceptive needs. In addition, awareness of sexually transmitted infections can be limited at this age.

THE COUPLE

The early months of a relationship may be characterised by frequent sex, with couples usually learning how to establish good communication and to adjust their sexual behaviour to suit each other's needs. Should this communication not occur, dysfunctional patterns may develop, potentially resulting in sexual problems and relationship difficulties.

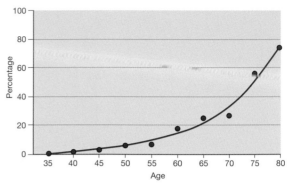

Fig. 19.5 Erectile dysfunction increases with age. (From Bancroft, J. (1989). Human sexuality and its problems (2nd ed.). Churchill Livingstone, with permission. Data from Kinsey, A. C., Pomeroy, W. B., & Martin, C. E. (1948). Sexual behavior in the human male. Saunders.

EARLY PARENTHOOD

The time it takes for sexual interest to return after childbirth is variable; in some women, it can be a year or more. Problems can result from a difficult birthing experience or postnatal depression but more commonly are due to fatigue and the difficulties of coping with the demands of the new baby.

MIDDLE AGE

When the novelty of a sexual relationship has worn off, sexual activity usually becomes less frequent, which may cause anxieties for some couples. Couples may feel they 'ought' to be having sex more often, resulting in guilt or anger. Stresses at work for both partners in combination with social commitments can make it difficult for them to find time to relax together. In the years before menopause, women often have menstrual problems. After menopause, there may be a reduction in sexual interest or a problem with vaginal dryness. These can usually be corrected by hormone replacement therapy.

OLD AGE

There is a decline in erectile function with age, which can be a manifestation of physical disease (Fig. 19.5). Postmenopausal women may experience low libido and vaginal dryness or atrophy. These factors can impact on the couple's sexual relationship.

The Functions of Sex

It is important to remember how much people differ from one another and how wide the range of normality may be. Sex can fulfill a multitude of functions, including some of the elements described here.

Reproduction

Reproductive sex is often limited to a short interval in a couple's relationship once conception has occurred. Couples who have fertility problems may find that this causes difficulty with their sex life or, conversely, may find that after they achieve pregnancy it is difficult to have sex for pleasure only.

Physical Exercise

Sexual activity is a form of physical exercise, which improves self-esteem and feelings of well-being but is also something to be mindful of in people with physical problems, such as cardiac disease.

Pleasure

Though sex is readily associated with pleasure, there are, in some cultures, taboos that prevent some people from enjoying sex.

Pair-Bonding

Enjoying sex means lowering one's defences, and sharing this experience strengthens the bond between partners. People who have had to build particularly strong defences – for example, after sexual or emotional abuse in childhood – may have difficulty in relinquishing them.

Asserting Masculinity or Femininity

People may use sexual activity to reassure themselves about their sexual identity.

Bolstering Self-Esteem

Satisfactory sex can improve one's self-esteem. However, for some, promiscuous behaviour to accomplish this can have negative consequences.

Achieving Power

Some people see the sexual relationship in terms of dominance and submission not within the realms of sadomasochism. This can apply to coitus itself or to the power to allow or deny access to sex. Rape can be seen as an example of this.

Reducing Anxiety or Tension

This can be helpful for most people but, in some cases, can cause relationship or personal problems through risk taking – for example, promiscuity or use of Internet pornography.

Material Gain

Prostitution is the most obvious form of sex for gain and is often the result of poverty (sometimes referred to as 'survival sex'). Marriage, even now, may also be a way of using sex to ensure financial security.

History Taking

Some sexual problems may present as another symptom, such as pelvic pain, or are discovered fortuitously, for example, when a routine enquiry is made about contraception. It is not possible to take a detailed sexual history from every person, whatever their symptoms. However, it is reasonable, particularly in a gynaecological clinic, to ask one or two questions about sex as a routine: for example, 'Do you have any trouble with intercourse?' or, if appropriate, 'Is this symptom worse after intercourse?'. An evasive reply may suggest that all is not well, which may require some further sensitive questioning.

Elucidating a sexual problem relies mainly on the history, although useful information may be obtained from examination or investigation. The interviewer should be comfortable with the subject, as the patient is likely to be embarrassed by talking about a sexual problem. A sympathetic but matter-of-fact approach may help to reduce this embarrassment. The vocabulary used must also be appropriate, using words that avoid being too technical on the one hand and appearing too crude on the other hand.

It is usually helpful to see both partners, but not necessarily together on the first occasion. A person may be more open if interviewed alone, but the partner may give quite a different version of the history. When treatment is planned, both partners should be involved, ideally.

The history needs to be thorough; if too intrusive, however, it may be off-putting. If a topic seems uncomfortable, the subject can be changed and revisited later. Sometimes, more than one interview is necessary, with sensitive topics being explored on the second occasion after a rapport has been established. Requesting a detailed account of a specific instance may be more helpful than asking general questions. For example, if the patient is asked 'How often do you have intercourse?' the reply is likely to depend partly on what the patient thinks is expected (e.g., 'About twice a week'). It may be better to ask, 'When did you last have intercourse?' and then, if the couple's last attempt was unsatisfactory, to ask in detail about what went wrong. Open questions should also be used, for example, 'How did you feel when that happened?'

Many patients, especially if talking about their sexual problem for the first time, find it difficult to put their feelings into words. It may be helpful to offer the occasional summary: 'What I think you're saying is that …' The patient will usually give a clearly positive response if the doctor has summed up the situation correctly. If the patient's response is more guarded, the doctor should be cautious about the conclusions drawn.

HUMAN SEXUALITY

There are several variations of human sexuality which should not be seen as problems unless they are presented as such by the patient. Some of the more common variations are detailed here.

Heterosexuality

The majority of people are heterosexual or 'straight' in that they are attracted to a sexual partner of the opposite biological sex.

Homosexuality

This refers to being attracted to a partner of the same gender. Homosexuality, or being 'gay', is widely accepted in most societies. However, in some cultures, there remains a degree of stigma which can be difficult for the homosexual person to cope with. This can result in abuse and even mental health problems in some cases.

Fetishistic Transvestitism

A transvestite is someone who enjoys dressing in the clothes of a different gender. This is associated with sexual excitement and is not associated with a desire to change one's gender. The vast majority of transvestites are biologically male and rarely present to services unless their behaviour causes relationship difficulties.

Sadomasochism

This is a spectrum of sexual behaviours encompassed in the term 'BDSM' (bondage, discipline, sadism and masochism), which involves mild to extreme pain being inflicted or received for sexual pleasure. It is unusual for these people to present to services unless they are traumatized either physically or psychologically by their practices or their behaviour results in injury to another person and possibly legal action.

Fetishism

Particular parts of the body (e.g., feet), articles of clothing (e.g., shoes) or materials (e.g., rubber or plastic) can become objects of sexual stimulation.

Paedophilia

This term refers to a sexual preference for children, usually of pre-pubertal age. This is an illegal practice and adults engaging in this behaviour should be reported to the police if it is apparent that they are engaging in it. This is an instance when medical confidentiality can be breached.

SEXUAL DYSFUNCTION

Sexual dysfunction may be due to psychological or relationship problems or may have an underlying medical or surgical cause. Sexual dysfunction is common, with 43% of women and 31% of men experiencing some form of sexual dysfunction during their lifetime.

The common disorders of sexual function can be classified according to the physiological stages described early in this chapter:
- Impaired desire
- Disorders of arousal
- Disorders of orgasm
- Dyspareunia

The causes of sexual dysfunction can be classified into physiological or psychological factors. However, it is hard to make a distinction between the two, as they often co-exist. For example, painful intercourse due to a physical cause such as a herpetic lesion may lead to secondary anxiety in both partners. However, anxiety due to sexual abuse in childhood may lead to spasm of the pelvic floor muscles. Treatment often needs to be directed towards physical and psychological causes at the same time.

A list of pathological causes of sexual dysfunction is given in Box 19.1. These causes are more common in

BOX 19.1 PATHOLOGICAL CAUSES OF SEXUAL DYSFUNCTION

Medical Disorders

- Acute and chronic illness
- Psychiatric illness
- Cancer–especially gynaecological
- Neurological problems, for example, spinal cord injuries, multiple sclerosis, neuropathy
- Endocrine, for example, diabetes
- Cardiovascular, for example, myocardial infarction
- Respiratory
- Arthritic
- Renal, for example, dialysis
- Gynaecological, for example, vaginitis

Surgical Procedures

- Mastectomy
- Colostomy
- Gynaecological–oophorectomy, episiotomy, vaginal repair
- Amputation

Drug Effects

- Anticholinergics
- Anticonvulsants
- Antihypertensives
- Anti-inflammatories
- Hormones
- Hypnotics and sedatives
- Major tranquillizers, for example, antipsychotics
- Alcohol
- Opiates
- Antidepressants

BOX 19.2 PSYCHOLOGICAL FACTORS IN SEXUAL DYSFUNCTION

Predisposing

- Repressed family attitudes to sex
- Poor sex education
- Sexual or physical trauma

Precipitating

- Psychiatric illness
- Childbirth
- Infidelity
- Partner's sexual dysfunction
- Relationship problem–may be cause or effect

Maintaining

- Anxiety
- Poor communication
- Lack of foreplay
- Depression
- Poor information

an ageing population. Psychological causes of sexual dysfunction are given in Box 19.2.

Female Sexual Dysfunction

IMPAIRED AROUSAL/DESIRE

This is a common presentation to specialist sexual medicine clinics, although it is not as frequent a symptom in routine gynaecology clinics. The woman reports that she is just not interested in sex. Such 'loss of libido' may be primary or secondary.

Primary

Some women have never felt interested in sex. In these cases, there is usually impairment of arousal and orgasm as well. In fact, the latest *Diagnostic and Statistical Manual of Mental Disorders*, Fifth Edition (*DSM-5*)

has not separated disorders of arousal and desire, as it is difficult to distinguish between these interrelated concepts. The underlying cause is often psychological. Sometimes, women may try to choose a partner who also has an apparently low sex drive to match their level of desire.

Secondary

More commonly, loss of libido follows an interval of apparently normal sex drive, during the woman's teens or early 20s, or early in the relationship with her partner. Loss of interest in sex may occur after childbirth, when both parents devote all of their attention to the baby, often combining parenting with a return to paid employment. If there has been postnatal depression, this will exacerbate the problem.

Other causes include:

- Depression
- Bereavement
- Menopause
- Medical causes or drugs (see Box 19.1)
- Gynaecological investigation, for example, for an abnormal cervical smear
- Loss of self-esteem, for example, problems at work

Sometimes, the secondary loss of libido has no obvious specific cause. A woman who has suffered sexual or physical abuse in childhood, or who has had a sexually repressed upbringing, may go through a phase of normal or increased sexual activity in her teens and 20s and then present with loss of libido due to the long-term effects of childhood experiences.

Often, a partner reacts to the woman's loss of interest by making persistent sexual demands and then, after some years, gives up approaching her for sex. Loss of desire can be due to, or cause, relationship difficulties. Counselling will be directed towards improving communication between the partners. A specific cause, such as childhood abuse, may require specialist referral. Hormone therapy is appropriate for postmenopausal women but not for those who still have a normal menstrual cycle.

ORGASMIC DYSFUNCTION

Inability to achieve orgasm is usually associated with lack of interest in sex, but sometimes can be an isolated symptom in a woman who has an otherwise satisfactory sex drive and is able to experience normal arousal. However, orgasmic dysfunction may result in extreme frustration and distress.

Primary

This refers to a woman who has never been orgasmic. Inability to achieve orgasm despite adequate arousal may be due to inexperience of the person or the partner or unrealistic expectations. For example, reading erotic fiction may have led the couple to believe that orgasm occurs automatically on penetration. Often, education and reassurance about normal sexual behaviour is all that is required in these circumstances. Sometimes, the cause is more deep-seated – possibly because of childhood/cultural repression resulting in the woman not being able to let go of her defences. Psychological counselling may be helpful in these cases.

Secondary

Secondary orgasmic dysfunction follows an interval of adequate sexual functioning. It is usually associated with reduced desire or arousal, as discussed in the previous section, and has similar causes.

Situational Orgasmic Dysfunction

Some women can achieve orgasm through masturbation but not coitus, or with one partner but not with another. This can be an indicator of relationship difficulties.

BOX 19.3 CAUSES OF DYSPAREUNIA

Superficial Dyspareunia
- Infection, for example, candida, herpes
- Atrophic change, particularly after menopause
- Vulval skin disorders, for example, lichen sclerosus
- Vaginismus

Deep Dyspareunia
- Endometriosis
- Pelvic inflammatory disease
- Bowel dysfunction
- Pelvic mass
- 'Unexplained' pelvic pain

VAGINISMUS AND DYSPAREUNIA

Vaginismus is involuntary spasm of the pelvic floor muscles and perineal muscles, provoked by attempted penetration. It is also provoked by vaginal examination or by attempts to insert a tampon or the woman's own finger into the vagina. When severe, the conditioned reflex includes spasm of the adductor muscles of the thighs. The spasm results in intense pain and inability to have penetrative intercourse. In extreme cases, it can be so severe that penetration is physically impossible.

Dyspareunia is the experience of pain on intercourse and is the most common sexual problem presenting to the routine gynaecology clinic. It is usually classified into superficial and deep dyspareunia, but it is not always possible to make a clear distinction between the two (Box 19.3). With superficial dyspareunia, there is pain at the vaginal introitus or vestibule (vestibulodynia) on attempted penetration, often making full intercourse impossible. In deep dyspareunia, there is pain in the pelvis on deep penetration.

The separation between vaginismus and dyspareunia is increasingly seen as unfounded as the conditions are closely interrelated, with vaginismus being seen as a response to pain but also a cause of pain. The *DSM-5* has developed a category merging both conditions into 'genito-pelvic pain/penetration disorder', illustrating this overlap.

Primary

Primary vaginismus/dyspareunia is discovered during the first attempt at intercourse and persists thereafter. It may be due to apprehension that intercourse will be painful or due simply to failure to control the pelvic musculature. Persistent attempts at penetration cause more pain and a 'vicious cycle' is set up, reinforcing the vaginismus/pain cycle. There may also be deep-seated psychological problems, such as an inability to accept sexual maturity, sexual repression in childhood, childhood sexual abuse or fear of pregnancy.

Secondary

Symptoms may also follow a physically painful experience, such as a sexual assault, an obstetric problem at delivery, or an insensitive vaginal examination. It can sometimes also result from painful infections or other conditions, for example, lichen sclerosus. Therefore, an examination is essential in all patients with vaginismus/dyspareunia to exclude organic causes.

Examination of the vulva may reveal the inflammatory appearance of candidal infection, herpes lesions or the presence of atrophy or dystrophy. Careful examination may be necessary to reveal the localized inflammation of vestibulitis. Vulval and vaginal swabs should be taken for microbiological examination and treatment given if appropriate. The cotton-swab test elicits intense pain on light touch in the vestibular area and is indicative of vestibulodynia. If no cause is found for what appears to be superficial dyspareunia, it may be necessary to consider the causes of deep dyspareunia or psychological causes.

Bimanual examination may reveal a specific area of tenderness, for example, the cervix or on palpating the posterior fornix, the rectum, or one or other lateral fornix. Sometimes, however, the tenderness is more general and a specific site cannot be identified. Deep dyspareunia is often associated with other symptoms, such as dysmenorrhoea or persistent pelvic pain. The history should include questions about bowel habits. Bowel dysfunction is not uncommon and can be treated with a high-fibre diet. The timing of the pain in relation to the cycle should also be noted – it may occur just before ovulation or menstruation. Bimanual examination may reveal a pelvic mass.

The finding of a retroverted uterus is unlikely to be significant, as uterine retroversion is common. Occasionally, however, a sharply retroverted uterus can be the only site of tenderness. High vaginal and cervical swabs should be taken if there is any suspicion of pelvic infection. In most cases, laparoscopy is necessary to diagnose or exclude endometriosis or pelvic inflammatory disease.

When a specific cause is identified, the appropriate treatment is given. If laparoscopy is negative, a high-fibre diet may help even in the absence of obvious bowel symptoms. If no cause is found and the deep dyspareunia is not associated with other symptoms, the problem may be due to limited foreplay, leading to inadequate arousal and insufficient relaxation of the upper vagina. The couple should try allowing more time for arousal and may be advised to avoid positions in which penetration is particularly deep. Lubricants can be helpful and are worth trying in most instances.

If deep dyspareunia is associated with 'unexplained pelvic pain', treatment can be difficult and may require a combination of endocrine manipulation and psychological support.

Ongoing Care

Treatment of any underlying condition is important, for example, steroids for lichen sclerosus or topical estrogens for postmenopausal atrophy. Where no underlying cause is identified, most cases respond well to simple treatment involving training in relaxation and the use of vaginal dilators/trainers. The female should be helped to relax completely: vaginal examination should not be attempted until the adductor muscles of the thighs have fully relaxed. In severe cases, physiotherapy can be helpful. The patient can be taught to insert a small vaginal dilator or trainer. Once she is comfortable about inserting the small trainer regularly, she can progress to gradually larger sizes. During treatment, she is also taught pelvic floor exercises, which help her to gain control of the muscles. It may take several weeks or months before full control is achieved.

Attempts at intercourse should be discouraged until the larger-sized vaginal dilators can be inserted with ease. This can take a long time and requires the patient to be highly motivated. In most instances, satisfactory intercourse follows. An alternative to vaginal trainers is for the woman to use her own finger and then for the partner to insert one and then two fingers into the vagina. For most couples who present to the clinic, however, they are reluctant to do this and prefer the dilators. If primary vaginismus is due to more deep-seated problems, treatment may take many months and the prognosis is not as promising. Psychosexual counselling may be appropriate in these cases. In cases of vulvodynia, techniques such as mindfulness have proven to be effective.

For treatment-resistant cases, botulinum toxin (Botox) injected into the pelvic muscles can be very effective to prevent vaginal muscle spasm. The use of topical anaesthetic agents can help to relieve the pain of vestibulodynia.

Male Sexual Dysfunction

Male sexual dysfunction can be classified as impairment of desire, arousal (erection) or ejaculation.

IMPAIRED DESIRE

In the male, libido is dependent on normal testosterone levels. Thus, serum testosterone should be checked in men complaining of lack of libido. If the level is normal, testosterone supplements are unlikely to help. Further enquiry may then elicit contextual factors, for example, work stress, relationship difficulties, and the like, which may impact on desire. This condition is a lot less common than in females.

ERECTILE DYSFUNCTION

Inability to achieve or maintain a satisfactory erection ('impotence') is the most common sexual problem among males. It may be associated with impaired desire, but desire usually is normal and, therefore, frustration is common.

Erectile dysfunction can be due to psychological factors; however, it is important to exclude organic causes. Erectile dysfunction is often the first sign of cardiometabolic disease and all patients who present with this symptom should have their cardiovascular risk status assessed. If a physical cause is found, treatment and modification of risk factors may resolve the problem. The patient may also not accept a diagnosis of a psychological cause until all possible physical causes have been excluded (Box 19.4).

In addition to a full sexual history, the man should be asked about the duration of the problem, whether it is primary or secondary, and whether it is situational (i.e., does he get 'early morning' erections or can he get an erection by masturbation but not with his partner). Situational erectile dysfunction is usually indicative of psychological causation. Enquiry should be made

BOX 19.4 PHYSICAL CAUSES OF ERECTILE FAILURE

Endocrine Disorders
- Hypogonadism. Disorders causing reduced plasma testosterone may cause erectile failure, but these usually cause loss of libido as well.
- Diabetes may cause impotence. The incidence of erectile failure at age 50 years is 40% amongst diabetic men, and only 5% amongst non-diabetic men. The mechanism may be either diabetic neuropathy or vascular disease.

Neurological Disorders
- Multiple sclerosis
- Spinal injury causes erectile failure; however, after the initial phase of 'spinal shock', reflex erectile ability may return if the sacral segments of the spinal cord are intact.

Vascular Disorders
- There is a decline in sexual activity after myocardial infarction and, interestingly, before a heart attack. Erectile dysfunction is an important warning of likely cardiovascular disease and is often the first sign (perhaps because they share a common disease process and many risk factors).
- Hypertension is associated with erectile dysfunction.

Drugs
- Antihypertensives
- Antipsychotics

Psychiatric Illness
- Severe depression causes loss of sexual interest in over 60% of cases
- Severe anxiety

Surgery
- Prostatectomy need not cause impotence, particularly if it is by the transurethral or retropubic route. Radical prostatectomy usually causes erectile failure.

Physiological
- Ageing reduces the frequency of erections. Some men may also fail to understand the refractory period and may have unrealistic expectations of how soon erection can recur after orgasm.

about symptoms of general disease, including those listed earlier. Smoking history is also important.

Clinical examination should include a check for signs of systemic disease. The genitalia should be examined for abnormalities of the penis (such as hypospadias, Peyronie disease) or abnormally small testes. Serum testosterone, glucose and lipids should be checked as a matter of routine.

Therapeutic options include:
- Phosphodiesterase inhibitors (PDE5 inhibitors), for example, sildenafil (Viagra). Penile erection is

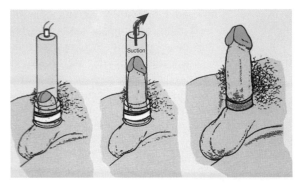

Fig. 19.6 The use of a vacuum device to manage erectile dysfunction.

due to relaxation of the smooth muscle around the cavernosal vascular spaces, allowing them to fill with blood. This is under the control of the autonomic nervous system, mediated by cyclic guanosine monophosphate (cGMP). These drugs are taken orally and enhance erection by blocking breakdown of cGMP. Alternatives to sildenafil are vardenafil (Levitra), which acts more quickly, and tadalafil (Cialis), which has a longer duration of action. Their success rate in treating erectile dysfunction is about 85%. Side effects are mild and transient and include flushing, dyspepsia, headache and disturbance of colour vision. These drugs must not be used by men who use nitrates or have severe cardiac disease, as they could lead to a life-threatening drop in blood pressure.

- Alprostadil (prostaglandin E_1 [PGE_1]). This drug also relaxes cavernosal smooth muscle but has to be injected directly into the corpora cavernosa. It is more effective than sildenafil in severe erectile failure. It is also available as a urethral pellet, but this is less effective.
- Other treatments used include vacuum devices (Fig. 19.6) and penile implants, the latter only when no other treatment has been effective.

EJACULATORY DYSFUNCTION

The most common type of ejaculatory dysfunction is premature ejaculation, affecting around one-third of all males. Retarded ejaculation is much less common and may be associated with deep-seated psychological issues. Painful ejaculation is relatively rare and is most commonly a symptom of prostatitis.

Premature ejaculation is normal in early sexual experiences. There are various definitions; the best guide is if the male feels he has insufficient control to satisfy his urge to ejaculate following penetration (usually within 2 minutes of penetration). Sometimes, ejaculation occurs before penetration or within a few seconds of penetration. The cause of premature ejaculation is unknown. However, when it occurs, it leads to anxiety and a vicious cycle of recurrence.

Treatment requires the cooperation of the partner; it can be difficult to help a male who presents for treatment without his partner's knowledge. If the couple have a good relationship, they can be instructed in the 'stop–start' technique. This is when the couple has sex until just before the point of orgasm, then 'stop' moving or withdraw the penis until the sensation passes, then 'start' again and repeat this. Practice with this technique helps to build a feeling of control. This can also be adopted during masturbation. The 'squeeze' technique – firm pressure on the glans at the level of the frenulum when an orgasm is imminent – may also help to retard ejaculation. Antidepressant drugs – selective serotonin reuptake inhibitors (SSRIs), for example, sertraline – are used off licence to delay orgasm and are very effective. More recently, an SSRI-like drug, dapoxetine, has been given a licence for treatment of premature ejaculation. A small amount of local anaesthetic applied to the frenulum before sex can also be helpful in some cases.

Care of People With Sexual Problems

The treatment of sexual problems can be divided into two categories:

- Counselling, which should be within the scope of any health care worker
- Sex therapy, which requires specialist training

COUNSELLING

Some problems can be helped by a single consultation or a few consultations. Simple counselling may include the items that follow, using the acronym PLISSIT.

Permission Giving

Patients can be embarrassed or nervous about discussing sexual problems. Therefore, it would be helpful for the clinician to open the discussion about sexual activity, for example, 'How is your sex life?' or 'Have these medications affected your sex life?' These kinds of questions enable patients and let them know that it is okay to talk about sexual issues.

Limited Information

An explanation of normal anatomy or physiology and sexual norms may also be helpful. The patient may be reassured by an examination, which shows that the genitalia are normal. The clinician may also recommend a book or website which explains sexual matters.

Specific Suggestions

Common-sense advice on sexual techniques may be helpful. Examples of this would be advice about foreplay, spending time with your partner, using sex toys (e.g., vibrators), suggesting different sexual positions, use of vaginal dilators/trainers or the 'stop–start' technique. The use of specific medication would also be appropriate, for example, PDE5 inhibitors for erectile dysfunction.

Intensive Therapy

Some patients may benefit from referral to intensive therapy, including psychological interventions, sex therapy and/or biomedical approaches.

SEX THERAPY

Some problems are more complex – for example, sexual abuse – and require specialist referral. Specialist treatment usually involves an average of about 12 sessions. Sexual therapy consists of behavioural elements and counselling. Both methods allow exploration of the sexual history in a nonthreatening and supportive environment. A behavioural approach offers practical solutions to sexual dysfunction supported by the counsellor, for example, the 'stop–start' technique. It also includes elements of education about sexual functioning. Counselling allows exploration of the reasons behind the sexual dysfunction so that the patient can develop a greater understanding of the difficulties in order to solve or accept them.

Conclusion

Sexual problems can be very distressing and may present to any clinician. Some problems can be treated easily with simple advice or prescribed medication, whilst others need more prolonged specialist treatment. A few may never respond to treatment. The main aim for a clinician is to be able to discuss the subject comfortably. This is not easy, as both parties need to overcome their embarrassment. With sexual problems, more than with many aspects of medicine, there are many sensitivities, but with experience and some knowledge, any doctor can develop skills in this area. Sexual medicine is a diverse and interesting area of work and can be very rewarding for both the doctor and the patient.

Key Points

- **Sexual problems are important and history taking requires considerable skill. The problems may present directly, in the guise of another condition, or may be discovered coincidentally.**
- **Normal sexual response has five phases: desire, arousal, orgasm, resolution and a refractory phase, during which further arousal does not occur.**
- **Sexual response varies with age and with different phases of a relationship.**
- **Sex has several functions in addition to reproduction, for example, the strengthening of the pair bond.**
- **The most common male problems include erectile dysfunction and premature ejaculation.**
- **The most common female problems include loss of libido, orgasmic dysfunction and sexual pain.**
- **Causes of sexual dysfunction may be medical or psychological. Psychological factors include predisposing factors (e.g., poor sex education or childhood abuse). Dysfunction is also more likely after childbirth or if there has been infidelity, anxiety or poor communication.**
- **Treatment involves counselling and education, hormonal therapy and relaxation exercises. Couple, group or psychotherapy is sometimes required.**

Chapter 20

Abortion

Janine Dorothea Simpson, Audrey Brown

Chapter Outline

Introduction

Induced abortion or termination of pregnancy has been carried out for thousands of years. The provision of abortion in a legal, medically supervised, and safe framework remains one of the most contentious issues in modern-day medicine. Many people have strongly held and often divergent opinions about abortion. Those who are pro-abortion maintain that they are 'pro-choice' and support the right of individuals to make their own decisions. They are sensitive to the difficulties of bringing an unwanted baby into the world and are aware of the impact on both the woman concerned and the society more broadly. Often, the decision to proceed with abortion is multifactorial, including socioeconomic concerns, health- or partner-related issues

or fetal anomaly. Termination of pregnancy for fetal anomaly is discussed in Chapter 25 (Fetal medicine).

Those who are anti-abortion, or 'pro-life', argue that the fetus is more than just part of the mother. They maintain that it is a life in and of itself and should be protected, even if that means limiting the mother's choices regarding her body.

There are many factors leading to unplanned pregnancy: contraception may have failed or perhaps was not used at all. Occasionally, intercourse without the woman's consent has resulted in pregnancy. Of course, a woman may have an unplanned pregnancy but be pleased to be pregnant and continue the pregnancy. Another may have planned to be pregnant but then her circumstances may have changed, and she feels unable to continue. Among women attending antenatal clinics, research demonstrates that only two-thirds of women had an intended pregnancy, with the rest either ambivalent or having an unplanned pregnancy. Although abortion should not be considered as a method of contraception, contraceptive failures do occur and access to abortion allows women complete fertility regulation.

The Royal College of Obstetrics and Gynaecologists (RCOG) views abortion care as a health care need and important public health intervention. It forms a large part of the gynaecology workload in the United Kingdom, and induced abortion is one of the most common gynaecological procedures. In Britain, 1 in 3 women will have had an abortion by the age of 45 years. Although doctors may have differing degrees of involvement in abortion services, most at some point in their career will come into contact with women who are seeking abortion. Thus, doctors need to be familiar with the legal framework and options open to these women.

Worldwide Perspectives

Unintended pregnancy and abortions are experiences shared by people worldwide, irrespective of country, income, region or the legal status of abortion. It is estimated that there were 121 million unintended pregnancies worldwide each year between 2015 and 2019 and that almost two-thirds resulted in abortion. This equates to 73 million abortions per year.

Unintended pregnancy rates are higher in countries that restrict abortion access. It is estimated that the percentage of unintended pregnancies has increased over the last 3 decades from 36% (1990–1994) to 50% (2015–2019). This highlights an unmet need for contraception services.

The World Health Organization (WHO) estimates that 45% of all abortions worldwide are unsafe, with almost all of these occurring in low-income countries with the most restrictive laws. Illegal abortions are often performed in unclean environments, by persons lacking skills, or are possibly self-induced.

Unsafe abortion is a significant cause of maternal morbidity and mortality, accounting for approximately 13% of maternal deaths worldwide. In contrast, abortion performed in appropriate conditions with trained staff is a very safe procedure, with extremely low morbidity and mortality. This highlights the importance of improved access to modern contraception, postpartum contraception, and comprehensive abortion care. Strong partnerships from many sectors at a global, regional and country level are required to achieve these objectives.

United Kingdom (UK) Legal and Ethical Issues

GREAT BRITAIN (ENGLAND, SCOTLAND AND WALES)

Abortion has been a criminal offence in Britain since the 19th century when legislation was passed to reduce legal access to abortion (The Offences Against the Person Act, 1861, England and Wales; Scottish Common Law). During this time, there was a rise in 'back street' unsafe abortions, often with use of poisonous or ineffective treatments (e.g., lead). This saw an increase in maternal deaths during 1923 to 1933, with approximately 15% attributed to illegal abortion.

In 1967, legislation was passed (The Abortion Act) to allow abortions where certain criteria were met. This was further amended in 1990 by the Human Fertilisation and Embryology Act (Box 20.1).

Medications that are used in the abortion process are the prostaglandin analogue misoprostol and

---

BOX 20.1 CIRCUMSTANCES IN WHICH AN ABORTION MAY BE CARRIED OUT UNDER THE ABORTION ACT 1967 (AMENDED 1991)

A. The continuance of the pregnancy would involve risk to the life of the pregnant woman greater than if the pregnancy were terminated.

B. The termination is necessary to prevent grave permanent injury to the physical or mental health of the pregnant woman.

C. The pregnancy has *not* exceeded its 24th week and continuance of the pregnancy would involve risk, greater than if the pregnancy were terminated, of injury to the physical or mental health of the pregnant woman.

D. The pregnancy has *not* exceeded its 24th week and continuance of the pregnancy would involve risk, greater than if the pregnancy were terminated, of injury to the physical or mental health of the existing child(ren) of the family of the pregnant woman.

E. There is a substantial risk that if the child were born it would suffer from such physical or mental abnormalities as to be seriously handicapped.

mifepristone, an anti-progestogen. Prior to 2017, misoprostol had to be administered within a National Health Service (NHS) hospital or approved clinic. A women's place of ordinary residence was approved for home misoprostol use up to 9+6 weeks' gestation in Scotland in 2017, followed by England and Wales in 2018. This allows women the option of having their medical abortion at home, where they can be as comfortable as possible. Safety data and qualitative research supported this change, which reduces repeat clinic appointments, time away from work, childcare issues and risk of symptoms on their way home from clinic after taking the medication.

Further amendments were made in 2020 to ensure that essential abortion services continued during the COVID-19 pandemic. In March 2020, England, then Scotland and Wales, approved the use of home mifepristone and telemedicine to avoid women attending hospital/clinics due to the risks associated with COVID-19 spread.

There are also attempts in Britain to decriminalise abortion care (to bring Britain in line with Northern Ireland) and introduce buffer zones around abortion clinics to stop anti-abortion protests outside clinics.

The 1967 Abortion Act, as amended in 1990, states that abortion can be performed if two doctors agree that the pregnancy can be terminated on one or more grounds (see Box 20.1). Most abortions (98%) are carried out under Clause C of the Abortion Act, where two doctors agree that continuing the pregnancy would carry greater risk to the physical or mental health of the woman than abortion. A smaller number of abortions (1%) are carried out to protect the health of existing children. Clauses C and D carry an upper gestational limit of 24 weeks.

Current methods of inducing abortion are now so safe that it is safer for the woman to have an early abortion than to continue to term and give birth. Of course, that does not mean that abortion should be recommended for all women. However, a clinician may positively consider a request for an abortion when a woman feels that her health or well-being (or that of her children) will be adversely affected by continuing the pregnancy.

Although this provision is uncommonly used, the Abortion Act also allows abortion to be performed in an emergency situation upon the single signature of the doctor performing the procedure. Such an emergency abortion can be carried out either to save the life of the pregnant woman or to prevent grave permanent injury to the physical or mental health of the pregnant woman.

NORTHERN IRELAND

Abortion was decriminalised in Northern Ireland in 2019, meaning that now it is seen as a health care rather than a criminal matter. Prior to this, the 1861 Offences Against the Person Act was in place, limiting abortion to the most exceptional cases (rape or fatal fetal anomaly were not included). This meant that in 2018, approximately 1000 women travelled to Britain for an abortion, often self-funded. Others purchased abortion pills online illegally.

In June 2018, the UK Supreme Court found this to be in breach of the European Convention of Human Rights. In July 2019, the UK Parliament voted in favour of an amendment to a parliamentary bill.

The relevant section of the Northern Ireland (Executive Formation etc.) Act 2019 came into force in October 2019, with 2 key components.

1. Decriminalise abortion and a moratorium on abortion-related criminal prosecutions from that date.
2. Place the UK Government under a duty to bring forward regulations and introduce a new legal framework for abortion by 31 March 2020.

The regulations are detailed in Box 20.2.

BOX 20.2 THE ABORTION (NORTHERN IRELAND) REGULATIONS 2020

The Abortion (Northern Ireland) Regulations 2020 allow for:
1. abortion on request until a gestation of 12 weeks (certification by one registered medical practitioner)
2. abortion in circumstances in which the continuance of the pregnancy would involve risk of injury to the physical or mental health of the pregnant woman which is greater than if the pregnancy were terminated until a gestation of 24 weeks (certification by two registered medical practitioners)
3. abortion in cases of severe fetal impairment or fatal fetal abnormality (no gestational limit)
4. abortion if the pregnancy poses a risk to life or grave permanent injury to the physical or mental health of the pregnant woman (no gestational limit)

UK Perspectives

The Abortion Act was passed in 1967, after which there was a rapid rise in the number of abortions carried out in England, Wales and Scotland due to the legal framework and increased reporting.

In 2019, just over 207,000 abortions took place in England and Wales, with a further 13,583 in Scotland. Women of all reproductive ages have abortions, although the highest rate is among women aged 20 to 24 years, with the largest increase seen recently in women over 35 years. Most terminations (80%) are carried out before 10 weeks of pregnancy, with only 8% performed above 13 weeks of gestation. In Britain, 1 in 13 pregnant women have conceived within 1 year of a previous birth. This suggests an unmet contraception need for women following pregnancy, particularly following childbirth. Deprivation is associated with increased abortion prevalence.

Personal Beliefs

The Abortion Act 1967 allows doctors the legal and professional right to opt out of participating in abortion care. However, guidance from the General Medical Council in the United Kingdom advises that if a doctor is unable to make a referral for abortion, then a timely referral of the woman to a colleague who does not hold similar views is obligatory. Direct self-referrals to abortion clinics are now favoured to avoid untimely delays.

However, every doctor has an obligation to treat in an emergency situation. Therefore, it is essential that abortion care is embedded in undergraduate and postgraduate education.

Often, conscience is not black and white and should be visualised on a spectrum with conscientious objection and conscientious commitment at opposing ends. In practice, this allows doctors to set the limits on what they opt in and out off. It is recognised that these limits can change over time. However, it is important that conscientious objection does not lead to conscientious obstruction, whether that be overtly (e.g., providing false information), or delaying referral in subtle ways (e.g., being judgemental), or stating one's moral objection to abortion.

It is important to be open and honest with colleagues about conscience to ensure a supportive work environment and optimal patient care.

Consultation and Counselling Before Abortion

When a woman is considering abortion, it is important that she is able to weigh the practical and emotional aspects of her decision to ensure that the best choice is made in her circumstances. The National Institute for Health and Care Excellence (NICE) guideline on abortion care recommends that the initial assessment should be available within 1 week of the request to avoid any unnecessary delays. The abortion should be provided within 1 week of the assessment if required. There is no compulsory time period for reflection prior to abortion. It is important to meet the needs of the local populations, and assessments may need to be carried out by telephone or video call if appropriate (as occurred during the COVID-19 pandemic).

The woman will require sympathetic but non-directional support so that she is able to explore her own feelings and to make her own informed decision. Many women with an unplanned pregnancy will make their decision within a few days of knowing that they are pregnant. Other women may remain undecided for some time. It is important that the decision to abort or continue the pregnancy is made freely by the woman and that she is not coerced by another party, for example, a parent or partner. For this reason, it is imperative to speak to the woman alone at some point during the consultation.

Psychological problems and rates of depression are not increased after abortion when compared with background population risk, but some women may experience coping problems and distress. The assessment process can help to identify these women and ensure that appropriate support is offered both before and after the abortion. Box 20.3 outlines risk factors for emotional problems.

BOX 20.3 FACTORS ASSOCIATED WITH COPING PROBLEMS AND DISTRESS AFTER ABORTION

- Women with a history of mental health problems
- Younger women
- Women from cultural or religious groups who do not believe in abortion
- Women with low self-esteem
- Women without a close supportive person to talk to
- Women undergoing later abortions
- Women in whom the pregnancy was initially planned
- Women who feel there is no choice, for example, due to financial pressures

Women who blame themselves for the pregnancy and subsequent abortion can struggle to come to terms with their decision. It can help to identify what went wrong that led to the pregnancy. Jointly agreeing on a contraceptive plan with the woman can return a sense of control to her and give her something positive for the future to take from the experience.

Clinicians are used to taking a structured gynaecological and sexual history, collecting factual information, such as date of last menstrual period. However, clinicians should also help the woman to express her emotional needs by using some basic counselling techniques:

- Ask open-ended questions, for example, 'How did you feel about the pregnancy?' rather than 'Were you upset when you found out?'
- Actively listen to the woman, for example, show interest in her views, and show understanding.
- Reassure her that her feelings are normal, for example, saying 'I understand that you are finding this difficult to talk about'.
- Encourage questions, for example, say 'What would you like to ask me about your choices?', rather than 'Any questions?'

Some women need practical information to make their choice, such as details about maternity leave, housing rights and so forth, or information about adoption. Timely referral to a social worker should be available.

Pre-Abortion Investigations

Once the woman has decided to proceed to abortion, there are a number of investigations which are usually performed to ensure that the abortion is as safe as possible:

- *Blood tests:* Rhesus status should be established for those over 10^{+0} weeks proceeding with either medical or surgical abortion. Anti-D immunoglobulin is not recommended for those opting for a medical abortion who are 10^{+0} weeks or less but can be considered with surgical abortions if rhesus negative. If required, the dose for anti-D immunoglobulin is 250 international units (IU) if <20 weeks and 500 IU if >20 weeks.

  Human immunodeficiency virus (HIV) and syphilis testing should be offered to all women. Other blood-borne virus (BBV) testing and haemoglobinopathy screening can be performed if indicated.

  Haemoglobin measurement is no longer routine unless symptomatic of anaemia, for example, dizziness, shortness of breath.

- *Estimation of gestation:* This can be performed by history, clinical examination or ultrasound. RCOG and NICE guidance state that routine ultrasound scanning to confirm gestation is not required. This supports the use of telemedicine. However, it is essential to provide when gestation is unclear, when ectopic pregnancy is suspected, or if requested by the person.

  Some women will not make the decision until they know the gestation of the pregnancy, that is, they may decide to abort an early pregnancy but would not wish to undergo a later abortion. Occasionally, women may request a scan photograph as a memento of the pregnancy. Ultrasound will sometimes show a non-viable pregnancy, which will then relieve the woman of a decision around abortion and may avoid an unnecessary intervention.

- *Prevention of infection:* The NICE suggests that routine antibiotic prophylaxis is not required with medical abortions but should be offered with surgical abortions. Prophylaxis may be appropriate for women at high risk of sexually transmitted infections (STIs) or who would find it difficult to access treatment at a later date if screening was performed.

  Some clinics offer routine STI screening (including *Chlamydia trachomatis* and *Neisseria gonorrhoea*) to all women. This provides a holistic opportunity to detect infection and carry out partner notification (contact tracing) when there is a positive test, thus preventing reinfection of the woman and onward transmission.

  If antibiotics are indicated, doxycycline 100 mg twice daily for 3 days should be considered in medical or surgical abortions. If metronidazole is used, it should not be routinely used in combination with broad-spectrum antibiotics, for example, doxycycline.

- *Cervical cytology*: If a woman is due cervical cytology within the national screening programme, then this should be offered opportunistically at the time of the clinic visit.
- *Provision of information*: Information given verbally should be supported with written information for the woman to take away, available in a range of languages and formats. This should include information about the types of abortion available, the risks and complications of abortion, and whom to contact if there are any problems after the procedure.
- *Venous thromboembolism (VTE) prophylaxis*: Pregnancy increases a woman's risk of developing VTE; this increased risk begins in the first trimester. All women should be assessed for VTE risk factors and thromboprophylaxis with low-molecular-weight heparin offered if appropriate (see Chapter 24, Maternal Medicine).

Methods of Abortion

Historically, a wide range of surgical and medical techniques has been used to induce abortion. Advances made in the past 3 decades in abortion techniques mean that safe and effective methods are now available at all stages of gestation. Medical methods have been increasingly used since the licencing of mifepristone in 1991. Both medical and surgical abortion can be offered up to 24 weeks, but availability varies in different geographical areas.

In England and Wales, around 73% of abortions are performed using medical methods, whereas in Scotland, 88% are medical. The most appropriate method depends on gestation, medical history and the woman's preference (Box 20.4).

MEDICAL ABORTION

Mifepristone is a synthetic steroid that blocks the biological action of progesterone by binding to its receptor in the uterus and other organs. It is taken orally. Between 24 and 48 hours later (usually 48 hours), a prostaglandin is administered, which can be given vaginally, buccally or sublingually. Bleeding usually starts within a few hours, followed by uterine contractions which expel the fetus and placenta. Most women experience period-like pains but there is much

---

BOX 20.4 ABORTION OPTIONS, DEPENDING ON GESTATION

Medical Abortion
- 'Early' medical abortion
  - up to and including 10^{+0} weeks
  - mifepristone plus single-dose misoprostol
- Medical abortion between 10^{+1} and 23^{+6} weeks
  - mifepristone plus misoprostol
  - several doses of misoprostol may be required
  - need to perform feticide intervention if over 22 weeks' gestation

Surgical Abortion
- Manual vacuum aspiration
  - under local anaesthesia
  - careful follow-up required
- Suction abortion
  - between 7 and 13^{+6} weeks
  - cervical preparation recommended
  - local or general anaesthesia
- Dilatation and evacuation
  - between 14 and 24 weeks
  - requires specially trained surgeon

Note: Providing a choice of abortion method increases women's satisfaction.

---

variation, with some women needing no pain relief while others (about 10%–20%) require opiates. Bleeding usually continues for about 10 days after medical abortion.

Early Medical Abortion (Up to and Including 10 Weeks' Gestation)

When a woman is less than 7 weeks' pregnant, medical abortion is the most effective type of termination, with a lower failure rate than early surgical abortion. This can be performed at home, an approved clinic or hospital setting, depending on preference and individual circumstances.

If the woman chooses to be at home, analgesia and a follow up human chorionic gonadotrophin (hCG) urine test with written instructions should be provided. This is often performed by the woman 2 to 3 weeks following abortion. Contraception should also be issued and inserted or commenced immediately if required.

The usual regimen is mifepristone 200 mg orally followed by misoprostol 800 μg vaginally 24 to 48 hours later. If 9^{+6} days or less, both medications can be taken

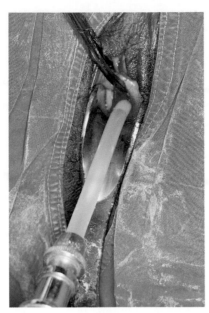

Fig. 20.1 Surgical termination of pregnancy at 10 weeks' gestation.

and administered in either the person's ordinary residence or a hospital or approved clinic setting. If 10+0 weeks, medication needs to be administered in a hospital or approved clinic setting due to the legal framework. This will require 2 clinic appointments. The woman can have the option of expulsion at home following misoprostol administration.

MEDICAL ABORTION (BETWEEN 10+1 AND 23+6 WEEKS)

In the past, surgical termination alone has been offered to women in the late first trimester. However, it is now recognised that medical abortion is an effective alternative to surgical termination in the late first trimester.

Traditionally, mid-trimester medical abortion was carried out using prostaglandins alone or in combination with an oxytocin infusion. With this regime, it would commonly take several days for the abortion to be completed. Giving mifepristone prior to prostaglandins significantly reduces the length of time taken for the abortion to occur.

Medical abortions at this gestation are often carried out in an inpatient setting. The usual regimen is:

- Mifepristone 200 mg orally followed by misoprostol 800 μg vaginally 36 to 48 hours later. Subsequent doses of misoprostol 400 μg, given every 3 hours vaginally, sublingually or buccally, are given until abortion occurs. Lower doses may be used at later gestations for women who have had a previous caesarean section.

SURGICAL ABORTION

Surgical abortion can be carried out under local or general anaesthesia (GA).

Surgical Abortion (7–13+6 Weeks)

Surgical abortion below 7 weeks' gestation has a higher failure rate than medical abortion at these earlier gestations.

Cervical priming should be offered, with the aim of reducing incomplete abortions for parous women and to aid cervical dilatation. It may cause bleeding and pain prior to the procedure.

The usual regime is:

- 400 μg misoprostol sublingually 1 hour prior to abortion
- 400 μg misoprostol vaginally 3 hours prior to abortion.

This can be performed by either manual vacuum aspiration (MVA) under local anaesthetic or by suction or vacuum aspiration using a flexible suction curette and a mechanical or electrical pump under GA. The suction curette is inserted into the uterine cavity after cervical dilatation, and the contents aspirated (Figs 20.1 and 20.2). Intrauterine contraception can be fitted after the products of conception have been expelled.

A women's choice may be influenced by the need to fast, or requirement to be discharged home with an adult following GA. She may find this difficult if she does not wish anyone to know that she has had an abortion.

Manual Vacuum Aspiration

Following cervical priming, a flexible suction curette is inserted into the uterus under local paracervical block after adequate cervical dilatation. This is often performed in an outpatient setting, with specialized staff supporting both the woman and clinician. The pregnancy is aspirated using a specialized double-valve syringe. It is very important to ensure that the abortion is complete, either by identifying the products of conception or by hCG follow-up. If it is the chosen method, post-abortion intrauterine contraception can be fitted after the products of conception have been expelled.

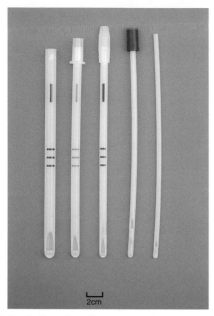

Fig. 20.2 A selection of suction curettes for surgical pregnancy termination.

TABLE 20.1	Abortion-Related Complications	
	Early Medical Abortion	Vacuum Aspiration
Failure to end the pregnancy	1 in 100	1 in 1000
Retained (non-viable) tissue	3–5 in 100	1 in 100
Infection	<1 in 100	<1 in 100
Haemorrhage	1 in 1000	1 in 1000
Cervical tear	–	1 in 100
Uterine perforation	–	1 in 1000

Complications of Abortion

Health care professionals should ensure that women have the information they require to make an informed choice and provide fully informed consent. However, the risk of complications is low and, indeed, an abortion is safer than continuing the pregnancy to term. Nevertheless, complications do occasionally occur. Thus, women should be given information about where to seek help if there are problems (Table 20.1).

RETAINED PRODUCTS OF CONCEPTION

Retained products of conception occurs in less than 5% of women. It is more common after medical abortion and when surgical abortion is carried out at either very early or later gestations. Some women with retained products will require (further) surgical evacuation of the uterus, particularly if there is heavy or prolonged bleeding. However, many women will pass the retained tissue spontaneously, without the need for further intervention. Antibiotics can be given to reduce the risk of secondary infection until the tissue is passed.

FAILURE OF ABORTION

Ongoing pregnancy after an abortion procedure is unusual, occurring in less than 1% of cases. Women should be advised of the importance of performing a follow-up hCG urine test (if medical abortion at home) or returning for follow-up if there was any doubt over completion at the time of the procedure or if there are continuing symptoms of pregnancy.

POST-ABORTION INFECTION

Pelvic infection can occur in up to 10% of women after termination. Women should be advised about signs of

Later Surgical Abortion (14–24 Weeks)

Cervical preparation followed by dilatation and evacuation (D&E) can be offered in the second trimester.

The usual regime is:
- 14^{+0} to 16^{+0}: osmotic dilators or misoprostol (buccal, vaginal, sublingual) or mifepristone (given the day before procedure)
- 16^{+1} to 19^{+0}: osmotic dilators or misoprostol (buccal, vaginal, sublingual)
- 19^{+1} to 23^{+6}: mifepristone (given day before procedure) *and* inserting osmotic dilators at the same time as mifepristone.

This is the method of choice in the United States but in the United Kingdom is offered by a limited number of doctors experienced in the technique. It may be necessary to dilate the cervix up to a diameter of 20 mm before the fetal parts can be extracted using special instruments. D&E has the advantage that the woman is under anaesthesia – thus, she is unaware of the procedure. There is evidence from the United States that women prefer D&E to medical methods, although some nurses and doctors can find the procedure distressing.

infection – such as pyrexia, pelvic pain and offensive vaginal discharge – and should return if concerned.

HAEMORRHAGE

Significant haemorrhage of over 500 mL at the time of termination occurs in less than 1 in 1000 early abortion cases, rising to 4 in 1000 when over 20 weeks' gestation.

TRAUMA TO THE GENITAL TRACT

Perforation of the uterus happens in about 1 in 1000 surgical cases and is more common with later-gestation abortions and with less experienced surgeons. Cervical trauma is also uncommon (<1 in 100) and is reduced by cervical preparation with prostaglandin. Uterine rupture has been described with mid-trimester medical abortion.

FUTURE FERTILITY

Women often ask about the chance of an abortion affecting their future fertility. There is no established positive association between previous termination of pregnancy and future infertility, ectopic pregnancy or placenta praevia. There may be a slight increase in risk of subsequent miscarriage and pre-term delivery with later abortion, although the evidence is unclear.

PSYCHOLOGICAL SEQUELAE

There is no evidence of lasting psychological harm to women undergoing abortion and, indeed, there is no difference in psychological sequelae if women abort or continue the pregnancy. Some women may be at higher risk of distress after the abortion; they can be identified at the time of pre-abortion consultation and offered greater support.

BREAST CANCER

There is no evidence that having an abortion increases the risk of breast cancer.

Abortion Aftercare

Women should be provided with appropriate information regarding symptoms and signs of complications and should be given a contact telephone number if they have concerns after the procedure. There is no need for routine follow-up when the completion of the abortion was confirmed at the time.

POST-ABORTION CONTRACEPTION

Over one-third of terminations are carried out on women who have had a termination in the past. Ensuring that there is adequate contraception available can reduce the chance of a further abortion. All methods of hormonal contraception (combined hormonal, progestogen pill, implant or injection) can be started on the day of surgical abortion, or on the prostaglandin treatment day of medical abortion, with immediate contraceptive cover.

Intrauterine contraception can be fitted immediately following abortion. This can be done at the end of the surgical procedure or following expulsion of the pregnancy with medical termination.

Women are usually advised not to use a diaphragm within 6 weeks of mid-trimester abortion in case refitting is required. Female sterilization is not usually performed at the same time as abortion. This is because simultaneous sterilization is associated with a higher sterilization failure rate and increased subsequent regret about being sterilized. Women who wish to be sterilized can be offered an interval sterilization, with provision of a bridging method of contraception in the interim.

Education and Training

Abortion care should be embedded into both undergraduate and postgraduate medical, nursing and midwifery curriculums. As mentioned earlier, 1 in 3 women in Great Britain will experience abortion by the age of 45 years. Therefore, all medical disciplines are likely to be involved with abortion assessment or post-abortion care.

Conclusion

Over 200,000 women undergo induced abortion each year in the United Kingdom. Women need to be well informed about pregnancy and abortion options and supported to make an informed choice. A choice between medical and surgical abortion should be offered. A range of contraceptive options should be made available to women at the time of termination.

Key Points

- **Unsafe abortion is a great threat to women's health worldwide and causes many maternal mortalities.**

- Induced abortion is a common, safe and effective procedure. In the United Kingdom, it is carried out under the terms of the Abortion Act 1967/The Abortion (Northern Ireland) Regulations 2020.
- Women considering abortion need information about options to guide their choice and non-directive support to ensure that they reach the most appropriate decision.
- A choice between medical and surgical abortion should be offered.
- A contraceptive plan should be agreed upon and in place immediately after the abortion.

Chapter 21

Contraception

Savita Brito-Mutunayagam, Susan Brechin

Chapter Outline

Introduction

A rights-based approach to sexual and reproductive health supports women to choose if and when they wish to have children, and if so, how many. This is central to women's empowerment, reducing poverty and achieving the United Nation's Sustainable Development Goals.

The growing use of contraception worldwide has led to a reduction in maternal and neonatal mortality and improvements in socioeconomic conditions.

Currently, the World Health Organization (WHO) recommends a 24-month inter-pregnancy interval after childbirth. It has been estimated that worldwide effective family planning could prevent 1 in 10 deaths among babies by helping women to space births at least 2 years apart, because a short inter-pregnancy interval of less than 12 months increases the risk of complications such as low birth weight, pre-term birth, stillbirth and neonatal death.

The Faculty of Sexual and Reproductive Health-care (FSRH) has developed the UK Medical Eligibility

TABLE 21.1 UK Medical Eligibility Criteria (UKMEC) Categories

UKMEC Category	Definition
UKMEC 1	A condition for which there is *no restriction* for the use of the contraceptive method
UKMEC 2	A condition for which the *advantages of using the method generally outweigh the theoretical or proven risks*
UKMEC 3	A condition in which the *theoretical or proven risks usually outweigh the advantages* of using the method[a]
UKMEC 4	A condition which represents an *unacceptable health risk* if the contraceptive method is used

[a]The provision of a method to a woman with a condition given a UKMEC category 3 requires expert clinical judgement and/or referral to a specialist contraceptive provider since use of the method is not usually recommended unless other methods are not available or not acceptable.

Criteria (UKMEC), which provide evidence-based recommendations to facilitate the safe use of contraception without imposing unnecessary medical restrictions. The categories used to define risk are summarized in Table 21.1.

Defining 'contraceptive failure' is not easy, as it depends on the population studied. Studies on a young population will suggest a higher failure rate than in an older age group, since fertility is higher in younger people. Therefore, caution is required when interpreting relevant figures. Contraceptive 'method' failure includes the inherent chance of pregnancy provided the method is used correctly. It is quantified in the unit per 100 woman-years (HWY), which represents the number of women who would become pregnant if 100 of them used that method of contraception for 1 year. Contraceptive user failure is the chance of pregnancy when the method is not used correctly (e.g., missed pills, late injections, drug interactions). If used correctly, hormonal contraceptives (combined hormonal method, progestogen-only pills [POPs], injectables, implant and intrauterine system) and the non-hormonal methods (copper intrauterine device [Cu-IUD], male and female sterilization) are more than 99% effective in preventing pregnancy. These methods, as well as emergency contraception (EC), barrier methods and fertility-awareness methods, are described in this chapter.

Methods of Contraception

Contraception can be considered as either hormonal (pills, patch, intravaginal ring, injectables, the subdermal implant and the levonorgestrel-releasing intrauterine system [LNG-IUS]) or non-hormonal (Cu-IUD, barrier methods, sterilization, lactational amenorrhoea method [LAM] and fertility-awareness methods). In the United Kingdom, oral contraception remains the most popular method, with a third of women on contraception using this as their primary method. Increasingly popular are the long-acting reversible contraceptive (LARC) methods, which include subdermal implants and both the Cu-IUD and LNG-IUS. LARCs are cost-effective in the prevention of pregnancy and there is no delay in return to fertility after discontinuing these methods.

Hormonal Contraception

COMBINED HORMONAL CONTRACEPTION (CHC)

CHC (pills, patch, and intravaginal ring) methods work primarily by inhibiting ovulation via the hypothalamo – pituitary – ovarian axis, leading to a reduction in luteinizing hormone (LH) and follicle-stimulating hormone. In addition, cervical mucus is less easily penetrated by sperm and the endometrium is thinned. Most data on the use and safety of CHC relates specifically to the combined oral contraceptive (COC) pill. This evidence is extrapolated to the transdermal patch and intravaginal ring, as they also contain estrogen and progestogen.

Most currently available COC pills contain ethinylestradiol (EE) and a progestogen (synthetic progesterone), which can be norethisterone (first generation); levonorgestrel (LNG, second generation); desogestrel, norgestimate and gestodene (third generation); or drospirenone, dienogest and nomegestrol acetate (fourth generation). The majority of COCs are usually a fixed-dose (monophasic) pill containing 20 to 35 μg of EE and a progestogen. There are no proven benefits of biphasic or triphasic COCs (doses of the constituent hormones of which are varied week to week) over a monophasic pill.

How to Take the Combined Oral Contraceptive Pill

Conventionally, a monophasic COC can be started up to and including day 5 of the menstrual cycle (or following termination of pregnancy) to provide immediate contraceptive protection. If started after this time, condoms or abstinence is advised for the next 7 days (or until 7 consecutive pills have been taken). Most COC packages contain 21 active tablets: one tablet is taken daily for 21 consecutive days, followed by a 7-day pill-free interval (PFI) or placebo pill week. For pills with placebo, 21 active pills are followed by 7 inactive pills with no pill-free week. A withdrawal bleed usually occurs in the PFI due to the withdrawal of hormones, which induces endometrial shedding.

Women should be encouraged to take COCs around the same time every day to support compliance. In general, one pill can be missed without requiring any further action as long as all of the other pills have been taken and continue to be taken correctly. Tailored regimens for taking CHCs are supported by the FSRH and detailed later in this chapter.

Contraindications to Combined Hormonal Contraception

Most of the available evidence relates to the COC, but this evidence can also be applied to the use of the combined patch and intravaginal ring. Women considering CHC should be informed of the potential risks and benefits associated with use. However, it is safe for most women most of the time (Table 21.2). COCs increase the risk of venous thromboembolism (VTE) above the background risk of 2 per 10,000 woman-years among women not using a COC. The COCs containing LNG, norethisterone or norgestimate have the lowest risk (5 – 7 per 10,000 women) and those containing drospirenone, desogestrel or gestodene have the highest risk (9 – 12 per 10,000 women). The risk is greatest in the first few months after initiating the COC and the risk falls to that of non-users within weeks of discontinuation. Nevertheless, when prescribed appropriately, the benefits of CHC use generally outweigh the risk of venous thrombosis, which is low overall and is lower than the VTE risk associated with pregnancy and the postpartum period (Table 21.3). A clinical history should identify any risk factors for VTE that fall within the UKMEC categories 3 or 4 for use of hormonal contraception. A personal history of VTE, current VTE, a family history of VTE in a first-degree relative under the age of 45 years, major surgery with prolonged immobilization, immobility

TABLE 21.2	Risks and Benefits Associated With Combined Oral Contraceptive (COC) Use
Disease	**Relative Risk With COC Use in Non-Smokers**
Potential harms (risks)	
Coronary artery disease	Very small increase
Ischaemic stroke	Two-fold increase
Venous thrombo-embolism	Three- to six-fold increase
Breast cancer	Any increased risk likely to be small and will vary with age
	No increased risk above background risk 10 years after stopping COC
Cervical cancer	Small increase after 5 years and a two-fold increase after 10 years
Benefits	
Ovarian cancer	Halving of risk, lasting for >15 years
Endometrial cancer	Halving of risk, lasting for >15 years
Colorectal cancer	Reduction

TABLE 21.3	Risk of Venous Thromboembolism (VTE)
Absolute Risk of VTE per 10,000 Woman-Years	**Circumstance**
2	For women not using combined oral contraceptive (COC) and not pregnant
9 – 10	For women using a COC
29	For women who are pregnant
300 – 400	For women who are immediately postpartum

and known thrombogenic mutations fall under these UKMEC categories. Non-smokers may safely continue to use CHC, including COC, to age 50 years if they have no contraindications for use. Deaths in COC users over 35 years of age are eight times more common in smokers than non-smokers. For women who continue to smoke (<15 cigarettes/day) at the age of 35 years, COC use is given a UKMEC category 3 (risks outweigh benefits) and if smoking ≥15 cigarettes/day, a UKMEC category 4 is given (unacceptable health risk).

The use of CHC may pose an unacceptable health risk (UKMEC 4) in women with current and/or history of ischaemic heart disease, stroke, vascular disease, hypertension, liver disease (severe cirrhosis, active viral hepatitis, tumours) or migraine with aura at any age, or for women within 6 weeks postpartum and breastfeeding. Notably, women who have recently given birth (between 3 and 6 weeks postpartum), who are not breastfeeding, and have no risk factors for VTE can safely start CHC.

Drug Interactions

Enzyme-inducing drugs increase the metabolism of estrogens and progestogens. This may, in turn, reduce the contraceptive efficacy of CHC. Women using enzyme-inducing drugs should switch to a method that is unaffected by their use (such as the Cu-IUD, the LNG-IUS or the progestogen-only injectable). Liver enzyme – inducing drugs include some antiepileptics (such as carbamazepine), some antiretrovirals, certain antibiotics (such as rifabutin and rifampicin) and the over-the-counter herbal medicine St John's Wort. These liver enzyme – inducing drugs can accelerate the hepatic breakdown of contraceptive steroids, potentially reducing the efficacy of the COC. Women using COC whilst also receiving liver enzyme – inducing drugs in the short term may continue to use this method if they consider a minimum 50-µg EE pill (such as a 30-µg pill plus a 20-µg EE monophasic) as a tricycling regimen with a PFI of 4 days. This should be used during treatment and continued for a further 28 days after treatment with the liver enzyme – inducing medication has stopped. The use of two patches or two rings is not recommended. For women using the very potent enzyme inducers rifampicin and rifabutin, an alternative method is always advised. Additional contraceptive precautions are not required when non-liver enzyme – inducing antibiotics are used.

Conversely, some medications may themselves be affected by hormonal contraceptive use. For example, women taking lamotrigine should be advised that there is a risk of reduced seizure control whilst on CHC along with the potential for lamotrigine toxicity in the CHC-free week; the risks of using CHC may outweigh the benefits in these women.

Follow-Up

A 12-month supply of COC can be provided at the first visit. However, for some women, a follow-up at 3 months may be appropriate to assess any problems and provide re-instruction if necessary. Blood pressure should be measured annually. Women should be encouraged to attend at any time if problems arise. The pill should be discontinued if any potentially serious side effects occur (e.g., chest pain, leg pain or swelling). Follow-up visits are also an opportunity to carry out other well-woman screening (e.g., blood pressure, cervical cytology, new risk of sexually transmitted infections [STIs]).

The COC should be stopped and an alternative method used at least 4 weeks before any major surgery when other than a brief period of immobilization is expected. The COC may be recommenced from 2 weeks after return to full mobility.

Combined Hormonal Contraceptive Patch

A combined transdermal patch (CTP) releases an average of 33.9 µg EE and 203 µg norelgestromin per 24 hours. The risks and benefits associated with transdermal patch use are as for the COC (see Table 21.2).

A patch can be applied to the abdomen, buttock or thigh on the same day each week for 3 consecutive weeks. This may be followed by a patch-free week during which time there is endometrial shedding and a withdrawal bleed. As per its licence, the transdermal patch is usually changed every 7 days, although a single patch will provide effective contraceptive protection for up to 9 days. As for the COC, the transdermal patch can be started up to and including day 5 of the menstrual cycle to provide immediate contraceptive protection. If started after this time, condoms or abstinence are advised for the next 7 days.

Combined Hormonal Intravaginal Contraceptive Ring

The risks and benefits associated with intravaginal ring use are as described for the COC (see Table 21.2). The intravaginal ring is associated with a low and stable serum concentration of EE of only 15 µg. As per its licence, the ring should be inserted into the vagina on the same day each month and is retained for 3 weeks. This may be followed by a ring-free week, during which time the endometrium sheds and there is a withdrawal bleed. Once inserted into the vagina by the woman, the ring sits above the pelvic floor and should not be felt by her and does not need to be removed during intercourse. The intravaginal ring can be inserted up to and including day 5 of the menstrual cycle to provide immediate contraceptive protection. If started after this time, condoms or abstinence are advised for the next 7 days.

'Tailored' CHC Regimens

Continuous dosing or extended regimens of CHC are becoming increasingly common modes of administration. Although these regimens are outside product licences, there is evidence and guidance to support use in such a manner. The conventional 21/7 CHC regimens for oral, transdermal and intravaginal methods, with their monthly withdrawal bleed, confer no health benefit over other patterns of CHC use. 'Tailored' CHC regimens, in which there are fewer (or no) hormone-free intervals (HFIs) and/or shortened HFI can be safely used to avoid withdrawal bleeds and associated symptoms and theoretically reduce the risk of contraceptive failure. Women should be given information about both standard and tailored CHC regimens to broaden contraceptive choice. Women should be advised that use of tailored CHC regimens is outside the manufacturer's licence but is supported by the FSRH, the United Kingdom. See Table 21.4 for standard and tailored regimens for use of CHC.

PROGESTOGEN-ONLY CONTRACEPTION

Progestogen-only contraception (pills, injectables, subdermal implant and the LNG-IUS) avoids the potential risks attributed to estrogen use. Most progestogen-only methods are associated with a disturbance in the bleeding pattern, which is often the main reason for discontinuation of these otherwise very effective methods. Other side effects have been reported (abdominal bloating, weight changes, acne, headaches and mood changes) but few have been objectively related to progestogen use.

Drug Interactions

The effect of liver enzyme-inducing drugs on the metabolism of progestogens is similar to that for estrogens. This reduces the efficacy of the POP or subdermal implant and alternative methods of contraception are recommended. However, the progestogen-only injectable depot medroxyprogesterone acetate (DMPA) and the LNG-IUS are not affected by liver enzyme – inducing medication and may be a good option for women in these circumstances.

Progestogen-Only Pills (POPs)

POPs containing LNG, norethisterone or desogestrel are currently available in the United Kingdom. Although POPs are suitable for most women, they are often used by women for whom a COC is contraindicated. All POPs thicken cervical mucus, thus preventing sperm penetration, which is the primary mode of action of POPs. Some POPs also inhibit ovulation, although not in every cycle: POPs containing norethisterone or LNG inhibit ovulation in up to 60% of cycles and the desogestrel POP inhibits ovulation in up to 97% of cycles. A POP should be taken at or around the same time every day *without* a PFI. A POP can be started up to and including day 5 of the menstrual cycle (within 5 days of a termination of pregnancy or up to day 21 postpartum) to provide immediate contraception. If started at other times, additional contraception, such as condoms, is required for the first 48 hours. A norethisterone or LNG-POP is late if

TABLE 21.4 Standard and Tailored Regimens for Use of Combined Hormonal Contraception (CHC), Monophasic Combined Oral Contraceptive (COC), Patch, and Ring

Type of Regimen	Period of CHC Use	Hormone-Free Interval (HFI)
Standard use	21 days (21 active pills or 1 ring, or 3 patches)	7 days
Tailored Use		
Shortened HFI	21 days (21 active pills or 1 ring, or 3 patches)	4 days
Extended use (tricycling)	9 weeks (3 × 21 active pills or 3 rings, or 9 patches used consecutively)	4 or 7 days
Flexible extended use	Continuous use (≥21 days) of active pills, patches or rings until breakthrough bleeding occurs for 3 – 4 days	4 days
Continuous use	Continuous use of active pills, patches or rings	None

taken ≥3 hours after when it was due to be taken; the desogestrel POP is late if >12 hours has elapsed. Contraception from intercourse prior to the missed pill is maintained but barrier methods are recommended until two consecutive pills have been taken, by which time the cervical mucus effect preventing sperm penetration is maximal again.

Progestogen-Only Injectable Contraception

The most widely used progestogen-only injectable in the United Kingdom is DMPA, which is licenced to be given as an intramuscular (IM) injection every 12 weeks. The FSRH recommends that the IM DMPA injection dosing interval can be extended up to 13 weeks ± 7 days (outside licence) and still provide effective contraception.

A subcutaneous DMPA (SC DMPA) preparation licenced for self-administration is also available. It is bioequivalent to IM DMPA and is administered at the same dosing interval of 13 weeks ± 7 days. SC DMPA is supplied in a pre-filled injector and can be self-injected into the anterior thigh or abdomen. This self-delivered method provides an option for women who cannot or do not wish to attend regular appointments.

The primary mode of action of the progestogen-only injectable is inhibition of ovulation. Unpredictable bleeding is common in the initial months of use but usually resolves spontaneously and up to 70% of women experience no bleeding at 1 year of use. Women should be informed that there could be a delay of up to 1 year in the return of fertility after stopping the use of injectable contraceptives. This is possibly due to the serum levels of DMPA, which in some women can still be detected between 6 and 9 months after a single injection and, for some women, in concentrations sufficient to inhibit ovulation. Hormonal investigations should not normally be considered until amenorrhoea continues for up to 12 months after the last injection was given.

A reversible loss of bone mineral density occurs with DMPA use. Most of this bone loss is in the initial 2 years of use; thereafter, there is no further loss. There is no indication to consider dual-energy X-ray absorptiometry bone scans routinely in women using DMPA, even with long-term use. Serum concentrations of estrogen in women using DMPA are similar to concentrations seen in the follicular phase of the menstrual cycle; therefore, women are not hypo-estrogenic. There is no apparent increase in risk of fracture and, moreover, bone mineral density recovers after cessation of DMPA use. In women aged under 18 years, DMPA may be used as first-line contraception after other options have been discussed and considered unsuitable or unacceptable. Women can use DMPA up to the age of 50 years, at which time an alternative method should be considered. This is because of concerns about the impact on skeletal health and the theoretical risk of osteoporotic fracture in menopause. However, if a woman prefers to continue or start the method at the age of 50 years or over, this would not be an unacceptable health risk provided the benefits and risks have been assessed and explained. Women using DMPA who wish to continue use should be reviewed every 2 years to assess individual situations and to discuss the benefits and potential risks.

Weight gain is a recognised effect of DMPA use, particularly in women under 18 years of age with a starting BMI of ≥30.

Progestogen-Only Subdermal Implants

This is a single subdermal etonogestrel implant or rod made from a non-biodegradable polymer that contains an active slow-release progestogen formulation and is about the size of a matchstick. The implant is licenced to provide contraception for up to 3 years. Changes in bleeding patterns are common: infrequent bleeding is the most common pattern (in approximately one-third of women); around one-fifth of women experience no bleeding; and approximately one-quarter have prolonged or frequent bleeding. These bleeding patterns may not settle with time. Women who experience troublesome bleeding while using the progestogen-only implant and who are eligible to use CHC may be offered and respond to a COC taken cyclically or continuously for 3 months (outside of the product licence). There is no evidence of a causal association between the use of the implant and weight change, mood change, loss of libido or headache. Health care professionals who insert and remove progestogen-only implants must be appropriately trained. Insertion is intended to render the implant palpable beneath the skin. Barium sulphate is added to the implant so that if an implant cannot be palpated, an X-ray of the upper arm enables it to be located. The incidence of 'deep' insertion is around 1 in 1000 women: an ultrasound scan can be used to facilitate location and subsequent removal of deep implants lying above muscle.

Levonorgestrel-Releasing Intrauterine Systems

There are three intrauterine systems that contain different doses of LNG. Both offer highly effective and reversible contraception. They are T-shaped devices with an elastomer core containing LNG (Fig. 21.1A). The LNG-IUS works primarily by its progestogenic effect on the endometrium, preventing implantation. In addition, effects on cervical mucus reduce sperm penetration. Ovulation may be inhibited in some women. Systemic side effects due to absorption of LNG are often mild and usually settle in the first 3 months of use.

The 52-mg LNG-IUS is licenced for 5-year use as contraception (and/or as a treatment for heavy menstrual bleeding). Failure rates for 5-year use are low (1%). Irregular bleeding with the 52-mg LNG-IUS is common in the first few months after insertion but often settles by 6 months after insertion. Menstrual loss is reduced by an average of 90% at 12 months, with 20% of women experiencing amenorrhoea. For women who have the device inserted after the age of 45 years, the 52-mg LNG-IUS may be continued until menopause is confirmed or until the age of 55 years, at which time the large majority of women are postmenopausal.

The 13.5-mg LNG-IUS is a smaller device with a lower dose of LNG. It is licenced for contraception for a duration of 3 years. The device contains a silver ring, which distinguishes it from other intrauterine devices on ultrasound scan or X-ray. Women using the 13.5-mg LNG-IUS are less likely to experience amenorrhoea in comparison with those using the 52-mg LNG-IUS.

The 19.5-mg LNG-IUS device provides contraception for 5 years. The T-frame dimensions of the device are identical to those of the 13.5-mg LNG-IUS; it also contains a silver ring which improves visibility on imaging. The contraceptive effectiveness of the 19.5-mg LNG-IUS appears to be comparable to other LNG-IUS devices. Women using the 19.5-mg LNG-IUS report a decrease in menstrual bleeding over time. Limited evidence suggests that those using the 19.5-mg LNG-IUS are more likely to experience amenorrhoea than those using the 13.5-mg LNG-IUS device and are less likely to experience amenorrhoea

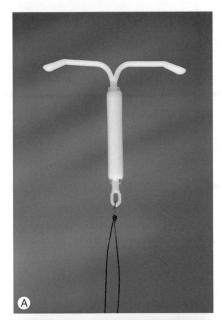

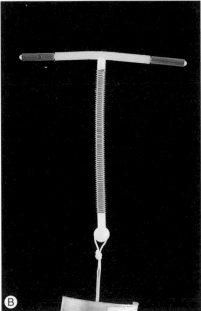

Fig. 21.1 Intrauterine contraception (IUC). (A) Levonorgestrel-releasing intrauterine system. **(B)** Copper intrauterine device.

than those using the 52-mg LNG-IUS, reflecting an anticipated dose – response effect.

The potential adverse effects and complications associated with insertion of the LNG-IUS are as for a Cu-IUD (see later discussion).

Non-Hormonal Contraception

COPPER INTRAUTERINE DEVICES

Copper is toxic to ova and sperm – the Cu-IUD works primarily by inhibiting fertilization. In addition, the endometrial inflammatory reaction generated by the Cu-IUD has an anti-implantation effect and alterations in cervical mucus inhibit sperm penetration. Failure rates for Cu-IUD contraception used for up to 5 years are low (2% with a 380-mm² Cu-IUD). Banded Cu-IUDs, which have 380 mm² of copper in the vertical stem and copper sleeves on the horizontal arms, are the most effective IUDs available and are recommended to be used as a first-line device (Fig. 21.1B). Some banded devices available in the United Kingdom can be used for up to 10 years.

The intrauterine ball (IUB) is a novel copper device that is distinct in its three-dimensional spherical shape, consisting of several copper pearls. It is thought to have an elasticity that allows it to conform to the uterus. This device is not widely available in the United Kingdom at present but may become so in the near future.

Spotting, light bleeding or heavier or prolonged bleeding is common in the first 3 to 6 months of Cu-IUD use, but this may settle. There are few contraindications to use of intrauterine contraception (IUC; Table 21.5). The management of common problems associated with Cu-IUD and LNG-IUS use is outlined in Table 21.6.

THE ADVERSE EFFECTS AND COMPLICATIONS ASSOCIATED WITH INSERTION OF INTRAUTERINE CONTRACEPTION

The term 'intrauterine contraception' includes both LNG-IUS and Cu-IUD. There are few contraindications to use of IUC (see Table 21.5). The management of common problems associated with IUC use is outlined in Table 21.6. Clinicians who insert IUC should be appropriately trained and able to maintain competency. Discomfort during and/or after insertion of IUC and the need for pain relief during insertion should be discussed with women in advance and analgesia administered when appropriate. Emergency equipment must be available in all settings where IUC is being inserted and local referral pathways must be in place for women who require further medical input.

Expulsion and Perforation

The risk of expulsion with IUC is around 1 in 20 and is most common in the first year of use, particularly within 3 months of insertion. The risk of uterine perforation associated with IUC is up to 2 per 1000 insertions and is approximately six-fold higher in breastfeeding women. Most perforations occur at the time of insertion, but a delayed 'migration' is a recognised phenomenon. Perforation at the time of insertion may be detected because of acute pain or it may be detected later, if pregnancy occurs. Most commonly, perforation is identified following the investigation of 'missing threads', although the most common reason for missing threads is that they have curled up in the endocervical canal in the presence of a normally placed device. The management of suspected perforation and missing threads is outlined in Table 21.6. If the device is not in the uterine cavity, an abdominal X-ray will identify the IUC if it is lying within the peritoneal cavity (Fig. 21.2), where it may cause adhesion formation and usually is removed by laparoscopy or laparotomy.

Pelvic Infection

There is an increased risk of pelvic infection in the 20 days following insertion of IUC. Thereafter, the risk is the same as for the population not using IUC. The risk of acquiring pelvic inflammatory disease (PID) is related to the insertion procedure and background risk of STIs. A relevant history (including sexual history) should be taken to identify those at higher risk of STIs. Women aged <25 years, or 25 and over with a new sexual partner or more than one partner in the last year, or those with a regular partner who has other partners are at a higher risk of STIs. For these women (or for women who request STI testing), a self-administered low vaginal swab dual test for *Chlamydia trachomatis* and *Neisseria gonorrhoeae* should be taken in advance of insertion. If results are unavailable before insertion, prophylactic antibiotics should be considered for the higher-risk group (to at least cover *C. trachomatis*).

Pregnancy

A pregnancy due to an IUC failure is rare. However, if it occurs, the chance of having an ectopic pregnancy is higher than in those without a device (see Table 21.5).

TABLE 21.5 UKMEC Categories in Which Risks May Outweigh Benefits or Pose an Unacceptable Health Risk for Use of IUC

UKMEC Category 3 (Risks Outweigh Benefits)	UKMEC Category 4 (Unacceptable Risk)	Where Cu-IUD and LNG-IUS are Given Different UKMEC Categories
Between 48 hours and <4 week postpartum	Postpartum sepsis	A UKMEC category 1 is given for a Cu-IUD and a category 3 is given for the LNG-IUS due to the progestogen content for the following medical conditions: Continuation of LNG-IUS if a new diagnosis of ischaemic heart disease or stroke is made Having an LNG-IUS if there is a past history of breast cancer Severe decompensated cirrhosis Hepatocellular adenoma Malignant hepatocellular carcinoma
Initiation following a complicated organ transplant: graft failure (acute/chronic), rejection, cardiac allograft vasculopathy	Post-abortion sepsis	A UKMEC category 1 is given for a Cu-IUD and category 4 is given for the LNG-IUS due to the progestogen content for the following medical condition: Current breast cancer
Initiation in long QT syndrome	Initiation of the method in women with unexplained vaginal bleeding	
Initiation in women with HIV whose CD4 is <200	Gestational trophoblastic neoplasia when serum human chorionic gonadotrophin (hCG) concentration persistently elevated or malignant disease	
Gestational trophoblastic neoplasia when serum hCG concentrations are decreasing	Initiation of the method in women with cervical cancer awaiting treatment or in women with current endometrial cancer	
Initiation in women with radical trachelectomy	Initiation of intrauterine methods in women with current PID or purulent cervicitis or gonorrhoea	
Uterine fibroids or uterine anatomical abnormalities distorting the uterine cavity	Initiation in women with symptomatic chlamydia infection	
Initiation in women with asymptomatic chlamydia infection	Initiation of intrauterine methods in women with known pelvic tuberculosis	
Continuation of intrauterine methods in women with known pelvic tuberculosis		

Note: Liver enzyme – inducing drugs are not thought to reduce the contraceptive efficacy of a Cu-IUD or the LNG-IUS.
Cu-IUD, Copper intrauterine device; *HIV*, human immunodeficiency virus; *IUC*, intrauterine contraception; *LNG-IUS*, levonorgestrel-releasing intrauterine system; *PID*, pelvic inflammatory disease; *UKMEC*, UK Medical Eligibility Criteria.
From Faculty of Sexual and Reproductive Healthcare, UK Medical Eligibility Criteria 2016.

TABLE 21.6   Managing Common Problems Associated With Intrauterine Contraception (IUC)

Problems Associated With IUC	Management
Suspected perforation at the time of insertion	The procedure should be stopped and vital signs (blood pressure and pulse rate) and level of discomfort monitored until stable. An ultrasound scan and/or plain abdominal X-ray to locate the device if it has been left in situ should be arranged as soon as possible.
'Lost threads'	Advise women to use another method (condoms or abstinence) until medical review. Consider the need for emergency hormonal contraception. If no threads are seen and uterine placement of the intrauterine method cannot be confirmed clinically, an ultrasound scan should be arranged to locate the device and alternative contraception recommended until this information is available. If an ultrasound scan cannot locate the intrauterine method and there is no definite evidence of expulsion, a plain abdominal X-ray should be arranged to identify an extrauterine device. If the intrauterine method is not confirmed on an ultrasound scan, clinicians should not assume that it has been expelled until a negative X-ray is obtained (unless the woman has witnessed expulsion). Hysteroscopy is not readily available in all settings but can be useful if the ultrasound scan is equivocal. Surgical retrieval of an extrauterine device is advised.
Abnormal bleeding	Gynaecological pathology and infections should be excluded if abnormal bleeding persists beyond the first 6 months following insertion of IUC. Women using the LNG-IUS who present with a change in pattern of bleeding should be advised to return for further investigation to exclude infections, pregnancy and gynaecological pathology. For women using a Cu-IUD, non-steroidal anti-inflammatory drugs can be used to treat spotting, light bleeding, or heavy or prolonged menstruation. In addition, antifibrinolytics (such as tranexamic acid) may be used for heavy or prolonged menstruation.
Pregnancy	Most pregnancies in women using IUC will be intrauterine, but an ectopic pregnancy must be excluded. Women who become pregnant with an intrauterine contraceptive in situ should be informed of the increased risks of second-trimester miscarriage, pre-term delivery and infection if the intrauterine method is left in situ. Removal would reduce adverse outcomes but is associated with a small risk of miscarriage. If the threads are visible or can easily be retrieved from the endocervical canal, the intrauterine contraceptive should be removed up to 12 weeks' gestation. If there is no evidence that the intrauterine method was expelled prior to pregnancy, it should be sought at delivery or termination and, if not identified, a plain abdominal X-ray should be arranged to determine whether the intrauterine method is retained.
Suspected pelvic infection	For women using IUC with symptoms and signs suggestive of pelvic infection, appropriate antibiotics should be started. There is no need to remove the intrauterine method unless symptoms fail to resolve within the following 72 hours or unless the woman wishes removal. All women with confirmed or suspected PID should be followed up to ensure: resolution of symptoms and signs, their partner has also been treated when appropriate, completion of the course of antibiotics, STI risk assessment, counselling regarding safer sex and partner notification.
Presence of *Actinomyces*-like organisms (ALOs)	IUC users with ALOs detected on a swab who have no symptoms should be advised that there is no reason to remove the intrauterine method unless signs or symptoms of infection occur. There is no indication for follow-up screening. If symptoms of pelvic pain occur, women should be advised to seek medical advice. Other causes of infection (in particular, STIs) should be considered and it may be appropriate to remove the intrauterine method.

Cu-IUD, Copper intrauterine device; *LNG-IUS*, levonorgestrel-releasing intrauterine system; *PID*, pelvic inflammatory disease; *STI*, sexually transmitted infection.

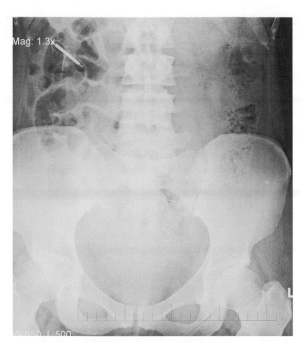

Fig. 21.2 The intrauterine device has perforated the uterus and attached itself to the omentum.

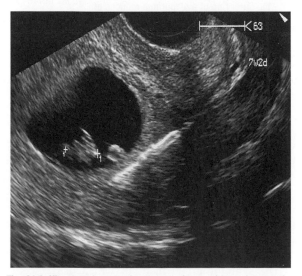

Fig. 21.3 Ultrasound scan of a 7-week fetus with an intrauterine device visible low in the uterine cavity.

Compared with using no contraception, the risk of ectopic pregnancy is reduced with the use of an IUC. If the pregnancy is intrauterine, there is an increase in the risk of spontaneous miscarriage and pre-term labour (Fig. 21.3). Removal of the IUC reduces these

risks and should be carried out as soon as is practical, ideally before 12 weeks' gestation, provided the threads are easily seen. If they are not present, no attempt at retrieval should be made (see Table 21.6).

BARRIER METHODS

Barrier methods of contraception aim to prevent sperm gaining access to the female upper reproductive tract. Barrier methods offer advantages in terms of safety and reversibility, but their efficacy is dependent upon consistency and quality of use. The failure rates can be low when they are used correctly by well-motivated couples.

Male and Female Condoms

Used consistently and correctly, male condoms are up to 98% effective at preventing pregnancy and female condoms are up to 95% effective. Failure rates with 'real life' use can be much higher, at 18%, and failures are often not recognised at the time. In general, evidence supports the use of condoms to reduce the risk of STI transmission. However, even with correct and consistent use, transmission may occur. The consistent and correct use of male and female condoms is recommended to reduce the risk of transmission of genital human papillomavirus (HPV).

Men and women with latex sensitivity or allergy can use polyurethane or deproteinized latex condoms. Condom users should be made aware of the risk of pregnancy, the option of EC, and the risk of acquiring STIs should a condom fail. Condoms lubricated with non – spermicidal lubricant are recommended. Non-oil-based lubricants are recommended, as they can be used safely with latex and non-latex condoms.

The female condom is a polyurethane sheath, its open end attached to a flexible polyurethane ring, which sits at the vaginal entrance and is available in one size.

Female Diaphragms and Caps

When used consistently, correctly and with spermicide, diaphragms and cervical caps are estimated to be between 92% and 96% effective at preventing pregnancy. These methods require a relatively high degree of user motivation. Failure rates are comparable with those observed with the male condom. The diaphragm is a soft dome, the edge of which contains a supporting metal spring to exert a slight pressure on the vaginal walls. It is inserted to lie diagonally across the vagina between the back of the symphysis pubis and the posterior fornix. Diaphragms are available in different diameters, ranging from 55 to 95 mm in 5-mm increments. It is important that the diaphragm cover the cervix after fitting – a vaginal examination by a suitably trained health care professional is essential to ensure that the correct diaphragm size is used. Women may purchase a silicon diaphragm in a single size designed to fit most women (approximately 80%) for which no fitting is required by a health care professional. Cervical caps depend on suction to hold the cap over the cervix; three sizes are currently available in the UK. Correct fitting will be facilitated by a healthcare professional

There is limited evidence on the use of diaphragms and cervical caps for reducing the risk of STIs or the development of cervical intraepithelial neoplasia. Women with sensitivity to latex can use silicone diaphragms or cervical caps. For women with a history of toxic shock syndrome, the use of diaphragms and cervical caps is not recommended. Guidance on the correct use of diaphragms and caps is outlined in Box 21.1. It is usually recommended that diaphragms and caps are used with a spermicide.

Spermicide

The use of spermicide alone is not considered to provide effective contraception. Nonoxinol-9 (N-9) is the main spermicide commercially available in the United Kingdom. N-9 is a surfactant, which disrupts cell membranes. Epithelial disruption in the vagina and rectum has been identified in association with N-9 use in human and animal models. Repeated and high-dose use of N-9 is associated with an increased risk of genital lesions, which may increase the risk of human immunodeficiency virus (HIV) acquisition. Thus, the WHO recommends that women at high risk of HIV infection should not use N-9. The risks of using a diaphragm or cervical cap (with N-9) in women with a high risk of HIV or those with HIV or acquired immune deficiency syndrome generally outweigh the benefits (UKMEC 3).

Fertility-Awareness Methods

Women who choose to use fertility-awareness methods should be made aware of the different fertility indicators and the failure rate of different combinations in

BOX 21.1 INSTRUCTIONS FOR WOMEN USING A DIAPHRAGM OR CERVICAL CAP

- Initial assessment of diaphragm and cervical caps should be done by a suitably trained health care professional.
  - Before the woman relies on the method for contraception, she should be asked to return for assessment whilst wearing the diaphragm/cap.
- All methods can be inserted any time before intercourse.
- The use of spermicide is recommended when using diaphragms and cervical caps.
- If intercourse is repeated or occurs ≥3 hours after insertion, more spermicide is required and should be inserted with an applicator or as a pessary without removing the diaphragm or cervical cap.
- The diaphragm or cervical cap must be left in situ for at least 6 hours after the last episode of intercourse. Sperm in the lower reproductive tract are unlikely to be alive after 6 hours.
- Oil-based lubricants can damage latex; thus, women should be advised to avoid their use when using latex diaphragms or cervical caps.
  - Water- or silicone-based lubricants are recommended when using latex diaphragms and caps.
- Women should be advised to check the diaphragm or cervical cap regularly for tears, holes or cracks.
- There is no evidence that a change in colour or shape of the outer ring of a diaphragm reduces efficacy.
- Women should be advised on the use of emergency contraception should female barrier methods be used incorrectly.
- Women should be advised to attend for a review of contraception if they have
  - any problems with the method
  - had a pregnancy

order to decide on the most appropriate method for them. The use of single fertility indicators is not recommended, as the typical pregnancy rate at 1 year is approximately 24%. Combining fertility indicators is considered more effective than using single fertility indicators alone. The term 'natural family planning' is used to describe fertility-awareness indicators used in conjunction with abstinence.

The symptothermal method (which uses a combination of monitoring cervical secretions and basal body temperature with a calendar calculation to identify the fertile window) has been shown to be an effective method of contraception when used consistently and correctly, with fewer than 1 in 100 women becoming pregnant over 1 year. There are several commercially available fertility-monitoring devices that are designed to identify the period of fertility, usually by measuring urinary LH. However, because these methods are primarily designed to identify the most fertile window, they may underestimate the time of risk of pregnancy for women who do not wish to become pregnant. There are also fertility-awareness applications for mobile phones that require women to enter information such as body temperatures, ovulation test results and date of menstruation prior to informing them of their fertile period that month. More rigorous research is required before conclusions can be drawn regarding the effectiveness of these devices and applications.

The LAM can provide very effective contraception (98%) if the woman is fully breastfeeding (day and night 'on demand') with no supplementary feeds, she is less than 6 months postpartum, and she is amenorrhoeic. Women using LAM should be advised that the chance of pregnancy is increased if the frequency of breastfeeding decreases (stopping night feeds, introducing supplementary feeding, use of pacifiers/dummies), when their period returns or when more than 6 months postpartum. Ideally, they should be supported to commence another method of contraception prior to this occurring (Fig. 21.4).

Emergency Contraception (EC)

EC can be used:
- After unprotected sexual intercourse (UPSI)
- After 'accidents' with a barrier method (e.g., burst condom or diaphragm removed too early)
- If pills are missed, injectable methods are late or an intrauterine method is expelled.

It can be difficult to accurately assess an individual woman's risk of pregnancy. A woman who has a single act of UPSI mid-cycle has an approximately 20% to 30% chance of pregnancy. The risk reduces to 2% to

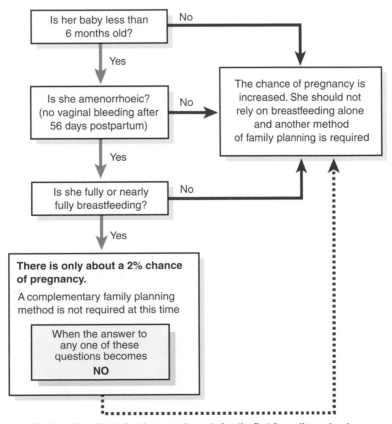

Fig. 21.4 Use of lactational amenorrhoea during the first 6 months postpartum.

3% before day 10 and after day 17 (in a regular 28-day cycle). Other factors have an effect on pregnancy risk, such as the age of the woman.

Three methods of EC are currently available: the Cu-IUD, oral levonorgestrel emergency contraception (LNG-EC) and oral ulipristal acetate emergency contraception (UPA-EC).

The most effective emergency method of contraception is the Cu-IUD – women should be offered this option. Unlike the Cu-IUD, oral EC does not provide contraception for the remainder of the cycle and effective contraception or abstinence is advised after it is taken. The Cu-IUD is the only method of EC that is known to be effective after ovulation has occurred. Women who experience vomiting within 3 hours of administration of the oral methods (LNG-EC and UPA-EC) will require a repeat dose or may wish to consider a Cu-IUD.

THE CU-IUD

EC providers should be aware that a Cu-IUD can be inserted up to 5 days after the first UPSI in a natural menstrual cycle or up to 5 days after the earliest likely date of ovulation, that is, up to day 19 in a woman with a regular 28-day cycle. Almost 99% of expected pregnancies can be prevented. It is for this reason that women of any age may opt for this method of EC. The copper is immediately toxic to ovum and sperm, thus making it effective immediately after insertion. The LNG-IUS is not effective as EC and should not be used for this indication.

ULIPRISTAL ACETATE

The progesterone receptor modulator UPA (30 mg) is licenced to be used up to 5 days (120 hours) after UPSI. The primary mode of action of UPA is to inhibit or delay ovulation. UPA-EC is significantly more effective than LNG-EC at preventing pregnancy when taken up to 5 days after UPSI. This is likely to be due to UPA-EC's ability to delay ovulation even after the start of the LH surge, a time when LNG-EC is no longer effective. Therefore, UPA-EC should be the first-line oral EC for a woman who has had UPSI within the last 5 days, if the UPSI is likely to have taken place during the 5 days prior to the estimated day of ovulation. Studies estimate that UPA-EC can reduce the chance of pregnancy by 60% to 80%.

Use of UPA can cause delay in the onset of menstruation and cause menstrual irregularities (similar to LNG-EC). For women using a liver enzyme – inducing drug, UPA is not recommended. Use of UPA is not recommended for women with severe asthma controlled by oral glucocorticoids. Women who are currently breastfeeding should be advised to express and discard breastmilk for 1 week after they have taken UPA-EC.

Following UPA administration, women should be advised to wait 5 days before starting suitable hormonal contraception. This is because hormonal contraception may reduce the efficacy of the UPA-EC. Women should be made aware that they must use condoms reliably or abstain from sex during this 5-day period and then until their contraceptive method is effective again (e.g., 2 days for the POP and 7 days for other hormonal methods).

If a woman has already taken UPA-EC in a cycle, UPA-EC can be offered again after further UPSI in the same cycle, provided ovulation has not occurred. Evidence suggests that UPA-EC does not disrupt an existing pregnancy and is not associated with fetal abnormality.

LEVONORGESTREL EMERGENCY CONTRACEPTION

LNG-EC is effective up until 72 hours after UPSI. The 1.5-mg oral tablet inhibits ovulation, delaying or preventing follicular rupture and causing luteal dysfunction. If taken prior to the start of the LH surge, LNG-EC inhibits ovulation. In the late follicular phase and once ovulation has occurred, LNG-EC becomes ineffective. If taken within 72 hours of a single episode of UPSI, LNG-EC is thought to prevent between 60% and 80% of expected pregnancies. For women using liver enzyme – inducing drugs, a single 3-mg tablet of LNG can be considered. However, women should be informed that the effectiveness of this approach is unknown.

After taking LNG-EC, women can start hormonal contraception immediately. Women should be made aware that they must use condoms reliably or abstain from sex until their chosen method of contraception becomes effective (2 days for POP and 7 days for other hormonal methods). If a woman has already taken LNG-EC in a cycle, LNG-EC can be used again after further UPSI, provided ovulation has not occurred.

Sterilization

Counselling and advice on sterilization procedures should be provided to women and men within the context of a service providing a full range of information and access to other methods of contraception. This should include information on the advantages and disadvantages and relative failure rates. Failures can occur with all methods of sterilization and a pregnancy can occur several years after the procedure. Women should be informed that other female methods of contraception such as IUD and subdermal implants are as, if not more, effective than sterilization and may confer non-contraceptive benefits. Men and women seeking sterilization counselling should be informed of the different methods of sterilization available, including laparoscopic tubal occlusion in women and vasectomy in men.

FEMALE STERILIZATION

Laparoscopic sterilization is still the most common method of female sterilization in the United Kingdom. It is usually achieved with titanium clips placed on the fallopian tubes under general anaesthesia. All women must be informed of the risks of laparoscopy, including those of visceral and vascular injury necessitating additional surgery. The lifetime risk of failure is estimated to be 1 in 200 for laparoscopic sterilization. Laparoscopic sterilization is intended to be permanent but can be reversed. However, women should be informed that reversal has variable success rates. Sterilization by ligation of the fallopian tubes can be performed at laparotomy. It can also be performed at the time of caesarean section (when the failure rate is slightly higher), but only if there has been appropriately documented pre-procedure counselling.

Hysteroscopic female sterilization involves tubal cannulation and occlusion of the fallopian tubes from within the uterine cavity using flexible micro-inserts. The micro-inserts cause fibrosis, resulting in the permanent occlusion of each tube after approximately 3 months. The procedure is performed under local anaesthetic. It is irreversible and has a similar failure rate to laparoscopic tubal occlusion. Tubal occlusion can be confirmed by transvaginal scan or hysterosalpingography. Hysteroscopic approaches to female sterilization are no longer available in the United Kingdom.

Compared with women using no method of contraception, the risk of ectopic pregnancy is not increased after sterilization. However, women should be informed that if pregnancy occurs, the resulting pregnancy has a higher chance of being ectopic because tubal anatomy is distorted.

There is no causal effect between female sterilization and the development of heavy menstrual bleeding. There is evidence to suggest an association between tubal occlusion and subsequently undergoing a hysterectomy, but there is no evidence of causation.

VASECTOMY

Vasectomy is ligation of the vasa deferentia for the purpose of excluding spermatozoa from the ejaculate. The procedure is usually performed under local anaesthesia. Vasectomy is intended to be permanent but men should be given information on the success rates associated with reversal. Following vasectomy, an effective contraceptive must be used until azoospermia has been confirmed by semen analysis. It can take up to 20 ejaculations to clear any sperm ahead of the now blocked vasa deferentia. Twelve weeks postvasectomy is the optimal timing to schedule the first post-vasectomy semen analysis.

There is no increase in the risk of testicular cancer or heart disease associated with vasectomy. The possible association of an increased risk of being diagnosed with prostate cancer is currently considered not to be causal. Men should be informed about the possibility of chronic testicular pain after vasectomy. Serum testosterone concentrations, libido, and the colour, consistency and volume of the ejaculate are unaffected by undergoing a vasectomy. Vasectomy is highly reliable, with a failure rate of 1 in 2000.

Key Points

- **By reducing unintended pregnancies and abortions, and facilitating safe inter-pregnancy intervals, effective contraception provides health and socioeconomic benefits to women, their children and the communities they live in.**
- **Medical eligibility criteria can be used to ensure the safe provision of contraception to women and men without imposing unnecessary medical restrictions.**

- Efficacy of contraception is measured by failure rate expressed as pregnancies per hundred women-years.
- Consistent and correct use of contraception is important to maintain efficacy. Methods that reduce the risk of user failure, such as long-acting methods (implant, injectable and intrauterine), are more effective than those that rely on user input (pill taking or patch use).
- The combined hormonal methods (pill, patch, vaginal ring) contain estrogen and a progestogen. These methods may be unsuitable for some women, such as those with cardiovascular disease (e.g., myocardial infarction, stroke, hypertension, VTE), smokers aged ≥35 years, women with migraine with aura, and women with breast cancer.
- Progestogen-only contraception consists of pills, injections, implants and the LNG-IUS. They are useful for women with contraindications to estrogen use and can also be used as a first-choice contraceptive.
- The LARC methods, which include intrauterine methods and subdermal implants, can be used by women of any age. They are the most cost-effective contraceptive options, with high levels of satisfaction and low discontinuation rates.
- Barrier methods are less effective than other methods. Male and female condoms will provide some protection against STIs.
- EC can reduce the risk of unplanned pregnancy following UPSI or contraceptive method failure.
- Male and female sterilization provides effective permanent contraception. Vasectomy has lower failure rates than female sterilization and can be performed without general anaesthesia.

Chapter 22

Ethical Issues

David Obree, Elizabeth A. Layden

Chapter Outline

Introduction

Ethics (Box 22.1) is the philosophical study of human conduct. It is not what we do or what we can do, it is what we 'should' do and, therefore, what we 'should not' do. In the subset of medical ethics that is clinical ethics, attention is focussed on the individual patient, such that resolution is case and patient specific (Fig. 22.1). What follows is a general discussion of the issues at stake, to be interpreted for each individual within the cultural and legal context of geographical region.

Each clinical discipline within medicine has both distinct and shared ethical challenges. Often, the issues are straightforward and easily resolved by attention to professional guidelines or by balancing best interests, autonomy and justice (see Fig. 22.1). In certain areas, such as paediatrics and

end-of-life care, the involvement and expectations of parents and families amplifies the emotional context, adding further tension to ethical decision-making.

Arguably, however, no area of medicine is more ethically challenging than that of obstetrics and gynaecology. Pregnancy brings its own emotional complexity, less so when the interests of the mother and fetus (or embryo) are aligned and more so when those interests are competing and where unconnected parties' moral claims add to the conflict. Emerging medical technologies to prevent or enhance reproduction have created new dilemmas, often attracting the attention of governments and resulting in variation between region-specific legislation. At the same time, progressive liberal social attitudes have developed against traditional positions (often derived from religious teachings), meaning that clinicians have to keep abreast of changing social norms and terminology, not least of which currently involves the area of gender identity and transgender politics.

This chapter will explore the ethical dilemmas which present in obstetrics and gynaecology to identify competing values and priorities, asking whose interests we should consider – woman, doctor, partner, baby, the state and the views of third-party groups such as women's rights, pro life and religious campaigners. Also included, a discussion framed by pregnancy not being a disease but rather a natural process, although one that may require the closest medical attention to avoid harm.

BOX 22.1 ETHICS AND MORALITY

> How is ethics related to morality? In general usage, we sometimes think of morality as our internal value system and ethics as the externalisation, study or codification of that morality. While some philosophers make a distinction between the two terms, in most ethical discourse they are interchangeable: if something is unethical it is immoral and if something is moral it is ethical, to the point that if you see someone say or write that such and such is morally 'and' ethically wrong, that is a tautology. This also reflects the etymological origins of the terms 'ethos' and 'ethikos' from Greek and 'mores' and 'morales', the Latin translation.

Conception

This section considers the right to conceive and the role of artificial reproductive technologies (ARTs), the right to de-conceive and the moral issues around abortion, beginning with contraception. For some, the latter may be the least controversial of the three topics. However, there is a legacy of dissent, notably from religious groups, and some recent positions relating to overpopulation and climate change.

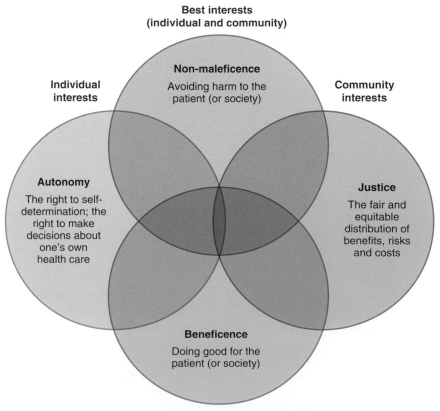

Fig. 22.1 The four principles of medical ethics. The four principles (or pillars) of medical ethics were described by Beauchamp and Childress in 1979 and have been influential in medical ethics discourse worldwide. Although non-maleficence and beneficence were originally discussed as principles for individual patients, with an increasing emphasis on public health ethics these two principles can also be applied to society, where they overlap with the principle of justice. It is sometimes easier to conflate beneficence and non-maleficence and use the less clumsy term 'best interest'.

Contraception

Moral objections to contraception have been generated principally by religious groups (including Catholicism, Orthodox Judaism and Baptist teachings), commonly asserting that sex should be for procreation, not pleasure, and that facilitating sex without the risk of procreation increases the likelihood of sex outside marriage, a further moral insult. Secular groups who oppose contraception may base objections on the premise that it 'interferes with nature'.

THE PILL AND WOMEN'S PROCREATIVE AND SOCIAL FREEDOM

The advent of the first effective (women-controlled) oral contraceptive in the 1960s, 'the pill', has had a historic impact on women's societal options. Pregnancy often leaves a woman dependent on others for financial support; being able to control fertility has facilitated an epoch of economic and educational independence, with an increase in the numbers of women entering higher education and obtaining professional qualifications. The subsequent delay in the age of first pregnancy due to career development means that mothers are raising children at an older age than women of previous generations. Medical advances have not been able to correct the discrepancy between the best biological age for women to have children and the best social age for supporting and parenting them, a problem that can be exacerbated by the absence of supportive social welfare systems. Such problems are persistent in countries where contraception is more difficult to access and where there is an associated undercurrent of gender inequality and socioeconomic deprivation.

BARRIER METHODS OF CONTRACEPTION

The controversial religion-based resistance to condom use in the face of rapidly spreading human immunodeficiency virus in Africa has diminished following concessions by the Catholic Church to allow barrier methods for disease prevention. The principle of 'Double Effect' underlies this position, the intent to prevent transmission of disease is acceptable, while for contraception it remains unacceptable. There is no practical difference between using condoms for disease prevention and using condoms for contraception. However, for some, there is a moral difference.

CONTRACEPTIVE METHODS THAT ALLOW FERTILIZATION BUT PREVENT IMPLANTATION

Stronger objections remain to contraceptive methods that allow fertilization but prevent implantation. For the 'life begins at fertilization' adherents, this is considered another form of abortion. For others, it is the loss of undifferentiated cells before pregnancy has started. Provision of emergency contraception (the 'morning-after pill') has been the target for conscientious objection to prescribing or dispensing by doctors and pharmacists (see page 245). However, the morning-after pill works primarily by suppressing ovulation; it is the copper intrauterine device (Cu-IUD) which has a potential post-fertilization effect in preventing implantation when used as emergency contraception. Other contraceptives have multiple effects, which may include reducing the chance of implantation (see Chapter 21).

STERILIZATION

Surgical sterilization (vasectomy) is the most robust contraceptive intervention for men, with a few ethical issues warranting a mention: responsibility for failure, awareness of the risk of sexually transmitted infections, and whether the female partner has been informed of the diminished reproductive status of her partner. In some countries, women can be sterilized only if they have their husband's consent; parallel requirements for wives to consent to their husband's sterilization are very rare. As most non-barrier forms of contraception are not visible to a person's partner, disclosure of the presence or absence of contraceptive measures is morally incumbent on both parties as a matter of mutual respect.

Awareness of the role of overpopulation in climate change may have precipitated an increase in younger women requesting sterilization. This is often resisted by clinicians aware of the high rate of subsequent regret and request for reversal of sterilization for women who have been sterilized in their 20s, along with a 'pro-natalist' assumption that humans should reproduce. In practice, young women tend to be counselled against sterilization and encouraged to look at other reliable, and more easily reversible, methods. In contrast, there may be a lack of counselling before in vitro fertilization (IVF), in which the negatives of having children are not mentioned, as an implicit assumption may be made that those seeking IVF have already decided to have children.

Although overpopulation and pollution caused by unfettered human consumption are a target for the majority of climate change activists, there is some controversy about forced contraceptive initiatives in countries where the environmental impact is less or in the context of externally enforced population control with eugenic intent. Concerns have been raised that controlling population growth can be an infringement of reproductive freedom rights. Sterilization without consent was not uncommon in the first half of the 20th century, particularly for adults who lacked capacity, justified on the basis of an alleged societal interest in preventing 'unfit persons' from reproducing – a form of negative eugenics. It is estimated that more than 400,000 individuals were involuntarily sterilized in Nazi Germany and more than 60,000 in the United States. These measures are ethically unjustifiable, particularly now given the increased availability of reversible, less restrictive options for avoiding pregnancy. Many countries now require independent review of cases in which non-therapeutic sterilization is proposed for someone who lacks capacity. In the United Kingdom, for instance, all such cases require a court hearing.

De-Conception Issues – Abortion

When a woman is seeking to conceive, it can be assumed that the interests of the mother and the fetus are aligned and that both will benefit from the term birth of a healthy baby. If the woman has been seeking to avoid conception, ethical difficulties arise if conception has already occurred, as there are varying sensibilities and representations relating to termination of pregnancy (Table 22.1). This section discusses ethical issues to supplement the practical and legal issues discussed in Chapter 20.

THE MORAL STATUS OF THE FETUS

The moral status of the fetus has been the subject of debate for centuries and remains central to the clinical and ethical challenges which confront obstetricians and gynaecologists in their daily practice.

If a fetus has moral status from conception equal to that of its mother, abortion would be morally unacceptable. This is the basis of the 1967 UK Abortion Act's provisions for conscientious objection (see page 226) and the recent challenges to the precedent established in the 1973 case of Roe vs Wade by the US Supreme Court. If, however, the fetus acquires moral status only at birth, abortion should be unrestricted on the basis of a woman's right to autonomy. Many regard the moral status of the fetus as a continuum, in which increasing moral status is acquired with increasing gestational age and fetal development, a view that is represented in many jurisdictions which allow termination up to a certain point in pregnancy.

The threshold of fertilization ('life begins at conception') has the advantage of being a clear position but disregards the difference between a fertilized ovum, a single cell and a baby born at term. Other problems with this definition include the difficulty of ascertaining when fertilization has occurred and the fact that most fertilized ova will not develop into a baby since they will not implant or will stop developing at an early stage.

The other unambiguous threshold is birth, which is uncomplicated to recognise, ethically supportable (as prior to this, the fetus does not exist independently of its mother), and easy to enforce. Most legal systems recognise birth as conferring legal 'personhood' on the fetus, although the legal status of the in utero fetus varies widely.

The point on the continuum between fertilization and birth at which the fetus is considered viable is crucial – that is, the point at which the fetus, if born, could survive independently outside the uterus. However, the gestation at which a baby would be expected to survive varies widely internationally depending on the availability of advanced neonatal care interventions (see Chapter 43) and whilst there is not a universal threshold of gestational viability, in advanced health care settings it can be as low as 22 weeks. Practical and moral difficulties arise when major fetal anomalies, including those not compatible with survival after birth, are not diagnosed until after the viability threshold has passed (see Chapter 25).

The advent and increasing sophistication of medical imaging technology means the fetus can now have a pre-birth social identity, as ultrasound pictures have

TABLE 22.1 Stages of Pregnancy

Gestation (Approx.)	Stage of Development	Ethical or Legal
2 weeks (post last menstrual period (LMP))	Fertilization – sperm fertilizes an ovum	'Life begins at conception', subscribed to by some Christian, Buddhist and Hindu groups. Catholic teachings regard abortion after this stage as morally unacceptable.
2–4 weeks	0–14 days after fertilization. Potential for embryo division to result in twin pregnancy.	In the United Kingdom, the use of embryos for research is restricted to embryos within 14 days of fertilization.
3–4 weeks	Implantation – the fertilized egg attaches to the lining of the uterus.	Pregnancy begins, in Islamic tradition.
4 weeks	Positive pregnancy test (hCG)	Earliest point pregnancy can be confirmed
6–7 weeks	Fetal heartbeat visible on ultrasound scan	Objective confirmation of ongoing pregnancy
7–8 weeks	40 days after fertilization	The embryo becomes a 'potential person' in Jewish tradition, which generally regards abortion after this point acceptable only to save the life of the mother. Groups within Judaism differ on the acceptability of other reasons for abortion. Some Islamic groups believe that the human spirit enters the embryo at this stage of gestation.
10+ weeks	Time frame for cell-free fetal DNA screening	Can be used to determine fetal sex
11–14 weeks	Time frame for combined ultrasound and biochemical screening	
11–14 weeks	Time frame for chorionic villus sampling (diagnostic genetic testing)	
12 weeks		Some Protestant Christian groups regard abortion after this stage of gestation as morally unacceptable.
15+ weeks	Time frame for amniocentesis (diagnostic genetic testing)	
17–19 weeks	120 days after fertilization	The human spirit enters the fetus in the majority of Islamic teachings, which generally regard abortion after this stage of gestation permissible only if it is to save the life of the mother.
18–22 weeks	Fetal movements felt by mother	Traditional point of 'ensoulment' (the fetus acquiring a soul) in early Christian teachings, now discarded.
18–24 weeks	Significant structural congenital anomalies likely to be identifiable on ultrasound scan	
23–24 weeks	Likely to survive outside the uterus if born in settings with advanced neonatal care	UK Abortion Act limit for some categories of termination. Terminations after this stage of gestation usually require feticide (see Chapter 20)
28+ weeks	Likely to survive outside the uterus if born in settings without advanced neonatal care	
Birth	After birth, the baby exists independently of its mother	The baby is now a separate person legally.

hCG = Human chorionic gonadotropin.

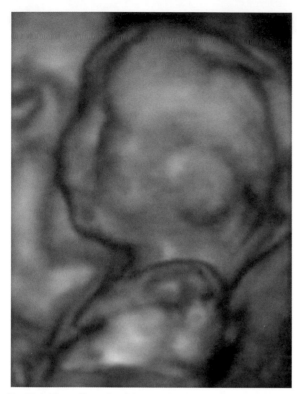

Fig. 22.2 Three-dimensional image of a fetal profile at 20 weeks' gestation.

become part of the anticipatory discussion between parents, family and friends, generating an enhanced emotional presence as the fetus makes its precocious entrance onto the social stage (Fig. 22.2).

WHY WOMEN CONSIDER ABORTION

Women consider abortion for a variety of reasons, either acting alone from a single driving concern or as one of a reinforcing web of personal and socioeconomic factors. Usually, but not always, the pregnancy is unplanned. Within the common reasons for seeking abortion (Box 22.2), some may attract censure from dissenting 'pro-life' (anti-abortion) groups. Nevertheless, it is important to recognise that from a national and social perspective, adequate social welfare services to support pregnant women and their children (paid maternity leave, affordable/subsidised childcare and housing, and free education for children, amongst others) can reduce the economic pressure towards abortion and unhindered access to affordable contraception (particularly long-acting reversible contraception (LARC)) reduces the rate of unintended pregnancies.

PATERNAL AND OTHER RIGHTS

The rights of the father of the fetus, who has contributed 50% of its genetic material but has no role in gestating the fetus, are limited in most countries. Some jurisdictions require a woman's partner to consent to an abortion. It is difficult to see an ethical mechanism for elevating the father's parental rights to a future child above the right of the mother to autonomy. This is more complicated in the context of surrogacy, in which the woman carrying the pregnancy may not be genetically related to the fetus but has chosen to carry the fetus for the intended parents (see later discussion).

Pregnancy can be dangerous and carries a risk of severe harm or death for the mother; many women still die every year as a result of pregnancy. Therefore, other parties' rights have to be weighted appropriately to reflect the uneven distribution of risk to the mother. Other parties may include the fetus, the father, the intended parents (in surrogacy) or family or guardians in situations in which the pregnant woman or girl lacks decision-making capacity.

Ethical debates around abortion should acknowledge that abortion can be a lifesaving procedure for the mother and that restrictive regulation of abortion increases the maternal mortality rate. This is because restricting access to safe abortion increases the rates of unsafe abortions (see Chapter 39) and because complications of pregnancy – such as haemorrhage, sepsis and pre-eclampsia, or exacerbation of existing maternal comorbidities (e.g., cardiac disease) by pregnancy – can necessitate termination of a (potentially much-wanted) pregnancy to save the life of the mother. It is hard to ethically justify a decision which leads to the death of both a woman and her fetus over the alternative outcome of the woman surviving on her own.

Assisted Conception

THE RIGHT TO CONCEIVE

The right to 'found a family' is recognised in the United Nations Universal Declaration of Global Rights, the European Convention on Human Rights and the 9th Amendment of the United States Constitution. As many parents will acknowledge, parenthood is a precious experience but not without negative aspects. There are financial, social and mental well-being sacrifices by parents, often unappreciated by their offspring, particularly during the challenging teenage years. It is always possible that some potential parents are better off not having children and, whilst it is not for clinicians to make such value judgements, awareness of the social care provisions for vulnerable children is paramount. For instance, in the United Kingdom, the requirement to consider the welfare of the future child is enshrined in the Human Fertilisation and Embryology Act 2008 (HFEA). HFEA regulates ART (see Chapter 5), restrictive criteria that do not apply to spontaneous conception and, therefore, are controversial to some observers.

STATE INVOLVEMENT/LEGISLATIVE INTEREST

IVF involves the creation of embryos ex utero; some of these embryos will never have the potential to implant and develop into a fetus. For those who believe that life begins at conception, this is morally unacceptable. Most countries legislate to control IVF. This legislation may be in relation to the welfare of the mother, the welfare of the future child or with regards to the embryos created (e.g., limiting or regulating the use of such embryos for research purposes). Assisted reproductive interventions are costly – both in terms of time and side effects for the parent(s) and in financial terms both for the parents and the

health care system. Where ART is state funded, the state has a vested financial interest. Where ART is not state funded but other medical treatment is, there may still be an indirect financial interest. Pregnancies conceived via IVF are more at risk for some complications, particularly multiple pregnancy with the associated risk of pre-term birth (with both short- and long-term health consequences), which increase health care costs for maternity and neonatology services.

SURROGACY

Surrogacy, in which a surrogate gestates and births a baby for another person or couple – the intended parent(s) – is ethically complicated. As pregnancy and birth involve physical effort and carry a risk of harm, surrogacy can be viewed as a form of occupational service warranting remuneration or as an altruistic act in which the reward is the (presumed) happiness of the intended parents and their future child. Opponents of paid surrogacy argue that commodification of reproduction ('buying babies') is ethically dubious. Proponents argue that there is a simple equivalence to traditional work and, thus, it is morally wrong to expect surrogates to do this work without being paid. Proponents also argue that financial reward increases the number of available surrogates. This is further complicated by the gendered nature of the labour and the risk of exploitation of women living in poverty or those who are vulnerable (predominantly in settings where paid surrogacy is acceptable), especially in the context of international surrogacy.

Additional ethical complexity surrounds the balance of rights between the autonomy of the surrogate and the rights of the fetus (as represented by the intended parents), which are potentially not as well aligned as they would be for a woman pregnant with her own child. Here, the parental rights over the future child are due consideration. In some countries, the intended parents have parental rights over the child from birth (or before). In other countries (including the United Kingdom), the parental rights to a child legally remain with the person who gives birth to the child (and, if she is married, her spouse) until the child is at least 6 weeks old, after which parental rights can be transferred (reforms to the

UK law have been proposed, but not yet enacted.) Cases have occurred in which surrogates changed their mind after birth, did not give the baby to the intended parents and raised the child themselves. There is very wide global variation on surrogacy law regarding remuneration and parental rights in particular, and international surrogacy arrangements can be extremely complicated.

Pregnancy and Birth

PREGNANCY

Prenatal testing (see Chapter 25) can be used to identify fetal anomalies but also, more controversially, fetal sex. Disability rights groups have raised concerns that earlier antenatal (or, in the case of pre-implantation genetic diagnosis, pre-pregnancy) diagnosis of fetal anomalies encourages termination of what are perceived to be 'imperfect' embryos or fetuses and that this heightens bias against children and adults with disabilities. This is an increasing and challenging issue as developments in the accuracy and scope of prenatal testing improves the range of pre-birth diagnoses. Termination of pregnancy for fetal anomalies not compatible with extra-uterine life is regarded as ethically acceptable in many countries. However, for 'minor' anomalies, this debate is more complicated. Conversely, some antenatal diagnoses benefit the fetus by permitting either in-utero intervention (such as intrauterine transfusion for fetal anaemia or surgery for spina bifida) or by allowing antenatal planning, for instance, for fetal cardiac anomalies in which antenatal identification allows optimisation of neonatal care (including location of birth) with improved outcomes. Even where there are no specific interventions available, some women and their families benefit from antenatal diagnosis, as it allows them to be psychologically prepared in advance of their child's birth.

Cell-free fetal DNA analysis can, from around 10 weeks' gestation, screen with a high degree of accuracy for fetal sex. In many jurisdictions, this will overlap with the time frame in which termination of pregnancy is considered acceptable for non-medical indications. In some regions, there are particular social and cultural pressures to have male rather than female children, resulting in selective termination of female fetuses. Ethically, this can be challenging, as preventing this infringes on the woman's autonomy. In some settings, this places her at risk for negative social or familial consequences, but permitting it perpetuates cultural gender discrimination and results in skewed gender ratios, which have negative macro societal effects.

As with abortion, partners and other family members may hold strong views on antenatal decision-making and, where there in an intention to continue with a pregnancy, advocates for fathers' rights support the right for fathers to contribute to these decisions. Obstetricians and midwives have a direct responsibility to the pregnant woman, who has a right to confidentiality and, in most countries, the legal right to make her own decisions.

Further morally complicated situations arise when a pregnant woman is undertaking activities which pose a risk to the fetus. Commonly considered examples of this are maternal use of illicit drugs or of legal, but potentially deleterious to the fetus, substances such as alcohol and tobacco. In some jurisdictions, criminal sanctions are imposed (for 'endangering the unborn child'). However, these usually result in worse maternal and perinatal outcomes than less punitive approaches and, thus, are difficult to justify ethically. Other related cases include maternal occupations or recreations which pose potential risks to the fetus, such as biological hazards (working with very young children or people with infectious diseases), environmental hazards (ionising radiation, chemicals) or physical hazards (heavy lifting, contact sports). These cases are less frequently considered, perhaps due to the greater social stigma associated with use of illicit drugs, alcohol and tobacco in pregnancy.

BIRTH

The majority of births will progress smoothly and result in a happy outcome without the need for intervention. Unfortunately, complications during labour or birth sometimes threaten the health or life of the woman, the baby, or both.

Where women are at higher risk of complications, this can be identified and discussed antenatally. It is also important to explore any pre-existing beliefs which may make management of complications more difficult – for instance, a woman who declines a particular procedure, such as operative vaginal birth, or blood transfusion. As consent is a process, rather than a snapshot, all exploratory dialogue should be documented and updated. Discussions may form the basis of a more formal 'birth plan' shared by the health care team. Whilst birth plans are based on the ideal wishes of the mother, they also should address her wishes in the event of non-ideal occurrences, for example, whether she would still decline an intervention if she or her baby were at immediate risk of dying without the intervention. It is preferable to discuss these issues calmly in an antenatal context rather than for the first time when someone is in labour and potentially distracted by pain. Should an emergency occur, there may be no time to have a challenging and detailed discussion; as such potentially coercive environments are not conducive to a reliable consent process, anticipatory discussion is far more appropriate. With this in mind, health care teams should encourage mothers to take a flexible view of birth plans in the context of clinical reality, as unrealistic or rigid promises invite disappointment when unfulfilled.

Gender

GENDER IDENTITY

It may soon be possible for a transgender woman to overcome her absence of a uterus via a uterine transplant, and become pregnant, utilising her own stored sperm and the eggs of a donor woman. This pregnancy could even be a surrogacy, perhaps on behalf of the egg donor. Sex and gender identity terminologies are challenges to both medical and linguistic norms, which have historically binarised male and female, man and woman, father and mother.

Consensus on a universal descriptive framework for gender remains elusive, with a political preference for self-identity which extends beyond gender to include sex, traditionally determined by physical characteristics, or chromosomal and hormonal criteria. This may cause confusion for the medical team when a person identifies outside one's anatomical or physiological birth identity, risking misdiagnosis and inappropriate treatment (e.g., not receiving sex-specific screening tests). However, for the individual, this risk may be an acceptable trade-off and preferable to misgendering. In clinical

practice, enquiring about a person's preferred pronouns (and title, if this is gendered) and using these when speaking to (or of) them is simple and important. Legal issues surrounding gender identity vary widely across different jurisdictions; space precludes discussion of these here.

Surgical Manipulation for Non-Medical Reasons

Clinicians may be confronted by requests for morally challenging procedures such as female genital mutilation (FGM), labiaplasty or hymenoplasty. Cultural relativism allows tolerance of practices that another group might find repulsive, an 'each to their own approach'. However, FGM (see page 181) involves physical and mental trauma to young girls and women, such that FGM, or procuring it abroad, is illegal in most countries. Although attempts have been made to justify 'medicalised FGM' as a harm reduction measure, with proponents arguing that procedures performed in an aseptic environment by a health care provider are less dangerous to the victims than FGM performed in non-sterile conditions, this remains morally dubious. This is reflected in the international recognition of all forms of FGM as human rights violations.

Requests for hymenoplasty or labiaplasty are more likely to come from consenting adults with capacity. Nevertheless, the demand for such services raises questions about what is medical, what is cosmetic and the origins of such requests. In particular, a clinician refusing a request for a hymenoplasty may be putting a young woman at risk for severe familial repercussions. However, acquiescence perpetuates controversial traditions linked to oppressive and patriarchal cultures. Labiaplasty may occasionally be medically indicated but may also be requested from a desire to achieve an imagined anatomical norm and in some countries may be illegal under FGM legislation.

Conclusion

The nexus of competing interests and tightly held values that occurs in obstetrics and gynaecology has been intensified by rapidly developing biotechnology and social progressiveness. The discipline has become rich in ethical, political and legal considerations, in which the rational may compete with the sentimental. In this environment, health care workers' own values may be challenged or may have to be suspended in the interests of their patient. It is here that teamwork plays an important part, exploring the ethical context of each situation in search of an objective consensus. There may also be a professional responsibility for clinicians to engage in the wider societal debates and health care policy decisions that affect the procreative lives of women around the world.

Key Points

- The discipline of obstetrics and gynaecology has particularly complex ethical challenges, with moral, legal, political and social considerations.
- Advances in medical technologies and changing social attitudes have created new ethical complexities.
- Ethical decision-making in medicine needs to balance best interests, autonomy and justice.

Obstetrics

Section Outline

Chapter 23

Antenatal and Postnatal Care

Judy Ormandy

Chapter Outline

The Aim of Antenatal Care

The aim of antenatal care is to maximise the chance of a positive outcome from a pregnancy: a healthy mother and a healthy baby or babies. This will involve regular contact between a pregnant woman and health care professionals.

The aims of antenatal care are to:
- Optimise maternal and fetal health
- Offer women maternal and fetal screening
- Make medical and social interventions where indicated
- Improve women's experience of pregnancy and birth
- Prepare women for motherhood

Antenatal care may be one of the few occasions that a woman has regular contact with health care providers. Thus, it is an ideal opportunity to promote positive health behaviours and provide education and guidance.

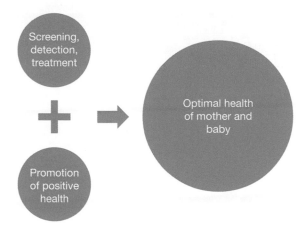

Fig. 23.1 The dual purpose of antenatal care.

Models of Antenatal Care

Models of antenatal care, and maternity care more generally, vary widely across the world (Fig. 23.1). The model of antenatal care includes how often the care is given, who provides the care, and where the care is located. It is determined by a range of factors, including patient history and preference, resource level, and organisation of care.

In middle- and high-income countries, the pattern of antenatal appointments is generally around 10 appointments for a woman in her first pregnancy and seven for a woman in a subsequent pregnancy. In low-income countries, the number of contacts is often much lower, though the World Health Organization (WHO) recommends a minimum of eight antenatal contacts.

The providers of antenatal care also vary considerably between countries and within countries. Antenatal care may be provided by midwives, general practitioners, and obstetricians. Healthy women without any significant risk factors or obstetric problems may receive all of their care from midwives. Women with risk factors, health problems, obstetric problems, or poor obstetric history will also receive some of their antenatal care from obstetricians. Continuity of carer during the antenatal period is associated with improved obstetric outcomes and increased maternal satisfaction.

The First Trimester

Ideally, the first contact between a health care professional and a pregnant woman occurs soon after the confirmation of pregnancy. We aim for women to have their first 'booking' appointment by 10 weeks' gestation.

The aims of this booking appointment are to:
- Identify risks
- Screen for abnormalities or illness
- Provide key health-promotion messages
- Develop a rapport and encourage future attendance by ensuring that the woman has a positive first experience of maternity care.

At the booking appointment, the gestation of the pregnancy should be determined through establishment of the first day of the last menstrual period and abdominal examination. Initial observations of the mother will assist with care planning and identification of any later deterioration.

Several risk factors increase the probability that problems or complications may emerge for the mother or fetus in pregnancy, during labour and childbirth, or postnatally. Being under 18 or over 40 years of age increases the risk of developing some problems during pregnancy, as does having had more than six previous births or having a first pregnancy.

Women may have underlying health conditions for which they take medication. The health care professional should identify what medication is currently being taken (both prescription and 'over the counter' medicines) and assess the risks and benefits of continuing the medication in pregnancy. Some women will need to keep taking their regular prescribed medications; they should be given accurate advice regarding this. Risk factors should be recorded and considered when planning care (Table 23.1).

If risk factors are identified, the health care professional should follow local referral pathways to ensure that women receive the appropriate surveillance, treatment, advice, or support to reduce the impact of the risks identified. Some interventions, such as aspirin to reduce the risk of pre-eclampsia or fetal growth restriction (FGR) in high-risk women, should be commenced in the first trimester.

Some family history and previous personal history risks will require additional screening appointments and multidisciplinary care planning. A personal history of postpartum psychosis has a recurrence risk of 1 in 2 to 4 (background risk of 1 in 500), and a family history of inherited blood disorders will require

TABLE 23.1   Risk Factors to Be Identified at First Appointment Through Discussion With Mother and Reference to Previous Medical or Obstetric Notes

Personal History and Current Health	Family History	Obstetric History Previous Pregnancies	Current Pregnancy
History of subfertility and fertility treatment	Pregnancy related—first-degree relative with a congenital abnormality or genetic abnormality, pre-eclampsia, venous thrombosis	Miscarriage at > 14 weeks, stillbirth or neonatal death	Hyperemesis
Medical condition, including diabetes, thyroid problems, epilepsy, asthma, heart disease, hypertension, renal disease, cancer	Medical conditions—diabetes, heart disease, inherited conditions, e.g., sickle cell anaemia, cystic fibrosis	Recurrent miscarriage (two consecutive first-trimester losses)	Vaginal bleeding
Surgical history—gynaecological procedures, treatment to the cervix, breast surgery, abdominal surgery	Mental health—first-degree relative with postpartum psychosis, schizophrenia, bipolar disorder, severe postnatal depression or depression	Premature birth or small-for-gestational-age infant	Abdominal pain
Raised body mass index (BMI) or very low BMI		Pregnancy-related hypertension, gestational diabetes, rhesus isoimmunisation antepartum haemorrhage	Findings from pregnancy ultrasound
Mental health—bipolar disorder, postpartum psychosis, schizophrenia, depression, postnatal depression, anxiety disorders, eating disorders		Induction of labour—indication	
Lifestyle—alcohol, smoking, non-prescription and prescription drug use		Operative birth (caesarean section or instrumental vaginal delivery), shoulder dystocia, breech birth	
Social difficulties—domestic abuse, financial difficulties, previous child-protection concerns		Postpartum haemorrhage, retained placenta, obstetric anal sphincter injury	

relevant counselling and screening. Medical conditions such as diabetes, thyroid conditions, and epilepsy will require multidisciplinary care planning and monitoring throughout the pregnancy (see Chapter 24). Previous obstetric complications or interventions, such as a caesarean section or shoulder dystocia, require discussion of choices relating to birth.

Identifying lifestyle risks may prompt referral for smoking cessation support or dietetic support to promote healthy eating. Identifying mental health risks,

such as a personal history of bipolar disorder, will require liaison with mental health services to ensure that a coordinated plan of care is in place during pregnancy and immediately after birth. Social difficulties will require a liaison with local social care or voluntary sector organisations.

At the first antenatal appointment, the health care professional will undertake a general physical examination, including calculation of the woman's body mass index (BMI), blood pressure measurement, and heart rate. In areas with a high incidence of cardiac and respiratory conditions, auscultation of heart and lung sounds is recommended. An abdominal examination will be undertaken to identify the uterine size and any abnormal masses or surgical scars.

Urinalysis should be undertaken for the presence of protein and glucose; proteinuria prompts testing for urinary tract infection, persistent glycosuria prompts testing for diabetes. Cervical screening is not routinely required but can be safely done in pregnancy, and contact with health professionals in pregnancy can provide an opportune time to address overdue cervical screening.

Further screening will differ between different countries, depending on local disease patterns and resources, but often includes:

- Full blood count to screen for maternal anaemia and thrombocytopenia
- Blood group to determine the ABO and rhesus status of the mother and to identify any red cell antibodies
- Rubella status to identify those mothers who are not immune. This has been discontinued as part of routine care in the United Kingdom since 2016 due to the high population coverage provided by the measles-mumps-rubella vaccine but remains part of routine care in Australasia.
- Haemoglobin (Hb) electrophoresis to screen for conditions such as thalassaemia and sickle cell anaemia
- Hepatitis B status. Women who are identified as positive for hepatitis B can have medication in the third trimester to reduce the risk of vertical transmission if they have a high viral load. The baby should also receive immunoglobulin and vaccination at birth.
- Syphilis. Syphilis rates are unfortunately increasing. Untreated syphilis in pregnancy is associated with miscarriage, stillbirth, and congenital syphilis (see pp. 204, 306).
- Human immunodeficiency virus (see p. 206).
- Hepatitis C screening should be considered for women at risk, such as intravenous drug users.
- Swabs for chlamydia should be offered to those at risk, such as women aged under 25 years.
- HbA1c can be used to assess for underlying type 2 diabetes. This is not routine in the United Kingdom but is in Australasia.

A clear process should be in place and shared with the woman about how and when she will receive test results following this first appointment.

Many women experience some discomfort or symptoms that may cause them to be concerned during the early stages of pregnancy. These include nausea and vomiting ('morning sickness'), some lower abdominal discomfort, frequency of micturition, vaginal 'spotting' (small amounts of bleeding per vagina), and breast tingling or discomfort. The health care professional should ask women about symptoms to identify when normal and transient discomforts appear to be more serious.

The booking appointment should include discussion about a woman's options for screening for chromosomal and structural fetal anomalies. Screening approaches vary in different countries. Screening for Down syndrome (T21) and/or Edwards (T18) and Patau syndrome (T13) usually includes a nuchal translucency scan between 11 and 14 weeks, combined with maternal blood tests for pregnancy-associated plasma protein A (PAPP-A) and human chorionic gonadotrophin (hCG) to provide a combined test. The nuchal translucency scan also allows for confirmation of pregnancy dating and fetal number and an early assessment of fetal anatomy. Women who miss this test can have a 'quadruple test' between 15 and 20 weeks' gestation, when blood is tested for alpha-fetoprotein, inhibin A, estradiol, and hCG to calculate the chance of the baby being affected by T21 (but not T13). Women should be advised that initial screening will not provide them with a conclusive diagnostic answer about the presence or absence of an abnormality but will present them with information on the risk of abnormality, enabling them to make a further decision about diagnostic testing (chorionic villus sampling or amniocentesis). Non-invasive prenatal screening tests (NIPTs) can be performed from 10 weeks' gestation onwards. A sample of maternal blood is taken, and the cell-free fetal DNA is extracted and analysed. Some of this comes from the baby's placenta, which allows testing for trisomy 21, 13, and 18 and fetal sex. NIPT has a much higher sensitivity and specificity than combined testing but remains solely a screening test; a positive result should be confirmed by diagnostic testing. Women may choose to use NIPTs as first-line testing or to proceed to NIPTs if the combined testing result is high risk (see Chapter 25).

Some women will choose not to undergo screening for fetal abnormality, as they would not terminate a pregnancy if an abnormality were found and feel they would not benefit from knowing about any conditions prior to the birth. Other women may choose to have screening, as they may wish to decide not to continue with a pregnancy if an abnormality is found, or they may wish to have time to prepare for a baby with additional needs. The morphology scan or fetal anatomy scan performed between 18 and 22 weeks allows for assessment for fetal anomalies and placental position.

For a significant proportion of women, pregnancy is the first time that they have regular contact with health services. It is important to make this contact as positive as possible to ensure that women feel motivated to return for regular appointments and are confident to seek help should problems arise.

All health care professionals should treat the woman with respect at this first appointment:

- Introduce yourself by role and name.
- Ask the woman what she prefers to be called, and call her by that name.
- Ensure that the woman's conversation with you is private and cannot be overheard by other women attending for care.
- Provide enough time to complete the appointment adequately.
- Explain the purpose of the appointment and the questions being posed.
- Ensure that the woman is able to communicate effectively with the health care professional. Provide an interpreter when required. Ideally, this interpreter will not be a family member or friend.
- Offer the woman evidence-based information to assist her in coming to an informed choice on care options or screening.
- Ask for verbal consent before undertaking any physical examination or taking a blood sample.
- Offer the woman and her partner (if present) the opportunity to ask any questions they have regarding the pregnancy, any problems, or the care planned.
- Explain the plan of care for the remainder of her pregnancy and the importance of attending regularly for antenatal care to monitor her and the baby's health and well-being.
- Ensure that services are culturally appropriate.

When a woman is helped to feel relaxed and comfortable during this first appointment, she will be more likely to share concerns with her healthcare professional and to attend future appointments.

Motivational interviewing or brief intervention approaches can be helpful in exploring a woman's readiness to make positive health behaviour changes, such as giving up smoking, drinking alcohol, or using illicit drugs; eating healthily; and being more physically active. The health care professional can best support women to make positive changes through providing clear information about the impact of particular behaviours on maternal and fetal health, while remaining non-judgemental in approach. Pregnancy is a time when women are making many changes in their lives; brief interventions, including advice and support, can have a big impact.

SMOKING, ALCOHOL, AND ILLICIT DRUG USE

The health care professional should screen for alcohol intake, smoking, and use of illicit drugs during pregnancy.

Smoking in pregnancy is linked to miscarriage, premature birth, small-for-gestational-age babies, stillbirth, sudden unexpected death in infancy (SUDI), and increased hospital admissions in the first year of a baby's life.

Alcohol, including 'binge drinking', is related to a spectrum of potential problems categorised as fetal alcohol spectrum disorder (FASD). It is estimated that as many as 1 in 100 babies are born with effects from alcohol. A safe level of alcohol use in pregnancy has not been determined, although the risk of FASD increases with increasing alcohol intake. The best advice is that 'there is no known safe level of alcohol intake in pregnancy', and women should avoid alcohol in pregnancy. FASD has a lifelong impact on the affected person, including learning and behavioural difficulties.

Illicit drugs (marijuana, opiates, cocaine, and methamphetamines) increase the risk of adverse pregnancy outcomes, although it is often difficult to separate outcomes from confounding factors such as cigarette smoking and socioeconomic deprivation. Marijuana use in pregnancy is associated with an increased risk of pre-term birth and poor neonatal outcomes. Pregnancy can provide an opportunity to start women on opioid replacement therapy to try to stop illicit drug use.

DIET

The health care professional can provide helpful information about a healthy diet during pregnancy, including eating plenty of fruit and vegetables, good food hygiene, and foods to avoid, such as unpasteurised milk. Vitamin and mineral supplements are a helpful addition to a balanced diet for pregnant women. The WHO recommends that all women take 400 µg folic acid supplements for the first 12 weeks of pregnancy to reduce the risk of neural tube defects (national guidance on the dose of folic acid may vary, e.g., in Australia 500 µg, in New Zealand 800 µg, and in the United States 600 µg). In the United Kingdom, 5 µg daily vitamin D supplements are also recommended for all pregnant women. Routine iodine supplementation is recommended in Australasia. Women should be advised to avoid vitamin A supplements, as they may be teratogenic.

PHYSICAL ACTIVITY AND EXERCISE

It is beneficial for women to be physically active during pregnancy. Advice about physical activity in pregnancy is the same as for all adults, that is, five periods of moderate physical activity for around 30 minutes each week. Moderate physical activity includes walking, swimming, gardening, and yoga. Physical activity and exercise are helpful in maintaining and improving physical and mental health in pregnancy and may help to relieve some of the discomforts of pregnancy. Exercise that risks abdominal trauma (e.g., contact tackle sports) should be avoided after the first trimester, and scuba diving is contraindicated in pregnancy.

SOCIAL AND ENVIRONMENTAL FACTORS

Health care professionals should ensure that, on at least one occasion during the pregnancy, they have some time alone with a woman in order to enquire about the woman's home situation and whether she is experiencing domestic violence or abuse. Violence against women in their own homes can begin or escalate in pregnancy. If a woman discloses violence or abuse, the health care professional should offer the woman support and appropriate onwards referral.

Health care professionals have a responsibility to consider the welfare of the woman, her new baby, and any other children in the family by assessing for issues of concern in the woman's life. These issues include domestic abuse, substance misuse, involvement with the judicial system, homelessness, and poverty. Health care professionals should talk to the woman about the need to make referral for social support through social services and/or voluntary sector organisations. Health care professionals should familiarise themselves with their local safeguarding and child-protection procedures.

Pregnant women who are recent migrants, asylum speakers or refugees, or who have difficulty reading or speaking the local language may face additional challenges in making full use of antenatal care services. Health care professionals should help support these women to obtain appropriate pregnancy care by using interpreters when required, using a variety of means to communicate with women, and educating women about antenatal care services and how to use them.

VACCINATIONS

It is recommended that pregnant women receive a pertussis booster each pregnancy from the second trimester onwards to provide some protection to the baby until it can receive its vaccinations. Influenza vaccine is recommended in at any gestation of pregnancy, given the association of influenza with severe maternal illness and perinatal complications. Tetanus immunisation is recommended, if the woman has not already received a full course, to reduce the risk of neonatal tetanus.

The Second Trimester (12–26 Weeks)

Antenatal care during the second trimester includes follow-up on results from initial blood tests, fetal anomaly screening at 18 to 22 weeks, and instigating any treatment or further surveillance indicated by these results.

At each antenatal appointment throughout the second trimester, the following should be assessed and recorded:

- Maternal blood pressure
- Maternal urinalysis
- Enquiry about any pain or vaginal loss
- Auscultation of the fetal heart from 18 weeks.

The health care professional should enquire about the woman's well-being, both physical and emotional, at each appointment. Many women experience symptoms that cause them discomfort or concern during pregnancy. Through discussing the impact of symptoms on a woman's life, the health care professional can identify when problems are of concern and require further investigation and possible follow-up (Table 23.2).

The Third Trimester (26 Weeks–Term)

At each antenatal contact, women should continue to have their blood pressure and urinalysis checked and clearly recorded in her maternity records. The following should also be assessed.

ABDOMINAL EXAMINATION

This examination will include inspection, palpation, and auscultation of the fetal heart using a hand-held Doppler device (or, occasionally, a Pinard stethoscope). If the fetal heart cannot be heard in this way, an ultrasound scan should be undertaken to assess fetal well-being.

PRESENTATION

Examination and palpation of the uterus will identify the presentation, position, and descent of the fetus into the pelvis. Further information about malpresentations can be found in Chapter 34, pp 408.

TABLE 23.2 Common Problems or 'Minor Disorders' of Pregnancy	
Condition	**Advice, Possible Treatment**
Nausea and vomiting	Investigate severity through history-taking. If more than occasional, monitor weight, dehydration (ketones on urinalysis), consider hospitalisation; exclude urinary infection as cause; advise woman to eat little and often. Antiemetics can be safely prescribed.
Heartburn	Antacids; monitoring of diet to identify which foods worsen or improve symptoms; advise woman to eat little and often. If persistent and not relieved by common treatments, consider treatment with H_2 antagonists.
Haemorrhoids	Over-the-counter treatments; woman needs to avoid constipation through remaining well hydrated and eating plenty of fruit and vegetables.
Constipation	Over-the-counter treatments; woman needs to avoid constipation through remaining well hydrated and eating plenty of fruit and vegetables, and increase fibre in diet.
Pelvic girdle pain, sciatica, back pain	Avoid over-abduction of hips; refer for physiotherapy—use of prescribed exercises to relieve pain, improve mobility, and strengthen muscles. Maternity belts can be helpful. In more severe cases, walking aids may be required.
Anaemia	Usually iron deficiency; thus, prescribe an iron supplement; improve intake of iron-rich foods; and monitor improvement.
Carpal tunnel syndrome	Monitor severity; exclude pre-eclampsia; refer for physiotherapy; wrist splints may be helpful.
Bleeding gums	Gingivitis or gum disease is more common due to hormonal changes in pregnancy. Careful oral hygiene and dental check-up recommended.
Fatigue	Fatigue is common in pregnancy, particularly the first trimester. Screen for anaemia; encourage physical activity to improve sleep quality.
Itching	Itching is quite common in pregnancy due to hormonal changes and stretching of the skin. However, severe itching, particularly after 30 weeks, can indicate obstetric cholestasis, which requires confirmation by testing of liver function and bile acid levels.
Rashes	• Polymorphic eruption of pregnancy (1:240 pregnancies); presents with abdominal urticaria and papules in striae with periumbilical area sparing, sometimes extends to the proximal limbs. Treat with antihistamines and topical steroids. It is more common in nulliparous women.
	• Pemphigoid gestationis (1:10,000 pregnancies); pruritic erythematous papules, plaques, and wheals spreading from the periumbilical area to the breasts, thighs and palms, associated with fetal compromise. Treat with antihistamines, topical steroids, and systemic steroids.
Vaginal discharge	A heavier discharge is normal during pregnancy. However, if the discharge is malodorous or accompanied by itching, a vaginal swab for culture is appropriate. In later pregnancy, ruptured membranes should be excluded (see Chapter 44).

EVALUATION OF FETAL GROWTH

At each appointment from 24 weeks onwards, the health care professional should measure from the symphysis pubis to the fundus of the uterus and plot the measurement (symphysis-fundal height [SFH]) on a growth chart. Customised charts such as Gestation-Related Optimal Growth (GROW) charts take into account a woman's height, weight, ethnicity, and parity to calculate a baby's growth potential. When the SFH measurement falls outside the normal range or is static over a few weeks, an ultrasound examination should be offered (see Chapter 27).

ENQUIRY ABOUT FETAL MOVEMENTS

Each woman should be encouraged at each appointment to become familiar with the individual pattern of her baby's movements. Movements will generally increase in frequency and strength until 32 weeks. Then, movements are likely to remain relatively stable until the birth. There should not be a reduction in movements closer to the birth, though the size of the movements may change. Women should be advised that the baby's movements are a sign of the baby's well-being. If they become aware of any reduction in the baby's normal pattern of movements, they should lie down for an hour to rest and focus on the baby's movements. If the movements continue to be reduced, they should seek advice from a health care professional on that day. Reduced fetal movement can be an indicator of fetal hypoxia and is a risk factor for intrauterine death.

A woman's description of reduced fetal movements is important and should be responded to by a face-to-face consultation with fetal heart rate monitoring by cardiotocography (CTG) and the selective use of ultrasound.

POLYHYDRAMNIOS (INCREASED AMNIOTIC FLUID VOLUME)

Palpation and measurement may identify polyhydramnios. Where polyhydramnios is suspected during routine antenatal care, the woman should be referred for an ultrasound scan.

Polyhydramnios is diagnosed with ultrasound and may be described by a single pool >8 cm in depth and/or an amniotic fluid index (AFI) >90th centile for gestational age. The AFI is a measurement of the maximum depth of amniotic fluid in the four quadrants of the uterus.

Polyhydramnios occurs in 0.5% to 2% of all pregnancies and is associated with maternal diabetes (pre-existing or gestational), congenital fetal anomaly (such as oesophageal atresia), and multiple gestations. It may be also be idiopathic.

Polyhydramnios is associated with an increased risk of:
- Placental abruption
- Malpresentation
- Cord prolapse
- A large-for-gestational-age infant (association with diabetes)
- Requiring a caesarean section
- Postpartum haemorrhage
- Premature birth and perinatal death.

When polyhydramnios is confirmed by ultrasound, diabetes must be excluded. Amnioreduction (aspiration of amniotic fluid) for maternal comfort is not commonly needed and, if performed, quickly reaccumulates. Increased antenatal fetal surveillance is important during the remainder of the pregnancy and during labour. Following birth, a paediatrician should examine the baby for congenital anomalies, particularly oesophageal atresia.

OLIGOHYDRAMNIOS (REDUCED AMNIOTIC FLUID VOLUME)

Abdominal palpation and measurement may suggest oligohydramnios. Oligohydramnios is unlikely to be specifically suspected by clinical palpation but may contribute to a smaller than expected SFH measurement. When oligohydramnios is suspected, the woman should be referred for ultrasound. Oligohydramnios is diagnosed by ultrasound when the AFI is <5 cm or a single cord-free pool of <2 cm. Oligohydramnios affects 1% to 3% of pregnancies and is associated with poorer perinatal outcomes. Oligohydramnios usually presents in the third trimester of pregnancy and is associated with prolonged pregnancy, rupture of the membranes, fetal growth restriction, and, rarely, fetal renal congenital abnormalities (when oligohydramnios may be present from mid-trimester onwards). Oligohydramnios may indirectly cause fetal hypoxia as a consequence of cord compression.

IDENTIFYING OTHER ANTENATAL COMPLICATIONS

Regular antenatal contacts facilitate screening for potential or emerging conditions during the third trimester.

Hypertension and Pre-Eclampsia

At each antenatal contact during the third trimester, blood pressure measurement and urine testing for proteinuria is undertaken. Each appointment will also include enquiry about symptoms that may be indicative of hypertension. Enquiries should be made about headache; visual disturbances; severe upper abdominal quadrant pain; and significant facial, hand, or ankle oedema (see Chapter 28).

Screening for Anaemia

Blood should be taken to assess each woman's full blood count in the third trimester to identify anaemia and abnormal platelet numbers. Iron requirements increase in pregnancy due to the demands of the growing fetus and placenta, increased erythrocyte mass, and expanded maternal blood volume. There is a physiological fall in Hb as pregnancy advances and the maternal plasma volume increases. Anaemia in pregnancy is defined by the WHO as an Hb concentration of less than 110 g/L at any stage of pregnancy, while UK antenatal guidelines define anaemia as less than 110 g/L in the first trimester or 105 g/L in the second or third trimester. Iron supplements may lead to gastrointestinal side effects and have no proven benefits in women who are not iron deficient. In women with thalassemia, iron therapy should be commenced only when the ferritin is low. Oral iron is well absorbed; an intravenous iron infusion should be reserved for when there is inadequate response to oral iron, when there are concerns regarding compliance, or there are prohibitive side effects with oral supplements. In addition to screening for anaemia, women are offered further screening for red cell antibodies at 28 weeks.

Impaired Glucose Tolerance and Diabetes

Testing for gestational diabetes is offered at around 28 weeks. The exact screening and testing protocol differ in different regions. Local guidelines should be followed—some areas offer universal screening, and others a risk factor–based approach. HbA1C is not useful for diagnosing gestational diabetes (see Chapter 24).

Mental Health Problems

The perinatal period is a high-risk time for mental illness to develop or deteriorate. Suicide is a leading cause of maternal mortality worldwide. An important aspect of antenatal care is screening for pre-existing and emerging mental health problems throughout the pregnancy.

Most psychotropic medications are relatively safe in pregnancy. The decision as to whether to continue them or utilise them should be made on an individual basis, weighing risks versus benefits, remembering that unstable mental illness is the greatest risk to infant outcomes. Women who discontinue these medications during pregnancy can be at high risk of relapse in late pregnancy and the postnatal period. Women with previous psychosis, with bipolar disorder, and those unresponsive to treatment are particularly high risk and should be referred to perinatal mental health teams. Women on mood stabilisers, such as lithium may be at higher risk of fetal cardiac abnormalities, although the absolute risk remains low. Sodium valproate is generally not used in women of child-bearing age, as it is teratogenic and associated with fetal anomalies and lower IQ in children exposed to it in utero. However, because of the risk of psychiatric decompensation if it is stopped, urgent psychiatric review and advice should be sought.

Some women develop mental health problems for the first time in pregnancy, including depression, anxiety disorders, such as obsessive-compulsive disorder (OCD), and panic attacks. Health care professionals should ask women about their emotional well-being at each antenatal contact. Open questions should be used to encourage women to be honest if they are feeling low, hopeless, or very anxious. Mental health problems that develop during pregnancy should be monitored, and women should be offered additional support. Antenatal depression is a significant risk factor for postnatal depression. Suicide is one of the leading causes of maternal death; thus, effective screening and multidisciplinary care is vital to reduce the impact of mental illness.

PROLONGED PREGNANCY

Prolonged pregnancy is defined as a pregnancy beyond 42 weeks' gestation. The risk of intrauterine death, intrapartum hypoxia, and fetal dysmaturity increase significantly beyond 42 weeks. To reduce these risks, induction of labour is generally offered between 41 and 42 weeks' gestation. Prior to formal induction of labour, women should be offered a vaginal examination for membrane sweeping to encourage spontaneous labour.

Some women may not wish to be induced, as they are concerned about the medical interventions involved and the resulting restrictions on their choices during labour and birth. They should be informed that an induction of labour at 41 weeks will reduce their chance of requiring a caesarean section. Women who decline induction of labour should be offered increased antenatal monitoring, typically consisting of a twice-weekly CTG and the ultrasound estimation of amniotic fluid volume. Early ultrasound dating of gestational age reduces the prevalence of post-term pregnancy compared with pregnancies dated with menstrual cycle dating.

Antenatal Summary

For healthy women without significant risks or complications, antenatal care may be predominantly or completely provided by midwives. For women with health problems or at increased risk of complications, antenatal care is generally provided by a multidisciplinary team including midwives, general practitioners, obstetricians, and other specialists.

Antenatal contacts should be planned to provide women with regular appointments that are accessible to them, as near as possible to where they live. Antenatal care systems should be designed to maximise the opportunity for women to get to know the health care professionals caring for them.

All antenatal contacts should aim to identify risks and needs for the woman and the baby through history-taking, physical examination, and offering screening tests. Each contact is an opportunity for the health care professional to encourage women to ask questions and to provide education and information. Each contact is an opportunity to promote positive physical and mental health. Care should acknowledge women's physical, emotional, and social context, and should be responsive to changing needs.

Postnatal Care

The aim of postnatal care is to monitor and promote the health and well-being of the mother and baby during the first 6 weeks after birth.

Postnatal care aims to:
- Monitor the well-being of the mother and newborn(s)
- Identify any emerging problems, and initiate appropriate review or treatment
- Support parents in the early days of parenting through the provision of advice and guidance.

Models of Postnatal Care

Approaches to postnatal care vary considerably between different countries. Midwives may provide the majority of postnatal care in maternity units and the woman's home. Obstetricians provide elements of care in the immediate postnatal period, particularly if there have been complications during the birth or complications develop.

Immediate Post-Birth Care

Immediately following the birth, if the baby does not require resuscitation, the mother and baby should be supported to have uninterrupted 'skin-to-skin' contact. Placing the newborn onto the mother's chest next to her skin supports the physiological transition of the newborn from intrauterine life and provides an important opportunity for 'bonding'.

'Skin-to-skin' contact supports neonatal thermoregulation and respiratory regulation and increases the rate of successful breastfeeding. Babies are often very alert during the first hour after birth. Being held close and hearing the familiar voice of the mother can calm the baby and allows the mother to spend time to get to know and feel close to her baby. Close physical contact with the baby stimulates the production of the hormone oxytocin, which increases uterine contraction, milk production, and feelings of love and protectiveness towards the baby.

Care should be taken to ensure that the baby is kept warm during this time. The room should be at a comfortable temperature; the baby should be gently dried and covered with a towel or blanket on the mother's chest.

Routine oral suction of the baby should not be undertaken, as this may stimulate the vagal nerve and negatively impact the establishment of normal respirations.

If the mother is rhesus negative, blood should be taken from the umbilical cord to identify the baby's blood group. If the baby is rhesus positive, the mother should receive anti-D immunoglobulin to prevent rhesus isoimmunisation (see Chapter 25).

Following birth by caesarean section, the care outlined in Table 23.3 is appropriate. In addition, however, the mother requires a period of observation in the recovery area of the birthing suite or operating theatre.

Postnatally, carers should ensure that parents feel informed about feeding the baby; providing care, including changing clothing, nappies, and washing; and safe sleeping arrangements. Most women will choose to stay in hospital initially to recuperate and to ensure establishment of lactation. If the woman and baby are well with normal observations following a normal vaginal birth, it is possible for them to return home within 6 hours of birth in a hospital or birth centre. Prior to returning home, it is advisable that both the baby and mother have passed urine and that the baby has fed.

Before discharging a woman and her baby home, caregivers should identify whether there are any risks or concerns, including a raised risk of postpartum psychosis or severe depression, potential child protection issues, or significant social concerns. When such concerns are present, a care plan should normally be devised before the birth. If no such plan has been devised, a consultation with the appropriate multidisciplinary team, including mental health specialists and social workers, should be undertaken before the mother and baby leave the hospital or birth centre.

Postnatal Follow-Up in the First 10 Days

This varies in different regions. For instance, in the United Kingdom, women are visited on at least three occasions by a community midwife in their own home during the first 10 days after the birth. The aims of these visits are to identify physical or emotional problems and support the mother with feeding and parenting.

During these visits, the mother and birth partner should be given the opportunity to discuss their baby's birth with the midwife caring for them. A proportion of women (and birth partners) experience birth as 'traumatic' and may develop symptoms of post-traumatic stress disorder (PTSD). It is important to enable parents to be open about their feelings about the birth and identify when further support may be required.

TABLE 23.3 Care in the First Hours After Vaginal Birth	
Neonate	**Mother**
Assessment of condition (represented by the Apgar score) at 1, 5, and 10 minutes—resuscitation only if indicated	Observation of vaginal blood loss, palpation of uterine fundus to identify if contracted
'Skin-to-skin' contact	Examine for perineal, labial and vaginal trauma, with repair as required. Offer analgesia.
Clamp and cut the umbilical cord—1–3 minutes after birth, unless the baby requires resuscitation	Support mother to hold baby skin-to-skin and, when she wishes, offer the breast to the baby
Measurement and recording of birth weight, length, head circumference, temperature	Observations—general well-being, colour, respirations, pulse, blood pressure, temperature
Initial physical examination of the neonate to identify any abnormalities—this should include examination of the head and facial features, the palate, limbs, digits, spine, and external genitalia	Offer something to eat and drink
A record should be made of the neonate's first micturition and first feed	A record should be made of the mother's first micturition after the birth
Discussion with parents about administration of vitamin K and administer with consent	Categorisation of the mother's risk of venous thrombosis and commencement of prophylactic measures as appropriate

At each visit, the midwife should ask the mother about her emotional well-being. Suicide is a leading cause of maternal death, with the first 6 weeks after the birth the period of highest risk. All health care professionals caring for women in the postnatal period should be aware of the signs and symptoms of postpartum depression and/or psychosis.

A physical examination should be undertaken at each visit:

- Pulse, blood pressure, and temperature as indications of haemorrhage, anaemia, or sepsis
- Abdominal examination is undertaken to establish that the uterus is involuting and non-tender. On the first day after birth, the uterine fundus should be palpable at the umbilicus. It gradually reduces in size until, by the 10th to 14th day, it is no longer palpable above the symphysis pubis.
- Perineal examination, checking for signs of wound breakdown in women who have experienced perineal trauma and/or required suturing. Cool gel packs may be applied intermittently, although ice packs are not recommended. Simple analgesia can be prescribed, and local anaesthetic gels or sprays may alleviate discomfort. Salt water, or 'sitz', baths can be soothing.

Contraception should be discussed (see Chapter 21). A physical examination of the baby should be undertaken (Chapter 43). The parents should feel enabled to raise any concerns and for the midwife to provide advice.

Caregivers should ensure that parents are confident with parenting skills, including feeding, winding, changing clothes and nappies, and washing the baby.

It is important to discuss safe sleeping with all new parents. Premature babies, low-birth-weight babies, bottle-fed babies, and babies with parents who smoke are at higher risk of SUDI or 'cot death'. All babies should be laid down to sleep on their backs. They should sleep in a flat, clear space. The room should be at about 18°C to 20°C. Bed sharing should be discouraged, especially when parents smoke, drink alcohol, or take sedative drugs.

Late Postnatal Examination

This usually takes place around 6 weeks after the birth and is an opportunity for the health care professional to spend time with the mother to review the birth, address any questions, and place these in context for possible future births. This is likely to be particularly important when a mother has required medical intervention during the pregnancy or birth.

The health care professional should ask the mother about physical symptoms, including perineal pain, pain during sexual intercourse (if resumed), faecal or urinary incontinence, vaginal bleeding, or breast pain. The maternal Hb concentration may be determined, and cervical cytology should be performed if due. Contraceptive requirements and preferences are revisited, and a plan for contraception should be instigated.

Postnatal Problems

PHYSICAL PROBLEMS

Anaemia

The incidence of postnatal anaemia is 25% to 30%. It is reasonably simple to treat non-symptomatic anaemia with oral iron supplements, reserving blood transfusion for those with significant symptoms and usually with an Hb concentration <70 g/L.

Bowel Problems

Constipation is reported by up to 20% of women in the puerperium and is due to a number of factors, including fear of defaecation in the presence of perineal trauma, reduced mobility, oral medications (such as iron or codeine), or narcotic analgesia received in labour. Haemorrhoids commonly affect pregnant women, which often persist after birth.

Breast Problems

Two-thirds of women will have a problem with their breasts, including nipple pain, nipple cracks, bleeding from the nipple, breast engorgement, mastitis, and breast abscesses. For women who are not breastfeeding, breast engorgement generating symptoms of discomfort is common. For breastfeeding women, problems can be reduced by good advice regarding positioning of the baby's mouth. If mastitis occurs, it is usually the result of a blocked mammary duct and frequently requires antibiotic treatment, principally aimed at *Staphylococcus aureus*.

Perineal Breakdown

This is not uncommon, but long-term problems are fortunately uncommon. If the wound is clean, perineal resuturing may be considered. There are usually signs of infection. In this situation, it is advisable to allow healing by secondary intention and to prescribe antibiotics. Swabs for culture should be taken.

Incontinence

Following a vaginal birth, at least 20% of women suffer from urinary incontinence if assessed 3 months after birth. This is mostly from neurapraxia (impaired pudendal nerve function due to compression at the time of delivery) and usually improves and resolves spontaneously. However, a small percentage of women will not fully regain urinary continence and will require additional help from a physiotherapist or gynaecologist.

Inability to control flatus or faeces occurs in around 5% of women after birth. However, as it is embarrassing, women may be reluctant to mention it. According to endo-anal ultrasound studies, up to 35% of primiparae undergoing a vaginal birth have damage to the anal sphincters (obstetric anal sphincter injury [OASI]), although such damage may be asymptomatic (Fig. 23.2). Both OASI and nerve damage following spontaneous or instrumental delivery contribute to the problem. Investigation and treatment of symptoms

is warranted, particularly if they persist beyond the initial postnatal weeks.

Puerperal Pyrexia

This is defined as a temperature of >38°C on any occasion in the first 14 days after birth. Pyrexia is usually due to urinary or genital infections (including endometritis, the 'classical' cause of puerperal sepsis) but may also be related to infection in the chest or breast. Deep venous thrombosis (DVT) and pulmonary thromboembolism should be considered as a cause of pyrexia. After a clinical examination including breasts, legs, perineum, chest, and abdominal palpation of the uterus, a mid-stream specimen of urine, endocervical/vaginal and wound swabs, as appropriate, and blood cultures are sent for microbiological analysis. A chest infection necessitates physiotherapy, and sputum should also be sent for culture.

Sepsis represents a major cause of maternal morbidity and mortality, and it is important to be vigilant to the possibility of infection in the postnatal period (see pp. 430). Risk factors for puerperal sepsis include maternal obesity and delivery by caesarean section. If the mother is unwell (pyrexia, tachycardia, hypotension, occasionally hypothermia, confusion),

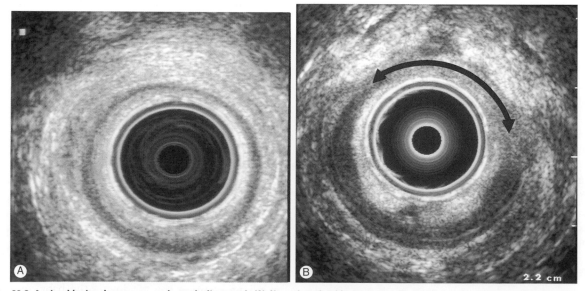

Fig. 23.2 Anal sphincter damage on endo-anal ultrasound. (A) Normal anal sphincter scan. **(B)** Anterior anal sphincter defect between the 10 o'clock and 3 o'clock positions.

treatment should be started with broad-spectrum antibiotics and fluid resuscitation without delay, with further investigation as necessary, in conjunction with advice from specialists in microbiology. Mastitis and breast abscess are particularly common in the puerperium and may be overlooked. Antibiotic therapy may be required for breast infections; however, breastfeeding or hand expression should continue when possible. A breast abscess may require surgical incision and drainage.

Secondary Postpartum Haemorrhage

See page 323.

Venous Thromboembolism (VTE)

The puerperium is the period in which women are at the highest risk of developing VTE. Women should be assessed as to their risk of VTE and low-molecular-weight heparin (LMWH) prescribed appropriately. Risk factors include medical comorbidities, obesity, pre-eclampsia, caesarean section, increasing age, and parity. Women who are classified as high risk will require 6 weeks of LMWH. It is important to encourage early mobilisation and avoid dehydration. VTE can present as a DVT or pulmonary embolus (PE). Signs and symptoms of DVT include swelling, redness, and pain in the leg or calf but may be asymptomatic, whereas a PE is typically accompanied by dyspnoea, chest pain, and, sometimes, cardiorespiratory collapse. Prevention is ideal. However, if VTE occurs, prompt diagnosis and treatment are essential. VTE remains a leading cause of maternal mortality in countries with low maternal mortality rates.

Superficial thrombophlebitis affects about 1% of women. There is a painful, erythematous, and tender (usually varicose) vein. Treatment is with support stockings and anti-inflammatory drugs.

Mental Health Problems

Around 50% of women will experience transient feelings of tearfulness and emotional lability in the first few days after birth. These are often described as the 'baby blues'. These differ from postnatal depression and psychosis in that they rapidly resolve. New mothers should be encouraged to talk about their feelings and given support and reassurance.

Talking about the 'baby blues' provides health care professionals with an opportunity to discuss the symptoms of a range of more serious mental health problems that may occur postnatally:

- 10% of new mothers are likely to develop a depressive illness. Of these, one-third to a half will be suffering from a severe depressive illness.
- 2% of new mothers will be referred to a mental health team.
- 2 per 1000 (0.2%) will suffer from postpartum psychosis.
- Postnatal depression may develop at any time during the first year after the baby's birth but generally peaks around 3 to 4 months postnatally.
- Untreated, postnatal depression can have a significant detrimental impact on the developing mother–infant relationship.
- Women may be reluctant to disclose their true feelings of depression to health care professionals after the birth if they are afraid that their baby will be taken from them.
- Postpartum psychosis generally has an earlier, more acute onset, often within the first few days after the birth.
- Maternal suicide is one of the leading causes of maternal death. Whenever assessing a woman with postnatal mental illness, it is essential to assess the safety of the woman and her baby (and any other children in her care).

Signs and Symptoms of Postnatal Depression

Cognitive

- Clouded thinking, difficulty making decisions or choices
- Lack of concentration/poor memory
- Avoidance—physical/psychological
- Fear of rejection by partner
- Worry about welfare of partner/baby
- Thoughts of harming the baby
- Suicidal ideation
- Broken sleep and early-morning awakening
- Feeling hopeless on waking
- Loss of appetite, and loss of weight
- Extreme tiredness, and lack of vitality
- Loss of pleasure ('not loving the baby' or 'not being a proper mother')

Emotional

- Persistent low mood for up to 10 to 14 days
- Feelings of inadequacy, failure
- Exhaustion, emptiness, sadness, tearfulness
- Lack of love for the baby/distance from the baby/dislike of the baby
- Guilt, shame, worthlessness
- Confusion, anxiety, panic
- Irritability, anger
- Fear for/of the baby
- Fear of being alone or going out
- Feelings of being on the outside—distanced from those around her

Behavioural

- Lack of interest/pleasure in usual activities
- Sleep disturbances/appetite changes
- Decreased energy/motivation
- Social withdrawal
- Poor self-care/inability to cope with routine tasks

Postpartum Psychosis

Many women who develop postpartum psychosis will have previously been well without obvious risk factors, but some women will have particular risk factors:

- Similar illness with a previous child
- Women with known bipolar affective disorder or previous psychosis
- Family history of bipolar illness or postpartum psychosis.

Postpartum psychosis most commonly occurs within the first 2 weeks of birth and may rapidly deteriorate. Earliest signs are:

- Perplexity, fear (even terror), restless agitation, insomnia
- Purposeless activity, uncharacteristic behaviours, disinhibition, irritation, fleeting anger, resistive behaviours
- Fear for her own or baby's health and safety or identity

- Elation and grandiosity, suspiciousness, depression or ideas of horror.

As the condition develops, there is generally a combination of mania, depression, and psychotic symptoms.

Early recognition and diagnosis are key. A woman's partner or family are likely to be the first to pick up on unusual behaviour. It is important for health care professionals to listen to family members' concerns. If treated, postpartum psychosis has a very good recovery rate. Treatment will usually include:

- Admission to a 'mother and baby' unit
- Antipsychotic or mood-stabilising drugs initiated to reduce disturbance of the mother–infant relationship. Other medication, such as antidepressants, may also be indicated.
- The psychiatrist will ensure suitable drug therapy if breastfeeding.
- Community follow-up with the perinatal mental health team
- Once recovered, discussion with the woman about risk of future illness and ways of reducing risk following a future pregnancy.

Key Points

- **The aim of antenatal care is to maximise the chance of a positive outcome from a pregnancy: a healthy mother and a healthy baby or babies.**
- **Antenatal care involves providing as much support as possible, along with a screening programme to identify maternal and fetal problems at an early stage.**
- **The puerperium is a time of major physiological change and a time of major personal upheaval.**
- **Postnatal checks are useful to assess both the mother and baby. The main maternal complications are sepsis, haemorrhage, thromboembolic disease, and depression.**

Chapter 24

Maternal Medicine

Catherine Nelson-Piercy, Kirun Gunganah

Chapter Outline

Introduction

Medical disorders are relatively common in pregnancy and often have no implications for the mother or her baby. However, the alteration in maternal physiology which occurs during pregnancy may affect the medical condition, or the medical condition itself may affect the pregnancy and the baby. Treatment options for the mother may be limited by concerns for fetal welfare. Therefore, there is the potential for difficult clinical decision-making.

The following conditions will be considered, but see also hypertension (Chapter 28) and infection in pregnancy (p. 430).

- Diabetes mellitus
- Venous thromboembolic disease
- Cardiac disease
- Connective tissue disease
- Epilepsy
- Hepatic disorders
- Renal disorders
- Respiratory disorders
- Thrombocytopenia
- Thyroid disorders.

Diabetes Mellitus

Diabetes mellitus may be diagnosed before pregnancy (pre-existing) or may be discovered for the first time during pregnancy. Discovery during pregnancy is rare for type 1 (insulin-dependent) diabetes but not uncommon for type 2 (non-insulin-dependent) diabetes. In addition to these, a transient, self-limiting state of hyperglycaemia may occur in pregnancy as a result of maternal endocrine changes.

Glucose homeostasis is maintained by the balance between insulin, which reduces glucose levels by increasing cellular uptake, and other hormones, such as glucagon and cortisol, which increase glucose production through gluconeogenesis. In pregnancy, the placenta produces multiple hormones and cytokines, such as human placental lactogen, which increase insulin resistance and increase production of insulin, respectively. If there is maternal insulin resistance, and the pancreatic β islet cells are unable to produce sufficient insulin, the mother may develop a state of hyperglycaemia referred to as gestational diabetes mellitus (GDM).

Pregnant women with pre-existing poorly controlled diabetes mellitus in the first trimester at the time of organogenesis have an increased rate of fetal congenital abnormalities. The abnormalities are principally cardiac defects, neural tube defects, and renal anomalies. Although the mechanism of this teratogenesis is unclear, there is evidence that improved pre-pregnancy and early pregnancy blood glucose control reduce the risk of congenital abnormality.

Fetal glucose levels closely reflect those of the mother, with glucose crossing the placenta through facilitated diffusion. Maternal insulin does not cross the placenta; the fetus produces its own insulin from around 10 weeks' gestation. This insulin is recognised to have a significant role in promoting fetal growth. As maternal levels of glucose are higher in mothers with diabetes, fetal levels are also increased. In turn, there is increased fetal insulin production. This fetal hyperinsulinaemia often results in macrosomia (large babies) and organomegaly, as well as increased erythropoiesis and neonatal polycythaemia.

In addition to the risk of congenital abnormality, there is also a risk of unexplained intrauterine fetal death, possibly because fetal hyperinsulinaemia leads to chronic hypoxia and acidaemia. A macrosomic fetus may be more at risk of these complications because of its increased oxygen demands.

Because babies of women with diabetes are often macrosomic, labour and delivery may be complicated by shoulder dystocia. Neonates may also become hypoglycaemic if the mother is hyperglycaemic during labour, and there is an increased incidence of neonatal respiratory distress syndrome.

EFFECTS OF PREGNANCY ON DIABETES

Insulin requirement may be static or decrease during the first trimester. It typically increases during the second and third trimesters and may reduce slightly towards term. Improvement in glycaemic control or tight control in pregnant women with pre-existing diabetes may worsen diabetic retinopathy. The optic fundi should be assessed for signs of proliferative retinopathy, with laser treatment advised as necessary.

EFFECTS OF DIABETES ON PREGNANCY

The incidence of pre-eclampsia is increased. There is also an increased incidence of maternal infection, particularly of the urinary tract. Polyhydramnios, which probably results from fetal polyuria, may result in unstable lie, malpresentation, and pre-term labour.

SCREENING FOR GESTATIONAL DIABETES

This is a controversial subject, with variations in timing, diagnostic tests, and diagnostic criteria between centres and countries. The National Institute for Health and Care Excellence (NICE) UK guidelines recommend offering a 2-hour 75-g glucose tolerance test (GTT) at 24 to 28 weeks to women with risk factors, including a family history of diabetes; a raised body mass index (BMI; >30 kg/m^2); a previous macrosomic baby (>4.5 kg); those with previous GDM; or ethnic minorities with high prevalence of diabetes. For those with previous GDM, early self-monitoring or GTT should also be offered at booking.

In the UK guidance from NICE, the diagnostic criteria for gestational diabetes after 2-hour 75-g GTT is:
- Fasting blood glucose level ≥5.6 mmol/L
  or
- 2-hour blood glucose level ≥7.8 mmol/L.

MANAGEMENT OF GESTATIONAL DIABETES

As a first step, women should be offered treatment with dietary advice and exercise. Metformin and subsequent insulin therapy should be instituted if the target levels are not achieved. Lifestyle intervention and therapy should aim to keep the fasting glucose <5.3 mmol/L and 1-hour postprandial <7.8 mmol/L.

Women with GDM have an increased risk of developing diabetes mellitus in the subsequent 25 years. Recurrence of GDM in subsequent pregnancies is up to 75% (especially if treatment with insulin was required).

ANTENATAL MANAGEMENT OF ESTABLISHED DIABETES

At pre-pregnancy counselling, advice should be given about good glycaemic control, diet, smoking cessation, weight loss if BMI >27 kg/m^2, and high-dose (5-mg) folate supplements. Glycosylated haemoglobin should be checked when planning a pregnancy and in early pregnancy, aiming for levels below 48 mmol/L (6.5%).

Care in pregnancy should be in a joint diabetic and antenatal clinic, with frequent visits planned as required. Capillary blood glucose should be measured on average four times a day (fasting and 1 hour postprandial), aiming for tight control (e.g., with pre-prandial levels of 4.0–5.3 mmol/L and 1 hour postprandial levels of <7.8 mmol/L).

Insulin is commonly given as a short-acting analogue three times a day (with meals), with long-acting background insulin once or twice a day. Ketoacidosis should be avoided, as it is associated with an increased risk of perinatal mortality. All women with type 1 diabetes should be offered ketone testing strips and a ketometer, as they are at increased risk of developing diabetic ketoacidosis. In recent years, there has been increased use of technology, such as flash glucose monitoring, continuous glucose monitoring (CGM), and continuous subcutaneous insulin infusion (CSII) to aid pregnant women with type 1 diabetes achieve better glycaemic control and, hence, achieve better pregnancy outcomes.

Maternal kidney function and optic fundi should be assessed in early pregnancy. A detailed anomaly scan, including a fetal heart scan, should be offered at 18 to 22 weeks. The maternal abdomen should be examined for polyhydramnios, macrosomia, or fetal growth restriction (measurement of symphysis-fundal height). Serial ultrasound fetal biometry is also recommended.

CHILDBIRTH

Childbirth between 37 and 38^{+6} weeks by elective birth (induction of labour) is recommended for women with pre-existing diabetes and by 40^{+6} weeks for women with gestational diabetes if there are no complications. Concern regarding fetal macrosomia, and the potential for shoulder dystocia in particular, may necessitate a planned caesarean section.

If pre-term labour occurs, corticosteroids may be given as for the non-diabetic woman but will lead to deterioration in diabetic control unless insulin doses are increased appropriately or a variable-rate insulin infusion (VRII) is used.

The aim of a VRII is to maintain tight intrapartum glycaemic control, whether during labour or for caesarean section, to reduce the risk of neonatal hypoglycaemia. In the immediate postpartum period, insulin requirements rapidly return to pre-pregnancy levels and the previous subcutaneous (SC) insulin regime can be re-established. For women with GDM, insulin should be discontinued following delivery.

Venous Thromboembolic Disease

ANTENATAL

In pregnancy, the balance of the coagulation system is altered towards thrombus formation. There are increased levels of fibrinogen, prothrombin, and other clotting factors, together with reduced levels of endogenous anticoagulants. This tendency to clot formation is offset only in part by an increase in fibrinolysis. In addition to the clotting system changes, the gravid uterus causes a degree of mechanical obstruction to the venous system and leads to peripheral venous stasis in the lower limbs.

Venous thromboembolic disease appears to be rare in Africa and East Asia but is the most common direct cause of maternal mortality in the United Kingdom. In the United Kingdom, over 50% of maternal deaths from thromboembolism occur antenatally.

Over 80% of deep venous thromboses (DVTs) in pregnancy are left-sided, in contrast to only 55% in the non-pregnant woman. This difference may reflect compression of the left common iliac vein by the right common iliac artery and the ovarian artery, which cross the vein on the left side only. The gravid uterus lies over the right common iliac artery. Furthermore, over 70% of DVTs in pregnancy are iliofemoral rather than femoral popliteal compared with the non-pregnant rate of around 9%. Therefore, they are more likely than lower calf vein thromboses to give rise to pulmonary embolism.

Thromboembolism may be asymptomatic but usually presents with the traditional symptoms and signs, such as calf tenderness, breathlessness, and chest pain. It may also present with lower abdominal or groin pain. It is essential to make a definitive diagnosis, not just for management of the current pregnancy but because there are major implications with regard to the need for thromboprophylaxis in subsequent pregnancies.

D-dimers and clinical decision rules employed without pregnancy are not helpful in pregnancy. Radiological investigations are required if there is clinical suspicion. Duplex Doppler ultrasound is particularly useful for identifying femoral vein thromboses, although iliac veins are less easily seen (Fig. 24.1). It is safe and should be the first-line investigation. Venography or magnetic resonance venography is appropriate if Doppler studies give equivocal results, or negative results, despite strong clinical suspicion. Pregnancy is not a contraindication to carrying out a chest X-ray and/or a ventilation-perfusion ($\dot{V}/\dot{Q}$) scan – any radiation risks are outweighed by the benefits of accurate diagnosis (Fig. 24.2). A normal scan virtually excludes the diagnosis of pulmonary embolism. A computed tomography pulmonary arteriogram (CTPA) may also be appropriate, especially if the chest X-ray is abnormal or an alternative diagnosis is suspected. CTPA, despite involving less radiation to the fetus than $\dot{V}/\dot{Q}$ scanning, is associated with significant radiation to the maternal breasts, which may increase a woman's chance of developing breast cancer in later life.

Treatment of DVT or pulmonary embolism in pregnancy is with SC low-molecular-weight heparin (LMWH). Intravenous (IV) unfractionated heparin is appropriate in cases of massive (high-risk) and submassive (intermediate-risk) pulmonary embolus, and thrombolysis should not be withheld in pregnancy if indicated in these situations based on raised biomarkers (troponin and brain natriuretic peptide), clot burden, and right ventricular dysfunction on echocardiogram. LMWH therapy is interrupted for birth to allow for regional analgesia and anaesthesia, and to minimise the risk of haemorrhage. After delivery, the woman may choose to continue with SC LMWH or commence warfarin, continuing anticoagulation for 6 to 12 weeks, as decided by timing of onset and clinical severity of the thrombosis. Direct oral anticoagulants are contraindicated in breastfeeding women.

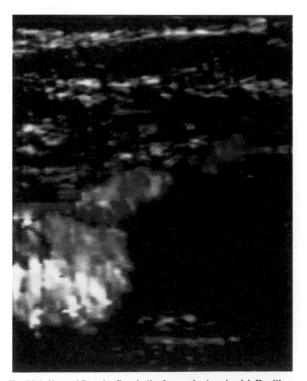

Fig. 24.1 Normal Doppler flow in the femoral artery (*red, left*) with no flow through the occluded femoral vein (*black, right*).

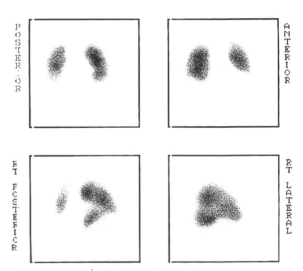

Fig. 24.2 Positive $\dot{Q}$ scan. Note the lack of perfusion in the right lower lobe. The ventilation scan was normal. (From Pitkin J, Peattie A, Magowan BA. *Obstetrics and Gynecology. An Illustrated Colour Text.* Churchill Livingstone, 2003.)

Women with a previous history of venous thromboembolism (VTE) – except women who have experienced a single episode of VTE provoked by major trauma who, in the absence of other risk factors, such as thrombophilia, may not require thromboprophylaxis (Box 24.1) – should be offered antenatal and postnatal (for 6 weeks) prophylaxis with LMWH.

ANTENATAL AND POSTNATAL RISK ASSESSMENT

The risks of thromboembolism should be assessed in all women at booking, at the time of any antenatal hospital admission, and postnatally (Box 24.2). Those at risk (previous thrombosis, thrombophilia, emergency caesarean section, or any two [postnatal] or three [antenatal >28 weeks] or four [antenatal throughout pregnancy] of the other risk factors) should be offered

BOX 24.1 HERITABLE THROMBOPHILIAS

- Antithrombin deficiency
- Protein C deficiency
- Protein S deficiency
- Factor V Leiden mutation
- Prothrombin gene variant

Acquired Thrombophilias

- Lupus anticoagulant and anticardiolipin antibodies

BOX 24.2 THROMBOEMBOLIC RISK FACTORS IN PREGNANCY AND POSTPARTUM

- Age >35 years
- Obesity (body mass index >30)
- Para 3 or more
- Gross varicose veins
- Current infection
- Pre-eclampsia
- Immobility (>4 days)
- Major current illness, for example, heart or lung disease, cancer, inflammatory bowel disease, nephrotic syndrome
- Caesarean section, particularly emergency caesarean section in labour
- Extended major pelvic or abdominal surgery, for example, caesarean hysterectomy
- Women with a personal or family history of deep vein thrombosis, pulmonary embolism, or heritable thrombophilia
- Women with antiphospholipid antibody (cardiolipin antibody or lupus anticoagulant)
- Paralysis of lower limbs
- Smoking, multiple pregnancy, and assisted conception (in vitro fertilization)

thromboprophylaxis with LMWH (e.g., enoxaparin 40 mg once daily). Admission to hospital is also a risk factor. Pregnant women admitted to hospital should usually be offered LMWH unless they have active bleeding or birth is imminent.

Cardiac Disease

Heart disease complicates less than 1% of all pregnancies but accounts for around 23% of maternal deaths in the United Kingtom. Rheumatic heart disease remains a significant problem in Africa, South Asia, and the Pacific Islands. It is also encountered with increasing frequency in other countries as a result of migration. There are increasing numbers of fertile women who have had surgery as children for congenital heart disease. Maternal mortality is highest in conditions in which pulmonary blood flow cannot be increased to compensate for the increased demand during pregnancy – particularly Eisenmenger syndrome, in which maternal mortality rates reach 20% to 40%.

Unfortunately, many symptoms and signs similar to those of heart disease occur commonly in normal pregnancy, making a clinical diagnosis difficult. Breathlessness and syncopal episodes are present in 90% of normal pregnancies, atrial ectopic beats are common, and up to 96% of normal women may have an audible ejection systolic murmur. Further investigation should be considered if the murmur is loud (>2/6), diastolic, if a precordial thrill is present, or if there are any other suspicious features, especially in migrant women.

If problems are discovered, a cardiologist with expertise in pregnancy cardiology should be involved during the antenatal period. If there is no haemodynamic compromise (e.g., congenital mitral valve prolapse), the prognosis is good, and there is often no requirement for cardiac follow-up. If there are potential haemodynamic problems, very close follow-up by a multidisciplinary team is mandatory, and a careful plan should be made for childbirth. Serious consideration of pregnancy termination is advisable in women with Eisenmenger syndrome, any cause of pulmonary hypertension, pulmonary veno-occlusive disease, in those with aortopathy with significant aortic dilatation, and in those with severely impaired left ventricular function. With atrial fibrillation, anticoagulation is required to prevent atrial clot forming and subsequent

BOX 24.3 SEVERE CARDIAC DISEASE AND BIRTH

- Labour should be conducted in a high-dependency or intensive care unit, possibly with central venous catheter and arterial line monitoring, aiming for a vaginal birth. Hypotension, hypoxia, and fluid overload should be avoided.
- Epidural analgesia may be used in most circumstances.
- For the third stage, oxytocin should be given slowly, rather than Syntometrine (a combination of oxytocin and ergometrine), because ergometrine can cause hypertension and bolus oxytocin can cause vasodilatation.
- Particular care is required in the immediate postpartum period, as the increased circulating volume following delivery of the placenta may lead to fluid overload and congestive heart failure.

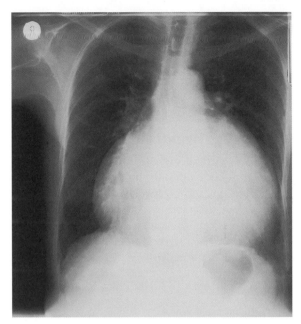

Fig. 24.3 Postpartum cardiomyopathy after the birth of twins in a mother aged 42 years.

embolic problems. If the maternal partial pressure of oxygen (PO_2) is decreased, the fetus is at risk from hypoxia and fetal growth restriction, thus, should be monitored closely.

Severe cardiac disease can cause problems at birth, particularly in those with prosthetic valves, aortic stenosis, mitral stenosis, left ventricular dysfunction, or pulmonary hypertension (Box 24.3).

Myocardial infarction is rare in pregnancy but is a common cardiac cause of maternal mortality. Peripartum cardiomyopathy is also rare (<1:5000) but carries a 5% mortality and is associated with hypertension in pregnancy, multiple pregnancy, high parity, and increased maternal age. It presents with sudden onset of heart failure and, on chest radiology or echocardiography, there is usually a grossly dilated heart (Fig. 24.3).

Connective Tissue Disease

These diseases are not uncommon and, as they often affect women during their childbearing years, they are not infrequently found in association with pregnancy. See also antiphospholipid syndrome (p. 78).

SYSTEMIC LUPUS ERYTHEMATOSUS (SLE)

There is an increased chance of an exacerbation of SLE (flare-up) occurring in pregnancy and during the postnatal period. Women should be discouraged from becoming pregnant when their disease is active, to minimise problems. Active lupus nephritis during pregnancy is associated with significant maternal and perinatal mortality and morbidity. In particular, it is associated with a risk of pre-eclampsia.

Lupus nephritis is associated with increased fetal loss rates from spontaneous miscarriages and pre-term birth. This is particularly so in those with antiphospholipid antibodies. There is an increased incidence of pre-eclampsia, which may be difficult to differentiate from a disease flare, as both are associated with hypertension and proteinuria. There is no increase in the rate of fetal abnormalities, although there is a 2% risk of fetal congenital heart block and 5% risk of neonatal cutaneous lupus associated with the presence of anti-Ro and anti-La antibodies (Fig. 24.4).

If lupus anticoagulant or anticardiolipin antibodies (antiphospholipid antibodies) are present, low-dose aspirin should be given. In women with a previous history of thromboembolic disease or adverse pregnancy outcome, LMWH is indicated. Careful monitoring of renal function is appropriate. Disease flares should be managed when possible with oral prednisolone. There should also be regular ultrasound fetal biometry owing to the increased risk of fetal growth restriction.

Epilepsy

A first seizure in the second half of pregnancy should be assumed to be eclampsia until proven otherwise. Around a third of pregnant women with epilepsy have an increase

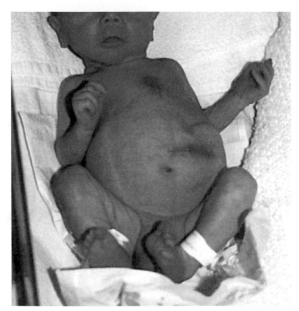

Fig. 24.4 Pacemaker in a baby with congenital heart block in association with anti-Ro antibodies.

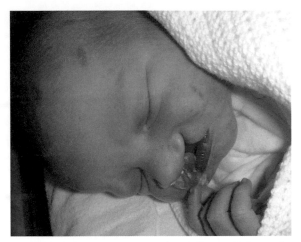

Fig. 24.5 Antiepileptic drugs are associated with neural tube, cardiac, and craniofacial anomalies.

in seizure frequency independent of the effects of medication. For women with epilepsy on treatment, the fall in antiepileptic drug (AED) levels due to dilution, reduced absorption, and increased drug metabolism may necessitate increased doses during pregnancy. This is particularly the case for lamotrigine. There is an increased incidence of fetal anomalies in association with the older AEDs (phenytoin 6%, carbamazepine 4% to 5% vs 3% in the general population; Fig. 24.5). Single-drug regimens are less teratogenic than multidrug therapy (Table 24.1), and sodium valproate carries the highest risk of teratogenesis (10%), as well as being associated with an increased risk of neurocognitive impairment, autism spectrum disorders, and attention deficit disorder. The risk of congenital malformations seems not to be increased with lamotrigine and levetiracetam.

Hepatic Disorders

There are a large number of potential causes of liver dysfunction in pregnancy (Tables 24.2 and 24.3). A history of a prodromal illness, overseas travel, or high-risk group

TABLE 24.1	Care of Women With Epilepsy in Pregnancy
Pre-pregnancy counselling	Monotherapy with AED ideal. Folate supplementation (5 mg/day) should be continued until at least 12 weeks.
AED dosage	AED doses adjusted on clinical grounds. There are fetal risks from AEDs as well as from not taking the drugs (from increased fit frequency).
	Increased doses recommended for lamotrigine therapy.
Detailed ultrasound scan at 18–22 weeks	Neural tube, cardiac, and craniofacial abnormalities, as well as diaphragmatic herniae, are more common.
Seizures	Most seizures in pregnancy will be self-limiting. If prolonged, however, rectal or IV diazepam or IV lorazepam, with or without ventilation, may be required.
Postnatal	The mother may breastfeed safely (drugs pass into the milk, but neonatal levels are low for most AEDs). Advice should be given about safe and suitable settings for feeding, bathing, and so forth. Carbamazepine, phenytoin, primidone, and phenobarbitone induce liver enzymes, reducing the effectiveness of the standard-dose combined oral contraceptives. Therefore, a higher-dose estrogen preparation or alternative form of contraception is required.

AED, Antiepileptic drug; *IV*, intravenous.

TABLE 24.2   Liver Disorders Specific to Pregnancy

Hyperemesis gravidarum	This may occasionally be associated with abnormal LFTs.
Intrahepatic cholestasis of pregnancy	Usually presents after 30 weeks' gestation, possibly due to a genetic predisposition to the cholestatic effect of estrogens. Pruritus affects the limbs and trunk, and it is often severe. There may be a positive family history in up to 35% of cases. Serum total bile acid concentration is increased early in the disease and is the optimum marker for the condition. Transaminases may be increased (<3-fold). Bilirubin is usually <100 µmol/L, and there may be pale stools and dark urine. There are no serious long-term maternal risks, but there is a risk of pre-term birth, fetal distress, and intrauterine fetal death. Birth at 37–38 weeks should be discussed with the woman, if bile acids are markedly elevated, in an effort to prevent fetal death.
HELLP syndrome	See page 342.
Acute fatty liver of pregnancy	This is very rare, is associated with increased maternal and fetal mortality, and may progress rapidly to hepatic failure. It usually presents with vomiting in the third trimester associated with malaise and abdominal pain, jaundice, thirst, and polyuria, and may cause hepatic encephalopathy. LFTs are elevated, urate is very high, and there is often profound hypoglycaemia. There may be hypertension and proteinuria. Coagulopathy, hypoglycaemia, and fluid imbalance should be corrected, and birth of the baby should be expedited. N-acetylcysteine should be administered. Following birth, there is a risk of postpartum haemorrhage and liver dysfunction may be prolonged. Hepatic encephalopathy may develop and liver transplant is occasionally necessary. If the woman recovers, there is no long-term liver impairment.

*HELLP, **H**aemolysis, **e**levated **l**iver enzymes, and **l**ow **p**latelets; LFT, liver function test.*

TABLE 24.3   Liver Disorders Coincidental to Pregnancy

Viral hepatitis	Serology should be performed for hepatitis A, B, and C, as well as for cytomegalovirus, Epstein-Barr virus, and toxoplasmosis (see p. 302).
Gallstones	Asymptomatic gallstones do not require treatment. Cholecystitis should be managed conservatively if possible.
Cirrhosis	In severe cirrhosis, there is usually amenorrhoea. If pregnancy occurs, and the disease is well compensated, there is usually no long-term effect on hepatic function. The main risk is bleeding from oesophageal varices.
Autoimmune chronic active hepatitis	Pregnancy does not usually have any long-term effect on liver function. Immunosuppressant therapy with prednisolone and azathioprine should be continued in those with autoimmune disease.
Primary biliary cirrhosis	This is variable in severity. The prognosis for mother and fetus is good in mild disease. It may present during pregnancy for the first time in a similar way to obstetric cholestasis.

*HELLP, **H**aemolysis, **e**levated **l**iver enzymes, and **l**ow **p**latelets; LFT, liver function test.*

for blood-borne illness may suggest viral hepatitis. Itch is suggestive of cholestasis. Abdominal pain is associated with gallstones, HELLP (**h**aemolysis, **e**levated **l**iver enzymes, and **l**ow **p**latelets) syndrome (p. 342), or acute fatty liver. Urea and electrolytes (U&Es), liver function tests (LFTs), blood glucose, platelets, and coagulation screen should be performed and blood sent for hepatitis serology. Liver autoantibodies may suggest pre-existing liver disease; anti-smooth muscle antibodies are a marker for autoimmune chronic active hepatitis, and antimitochondrial antibodies are a marker for primary biliary cirrhosis. A mild transaminitis is common in non-alcoholic steatohepatitis, which may be diagnosed for the first time in pregnancy. Abdominal ultrasound of the liver and gall bladder may show obstruction or gallstones. It is normal for the alkaline phosphatase level to increase in pregnancy (up to three- to four-fold increase).

Renal Disorders

In pregnancy, there is a physiological increase in the size of both kidneys as well as dilatation of the ureter and renal pelvis. This dilatation is greater on the right than on the left, in part because of dextrorotation of the uterus. There is also an increase in creatinine clearance owing to the increased glomerular filtration rate (maximal in the second trimester). In pregnancy, the normal serum urea is <4.5 mmol/L and creatinine <75 μmol/L.

INFECTION

Urinary tract infections (UTIs) occur in 3% to 7% of pregnancies. If untreated, they may lead to septicaemia and pre-term labour. Asymptomatic bacteriuria should be treated, since there is a 30% to 40% risk of developing a symptomatic UTI. Pyelonephritis should be treated with intravenous fluids, intravenous antibiotics, and analgesics.

OBSTRUCTION

Acute hydronephrosis is characterised by loin pain, ureteric colic, sterile urine, and a renal ultrasound scan showing dilatation of the renal tract greater than normal for pregnancy (Fig. 24.6). If the symptoms are not settling and the ultrasound scan does not demonstrate the cause of the obstruction, a limited IV urogram or magnetic resonance imaging should be considered. Treatment is with ureteric stenting or nephrostomy. There may be no obvious cause of obstruction, and complete resolution may occur following delivery. Renal tract calculi are associated with an increased incidence of UTIs but otherwise do not usually affect pregnancy (unless obstruction is severe).

CHRONIC KIDNEY DISEASE (CKD)

With CKD in pregnancy, the fetal prognosis is best if maternal renal function and blood pressure are optimised. If the plasma creatinine is <125 μmol/L (CKD stage 1–3a), the maternal and perinatal outcome is usually good. If pregnancy occurs with a creatinine >250 μmol/L (CKD stage 4–5), there is a high risk of deterioration in renal function as well as a lower chance of a successful pregnancy outcome. Between these levels, women should be advised that pregnancy may cause their renal function to deteriorate, and that there are also risks to the fetus (mainly fetal growth restriction and pre-term birth). Some renal diseases carry a poorer prognosis than others, and specialist advice is required.

Women with CKD should receive pre-pregnancy counselling. The woman should be seen frequently antenatally, particularly in the third trimester. Hypertension should be treated appropriately, U&Es, plasma albumin, urinalysis, and mid-stream urine samples checked at each visit, and a protein–creatinine ratio sent each month to quantify proteinuria. Close fetal monitoring is important. It is difficult to distinguish pre-eclampsia from increasing renal compromise, as both may present with hypertension, rising serum creatinine, and proteinuria. Newer tests using angiogenic markers for pre-eclampsia such as PlGF (placental growth factor) can be very useful in this context.

Pregnancy should be discouraged in women with CKD 4–5 (estimated glomerular filtration rate <30) or on dialysis, as the fetal prognosis is poor. Pregnancy in women who have had a renal transplant is increasingly common and usually successful with good allograft function. As with other causes of CKD, pregnancy and renal outcome is dependent on the baseline renal function.

Respiratory Disorders

Breathlessness due to the physiological increase in minute ventilation is a common symptom in pregnancy. Although there is an increased tidal volume from early pregnancy, the exact cause of the feeling of breathlessness is unclear. Investigation should be considered if the breathlessness is of sudden onset, associated with chest pain, or if there are clinical signs. It should be remembered that breathlessness can also be a feature of pulmonary thromboembolic disease and heart failure.

Asthma is a common condition. In most women, the disease is unchanged in pregnancy. Treatment

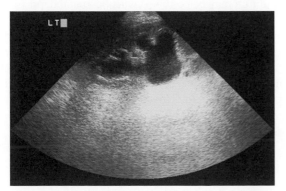

Fig. 24.6 Ultrasound of left kidney with ureteric obstruction and calyceal clubbing. There was a calculus in the lower-third of the ureter.

is the same as that outside pregnancy, and women already established on treatment should continue. Inhaled beta-sympathomimetics and inhaled steroids are considered safe. Oral steroids should be given if clinically indicated.

Thrombocytopenia

MATERNAL THROMBOCYTOPENIA IN PREGNANCY

In the second half of normal pregnancies, there is a mild thrombocytopenia (platelet count 100–150 × 10^9/L) in 8% of women, which is not associated with any additional risk to the mother or fetus. The platelet count may also be reduced in pre-eclampsia.

Autoimmune thrombocytopenic purpura is the most common cause of thrombocytopenia in early pregnancy (but can also arise in later pregnancy) and may be acute or chronic. Antiplatelet antibodies may cross the placenta and, rarely, cause fetal thrombocytopenia, although this seldom is associated with long-term morbidity. No treatment is required in the absence of bleeding, provided the platelet count remains above 50 × 10^9/L. If the platelet count falls below this level, steroids and/or immunoglobulin can be given. Specialist haematological advice is appropriate before considering treatment. Treatment may be warranted towards term to ensure that the platelet count is >70 to 80 × 10^9/L to permit regional analgesia/anaesthesia.

Thyroid Disorders

In total, 1% of pregnant women (in countries where testing is readily available) are affected by thyroid disease, with *hypo*thyroidism being more common than *hyper*thyroidism. The fetal thyroid gland secretes thyroid hormones from the 12th week and is independent of maternal control.

HYPOTHYROIDISM

This may present with fatigue, hair loss, dry skin, abnormal weight gain, poor appetite, cold intolerance, bradycardia, and delayed tendon reflexes. If untreated, there is an increase in the rate of spontaneous miscarriages and stillbirths compared with the euthyroid population, as well as a risk of fetal neurological impairment. There is

no fetal risk if the mother is treated and is euthyroid. Thyroid function should be regularly monitored, aiming to keep thyroid-stimulating hormone (TSH) and free thyroxine (T_4) within the normal range for pregnancy. If the woman is already on treatment and euthyroid at booking, the dose need not be increased. There is no evidence that treating subclinical hypothyroidism (normal T_4 with elevated TSH) either before or during pregnancy benefits pregnancy outcome.

HYPERTHYROIDISM

Thyrotoxicosis presents with weight loss, exophthalmos, tachycardia, and restlessness. It is usually due to Graves disease but may be secondary to a toxic thyroid adenoma or multinodular goitre. Untreated thyrotoxicosis is associated with high fetal mortality and a risk of maternal thyroid crisis when giving birth. Well-controlled hyperthyroidism is not associated with an increase in fetal anomalies, but there is a tendency for babies to be small for gestational age. Graves disease usually improves during pregnancy.

Carbimazole and propylthiouracil cross the placenta but are safe in pregnancy and potentially cause fetal thyroid suppression only in high doses. Radioactive iodine is contraindicated in pregnancy and surgery is indicated only for those with a very large goitre or poor compliance with oral therapy.

POSTPARTUM THYROIDITIS

This occurs following 5% to 10% of all pregnancies, usually with initial hyperthyroidism, followed by hypothyroidism, and then recovery. Because the hypothyroidism occurs at around 1 to 3 months, the condition may be confused with postnatal depression. Symptoms of hyperthyroidism may be treated with propranolol (antithyroid drugs). Hypothyroidism should be treated with thyroxine as above, withdrawing around 6 months after childbirth. Affected women may require long-term treatment or may develop subsequent hypothyroidism.

Key Points

- **Diabetes carries increased risks of congenital abnormality, macrosomia, and intrauterine death for the fetus. Good periconception and antenatal glycaemic control is the cornerstone of care.**

- Pregnancy-related venous thromboembolic disease is the most common direct cause of maternal mortality in many countries with low maternal mortality rates. Relevant symptoms should be appropriately investigated. Thromboembolic prophylaxis is important in both obstetrics and gynaecological practice.
- AED, particularly sodium valproate and polytherapy, increase the risk of fetal abnormality.

- Abnormal LFTs may be related to the pregnancy, incidental viral infections, or pre-existing liver disease.
- Asymptomatic UTIs in pregnancy should be treated.
- Well controlled thyroid disease poses little serious risk to the mother or fetus.

Chapter 25

Fetal Medicine

Lindsay Kindinger, Amrita Banerjee, Pranav P. Pandya

Chapter Outline

Introduction

Fetal medicine is a constantly evolving specialty. With improved understanding of scientific basis and development in technologies, numerous advances have been made in the past decade to provide more holistic and personalised perinatal care. Congenital anomalies are defined as being present at birth and include structural, chromosomal, and genetic anomalies. Fetal medicine involves the assessment of the unborn fetus mainly by ultrasound to allow monitoring of certain conditions, the diagnosis of congenital disorders, in utero therapy, optimisation of time and place of birth, and facilitating postnatal care. In some cases of serious or potentially serious underlying fetal conditions, termination of pregnancy (TOP) is discussed.

In the United Kingdom, approximately 2% to 3% of fetuses have congenital malformations, the most common of which are listed in Box 25.1.

BOX 25.1 SELECTED CONGENITAL ABNORMALITIES

Genetic Disorders
- Down syndrome (trisomy 21)
- Edwards syndrome (trisomy 18)
- Patau syndrome (trisomy 13)
- Triploidy
- Sex chromosome abnormalities
- XO (Turner syndrome)
- XXY (Klinefelter syndrome)
- XYY
- XXX
- Apparently balanced rearrangements (translocations or inversions)
- Unbalanced chromosomal structural abnormalities
- Gene disorders (e.g., fragile X syndrome, Huntington chorea, Tay-Sachs disease)

Structural Disorders
- Congenital heart disease
- Neural tube defects (e.g., anencephaly, encephalocele, spina bifida)
- Abdominal wall defects (e.g., exomphalos, gastroschisis)
- Genitourinary abnormalities (e.g., renal dysplasia, polycystic kidney disease, pyelectasis, posterior urethral valves, Potter syndrome)
- Lung disorders (e.g., pulmonary hypoplasia, diaphragmatic hernia, cystic fibrosis)

Congenital Infection
- Toxoplasmosis
- Rubella
- Cytomegalovirus (CMV)
- Herpes simplex virus
- Chickenpox
- *Erythrovirus*
- Human immunodeficiency virus
- Zika
- Hepatitis
- *Listeria monocytogenes*
- Syphilis
- Beta-haemolytic streptococci – group B

The aims of prenatal diagnosis are four-fold:

- To identify congenital anomalies at early gestation that are incompatible with life, or that are likely to result in significant disability to prepare the parents, involve other specialist clinicians, and offer the option of TOP if appropriate
- To identify conditions which may influence the timing, site, or mode of delivery
- To identify fetuses who may benefit from early neonatal/paediatric intervention
- To identify fetuses who may benefit from in utero treatment.

Principles of Screening

The goal of perinatal screening is to identify conditions that can have adverse outcomes for the mother, fetus, or both. Perinatal screening can be applied only to recognised conditions where a suitable test is available, treatment options (including TOP) are available and acceptable to parents, and the cost of case finding should be economically balanced in relation to possible expenditure on medical care as a whole.

Parents should be counselled that screening tests (particularly those for chromosomal anomalies) are not diagnostic and will identify only those at 'high or low chance' for a condition. Couples must understand that if they were placed in the 'high-chance' group, further tests would then be offered, and they should be aware of what that would involve. They should ideally also have given thought to what they would do should the pregnancy be affected. Whilst screening for fetal anomaly is offered to all couples in pregnancy, it is important to appreciate that after counselling, parents should be supported to make an informed choice and may decline the option of screening.

In the United Kingdom, the National Health Service (NHS) Fetal Anomaly Screening Programme provides information for health care professionals about the screening tests offered to each pregnant woman to enable her to make a personal informed choice about the tests. There are charities and support groups that can offer information, support, and advice for women with high-chance results.

Assessing the Chance of Anomalies

The majority of structural and chromosomal anomalies occur de novo in women with no predisposing risk factors. Maternal age, medical comorbidities, and family history of medical conditions are important to consider when assessing the risk of genetic or structural fetal anomaly. The likelihood of an autosomal trisomy, especially trisomy 21 (Down syndrome), increases with advancing maternal age. In some cases, however, there may be a family history of an inherited condition – for example, Duchenne muscular dystrophy, cystic fibrosis, and sickle cell disease. Consanguinity increases the chance of single-gene anomalies, especially relating to autosomal-recessive conditions. Structural anomalies are also slightly more likely to occur in those with a family history of the condition; in some instances, the chance may be higher still if the parents have had a previously affected child. A mother who has a child with spina bifida, for example, has up to a 5% chance of recurrence compared with a background prevalence of 0.4 to 0.5 per 1000 births in Europe. Mothers with pre-existing diabetes have a higher chance of cardiac and neural tube defects, whilst women with epilepsy are at increased chance of structural anomalies, especially if taking potentially teratogenic antiepileptic drugs.

Screening for Chromosomal Anomalies

FIRST-TRIMESTER COMBINED SCREENING TEST

In the United Kingdom, screening for chromosomal anomalies is offered to all eligible pregnant women to assess the chance of the baby being born with Down syndrome (trisomy 21 or T21), or Edwards syndrome (T18) or Patau syndrome (T13).

The test of choice is first-trimester combined screening. Women can choose:

1. Not to have screening
2. To have screening for T21 and T18/T13
3. To have screening for T21 only
4. To have screening for T18/T13 only

The combined screening test is performed between 11^{+2} weeks to 14^{+1} weeks of gestation, which corresponds to a crown rump length (CRL) of 45.0 mm to 84.0 mm (Fig. 25.1A). To calculate the chance of the pregnancy being affected by T21 or T18/T13, the combined test incorporates:

- Maternal age
- The measurement of the thickness of nuchal fluid behind the fetal neck (nuchal translucency [NT]; Fig. 25.1B)

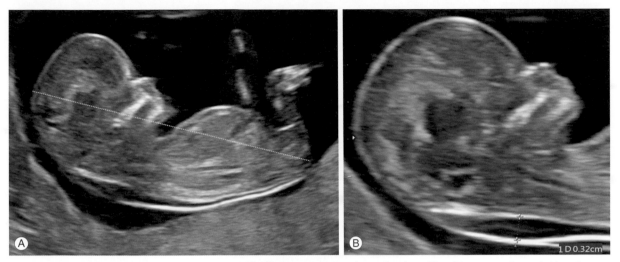

Fig. 25.1 The sagittal view required for a crown-rump length for accurate dating of gestational age (A) and to measure the nuchal translucency between the on-screen calipers (B).

- Maternal biochemistry, specifically free β-human chorionic gonadotrophin (β-hCG) and pregnancy-associated plasma protein A (PAPP-A)
- The gestational age calculated from the CRL measurement.

This combination of tests has a detection rate of 85% for Down syndrome when using a threshold risk of 1 in 150 for the definition of 'high chance'. This is associated with a 3% false-positive rate. In dichorionic twin pregnancies, each twin is given an 'individualised' chance. In monochorionic twins, the chance is calculated as an average of that allocated to both twins. As previously discussed, these screening tests can identify only those fetuses at increased risk of problems. For absolute certainty regarding whether a fetus is affected, an invasive diagnostic test will be required (see the amniocentesis and chorionic villous sampling [CVS] section later in the chapter).

SECOND-TRIMESTER QUADRUPLE TEST

For those in whom it is not possible to obtain a first-trimester screening test (such as when an NT measurement cannot be obtained in the first trimester due to poor fetal position or a pregnancy that is already beyond 14 weeks' gestation), a serological test for Down syndrome may be offered (but not for T18 or T13). The quadruple test incorporates maternal age and four biochemical markers measured between 14^{+2} weeks until 20^{+0} weeks: alpha-fetoprotein (AFP),

free β-hCG, estriol, and inhibin-A. The detection rate is 80%, lower than for the combined screening test (85%), with an associated 4% false-positive rate. Down syndrome is associated with low levels of AFP and unconjugated estriol and high levels of free β-hCG and inhibin A. A raised AFP should also prompt an ultrasound scan looking for a neural tube defect or gastroschisis (see later discussion).

NON-INVASIVE PRENATAL SCREENING TEST (NIPT)

NIPT is the analysis of cell-free fetal deoxyribonucleic acid (cffDNA) in maternal serum to screen for trisomies 21, 18, and 13. These are fragments of DNA that are released from the placenta into the maternal circulation. NIPT may be offered from 10 weeks of gestation, as by this stage, cffDNA makes up an average of 10% of cell-free DNA in the mother's blood and is detectable at serum testing.

NIPT is a far more sensitive and specific screening test than either the combined or quadruple test. However, it is more expensive and, therefore, is currently recommended by the NHS as an option for women who have been identified with a 'high chance' (>1 in 150) by either first-trimester combined or quadruple tests but who wish to avoid invasive diagnostic procedures. The detection rate for T21 is 99.7%, with an associated 0.01% false-positive rate. The detection rates for T18 and T13 are 97.4% and 93.8%, respectively, associated with a

0.13% false-positive rate. It is important to emphasise to women that NIPT is still a screening test, and those that are deemed to have a 'high chance' of T21, T13, or T18 are advised to undergo a diagnostic invasive test as detailed later.

There are several private providers offering NIPT screening for conditions above trisomies 21, 18, and 13. Some providers offer fetal sexing; screening for sex chromosome aneuploidies, such as Turner (45 X) and Klinefelter (47 XXY) syndromes; or microdeletions and duplications, such as DiGeorge syndrome (22q11 deletion). These indications are ethically controversial, lack scientific validation, and not supported by professional societies.

As cffDNA is produced by the placenta rather than the fetus, the accuracy of NIPT is influenced by a variety of factors. NIPT accuracy is reduced in twin pregnancies (NIPT cannot be offered to higher-order multiples), obesity, and at less than 10 weeks' gestation (due to insufficient fetal DNA in the maternal circulation). False-positive results can also be caused by confined placental mosaicism or a 'vanishing twin' (a twin pregnancy in which demise of one twin results in a singleton pregnancy) and maternal malignancy.

Screening for Structural Anomalies

Many structural anomalies may be reliably diagnosed on ultrasound scan. In the United Kingdom, it is recommended that all women should be offered a detailed ultrasound between 18^{+0} and 20^{+6} weeks' gestation to screen for major fetal anomalies. The fetal anomaly scan screens for 11 conditions at a minimum (Box 25.2).

The timing is such that it maximises the likelihood of obtaining satisfactory images whilst allowing those in whom major or lethal anomalies have been detected to consider a TOP. Despite highly skilled operators and optimal machinery, ultrasound scanning has its limitations. Some abnormalities may not be evident at this stage of gestation, thus, cannot be identified on routine scanning, and maternal obesity reduces the quality of images obtained. Therefore, it is essential to explain that whilst a normal detailed scan is reassuring, it cannot completely exclude all structural abnormalities.

Other problems associated with the routine anomaly scan include the fact that ultrasound is not selective

---

BOX 25.2   SELECTED CONGENITAL ABNORMALITIES SCREENED AT A MINIMUM

Anencephaly
Open spina bifida
Cleft lip
Diaphragmatic hernia
Gastroschisis
Exomphalos
Serious cardiac anomalies include the following:
- Transposition of the great arteries
- Atrioventricular septal defect
- Tetralogy of Fallot
- Hypoplastic left heart syndrome
Bilateral renal agenesis
Lethal skeletal dysplasia
Edwards syndrome (trisomy 18)
Patau syndrome (trisomy 13)

---

and minor abnormalities, or 'soft markers', may be seen. These markers are found in approximately 5% of detailed scans and include choroid plexus cysts (Fig. 25.2A), mild renal pelvic dilatation (Fig. 25.2B), echogenic cardiac foci, and hyperechogenic bowel. If the soft marker is noted in isolation, the chance of chromosomal problems is low. However, it is important to look for a structural defect, as in this situation, the chance of a chromosomal problem is likely to be increased.

Some fetal anomalies increase the chance of a chromosomal anomaly. Thus, the parents should be counselled by a fetal medicine specialist to discuss the option of invasive prenatal testing when appropriate. Screening for T21 is mainly performed by the combined or quadruple screening test. It is important to be aware that around two-thirds of fetuses with T21 will have a normal detailed scan, and the remaining third may demonstrate only minor defects not diagnostic for the condition. In contrast, over 90% of fetuses with T13 or T18 will have a major anomaly detected on a scan. Both T13 and T18 have a high chance of intrauterine demise or neonatal death, with few children surviving the first year of life.

Diagnosis of Chromosomal and Genetic Anomalies

If screening tests have identified a mother at 'high chance' of carrying a baby with a chromosomal or genetic anomaly, then she will be offered a diagnostic test, either CVS

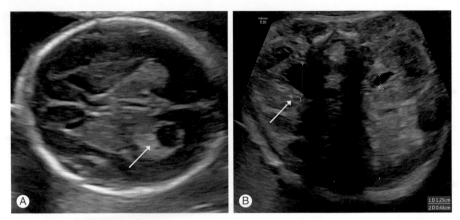

Fig. 25.2 (A) Unilateral choroid plexus cyst and (B) unilateral mild renal pelvis dilatation, both in karyotypically normal fetuses.

or amniocentesis, which aims to sample fetal cells. Both of these carry a small risk of miscarriage. Given the possibility of rhesus sensitization, rhesus-negative women require anti-D immunoglobulin.

CHORIONIC VILLUS SAMPLING (CVS)

CVS is typically performed between 11 and 14 weeks' gestation and involves passing a needle transabdominally, or occasionally transvaginally, under ultrasound guidance by an appropriately trained fetal medicine specialist to take a sample of placental tissue (villi). The risk of miscarriage is commonly reported to be 0.5%. At this early gestation, it is difficult to determine whether the miscarriage would have happened anyway due to an underlying genetic defect in the fetus or whether it is the result of the CVS.

AMNIOCENTESIS

Diagnostic amniocentesis may be performed from 15 weeks' gestation. It involves passing a thin needle transabdominally into the amniotic cavity, under continuous ultrasound guidance, to extract 10 to 18 mL of amniotic fluid. The risk of miscarriage is reported to be the same as CVS, at around 0.5%.

GENETIC TESTING

Traditionally, chorionic villi or amniocyte (fetal fibroblasts) culture was used to obtain karyotype results for both CVS and amniocentesis. This has been superseded by the following newer tests. Quantitative fluorescence polymerase chain reaction (QF-PCR) provides a more rapid assessment of the more common

aneuploidies. Fluorescently labelled markers are used to amplify specific regions of DNA to quantify the amount of DNA present in those regions. Results are available within 48 hours and are limited to the detection of T21, T13, T18, and 45X (Turner syndrome). Chromosome microarray analysis (CMA) has mostly replaced traditionally karyotyping. CMA provides a more detailed assessment of alterations in the genome. It can detect small gains and losses of genetic material, known as 'copy number variants' (CNVs). If fetal anomalies are present, microarray provides an additional diagnostic yield of 6% when the karyotype is reported as normal. Detected CNVs may be known to be pathogenic or, in up to 2% of cases, may be variants of unknown clinical significance (VOUS). In view of uncertainty, VOUS may lead to unnecessary parental stress and anxiety.

Whole-genome and exome sequencing for prenatal diagnosis are being explored largely in research settings and in highly specialised clinical genetics units. Whole-genome sequencing (WGS) involves sequencing or 'reading' the entire fetal genome. Exomes refer to the 1% to 3% of the genome that contains the vast majority of active genes. Whole exome sequencing (WES) therefore provides a more efficient yet still comprehensive genome assessment.

The NHS is the first national health care system to offer WES, providing an additional diagnostic yield of 8% to 10% when the microarray is reported as normal. At present, the utility of WGS and WES is limited by significant cost and the limited ability to correlate the significance of observed genomic variations with the phenotype being evaluated. As genome reference libraries expand, so will the capabilities of WGS and WES for prenatal diagnosis.

NON-INVASIVE PRENATAL DIAGNOSIS (NIPD)

NIPD is based on analysis of cffDNA circulating in the maternal plasma to identify specific monogenic disorders. Monogenic disorders affect around 1% of us; there are a few common scenarios when single-gene testing is used for prenatal diagnosis. This is undertaken when there is a known familial mutation for which the fetus is at risk or when prenatal ultrasound examination identifies features that are highly characteristic for a well-defined specific disorder.

NIPD is now offered for a small number of single-gene disorders, including achondroplasia, thanatophoric dysplasia, Apert syndrome, congenital adrenal hyperplasia, and cystic fibrosis. It can also be used for fetal sex determination when the pregnancy is at risk of a sex-linked disorder. NIPD offers definitive diagnosis and does not require an invasive test for confirmation of diagnosis, eliminating the risks associated with invasive procedures.

NIPD is most commonly employed to diagnose fetal rhesus D-antigen status for rhesus D-negative mothers. A fetus predicted to be rhesus D-negative by NIPD precludes the need for antenatal anti-D prophylaxis in the mother.

Chromosomal Abnormalities

DOWN SYNDROME (TRISOMY 21)

The overall incidence is approximately 1 in 1000 live births; however, this is known to increase with advancing maternal age:
- 20 years, 1 in 1500
- 30 years, 1 in 800
- 35 years, 1 in 270
- 40 years, 1 in 100
- 45 years, 1 in 50

All children born with Down syndrome (or Down's syndrome) have some degree of neurodevelopmental delay; however, this is extremely variable. Likewise, the physical characteristics commonly associated with the condition – including hypotonia, short stature, facial features with flat nasal bridge and protruding tongue, upward slanting eyes, broad hands and single palmar crease – manifest to differing degrees. Around 50% of those born with Down syndrome will also have a congenital heart defect, most commonly a septal defect. Down syndrome is also associated with gut mobility problems, hypothyroidism, and an increased risk of early-onset dementia. Life expectancy for those affected with Down syndrome has increased dramatically in the last 50 years, from 25 in the 1980s to 60 today. Of all cases, 95% are due to chromosomal nondisjunction, with 4% due to translocation, and the remaining 1% to mosaicism.

EDWARDS SYNDROME (TRISOMY 18)

The incidence is around 1 in 3500 live births, with the majority resulting from nondisjunction of chromosome 18. Clinical presentation is characterised by early-onset growth restriction, specific craniofacial features, including a small strawberry-shaped cranium, small facial features and low-set ears, and skeletal abnormalities, including overlapping fingers and prominent calcanei (rocker bottom feet). Major systemic abnormalities are common and include congenital heart disease, complex urogenital anomalies, and problems with the gastrointestinal system, such as omphalocele and oesophageal atresia. Approximately 68% die in utero; for those who survive to birth, the outcome is poor. Median survival is 2 weeks; up to 13.5% live to 1 year and 12.3% to 5 years.

PATAU SYNDROME (TRISOMY 13)

The incidence is low, ranging from 1 in 6500 to 1 in 29,000 live births. It is associated with multiple severe congenital abnormalities, which result in significant physical and mental impairment. Approximately 80% of children will have a severe heart defect. Significant brain defects, clefts of the lip or palate, kidney and urogenital anomalies, extra digits, omphalocele, and spina bifida are also common features. The majority of babies affected are stillborn, with survivors rarely expected to live longer than 1 week. Only 11.5% will survive the first year.

TRIPLOIDY

This describes the presence of an additional set of chromosomes acquired either from the mother (causing severe fetal growth restriction and fetal abnormality) or father (associated with a partial mole; see

Chapter 15) during fertilization, resulting in a total of 69 as opposed to the normal 46. Affected fetuses usually miscarry in early pregnancy and survival to birth is rare. There is no expected survival past the immediate neonatal period, with the affected fetus generally severely growth restricted and affected by multiple severe abnormalities.

TURNER SYNDROME (45,XO)

This affects around 1 in 2500 live-born girls. In most cases, it is due to the loss of the paternal chromosome, although some individuals have a mosaic pattern. Antenatally, Turner syndrome is associated with cystic hygroma (Fig. 25.3), cardiac defects, and non-immune hydrops, which results in many affected pregnancies miscarrying. If not identified antenatally, the majority of girls affected are diagnosed in infancy or childhood as a result of characteristic physical features. These include short stature, webbed neck, widely spaced nipples, and cubitus valgus. Other associated problems include renal dysgenesis, coarctation of the aorta, and ovarian failure, necessitating long-term hormone replacement therapy (HRT) requirements. Intelligence is largely unaffected, although there may be some impairment of non-verbal skills.

47,XXX

This is the most common female chromosomal abnormality, occurring in 1 in 1000 live births, although higher in pregnancies in women over 40 years. Those affected are phenotypically normal, with normal development of secondary sexual characteristics and fertility. There is often a delay in motor and speech development and an association with genitourinary problems, including premature ovarian insufficiency, requiring HRT.

KLINEFELTER SYNDROME (47,XXY)

This affects 1 in 1000 live births and is a frequent cause of male factor infertility. Those affected tend to be tall males with sparse body hair and gynaecomastia. Typically, the testes remain small; many cases are diagnosed during puberty as a result of this. There is some association with reduced intelligence quotient (IQ), hypothyroidism, cardiovascular disease, and type 2 diabetes.

JACOBS SYNDROME (47,XYY)

Incidence is around 1 in 1000 live births and is frequently undetected due to a lack of symptoms or fertility concerns. Characteristically, males are tall with acne. Whilst intelligence is in the normal range, there may be an association with behavioural problems, including impulsivity.

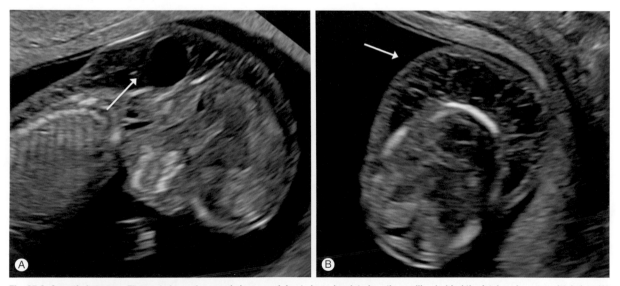

Fig. 25.3 A cystic hygroma. The nuchal translucency is increased due to large loculated cystic swelling behind the fetal neck on a sagittal view **(A)** and an axial view of the fetal neck and head **(B)**.

Single Gene Disorders

Single-gene disorders are those caused by a mutation in a single gene. There are over 6500 conditions in this group. These disorders are broadly classified into autosomal, in which the mutation is in a gene on a non–sex chromosome, or X-linked, in which the mutated gene is found on the X chromosome. A few common conditions are due to monogenic disorders; therefore, antenatal screening is offered to eligible women at their booking appointment.

HAEMOGLOBINOPATHIES

Thalassaemias and sickle cell disease are recessively inherited genetic conditions of the haemoglobin gene, which have serious health implications and require lifelong treatment. The NHS Sickle Cell and Thalassaemia Screening Programme recommends that all pregnant women be offered a blood test by 10^{+0} weeks of gestation to determine whether they carry a gene for thalassaemia and to differentiate those at high risk of being a sickle cell carrier. In low-prevalence areas, the family origin questionnaire (FOQ) information is used as an initial screening tool to assess a woman's eligibility for haemoglobin variant screening. All biological fathers are offered screening if the pregnant woman is a genetic carrier for sickle cell disease or thalassaemia.

When both parents are carriers, in each pregnancy, the risks to the baby are:

- 1 in 4 (25%) chance of being completely unaffected
- 2 in 4 (50%) chance of being a carrier
- 1 in 4 (25%) chance of inheriting the condition

Couples/women at risk of having a baby with sickle cell disease or thalassaemia major are referred to health care professionals who provide counselling and prenatal diagnosis. The diagnostic approach usually depends on the gestational age of the fetus. The fetal sample for prenatal diagnosis is usually obtained by CVS or amniocentesis.

CYSTIC FIBROSIS

This is an autosomal-recessive condition, with a UK incidence of around 1 in 2500. It is caused by mutations in the cystic fibrosis transmembrane conductance regulator gene on chromosome 7, which codes for a protein involved in chloride ion channel function. Alterations in this protein can lead to thickened mucous affecting the lungs, resulting in recurrent chest infections, pancreatic insufficiency, and malabsorption. Azoospermia in males is common, with subsequent subfertility. The prognosis in cystic fibrosis has significantly improved with the development of new drug treatments such as the combination of tezacaftor, ivacaftor and elexacaftor. If a couple are known to be carriers, there is a 25% risk of their baby being affected. Thus, it is reasonable to offer NIPD (assuming that both parents are CF carriers and have DNA from an affected or unaffected child) or invasive testing if they felt that they would not continue with an affected pregnancy.

HUNTINGTON DISEASE

This is an autosomal-dominant condition with a peak age of onset between 40 and 45 years. It is caused by a CAG trinucleotide expansion and can result in chorea, dementia, and neuropsychiatric disturbance. Generally, those affected deteriorate over time, and life expectancy tends to be about 20 years from the onset of symptoms. Given the lack of treatment, and the fact that the disease tends to manifest in later life, the ethical issues around testing the children of sufferers are complex. At present, testing is offered to those over 18 years who wish to proceed following genetic counselling. There is also the option for invasive prenatal testing, although this becomes even more complex if a member of the couple is at risk but does not wish to know.

DIGEORGE SYNDROME

This is due to a deletion in a small part of chromosome 22 (22q11 deletion). It affects 1 in 350 pregnancies and 1 in 2000 live births. Most are due to de novo mutations. Ultrasound findings include congenital heart abnormalities, kidney defects, and facial features, including a cleft palate. Those affected have a poor immune system, a higher incidence of learning difficulties, and, longer term, 1 in 4 will develop schizophrenia.

FRAGILE X SYNDROME

This results from an expansion in the CGG triplet repeat on the X chromosome, causing moderate neurodevelopmental delay. Unaffected individuals typically have 29 repeats; however, this is increased to up to 200 in those with a pre-mutation. These individuals are phenotypically normal; however, they are at risk of expansion to a full mutation. Full mutation is defined by over 200 repeats and is characterised by varying degrees of neurodevelopmental delay. The condition affects males more severely than females and is often associated with hyperactive behaviour and impulsiveness. Physical characteristics evolve with age and include a long, narrow face with a prominent jaw and forehead and enlarged testicles in males. Prenatal screening is possible; CVS can be used to identify the degree of amplification of the CGG repeats in potential offspring.

TAY-SACHS DISEASE

This is an autosomal-recessive condition characterised by a build-up of gangliosides in the central nervous system, resulting in progressive neurodegeneration, seizures, and blindness from the age of 3 to 6 months. The mutation is in the *HEXA* gene on chromosome 15 and can be tested for by measuring the level of hexosaminidase A in leucocytes. Sadly, most of those affected die before the age of 4 years.

People of Ashkenazi Jewish descent have a 1 in 25 chance of being a healthy carrier of Tay-Sachs disease, but it is rare in other groups. Descendants of Ashkenazi Jews can be referred for carrier testing and prenatal genetic counselling to provide an individualised risk of their offspring being affected by Tay-Sachs. If both parents are known carriers, prenatal diagnosis may be offered via CVS.

Structural Anomalies

NEURAL TUBE DEFECTS

The neural tube is formed from the closing of the neural folds, with both anterior and posterior neuropores closed by 6 weeks' gestation. Failure of closure of the anterior neuropore or posterior neuropore results in neural tube defects (NTDs). Spina bifida, anencephaly, and encephalocele are the three most common forms of NTDs (Fig. 25.4). The overall incidence of all NTDs is around 1 in 1000. Causes of NTDs are multifactorial, involving a combination of multiple genes and environmental factors. Known environmental factors include folic acid, diabetes, and maternal antiepileptic drugs.

ANENCEPHALY

This is characterised by the absence of the cerebral hemispheres and cranial vault, giving rise to prominent orbits and a typical 'frog-like' appearance on ultrasound. Most of those affected will be stillborn, with the remainder dying shortly after birth.

ENCEPHALOCELE

This describes the protrusion of the dura mater sac (with or without brain tissue) through a bony defect in the cranial vault (see Fig. 25.4). The majority are occipital. Prognosis depends on the presence on brain tissue within the sac and the degree of resultant herniation.

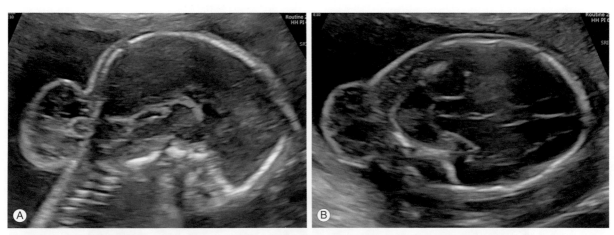

Fig. 25.4 Encephalocele. There is a defect in the posterior aspect of the skull, allowing brain tissue to herniate into the sac. This is visible on sagittal **(A)** and axial **(B)** planes of the head. Note the characteristic 'banana shape cerebellum' in **(B)**.

SPINA BIFIDA

This is the most common central nervous system malformation, resulting from the failure of closure of the neural groove. Lesions may be open or closed, closed defects having a skin covering, and open defects may take the form of a meningocele or myelomeningocele. In a meningocele, the meninges of the neural tissue bulge through a posterior wall defect. In a myelomeningocele, there is additional involvement of neural tissue. Scalloping of the frontal bones gives rise to the typical 'lemon' sign seen on ultrasound, and the descent of the cerebellum, pons, and medulla through the foramen magnum results in a 'banana' shape to the cerebellum, also visible on ultrasound (Fig. 25.4B). The extent of the associated disability depends on the site and size of the defect and can include abnormalities in lower limb neurology, including paralysis, with bladder and bowel dysfunction. Intelligence can be normal, although this is difficult to predict antenatally and depends in part on the degree of ventriculomegaly.

Recently, fetal surgery for open spina bifida has been offered to eligible women in highly specialised fetal medicine centres in the United Kingdom and around the world. Compared with postnatal spina bifida repair, in utero fetal surgery is associated with improved rates of ventriculoperitoneal shunt placement, hindbrain herniation, and independent walking at 30 months of age.

The protective effect of pre-conceptual folic acid is well established. All women planning pregnancy are advised to take 400 μg daily for at least 1 month prior to conception. Women at increased risk of neural tube defects – for example, those with type 2 diabetes, a raised body mass index, on antiepileptic medications, or a previous pregnancy with an NTD – are advised to take a higher dose, 5 mg daily.

VENTRICULOMEGALY

In a normal fetus, cerebrospinal fluid (CSF) circulates around the brain and through the lateral ventricles. When an accumulation of CSF occurs, this leads to dilatation of the ventricular system. The mean size of the lateral ventricles is 7 mm (Fig. 25.5A). Ventriculomegaly refers to an increase to 10.1 mm or more and is thought to affect up to 1% of pregnancies. Mild ventriculomegaly is considered when the lateral ventricles measure between 10.1 and 12 mm, moderate is between 13 and 15 mm, and severe ventriculomegaly is considered when the ventricles are greater than 15 mm (Fig. 25.5B).

Ventriculomegaly may be caused by congenital infection, obstruction from structural malformations, haemorrhage, or may be associated with chromosomal anomalies. Detection should prompt discussion regarding infection screen (so-called TORCH screen - toxoplasmosis, other (e.g. syphilis, zika), rubella, cytomegalovirus and herpes simplex virus) and possible invasive testing with CMA. Serial scanning should follow to look for the progression/regression of the ventriculomegaly and the possible development of anomalies, particularly in the brain. Fetal brain magnetic resonance imaging (MRI) in the second or preferably early third trimester may provide additional diagnostic information about the brain development which cannot be detected by ultrasound, for example,

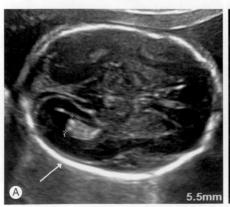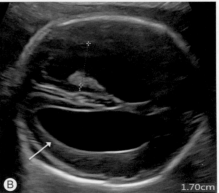

Fig. 25.5 A comparison of normal brain anatomy with normal-sized lateral ventricles (A) and severe ventriculomegaly (B).

migrational disorders. Normal development is common in the context of mild ventriculomegaly in over 90% of cases. Outcome is variable in severe cases and depends on the degree of the ventriculomegaly and the presence of other anomalies. It is associated with significant disability in approximately 50% of cases.

CYSTIC HYGROMA

Cystic hygromas are fluid-filled swellings at the back of the fetal neck, which are thought to develop as a result of a defect in the formation of lymphatic vessels (see Fig. 25.3). It is likely that the lymphatic and venous systems fail to connect, with lymph accumulating in the jugular lymph sacs. They are often associated with cardiac and renal anomalies, and may manifest alongside oedema, ascites, and pleural and pericardial effusions. They are also frequently associated with chromosomal anomalies. Thus, prenatal invasive testing should be discussed and offered to parents. 'Isolated cystic hygromas' may be corrected surgically after birth and have a good prognosis.

In cases of generalised fetal hydrops, defined as abnormal accumulation of fluid in two or more fetal compartments (including ascites, pleural effusion, pericardial effusion, and skin oedema), the prognosis is very poor.

FACIAL CLEFT

Facial clefts are the most common congenital anomalies of the face, affecting around 1 to 2 per 1000 live births. Facial clefts may either be isolated or associated with other structural or chromosomal anomalies (mainly, trisomy 13 and 18). Estimated distribution of facial clefts is 25% for cleft lip, 50% for cleft lip and palate, and 25% for isolated cleft palate. Adequate characterisation of the cleft is important to counsel parents appropriately on the severity of the defect and its likely association with chromosomal or syndromal anomalies. Thirty percent of cases are associated with any one of over 400 genetic and non-genetic syndromes. Chromosomal anomalies – mainly, trisomies 13 and 18 – are found in 1% to 2% of cases. However, unilateral cleft lip is not associated with chromosomal abnormalities. Isolated clefts are associated with low morbidity and mortality, and postnatal surgery generally provides a good cosmetic and functional outcome.

CONGENITAL HEART DISEASE

This is one of the most common congenital malformations in children, affecting just under 1% of live births. Most national screening programs now offer routine prenatal population screening. In most cases, there is no obvious cause. However, there are associated risk factors: family history; diabetes; maternal infection with rubella; and drugs, including some anticonvulsants, alcohol, and lithium. Antenatal detection rates vary. In the United Kingdom, about 60% of major abnormalities are identified on systematic evaluation of the heart, which should always include the four-chamber view and outflow tracts (Fig. 25.6A). These include atrioventricular septal defects (AVSD), transposition of the great arteries (TGA), tetralogy of Fallot (TOF), hypoplastic left heart (HLH) (see Fig. 25.6B and Box 25.2), and arrhythmias. Due to the frequent association with genetic and chromosomal abnormalities – including T21, T13, T18, and DiGeorge syndrome – invasive testing via amniocentesis should be offered.

DIAPHRAGMATIC HERNIA

Congenital diaphragmatic hernia has a prevalence of 1 in 4000 births. It is characterised by a defect in the diaphragm, most commonly on the left, through which the stomach, colon, liver, and even the spleen can herniate. The heart is pushed to the right, and the lungs are compressed. The incidence of aneuploidy and genetic syndromes is 15% to 30%, and there is an association with structural anomalies, including neural tube defects, congenital heart disease, and skeletal anomalies. The combination of liver herniation and ultrasound measurement of the observed to expected lung-to-head ratio (O/E LHR) is now widely used to individualise prognosis and counsel parents. Postnatal surgery is advised soon after delivery to reduce the hernia and correct the defect.

Fetal endoscopic tracheal occlusion (FETO) is a minimally invasive percutaneous procedure that is being offered to women antenatally in specialised centres, largely in a research setting. FETO aims to improve the outcome in a selected group of fetuses with the poorest prognosis and lowest probability of survival after birth.

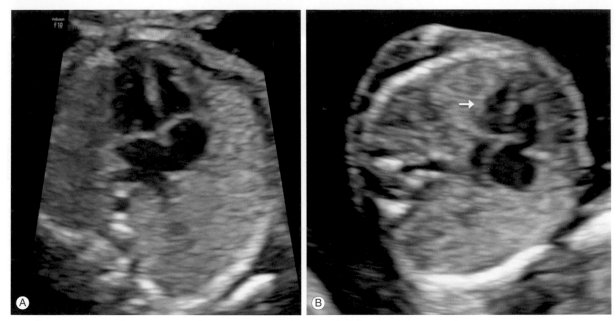

Fig. 25.6 A normal four-chamber view of the fetal heart (A) and a hypoplastic left heart (B).

ABDOMINAL WALL DEFECTS

Exomphalos (omphalocele)

This occurs following failure of the bowel to return to the abdominal cavity at 8 weeks' gestation, resulting in a midline defect through which the peritoneal sac protrudes (Fig. 25.7A,B). In some cases, the sac contains the small bowel or liver. Exomphalos affects approximately 1 in 2000 pregnancies. In 30% to 50% of cases, it is associated with chromosomal abnormalities, especially trisomy 18, and in conjunction with other structural abnormalities, in particular, cardiac and renal problems. Management should involve the offer of invasive testing and increased surveillance due to the increased risk of intrauterine death.

Gastroschisis

This occurs in 1 in 2500 to 3000 pregnancies and is associated with young maternal age, smoking, and recreational drug misuse (Fig. 25.7C). It is a paraumbilical defect through which the gastrointestinal organs herniate (usually bowel), allowing them to float freely in the amniotic fluid. There is no increased chance of chromosomal abnormality, and concurrent structural defects are rare. However, there is an association with

bowel atresia, and affected babies tend to be small for gestational age, requiring increased surveillance. With early surgical correction, the prognosis is good, although up to 5% of affected pregnancies will result in stillbirth.

GENITOURINARY ABNORMALITIES

Renal Tract Dilatation

Dilatation of the renal tract may be unilateral or bilateral and can occur at any level of the renal tract (Fig. 25.8). Renal pelvic dilatation (RPD), or pyelectasis, is usually due to a neuromuscular defect at the junction of the ureter and renal pelvis. It affects about 2% of pregnancies and presents with increasing pelvic dilatation in the presence of a normal ureter. The majority resolve spontaneously postnatally, although there is an association with postnatal urinary tract infections and reflux nephropathy. Thus, it is prudent to consider neonatal prophylactic antibiotics in those with marked dilatation and arrange postnatal radiological follow-up.

Severe RPD is defined as >15 mm and is most commonly caused by ureteric obstruction. It is unilateral

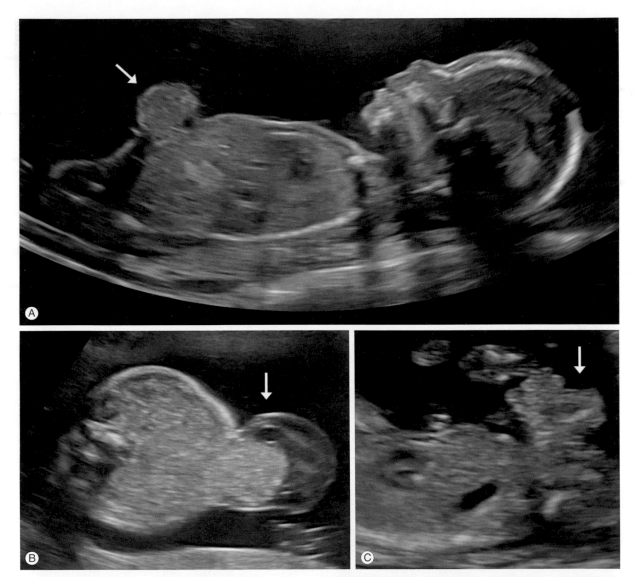

Fig. 25.7 A small isolated exomphalos enclosed within a sac is seen in sagittal (A) and axial (B) planes. In comparison, a gastroschisis with multiple loops of free bowel is seen in the amniotic fluid (C).

in 80% to 90% and affects males more commonly than females (see Fig. 25.2B). If the fetal bladder appears normal, the level of obstruction is proximal to the ureterovesical junction.

Bladder dilatation is most commonly caused by obstruction from posterior urethral valves, a condition exclusively affecting males, in which folds of mucosa at the bladder neck prevent urine from leaving the bladder. The result is progressive bladder dilatation with hydroureter and severe RPD. The kidneys may become dysplastic, and the resultant oligohydramnios can lead to problems with lung development (pulmonary hypoplasia). There is a potential need for vesico-amniotic shunting, whereby a stent is placed into the fetal bladder to relieve pressure by diverting urine out into the amniotic cavity. However, its use remains controversial due to associated complications and uncertain effects on long-term renal function.

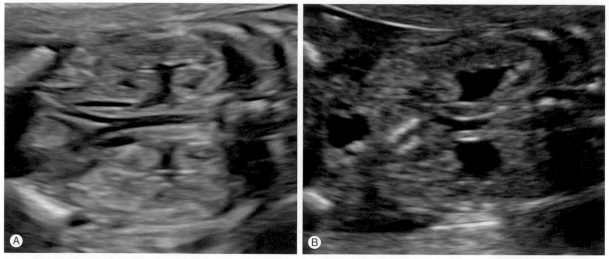

Fig. 25.8 A coronal view of normal kidneys (A) and bilateral mild renal pelvis dilatation (B). The renal cortex looks well preserved in both cases.

Multicystic Dysplastic Kidney Disease

This occurs in 1 in 1000 pregnancies and is characterised by the presence of multiple non-communicating cysts (Fig. 25.9). It may be unilateral, bilateral, or may affect only a small segment of kidney. If only one kidney is affected, and there is adequate amniotic fluid, then the prognosis is good. If the disease is bilateral, and especially if there is associated oligohydramnios, then the outcome is very poor, with a high perinatal mortality.

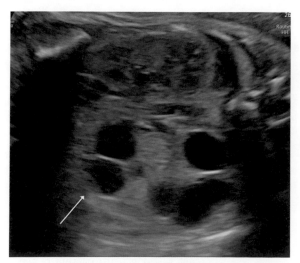

Fig. 25.9 A unilateral dysplastic kidney; note the fluid-filled cysts in the distal enlarged kidney.

Autosomal-Recessive Polycystic Kidney Disease (ARPKD) and Autosomal-Dominant Polycystic Kidney Disease (ADPKD)

ARPKD is characterised by the presence of multiple cysts of various sizes affecting the kidneys bilaterally. The condition has an autosomal-recessive inheritance, and expression is variable. Diagnosis is usually made in the antenatal period by the ultrasound findings of bilateral enlarged hyperechoic kidneys, an absent bladder, and oligohydramnios. Cysts may also be present in the liver and pancreas. Prognosis is poor and long-term survival rare. Prevalence is 1 in 30,000 births.

ADPKD is a relatively benign condition, which has an autosomal-dominant inheritance and is rarely diagnosed until adulthood. Prenatally, the kidneys are enlarged and hyperechogenic but smaller than in ARPKD. The renal pelvises can be visualized, and the bladder and amniotic fluid volume are normal. Nearly all babies have ultrasonically normal kidneys at birth. One in 1000 people carry the gene mutation.

Bilateral Renal Agenesis

Bilateral renal agenesis is a lethal condition affecting 1 in 3000 to 10,000 births. It is characterised by the ultrasound finding of an absent bladder and severe oligohydramnios due to the lack of any production of fetal urine. Confirmation of absent kidneys is often quite challenging due to difficult visualization of the fetal anatomy in the absence of amniotic fluid.

Without amniotic fluid, there is resultant pulmonary hypoplasia and limb deformities.

LUNG DISORDERS – PULMONARY HYPOPLASIA

Amniotic fluid is essential for the normal development of the fetal lungs. Without it, there is a 90% chance of pulmonary hypoplasia, especially with severe oligohydramnios prior to 22 weeks. Beyond 22 weeks and with greater levels of amniotic fluid, the risk is <30%. The causes of pulmonary hypoplasia are variable but most commonly relate to the underlying cause of oligohydramnios – in particular, pre-term pre-labour rupture of membranes and bilateral renal agenesis. More unusually, pulmonary hypoplasia can result from the compression effect on fetal lungs due to associated congenital anomalies, including diaphragmatic hernia and cystic lung lesions.

LETHAL SKELETAL DYSPLASIA

There is a wide range of rare skeletal dysplasias, with an overall prevalence of 1 in 4000 births. Sonographic evaluations of fetal skull, thorax, spine, long bones, and extremities are key to arriving at the correct diagnosis. However, there is considerable overlap between conditions. Lethal skeletal dysplasias are associated with a small thorax, which leads to pulmonary hypoplasia and neonatal death.

The vast phenotypic appearances of skeletal dysplasias relate to a wide variety of responsible genetic mutations. Some of these genetic mutations are detectable via microarray and WES, but many remain unknown. NIPD based on analysis of cffDNA in maternal blood is now possible for some of the more common skeletal dysplasias. This includes detection of mutations in the *FGFR3* (Fibroblast Growth Factor Receptor 3) gene, which are responsible for achondroplasia, an autosomal-dominant disorder commonly known as dwarfism, and thanatophoric dysplasia, which results in bowing of the long bones, a small chest with short ribs, and skull deformities.

PRENATAL CONGENITAL INFECTION

Maternal infections in pregnancy are important, as some have the potential to affect the fetus and may be potentiated by the relative immunosuppression of pregnancy. A number of infections are known to be teratogenic, especially if contracted early in pregnancy, whilst others have the potential to cause miscarriage, pre-term labour, severe neonatal sepsis, or long-term carrier states. It is worth remembering, however, that infection, in itself, does not necessarily mean that the baby will be affected.

Infection in general raises the maternal serological level of immunoglobulin G (IgG) and immunoglobulin M (IgM). Maternal IgG crosses the placenta, whilst IgM, a much larger molecule, does not. The fetus does not make IgM until after 20 weeks' gestation, and its presence in fetal or early neonatal blood implies infection, although its absence does not always exclude it. In 'high-risk' cases, the detection of pathogenic DNA in fetal blood or amniotic fluid by polymerase chain reaction has revolutionized the specificity of infection detection.

RISK FACTORS

Farm workers are at increased risk of infection with chlamydia and *Listeria*, both of which are associated with miscarriage. Toxoplasma may be acquired from cows, sheep, and cats, and certain foods have been implicated in congenital infection, as detailed in Table 25.1.

SPECIFIC INFECTIONS

Some specific infections in pregnancy are summarised in (Table 25.2).

VARICELLA-ZOSTER VIRUS (VZV/CHICKENPOX)

Having usually had chickenpox as a child, the majority of the antenatal population are seropositive for the VZV IgG antibody. Thus, primary infection in pregnancy is rare, affecting around 3 in 1000 pregnancies. If contracted in pregnancy, the illness tends to be more severe in the mother and may result in pneumonia, hepatitis, and encephalitis. Fetal congenital defects affect 1% to 2%, with no cases documented after 20 weeks. Fetal

TABLE 25.1	Foods That Carry Potential Infection Risks in Pregnancy
Soft cheeses	Unpasteurised milk and its products may contain *Listeria*. Those made from pasteurised milk are safe.
Raw eggs	Must be avoided, as there is a risk of salmonella (including puddings).
Meat or pâté	Undercooked meat may transmit toxoplasma or, rarely, *Listeria*.
Fruit	This should always be washed before eating, as it may be contaminated with salmonella, toxoplasma, or one of several intestinal parasites.

TABLE 25.2	Infections in Pregnancy				
Agent	Epidemiology	Maternal Features	Fetal, Neonatal, and Infant Features	Risk	Treatment/Prevention
Rubella	Person-to-person UK immunity now 97%, and congenital infection is rare	Asymptomatic or mild maculo-papular rash	Miscarriage, fetal growth restriction, ↓platelets, hepatosplenomegaly, jaundice, deafness, congenital heart disease, mental handicap, cataracts, microphthalmia, microcephaly, cerebral palsy	Risk of fetal defects: <12 weeks up to 85% 13–18 weeks up to 25%, no defect attributed to maternal infections occurring after 20 weeks' gestation	Consider termination of pregnancy (TOP) if <12 weeks Postnatal maternal vaccination if she is not immune
Toxoplasmosis (protozoan, *Toxoplasma gondii*)	From cats, uncooked meats, and unwashed fruits	May have fever, rash, and lymphade-nopathy, but most are asymptomatic	Hydrocephalus, chorioretinitis, intracranial calcification, ↓platelets	<12 weeks: transmission is 10%–25% 12–28 weeks: transmission is 30%–54% >28 weeks: transmission is 65%–80% Ultrasound abnormalities: 77.9% of infected fetuses at the first trimester, 20.4% of infected fetuses at the second trimester, and 0% of infected fetuses at the third trimester	Spiramycin can reduce the risk of transmission TOP can also be consid-ered, depending on risk of severe abnormalities
Cytomegalo-virus (CMV) (herpes virus)	Person-to-person	Nearly always asymptomatic	Hepatosplenomegaly, ↓platelets, fetal growth restriction, microcephaly, sensorineural deafness, chorioretinitis, hydrops fetalis, exomphalos, cerebral palsy	Transplacental transmission occurs in 30% of cases after primary infection and in 2% after non-primary infection 10% are symptomatic at birth, with a high associated mor-tality rate Sensorineural hearing loss and/or neurological sequelae is 32.4% after maternal infection in the first trimester and 0% in the second and third trimesters	CMV hyperimmune globu-lin and antiviral drugs valaciclovir are currently being investigated

Continued

TABLE 25.2 Infections in Pregnancy – Cont'd

Agent	Epidemiology	Maternal Features	Fetal, Neonatal, and Infant Features	Risk	Treatment/Prevention
Parvovirus B19 (erythrovirus)	Respiratory transmission	Erythema infectiosum (slapped cheek disease) May be asymptomatic	Aplastic anaemia, hydrops fetalis, myocarditis, intrauterine fetal death	Vertical transmission occurs in approximately 17%–33% The peak risk occurs at 17–24 weeks' gestation At <20 weeks, the estimated excess fetal loss rate during pregnancy is about 9% Non-immune hydrops fetalis occurs in up to 7% when infection occurs between 13 and 20 weeks' gestation	In utero fetal transfusion manages severe fetal anaemia
Chickenpox (varicella-zoster virus)	Person-to-person	Papules and pustules	Limb hypoplasia, skin scarring, fetal growth restriction, eye abnormalities, neurological abnormalities, and hydrops fetalis	Up to 25% vertical transmission, <2% have defects if <20 weeks. Defects are less common >20 weeks	Give zoster immunoglobulin to the mother if <10 days from contact Oral acyclovir if <24 hours of onset of rash and if the mother is 20+0 weeks of gestation or beyond (Acyclovir can be considered at <20 weeks)

varicella syndrome is rare and is characterised by limb deformity, microcephaly, and growth restriction. Maternal infection just prior to delivery may result in neonatal infection and, in some, clinical varicella. If delivery occurs within 7 days of maternal infection, or if the mother develops chickenpox within 7 days of giving birth, the neonate should be given varicella-zoster immunoglobulin with or without acyclovir.

CYTOMEGALOVIRUS (CMV)

CMV, a herpes virus, is the most common cause of congenital infection. The highest risk of fetal injury follows a maternal primary infection early in pregnancy.

CMV is highly prevalent but not clinically significant in young children and largely asymptomatic in adults. Person-to-person transmission is via mucosal sites (oral secretions, urine, and breastmilk). Thus, mothers of young children are at particular risk of infection. Transplacental transmission to the fetus increases with advancing gestation, occurring in 35% in the first trimester and 60% in the third trimester. Whilst vertical transmission is most prevalent in the third trimester, the fetus is at risk of being adversely affected by congenital CMV only if maternal infection – and, therefore, transmission – occurs before 15 weeks. Long-term sequelae – namely, neurodevelopmental delay and sensorineural hearing loss – are apparent in 32% after maternal infection in the first trimester compared with 0% in the second and third trimesters. Symptoms of congenital CMV are not always apparent at birth, presenting in the infant as late as 2 years of age. Overall, the risk of congenital infection is 30% of cases after primary maternal infection and in 2% after non-primary infection. Antiviral drugs, including valacyclovir, have shown promising results within research settings in the reduction of vertical CMV transmission and congenital CMV.

HERPES SIMPLEX VIRUS (HSV)

HSV is divided into two subgroups: type 1, which is generally associated with facial lesions, and type 2, which predominately affects the genitals. The management of genital herpes in pregnancy is dictated by the stage of gestation at presentation and whether the episode is primary or secondary. Women presenting with primary herpes up to 28 weeks should be treated with acyclovir to limit the duration of symptoms and be reassured that there is no association

with congenital abnormalities. Provided that mothers do not labour within 6 weeks of a primary infection, vaginal birth is advocated and encouraged. The maternal management of primary infection after 28 weeks is unchanged, although women often continue acyclovir until delivery. Birth, however, should be by elective caesarean section to avoid the potential risk of neonatal transmission. Secondary genital herpes presenting at any gestational stage is associated with a low risk of neonatal infection and vaginal birth is encouraged even in the presence of lesions during labour. If recurrent episodes occur during pregnancy, acyclovir suppression from 36 weeks should be considered.

RUBELLA

As a result of immunisation programmes, rubella is rare in the United Kingdom, with less than 2% of women susceptible. Infection during pregnancy may result in a collection of abnormalities known as congenital rubella syndrome, with transmission most common in the first trimester. Defects include pulmonary stenosis, patent ductus arteriosus, cataracts, neurodevelopmental delay, microcephaly, and sensorineural deafness. If primary infection has occurred in the first 12 weeks of pregnancy, the risk of congenital defects is high, and it is reasonable to discuss TOP.

PARVOVIRUS B19

Also known as slapped cheek or fifth disease, this is a highly contagious childhood illness. Maternal infection is often asymptomatic; diagnosis is made on serological testing, usually following contact with an infected child. Around 50% of the pregnant population will already be immune as a result of past exposure. Infection in the first 20 weeks of pregnancy can lead to serious adverse outcomes in the fetus. It is associated with risk of fetal anaemia and high-output cardiac failure resulting in hydrops (Fig. 25.10), and occasionally stillbirth. Middle cerebral artery (MCA) Doppler peak velocity measurements correlate well with the degree of fetal anaemia and can be used to identify those who would benefit from a therapeutic in utero transfusion (Fig. 25.11).

HEPATITIS

All women are screened for hepatitis B at booking, with the risk of transmission to the fetus depending

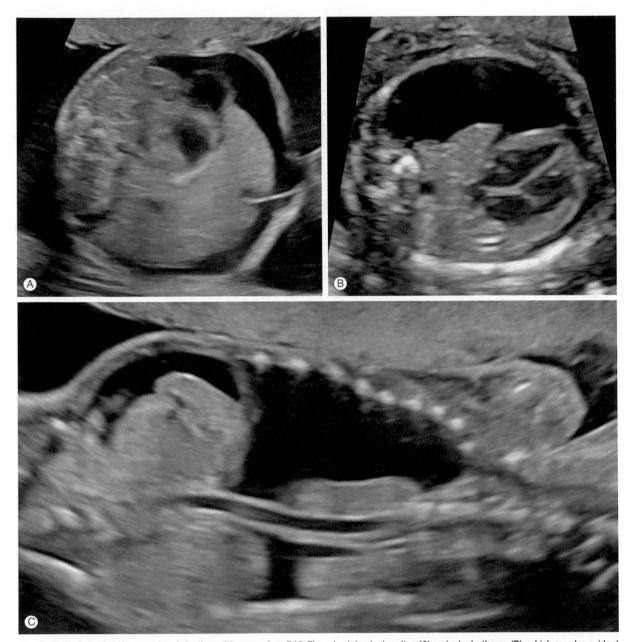

Fig. 25.10 Hydrops fetalis caused by infection with parvovirus B19. There is abdominal ascites **(A)** and a hydrothorax **(B)**, which are also evident on coronal views of the fetal body **(C)**.

on the antigen status. Vertical transmission is most likely to occur with acute infection or in the presence of hepatitis B e antigen (HBeAg), a marker of high infectivity. Ninety-five percent of cases of transmission occur during childbirth. Babies who are considered to be at high risk of acquisition should be given passive hepatitis B immunoglobulin for 24 hours after delivery, and then immunised. Those at lower risk are simply immunised. There is no routine antenatal screening for hepatitis C, although this should be considered

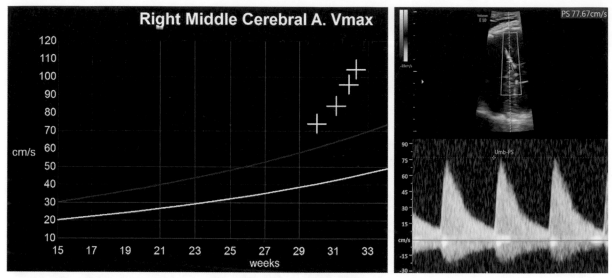

Fig. 25.11 Measuring the blood velocity in the fetal middle cerebral artery correlates well with the degree of fetal anaemia. This non-invasive assessment can be used to determine the need for in utero blood transfusion.

in high-risk women. The risk of vertical transmission is related to viral load; there is no evidence to suggest that treatment during pregnancy will reduce this risk. Hepatitis A is not known to cause any significant complication in pregnancy. Acute infection with hepatitis E in pregnancy is associated with fulminant liver failure and carries a mortality rate of up to 20% to 25% if infected in the third trimester.

LISTERIA MONOCYTOGENES

Listeria is a rare bacterial infection transmitted by food, usually soft, ripe cheese, pâté, cooked–chilled meats, and undercooked ready meals. Infection causes a non-specific illness with nausea and vomiting and bacilli cross the placenta. Fetal and neonatal infections can be severe, causing fetal loss, pre-term labour, neonatal sepsis, meningitis, and death. Diagnosis can be made following culture of blood, stool, CSF, or placental culture. Treatment is with penicillin.

BETA-HAEMOLYTIC STREPTOCOCCI – GROUP B

Group B streptococcus is a common vaginal commensal, occurring in around 20% of pregnant mothers and is transient in nature. If a woman is colonised with group B streptococci at term, there is a small chance that the bacteria could be transmitted to the baby during birth, leading to a serious neonatal infection.

Although some countries offer a screening program, the condition does not truly fulfil the recognised criteria for screening. In the United Kingdom, there is no formal antenatal screening programme. However, intrapartum antibiotics are offered to those known to be colonised and those with a previously affected baby.

SYPHILIS

Whilst congenital syphilis is rare in the United Kingdom, it is a significant cause of perinatal morbidity and mortality worldwide. Many of those infected will be unaware of it, and testing for syphilis at booking is part of the UK screening programme. The risk of fetal infection increases with gestation. The effects include miscarriage and stillbirth, along with hydrops and growth restriction. There may be deafness and abnormal neurological signs in later life. If diagnosed in pregnancy, syphilis should be treated with penicillin.

ZIKA

Zika virus disease is a mosquito-borne infection that has gradually spread from a narrow equatorial belt in Africa and Asia across to the Americas, leading to an epidemic in 2015 to 2016. It usually causes only a mild maternal illness, but epidemiological and pathological evidence suggest that it may also lead to fetal microcephaly and other fetal neurological problems referred to as congenital Zika syndrome. The diagnosis of Zika virus infection should be considered among individuals who experience symptoms suggestive of acute Zika virus infection within 2 weeks of leaving an area with active Zika virus transmission or within 2 weeks of sexual contact with a male sexual partner who has recently travelled to such an area. Testing of symptomatic individuals may be possible in some situations, but diagnosis of affected babies can be extremely difficult, especially as microcephaly may become apparent only in the third trimester or even postnatally.

COVID-19

The majority of pregnant women with COVID-19 (coronavirus disease 2019) infection are either asymptomatic or experience only mild or moderate symptoms. Amongst pregnant women, the highest risk of becoming severely unwell with COVID-19 appears to be for those who are 28 weeks pregnant or beyond, and women are often advised to take additional precautions beyond this gestational period. The symptoms of severe infection are no different in pregnant women; early identification and assessment for prompt supportive treatment is key. Current evidence from the United Kingdom suggests that symptomatic pregnant women who are infected with the SARS-CoV-2 (severe acute respiratory syndrome coronavirus 2) virus are more likely to be admitted to intensive care than non-pregnant women and undergo iatrogenic pre-term birth. Antenatal infection with COVID-19 is unlikely to be associated with vertical transmission, though there appears to be an increased rate of stillbirth.

Haemolytic Disease of the Fetus and Newborn (HDFN)

Haemolytic disease is likely to occur when maternal antibodies develop against fetal red blood cells. Red cells not infrequently cross from the fetus to the mother, either antenatally or at some intrapartum event. If they are antigenically different from the mother's red cells, there may be a maternal immune response with antibody production. IgG antibodies may cross in the opposite direction, back to the fetus, leading to haemolysis, anaemia, high-output cardiac failure, hydrops, and fetal death. There are numerous known red cell antigens, but the rhesus D antigen has traditionally accounted for a majority of

haemolytic disease of the fetus and newborn (HDFN). With the introduction of an anti-D prophylaxis programme for rhesus antigen–negative women, maternal rhesus alloimmunisation and HDFN are now rare.

THE BLOOD GROUP SYSTEM

Blood groups are determined by antigens on the erythrocyte cell wall. In the ABO system, the letter O is used to refer to those who lack both the A and B antigens. If the mother is group O and the fetus has paternally inherited the A or B antigen, the mother may, if exposed, develop antibodies to these fetal cells. In practice, these antibodies rarely cause significant haemolytic disease and no antenatal investigations are warranted.

The next most important system is the rhesus system, which comprises at least 40 antigens, the most important of which are C, D, and E. C and E have immunologically distinct isoforms, which are designated 'c' and 'e', but it seems unlikely that a 'd' isoform exists. If there is a 'd' antigen, it seems to have little if any immunogenic potential, and the notation 'd' is used to indicate the absence of 'D'. A parent contributes one or other antigen (e.g., C or c) to the offspring from each of these three alphabetically designated pairs. Therefore, an individual can be homozygous or heterozygous for any of the six (e.g., Cde/cDE, cde/cdE). Those who carry the D antigen, which is inherited as autosomal dominant, are referred to as rhesus D positive, whether in the homozygous or heterozygous form. Eighty-five percent of White, 92% of Black, and 99% of Asian ethnicities are rhesus positive.

Any of the rhesus antigens are capable of stimulating antibody formation, but the D antigen is by far the most immunogenic, followed by c and E. If a rhesus-negative mother has a rhesus-positive baby and is at some stage sensitised to the baby's red cells, there is a chance of anti-D antibodies developing against the fetal cells. These antibodies may cross back to the fetus and lead to fetal haemolytic anaemia.

There are other significant antigens in addition to the ABO and rhesus systems. Many of these (e.g., Ce, Fya, Jka, Cw) are poorly developed on the red cell surface and usually stimulate only low levels of antibody production, often of the IgM category (which does not cross the placenta). Some, however, will cause significant haemolytic disease. One notable exception is the anti-Kell antibody, which has the potential to cause significant fetal anaemia and, along with anti-RhD and anti-Rhc, are the most commonly reported antibodies in cases requiring intrauterine transfusion (IUT) Kell alloimmunisation differs from RhD alloimmunisation in that the anaemia is not solely due to haemolysis – erythroid suppression has an important role. In addition, past obstetric history cannot be relied on to predict the severity of disease in the current or subsequent pregnancies. Fortunately, the incidence of Kell alloimmunisation is low (0.1%–0.2%). Since only 9% of the White population is Kell positive, the majority being heterozygous, the number of cases of HDFN is small.

PATHOPHYSIOLOGY OF HAEMOLYTIC DISEASE

Exposure to a foreign antigen leads to an antigen-specific antibody response, initially of IgM antibodies, which do not cross the placenta. On subsequent exposure – for example, in a second pregnancy – the already primed B cells produce a much larger response, this time of IgG antibodies, which do cross the placenta. In the fetal circulation, an antibody–antigen complex is formed on the red cell membrane, which provokes phagocytosis of the cell by the reticuloendothelial system and results in fetal haemolysis. This will lead to anaemia unless there is sufficient compensatory haemopoiesis from the marrow, spleen, and liver.

Increasing anaemia causes progressive fetal hypoxia and acidosis, leading to hepatic and cardiac dysfunction. Generalised oedema of skin develops, as well as ascites and pericardial and pleural effusions (see Fig. 25.10). This syndrome is known as 'immune hydrops fetalis' and is potentially fatal.

Red cell haemolysis results in increased production of bilirubin, most of which passes across the placenta to the mother and is cleared by the maternal system. Therefore, the fetus does not become jaundiced antenatally. However, after delivery, its own liver is unable to metabolise bilirubin sufficiently quickly, and the neonatal bilirubin level rises. If untreated, the bilirubin can rise to levels which endanger the nervous system, and bilirubin deposition in the basal ganglia leads to a condition known as 'kernicterus'.

INCIDENCE

The incidence varies widely. Before the availability of anti-D prophylaxis, rhesus haemolytic disease was common in populations where there was a high prevalence of Rh(D)-negative individuals and where high parity caused an accumulation of alloimmunised women. In the United Kingdom, 17% of the population is Rh(D) negative, therefore, approximately 10% of pregnant women are at risk of developing anti D antibodies.

Since the effective use of prophylactic anti-D, the perinatal mortality from HDFN has fallen from around 46/100,000 to 1.6/100,000. Newly sensitised cases are detected at a rate of approximately 1/1000 maternities.

AETIOLOGY AND PREDISPOSING FACTORS

Transfer of fetal erythrocytes to the maternal circulation during pregnancy (fetomaternal haemorrhage) may occur without any obvious predisposing event. About 75% of women may be found to have fetal red cells circulating at some stage during the pregnancy or at the time of birth. Fetomaternal haemorrhage is more likely, however, with disruption of the placental bed. This may occur with:

- Miscarriage and ectopic pregnancy
- Invasive intrauterine procedures, for example, amniocentesis, CVS, fetal shunts
- External cephalic version
- Abdominal trauma
- Intrauterine death and stillbirth
- Antepartum haemorrhage
- Labour and birth, particularly with delivery of the placenta.

An immune response may, but does not inevitably, follow fetomaternal haemorrhage. The response depends in part on the volume of blood, its antigenic potential, and on maternal responsiveness. ABO incompatibility between mother and fetus may paradoxically offer some protection, as the transfused cells are likely to be haemolysed by circulating maternal antibodies, reducing the risk of immunisation. This observation illustrates the mechanism for the use of prophylactic anti-D immunoglobulin in that exogenous anti-D is used to bind and lyse any rhesus-positive fetal red cells that reach the maternal circulation.

PREVENTION OF HAEMOLYTIC DISEASE

The most effective preventive measure is the use of intramuscular anti-D to provide passive immunisation of non-sensitised women around the time of exposure.

For a rhesus-negative mother who has a potentially sensitising event (Box 25.3) before 12 weeks, anti-D

BOX 25.3 INDICATIONS FOR ANTI-D IMMUNOPROPHYLAXIS

First Trimester
- Ectopic pregnancy
- Surgical or medical termination of pregnancy
- Miscarriage or threatened miscarriage
- Evacuation of molar pregnancy
- Chorionic villous sampling

Second Trimester
- Amniocentesis
- Antepartum haemorrhage
- Abdominal trauma
- In utero therapeutic interventions (transfusion, surgery, insertion of shunts, laser)

Third Trimester
- Routine prophylaxis
- Abdominal trauma
- Antepartum haemorrhage
- In utero therapeutic interventions (transfusion, surgery, insertion of shunts, laser)
- External cephalic version
- Delivery
- Intraoperative cell salvage

Ig prophylaxis (minimum dose 250 IU) is indicated only following ectopic pregnancy, molar pregnancy, therapeutic termination of pregnancy, and, in cases of uterine bleeding where this is repeated, heavy, or associated with abdominal pain. For potentially sensitising events between 12 and 20 weeks' gestation, 250 IU of anti-D should be given as soon as possible after the event, and certainly within 72 hours. At more than 20 weeks, the minimum dose is 500 IU and a test for fetomaternal haemorrhage (FMH) is required. Following the birth of the baby, a sample of fetal cord blood should be rhesus-grouped and, if positive, a film made of the mother's blood for Kleihauer testing. The Kleihauer test estimates the volume of fetomaternal transfusion and allows an appropriate dose of anti-D to be calculated after a sensitising event or after birth.

Immunisation can occur as a result of silent FMH. Therefore, prophylaxis is likely to be more effective if anti-D is given to all non-sensitised rhesus-negative mothers routinely in the third trimester (either 500 IU at 28 and 34 weeks or a single larger dose early in the third trimester). This is standard practice in most areas.

PREDICTION OF AT-RISK PREGNANCIES

Routine Maternal Screening

All pregnant women at their first visit have serum sent for ABO and Rh(D) grouping to screen for irregular antibodies. The maternal serum level of any antibody discovered (usually anti-D) is used as an initial screening test for further action. There are regional variations; an example of when to check for antibody levels is shown in Table 25.3.

Having identified an irregular antibody in the maternal circulation, the next stage is to assess the likely rhesus status of the baby by establishing the genotype of the putative father and remembering that the D antigen is inherited as autosomal dominant. If the father is found to be d/d, it is likely that anti-D antibodies in a rhesus-negative woman have developed from exposure to some other source of incompatible red cells, for example, a previous blood transfusion or the fetus of a previous partner. Assuming confident paternity, the fetus will be unaffected and further specific action is unnecessary. If the father is homozygous for the D antigen, it follows that the fetus will also be rhesus D positive and will be at risk of HDFN. Where the father is believed to be D/d, half of his offspring will be rhesus positive. In this situation, it is important to establish the fetal blood group to determine whether the pregnancy is at risk. This can be done non-invasively by examining cffDNA present in a maternal blood sample. Accuracies of around 96% are reported for RhD genotyping. DNA amplification of amniotic fluid should be performed for fetal genotyping only if the woman is already undergoing amniocentesis for

TABLE 25.3	Possible Screening Programme for Antibodies in Haemolytic Disease of the Newborn
All pregnant women	Offer ABO and RhD (rhesus) group and antibody screen at booking and again at 28 weeks' gestation.
Patients identified with significant alloantibodies (e.g., anti-D-, c-, E-, or Kell-related)	Consider paternal or fetal genotyping. Frequency of further screening ± antibody titre and quantification depends on antibody and titre.

other indications. Non-invasive fetal genotyping using maternal blood is now possible for D, C, c, E, e, and K antigens.

Clinical Significance of the Antibody

Red cell antigens vary in their likelihood of stimulating an immune response, with the D antigen being the most immunogenic. Apart from c and Kell, most of the other antigens are less likely to lead to significant clinical problems. The D antibody titre in maternal serum and an actual quantification level can be measured. The level is recognised to correlate well with disease severity. Severe disease is rare if the maternal antibody level is <4 IU/mL, and additional specific intervention is probably not required. The risk of significant problems is only moderate between 4 and 15 IU/mL. Above 15 IU/mL, there is a risk of severe anaemia in 50% of fetuses. These higher levels call for further investigation, described later, and the management of these relatively uncommon cases should be centralised within specialised units. A sudden rise in levels, rather than a particular absolute level, is also likely to be significant.

An anti-c level of >7.5 IU/mL correlates with a moderate risk of HDFN, which warrants referral for a fetal medicine opinion. For anti-K antibodies, referral should take place once detected.

FETAL ASSESSMENT AND THERAPY

Clinical symptoms and signs of fetal haemolytic anaemia occur late, are easily missed, and are of little help in management. In advanced disease, fetal movements are reduced or even absent, and there may be fetal growth restriction. In severe cases, there may be fetal hydrops with signs of ascites, pericardial and pleural effusions, and oedema of the skin (see Fig. 25.10). Polyhydramnios, which is associated with fetal hydrops, may also be detected. Cardiotocography may reveal an unreactive pattern or even decelerations but, again, only in advanced disease. A sinusoidal fetal heart pattern is thought to be fairly specific for severe anaemia. These all represent the 'end stage' of the process of progressive fetal anaemia. It is critical in the management of known alloimmunised pregnancies to detect the fetus that will benefit from intrauterine therapy before the fetal condition is seriously compromised. A rise in antibody titre or quantification should prompt non-invasive monitoring, as described next.

Non-Invasive Testing

Fetal MCA Doppler studies correlate very well with the degree of fetal anaemia (see Fig. 25.11). Table 25.4 indicates the level for different antibodies at which there is a moderate or severe risk of anaemia. Once these levels are reached, MCA Doppler monitoring should be commenced. The peak systolic velocity of the MCA is measured and, if >1.5 multiples of the median for gestational age, is predictive of moderate to severe fetal anaemia in 100% of cases for a false-positive rate of 12%. The test is reliable up to 34 weeks' gestation. Once severe anaemia is predicted, intrauterine therapy should commence (see later discussion).

BIRTH

All babies with haemolytic disease should be born in a specialist unit with full neonatal intensive care facilities. If ultrasound assessment is normal, and the antibody level relatively low, a conservative approach with birth at term is appropriate. If premature birth is anticipated, maternal corticosteroid therapy is warranted. Babies in whom mild anaemia is suspected or who have been successfully treated with IUT can be born vaginally unless there are other obstetric indications for caesarean birth. For cases managed with serial IUTs, labour is induced at around 38 weeks' gestation. If a hydropic fetus requires birth, this should be by caesarean section. Experienced paediatric attendance at birth is essential; cord blood must be collected for assessment of haemoglobin, platelets, blood grouping, bilirubin, and direct Coombs testing. The neonate may require intensive support with measures to control anaemia, hyperbilirubinaemia, and any associated cardiorespiratory problems.

PROGNOSIS

For mildly affected fetuses who do not need intrauterine therapy, the outlook in experienced units is

TABLE 25.4	Risk of Fetal Anaemia According to Antibody Quantification/Titre	
	Antibody Level	
Risk of Fetal Anaemia	**Anti-D (IU/mL)**	**Anti-c (IU/mL)**
Low	0–4	0–7.5
Moderate	4–15	7.5–20
High	>15	>20

excellent. Survival rates for non-hydropic fetuses undergoing IUT are 94% compared with approximately 74% if hydrops is present.

Early reports suggested serious neurological impairments, including cerebral palsy, abnormal development, and hearing problems, especially in those children who were transfused in utero. Recent experience is very much more reassuring and suggests there are few if any additional risks beyond the well-recognised hazards of prematurity.

Advances in Fetal Therapy

Rapid development in the field of fetal medicine over the past few decades has allowed fetal therapy to be offered to parents of affected offspring in certain conditions. In utero therapy may provide immediate benefit (e.g., intrauterine transfusion) or may reduce associated fetal and long-term complications (e.g., surgery for spina bifida). However, fetal therapy may be associated with risks to the mother and fetus. Ongoing research in this field is needed to fully evaluate the safety, efficacy, and long-term outcomes of most interventions.

INTRAUTERINE TRANSFUSION

In women at risk of developing HDFN, intravascular fetal blood transfusions for severe fetal anaemia and hydrops have dramatically improved the outcome of these pregnancies. When the MCA-PSV (peak systolic velocity) demonstrates evidence of severe fetal anaemia, fetal blood sampling with the intention to transfuse should be undertaken.

Access to the fetal circulation is achieved by inserting a needle ideally into the intrahepatic portion of the umbilical vein or the baby's cord at its point of placental insertion. This enables an immediate haemoglobin (or haematocrit) estimation to be made and facilitates simultaneous transfusion of blood. Group O rhesus-negative blood is cross-matched to the mother's own serum prior to the procedure. If the haemoglobin/haematocrit is low, a calculated volume can be transfused during the same sampling procedure. Intrauterine transfusion carries the risk of cord haematoma, fetal bradycardia, intrauterine death, and further sensitisation of the mother-to-fetal red cell antigens. A procedure-related loss rate in the region of 1% to 2% has been reported. It is likely that multiple transfusions will be required owing to the relentlessly progressive anaemia that occurs in alloimmunised pregnancies.

FETAL SURGERY

Currently, open and laparoscopic fetal surgery is being offered in highly specialised fetal medicine centres in selected fetuses with a condition that is, without any intervention, either lethal or in which progressive loss of organ function can be prevented to improve quality of life postnatally.

Congenital Diaphragmatic Hernia

This is a potentially lethal condition. In moderate to severe cases, prenatal intervention aims to improve fetal lung development and subsequent outcomes post-delivery.

Advances in minimally invasive surgery have made FETO with a balloon possible. FETO is an invasive procedure that can be done under maternal local anaesthesia. Traditionally, removal of the balloon was undertaken at the time of caesarean delivery using an extrauterine intrapartum treatment (EXIT) strategy. However, recent data suggest that in utero reversal of tracheal occlusion could lead to morphologically better lung maturation. Therefore, elective intrauterine occlusion reversal is scheduled at 34 weeks' gestation, either by ultrasound-guided puncture or fetoscopy. Observational studies have shown that FETO leads to reduced early neonatal respiratory morbidity and an apparent increase in survival. However, data from current randomised controlled trials are still to come. One of the main associated complications is pre-term pre-labour rupture of the membranes and pre-term birth.

Spina Bifida

Open spina bifida is a multifactorial disease associated with significant lifelong neurological disability. A multi-centre randomised controlled trial, the Management of Myelomeningocele Study (MOMS), demonstrated that prenatal surgery significantly improves childhood neurological outcome compared with standard postnatal repair. Currently, open and laparoscopic fetal surgery for open spina bifida is being offered at highly experienced fetal therapy centres using a multidisciplinary team approach. Primary anatomical repair is undertaken; rarely, augmentation by patch may be required.

Potential benefits of surgery must be balanced against the risks of fetal and maternal morbidity. Fetal surgery is associated with significant maternal morbidity, including haemorrhage, pulmonary oedema, need for caesarean birth, and morbidity caused by uterine incision in current and subsequent pregnancies. Other obstetric complications related to prenatal surgery include pre-term pre-labour rupture of the membranes, pre-term birth, infection, and placental abruption, which increases perinatal morbidity. Clinical research is ongoing in this rapidly evolving field to develop ways to minimise the associated risks.

Chest and Bladder Shunts

Thoracocentesis and Pleuro-Amniotic Shunting

Fetal pleural effusions occur in 1 in 10,000 pregnancies. They can arise in isolation or can be secondary to structural malformations – frequently, heart defects, chromosomal anomalies, abnormal lymphatic drainage (chylothorax), anaemia, and viral infections. Severe pleural effusions can cause pressure on surrounding structures, including the heart and lungs, and result in hydrops (see Fig 25.10). Therapeutic prenatal interventions include thoracocentesis (a single needle insertion through the maternal abdomen to drain the fluid) and pleuro-amniotic shunting. Shunting is a more complicated invasive procedure, generally considered once re-accumulation of the pleural effusion is noted following a thoracocentesis. In the absence of hydrops or underlying genetic anomalies, the prognosis for babies undergoing a pleuro-amniotic shunt is good, with effective lung expansion occurring in 98% of cases.

Vesico-Amniotic Shunting

Lower urinary tract obstruction (LUTO) usually occurs due to presence of a posterior urethral valve or urethral atresia. It can lead to bladder dilatation (megacystis), damage to the developing kidneys, chronic renal failure, and fetal pulmonary hypoplasia. In utero therapy via vesico-amniotic shunting aims to decompress the pressure on the kidneys to prevent irreversible renal damage and restore amniotic fluid volume to prevent lung hypoplasia. However, vesico-amniotic shunting remains controversial due to the risk of complications, including blockage, dislocation, infection, fetal trauma, pre-term pre-labour rupture of the membranes, and pre-term birth, without any evidence for an improvement in neonatal or infant outcomes.

Ethical Considerations and Parental Support

The identification of a 'congenital anomaly' in pregnancy transforms what is usually a joyful and exciting experience into one that is fraught with anxiety and distress. Providing couples with accurate information in an understanding and tactful way is essential. This often requires input from senior obstetric staff, ideally those with fetal-medicine experience, as well as other specialties, including neonatologists, paediatric surgeons, microbiologists, clinical geneticists, and radiologists.

Detailed discussion and non-directional counselling are critical. It is important to remain completely neutral and avoid using expressions such as 'high risk' or 'severe handicap', which imply judgement. For example, 'the baby has a 95% chance of being unaffected' is a preferrable phrase to 'the risk of handicap is 5%'. When talking through diagnoses and options, it should not be assumed that all couples will request a termination of pregnancy, even in the presence of lethal abnormalities. Many couples opt to continue pregnancies in the face of severe anomalies, which have resulted in either intrauterine or early neonatal death, subsequently expressing the view that they found it easier to cope with their grief having held their child. Other parents make the difficult decision not to carry on with the pregnancy. More controversial still is the identification of conditions likely to cause long-term handicap and suffering for both the child and their parents. In this situation, the parents must decide what is acceptable to them; we can only advise, guide, and respect their final wishes, irrespective of our own personal opinions.

All discussions should be complemented with written information. Parents need time to absorb information – it is important that they are given time to reflect on the facts and to consider all options carefully. It can be extremely useful to arrange a follow-up appointment a few days after the initial visit. Indeed, it sometimes takes several appointments before they have come to a decision.

There are also various parent support networks and charities that provide an enormous amount of valuable information and advice, which may be of benefit depending on the parent's individual needs.

Termination of Pregnancy for Fetal Abnormality

In the United Kingdom, TOP under clause E of the Abortion Act (1967) allows the offer of TOP for fetal anomaly if two registered practitioners agree (see Chapter 20). Such a consultation requires sensitivity: not all couples will opt for prenatal TOP, thus, it is important that neonatal care is discussed as an alternative in such situations. If parents opt for a termination after 22 weeks' gestation, feticide should be offered. Beyond 24 weeks' gestation, the UK law regarding TOP is stringent; a multidisciplinary discussion is usually required, and a termination is agreed upon only if the fetus is deemed to have a significant risk of serious disability or a lethal condition.

Parents may initially be reluctant to see the baby after delivery but should be strongly encouraged to take the opportunity; other family members may also want this opportunity. Photographs and other mementos are extremely important.

Post-mortem examination should be discussed and encouraged, especially if the cause of the anomaly is unknown. If parents decline, they may accept a limited or minimally invasive post-mortem investigation with X-rays, MRI, micro-computed tomography scan, laparoscopy, clinical photographs, and specimens for genetic studies instead. Follow-up to discuss the results and their implications for subsequent pregnancy is also essential.

TOP is associated with significant parental grief reactions. Support following termination should be continued for as long as necessary.

Key Points

- Approximately 2% of newborn babies have a serious anomaly detectable at or soon after birth. Many of these can be diagnosed antenatally.
- There are a number of different strategies for prenatal screening programmes to detect chromosomal, structural, and genetic anomalies. Adequate verbal and written information is essential prior to undertaking screening.
- Parents are often confronted with difficult decisions. Explanations may need to be repeated and often involve multidisciplinary teams.
- Isoimmunisation occurs when maternal antibodies develop against fetal red blood cells. These antibodies cross to the fetus and may lead to haemolysis, anaemia, high-output cardiac failure, and fetal death. There are numerous known red cell antigens, but the rhesus D antigen accounts for more than 85% of HDFN.
- Treatment of severe haemolytic disease is highly specialised and requires referral to appropriately experienced units. Assessment involves the use of Doppler ultrasound; when fetal anaemia is suspected, fetal therapy with IUT is possible.
- Fetal surgery is currently being undertaken in various highly specialised fetal medicine centres for conditions that cannot await therapy after birth or when prenatal surgery changes the natural course of the condition and improves subsequent outcome.

Chapter 26

Obstetric Haemorrhage

Fiona Nugent, Andrew Thomson

Chapter Outline

Introduction

Obstetric haemorrhage is one of the leading causes of maternal mortality. Worldwide, approximately 300,000 women die during pregnancy and childbirth each year, and a quarter of these are caused by haemorrhage. Whilst most deaths occur in low-resource settings (primarily Sub-Saharan Africa and Southern Asia), deaths still occur in areas with low rates of maternal mortality, where around 8% of deaths are attributed to haemorrhage. Haemorrhage may be of rapid onset. It is important to recognize its severity promptly, institute effective therapy, and keep ahead of the blood loss via intravascular volume replacement.

Definitions

Vaginal bleeding associated with intrauterine pregnancy is divided into the following categories:

- Threatened miscarriage – up to 24 weeks' gestation
- Antepartum haemorrhage (APH) – from 24 weeks' gestation until the onset of labour
- Intrapartum haemorrhage – from the onset of labour until the end of the second stage
- Postpartum haemorrhage (PPH) – from the third stage of labour until 12 weeks after delivery.

Antepartum Haemorrhage

APH affects 3% to 5% of pregnancies. Placental abruption and placenta praevia are the most important causes of APH but are not the most common. The majority of cases of APH remain unexplained after clinical and ultrasound examination. The magnitude of APH can be usefully classified as follows:

- Minor APH is <50 mL and stopped
- Major APH is 50 to 1000 mL and no hypovolaemic shock
- Massive APH is >1000 mL and/or hypovolaemic shock.

CAUSES

APH is further classified according to the source of the bleeding. Around 50% of APH is caused by placenta praevia or placental abruption.

Local

There may be bleeding from the woman's vulva, vagina or cervix. Bleeding from the cervix is not uncommon in pregnancy and may follow sexual intercourse (post-coital bleeding). A cervical ectropion or benign polyp is often found; rarely, a diagnosis of cervical carcinoma is made. The passing of a blood-stained 'show', mucus along with a small amount of blood, may herald the onset of labour as the cervix becomes effaced.

Placental

Placenta Praevia

The term 'placenta praevia' was previously defined using transabdominal ultrasound scan as a placenta that lies wholly or partly in the lower uterine segment. A grading system, I to IV, was employed based on the relationship and/or the distance between the lower placental edge and the cervical internal os (Table 26.1, Fig. 26.1). The site of the placenta may also be described by its position, for example, anterior, posterior or lateral. More recently, and with widespread use of transvaginal ultrasound scanning, an alternative definition and classification has been widely adopted; the placenta is described as *low lying* when the placental edge is less than 2 cm from the internal os and *placenta praevia* when the placenta lies directly over and covers the internal os. Placenta praevia is more common among women who have previously given birth by caesarean, but the majority

TABLE 26.1		Traditional Classification of Placenta Praevia
Minor	I	Encroaches the lower uterine segment
	II	Reaches internal os of the cervix (marginal)
Major	III	Covers part of internal os (partial)
	IV	Completely covers the internal os (complete)

of women with placenta praevia have no discernible risk factors.

Women with pregnancies in which the placenta is low lying (less than 2 cm from the internal os) or praevia are recommended to give birth by caesarean section. Placental location is routinely determined at the time of the fetal anatomy scan at 18 to 22 weeks and may be found to be low lying or praevia at that stage (Fig. 26.2). As the uterus grows from the lower segment upwards, the placenta appears to move upwards with advancing gestation, with resolution of low-lying placenta in 90% of cases before term. This is not a reflection of placental migration; rather, it is simply a feature of uterine growth. When a low-lying placenta is detected on ultrasound scanning early in pregnancy, it is necessary to repeat the scan early in the third trimester and then review the woman's care if placenta praevia persists.

The risk of placenta praevia is of a sudden, unpredictable, major or massive haemorrhage. The woman's care may be either as an inpatient or outpatient. Factors that will affect this decision include distance and transport availability to a hospital where facilities for resuscitation and birth are immediately available, number of episodes of bleeding and their severity, haematology results, and willingness to accept blood and/or blood products. Elective birth by caesarean section is usually planned for 36 to 37 weeks but will be considered earlier if there is a history of vaginal bleeding or other risk factors for pre-term birth.

Caesarean section in the presence of placenta praevia should be directly supervised by, or performed by, a senior obstetrician since a large blood loss is frequently encountered owing to the relatively poor capacity of the lower segment of the uterus to contract and, in many cases, the need to incise through the placenta to deliver the baby.

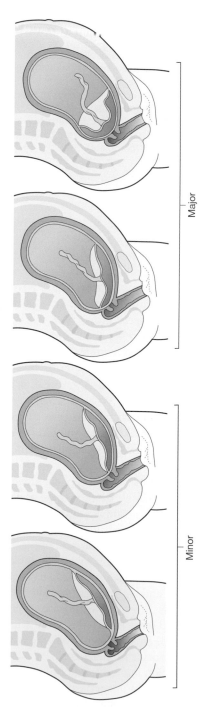

Fig. 26.1 Classification into 'major' and 'minor' placenta praevia depends on the distance of the placenta from the internal os of the cervix. In the presence of a caesarean section scar, an anterior placenta praevia may result in abnormal invasion (morbidly adherent placenta, placenta accreta).

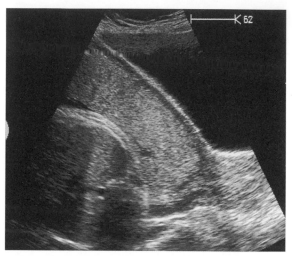

Fig. 26.2 Transabdominal ultrasound scan of an anterior placenta praevia extending to just beyond the internal os.

Placental Abruption

Placental abruption is defined as retroplacental haemorrhage (bleeding between the placenta and the uterus) as a result of some degree of placental separation prior to birth of the baby. The care of women with placental abruption depends on the amount of bleeding, presence or absence of maternal haemodynamic compromise, the maturity of the fetus and its condition. Separation of the placenta results in a reduced area for gas exchange between the fetal and maternal circulations, predisposing to fetal hypoxia and acidosis. It is crucial to remember that with placental abruption the amount of 'revealed' blood (bleeding from the vagina) may not reflect the total blood loss and that a woman may have considerable retroplacental bleeding without any external loss at all – a 'concealed abruption' (Fig. 26.3).

Recognised risk factors for placental abruption include a history of a previous pregnancy affected by placental abruption and maternal cigarette smoking (Table 26.2), but the majority of placental abruptions occur by chance in women without identifiable risk factors.

Light bleeding from the edge of a normally situated placenta does not normally compromise the fetus. A brief episode of inpatient observation and often surveillance of subsequent fetal growth with ultrasound fetal biometry is appropriate. Repeated episodes of placental abruption may lead to a decision to deliver early.

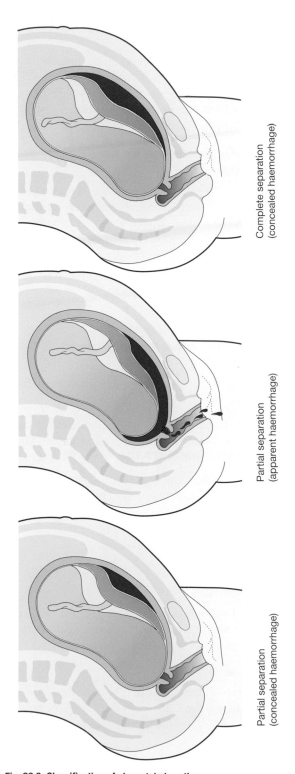

Complete separation
(concealed haemorrhage)

Partial separation
(apparent haemorrhage)

Partial separation
(concealed haemorrhage)

Fig. 26.3 Classification of placental abruption.

TABLE 26.2	**Risk factors for placental abruption**
Previous placental abruption	
Pre-eclampsia	
Fetal growth restriction	
Non-vertex presentations	
Polyhydramnios	
Advanced maternal age	
Multiparity	
Low body mass index	
Pregnancy following assisted reproductive techniques	
Intrauterine infection	
Premature rupture of membranes	
Abdominal trauma	
Smoking	
Drug misuse (cocaine and amphetamines)	

Major revealed haemorrhage is obvious, and urgent birth is usually required. A major concealed abruption is inferred from the degree of pain, uterine tenderness and evidence of hypovolaemic shock; again, urgent birth may be required. The decision between vaginal and caesarean birth is influenced by the degree of bleeding coupled with maternal and fetal conditions.

If intrauterine fetal death is diagnosed, vaginal birth is to be preferred, if safe to do so, although the woman's preferences should always be considered. However, in such a situation, it is likely that there will have been a major degree of blood loss. Hypovolaemic shock may develop and may progress to multisystem organ failure if not corrected. In addition, release of thromboplastins from the damaged placenta may lead to disseminated intravascular coagulation (DIC) with depletion of platelets, fibrinogen and other clotting factors. Therefore, waiting for the baby to be born vaginally carries risks, and caesarean birth may occasionally be indicated to minimise these systemic maternal risks. Deciding on the appropriate mode of birth is further complicated by the risks of carrying out an operation in the presence of DIC.

Less severe degrees of placental separation can still be associated with fetal compromise. The woman usually describes pain and frequent contractions, the contractions precipitated by irritation of the myometrium from the retroplacental clot. The fetal heart rate will often show a suspicious or pathological pattern, which may progress to a fetal bradycardia and fetal death unless birth of the baby is expedited. Placental abruption predisposes the mother to PPH.

Unexplained Antepartum Haemorrhage

In approximately half of cases, a specific cause for APH is not found. Bleeding with no explanation is the most common clinical scenario. In the absence of maternal or fetal compromise, it is managed expectantly. Unexplained APH, especially if more than one episode (recurrent unexplained APH), is a recognised risk factor for subsequent fetal growth restriction; additional ultrasound surveillance is recommended.

CLINICAL PRESENTATIONS

Bleeding can be spotting (minor staining of underwear or sanitary protection), minor, major or massive, and can occur with or without pain. Other than in circumstances of spotting that has stopped, admission to hospital is advised, as even minor bleeding may herald heavier bleeding.

An attempt should be made to determine the cause of the bleeding. In practice, history and initial examination are carried out simultaneously. It is relevant to ask when the bleeding started, how much blood has been lost and when the baby was last felt to move. Observation will tell if the mother is in pain, which suggests abruption or labour, and there may be visible blood on the bed, her legs or the floor. If the mother is pale, with low blood pressure and rapid pulse, there is probably hypovolaemic shock. With an abruption, the uterus is typically hard and tender ('Couvelaire' uterus) and the fetal heartbeat may be absent. There may be frequent contractions or continuous pain. When the bleeding is from a placenta praevia, the uterus is usually soft, the presenting part will usually be free and the fetal heartbeat is usually present. Subsequent care depends on the estimated severity of haemorrhage.

Minor Haemorrhage With a Soft Uterus and Normal Cardiotocography

An ultrasound scan should be arranged to determine the placental site (if not already established by an earlier scan) and, provided that the placenta is not praevia, a speculum examination should be performed to look for cervical effacement or dilatation, an ectropion or a cervical polyp. If all is normal, it is common practice to admit the woman at least until the bleeding stops. However, most clinicians will not admit the woman if the bleeding is minor and clearly seen to be coming from an ectropion. Women whose blood group is rhesus negative are advised to receive prophylactic anti-D.

If there is a placenta praevia and the pregnancy is at more than 36 to 37 weeks' gestation it is reasonable to arrange for birth by caesarean section. If less than this gestation, a conservative approach may be appropriate if the bleeding has settled.

Minor or Major Haemorrhage, but With a Hard, Tender Uterus

The diagnosis is probably a placental abruption (concealed and revealed). Clinical care revolves around maternal resuscitation, correction of hypovolaemia and coagulation defects and evaluation of the fetal condition by cardiotocography. Expediting birth is highly likely to be appropriate; the route of birth will be influenced by a number of factors, including evidence of fetal compromise and the presence or absence of maternal coagulopathy.

Antepartum Haemorrhage Requiring Maternal Resuscitation

Whether the diagnosis is placenta praevia or an abruption, such a massive APH is highly likely to prompt birth almost irrespective of gestational age.

Intrapartum Haemorrhage

Abnormal bleeding during labour should be distinguished from a 'show' that may occur during cervical dilatation. In a previously low-risk pregnancy, intrapartum bleeding is considered to be an indication for continuous electronic fetal monitoring.

CAUSES

Placental Abruption

Placental abruption (see earlier discussion) can occur during labour and should be particularly considered if the uterus does not relax between contractions.

Placenta Praevia

As the cervix dilates, the placenta separates from the uterine wall and typically painless bleeding occurs.

Uterine Rupture

Uterine rupture is relatively rare and is discussed on page 433 (obstetric emergencies).

Vasa Praevia

This is uncommon, with a prevalence ranging between 1 in 1200 and 1 in 5000 pregnancies. It occurs when the umbilical cord vessels run in the fetal membranes and cross the internal os of the cervix. These vessels may rupture spontaneously in early labour or may be ruptured at the time of amniotomy, which may lead to fetal exsanguination. It may be that the cord is inserted into the membranes rather than directly into the placenta (type 1 vasa praevia, Fig. 26.4) or that the vessels are running from the placenta to a separate succenturiate (accessory) placental lobe (type 2 vasa praevia). The condition typically presents as a pathological cardiotocography (CTG) or fetal death following a minor intrapartum haemorrhage. In the presence of an APH, diagnostic tests to differentiate fetal from maternal blood are seldom reliable and the baby is usually born urgently by caesarean section because of the fetal compromise. The diagnosis of vasa praevia is often only made retrospectively, by examination of the placenta and membranes. Although it is possible to diagnose the condition antenatally with colour flow Doppler ultrasound, routine screening for vasa praevia is not established practice, as there is concern there may be a high false-positive rate and no evidence of benefit is currently available. Risk factors for vasa praevia have been identified, with velamentous cord insertion and placenta praevia being the most common.

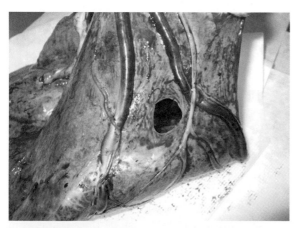

Fig. 26.4 Umbilical cord vessels running through the membranes. If these vessels overlie the internal cervical os, it is termed 'vasa praevia'.

Postpartum Haemorrhage

It is not possible to predict which women will have a PPH, and it is important to appreciate that a major haemorrhage can very rapidly lead to maternal death. Anticipation of PPH and an awareness of the relevant interventions is essential.

DEFINITIONS

There is inevitably some bleeding during the third stage of labour, usually around 200 to 300 mL following a vaginal birth.

- A primary PPH is defined as a blood loss of 500 mL or more within 24 hours of birth. The PPH is 'minor' if blood loss is 500 to 1000 mL with no hypovolaemic shock and 'major' if >1000 mL and continuing or associated with hypovolaemic shock.
- A secondary PPH is any excess vaginal blood loss between 24 hours and 12 weeks after the birth.

PRIMARY POSTPARTUM HAEMORRHAGE

Postpartum haemorrhage occurs in up to 18% of all births. It is more common in women of high parity (four deliveries or more), women over 35 years of age, women with a body mass index of over 35, multiple pregnancy, women with fibroids, placenta praevia and in those who have had a long labour or an instrumental birth. It may also follow an APH and is more likely in women with a past history of primary PPH. Women with risk factors for PPH are advised to give birth in a consultant-led unit.

Prevention

It is important to treat anaemia in the antenatal period (haematinic supplements), particularly if the woman has risk factors for PPH. It is recommended practice to give a uterotonic (typically, intramuscular [IM] oxytocin 10 IU) with delivery of the baby's anterior shoulder. This practice is described as 'active management' of the third stage and involves giving uterotonic drugs (usually, oxytocin alone or in combination with ergometrine) and controlled cord traction after signs of separation of the placenta. Active management of the third stage has been shown to reduce PPH by up to 50% by encouraging timely delivery of the placenta and uterine contractility.

Causes

There are a number of recognised factors that increase a woman's chance of having a PPH. These are listed in Table 26.3.

The causes of primary PPH are often referred to as the 'four Ts':

- *Tone*: Poor uterine contractility or atony. This is the most common cause of primary PPH (90%). Normally, contraction of the uterus in the third stage of labour causes compression of intramyometrial blood vessels, and bleeding from the placental site stops promptly (Fig. 26.5). If there is uterine atony, this compression does not occur
- *Trauma*: Bleeding may be from an episiotomy, a vaginal tear, cervical laceration (Fig. 26.6) or a rupture of the uterine wall. Lacerations of the genital tract are more common after an instrumental birth.
- *Tissue*: Retained placental tissue inhibiting uterine contractility. Placental tissue is considered retained if the placenta is not delivered in 30 minutes with active management or 60 minutes with physiological management and affects 2% to 3% of all vaginal births. The physical presence of placental tissue prevents effective uterine contraction and the partial placental separation results in bleeding from the placental bed.

TABLE 26.3	Risk Factors for Postpartum Haemorrhage
Pre-Existing Maternal Factors	**Pregnancy Factors**
High parity	Multiple pregnancy
Maternal age >35 years	Fetal macrosomia
Anaemia	Polyhydramnios
Raised body mass index	Previous postpartum haemorrhage
Uterine fibroids	Antepartum haemorrhage in current pregnancy
Coagulation disorders	Prolonged 2nd stage of labour
	Instrumental birth
	Retained placenta and placenta accreta
	Episiotomy and/or genital tract trauma
	General anaesthesia

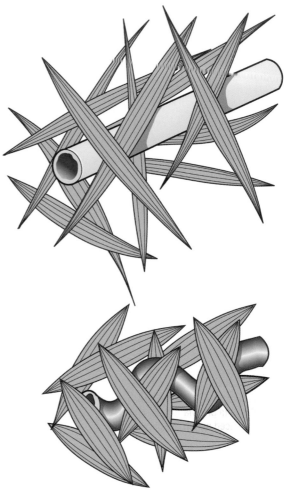

Fig. 26.5 Postpartum haemostasis is principally achieved by the contracting myometrial fibres constricting the blood vessels within the uterine wall.

Retained placental tissue is more likely in the presence of an abnormally invasive placenta, which is termed 'placenta accreta spectrum'. The severity of this condition ranges from invasion deep into the myometrium down to the serosa (known as an 'increta') or even through the uterine wall, invading surrounding pelvic organs such as the bladder (known as 'percreta'; Box 26.1, Table 26.4). Women with a placenta praevia overlying a previous caesarean section scar are at very high risk of this serious complication.

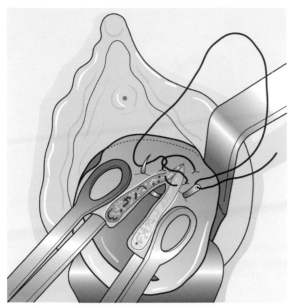

Fig. 26.6 Cervical lacerations may cause a primary PPH.

BOX 26.1 RISK FACTORS FOR PLACENTA ACCRETA

Spectrum

- Previous caesarean section
- Placenta praevia
- Advanced maternal age
- High parity
- Previous retained placenta
- History of dilatation and curettage or suction termination of pregnancy
- Previous postpartum endometritis

- *Thrombin*: Coagulopathy, usually DIC. DIC can occur in association with a number of different causes, including maternal sepsis, placental abruption and PPH, in which the blood loss causes the DIC and the DIC exacerbates the blood loss.

It should be acknowledged that multiple causes may be present, necessitating a systematic approach to the woman experiencing a primary PPH, for example, uterine atony in association with retained placental tissue.

Clinical Presentation

The bleeding is usually obvious. Occasionally, however, an atonic uterus can fill up without obvious

TABLE 26.4	Classification of Abnormal Placental Attachment	
Type	**Incidence**	**Pathology**
Placenta accreta	75%–78%	Invades superficially into the myometrium.
Placenta increta	17%	Invades deep into the myometrium.
Placenta percreta	5%–7%	Invades through the myometrium and penetrates the outer serosal layer of the uterus. It may invade adjacent structures, including bladder and bowel.

external loss, and the first sign of the PPH is hypovolaemic shock. A less dramatic, prolonged trickling of blood may go unnoticed, the significance of which may not be initially appreciated. With blood-soaked pads and bedding, it is common to underestimate the loss.

The key questions are:

1. Has the placenta been delivered and is it complete?
2. Is the uterus firmly contracted?
3. If so, is the bleeding due to trauma?

Care of Women With Primary Postpartum Haemorrhage

A reassuring presence is important. PPH is a common obstetric emergency but it is stressful to the mother and her birth partner. It is important to ensure that appropriate numbers, skill mix and expertise of staff are in attendance or are en route.

Assessment

- Measure the loss by weighing pads.
- Determine the pulse and blood pressure.
- Palpate the abdomen to assess the size and tone of the uterus.

Treatment and Interventions

Depending on the degree of haemorrhage, the following measures are often undertaken simultaneously. It is important that a multidisciplinary team approach is adopted in the woman's care.

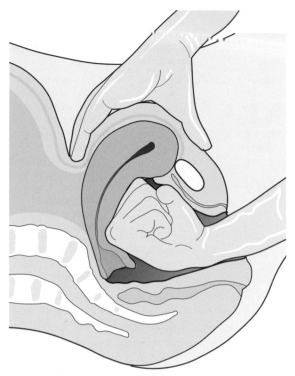

Fig. 26.7 Bimanual compression is often effective in the initial management of primary PPH.

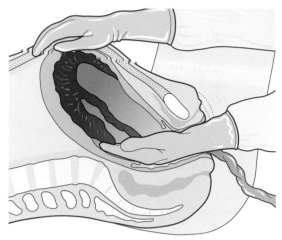

Fig. 26.8 A cleavage plane is identified with the fingers, which then continue along the plane until the placenta is fully separated from the uterine wall.

- If the uterus is atonic, a contraction can be 'rubbed up' by abdominal massage. Bimanual compression may also be performed (Fig. 26.7).
- Intravenous (IV) access should be established with two wide-bore cannulae and blood taken for haemoglobin concentration, platelet count, blood clotting and a red cell cross-match (the number of units depends on volume lost).
- An IV bolus of oxytocin 5 IU should be given to further contract the uterus, followed by an oxytocin infusion (usually 40 IU in 500 mL isotonic crystalloids at 125 mL/h).
- The woman's bladder should be emptied and an in-dwelling catheter left in situ to monitor the urinary output.
- Crystalloid and/or colloid up to 3.5 L should be rapidly infused to maintain the circulating volume. With rapid blood loss, O rhesus-negative blood may need to be given.
- If the placenta has not been delivered, a gentle attempt at umbilical cord traction should be tried. If still retained, a regional block or general anaesthetic will be required for a manual removal of the placenta (where a hand is passed into the uterus through the cervix to strip off the placenta under aseptic conditions (Fig. 26.8)). The procedure must be covered with antibiotics, as there is a significant association between manual removal of the placenta and postpartum endometritis.
- Further oxytocics can be given, for example, further boluses of IV oxytocin, IM ergometrine, IM carboprost and/or rectal misoprostol (carboprost and misoprostol are synthetic prostaglandin analogues).
- The antifibrinolytic drug, tranexamic acid 1 g IV, has been shown to improve outcomes in women undergoing PPH.
- Bleeding from genital tract lacerations should be diagnosed promptly by examination (often under regional block or general anaesthesia) and bleeding arrested by application of clamps and suturing.

If the haemorrhage continues, an arterial line should be considered and inserted by the anaesthetist, and a blood transfusion commenced. The coagulation defects of DIC should be corrected with fresh frozen plasma or cryoprecipitate following consultation with a haematologist. Additional techniques to stop haemorrhage due to atony are aimed at either maintaining compression of the uterus or applying pressure directly to the placental bed.

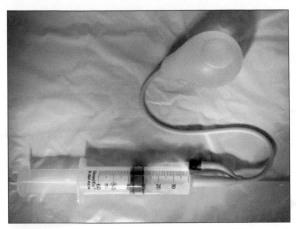

Fig. 26.9 An intrauterine balloon often provides effective uterine tamponade in atonic PPH.

A 'brace' suture involves an additional laparotomy (unless the haemorrhage is following a caesarean section) and the placing and tying of sutures around the uterine body in order to maintain compression. The most commonly known type of brace suture is called a 'B-Lynch' suture.

Placement of an intrauterine balloon does not require a laparotomy and works by applying pressure directly to the placental bed (Fig. 26.9). Balloon insertion is effective in the majority of cases in which it is considered appropriate.

Hysterectomy may be indicated, especially if there is an abnormally invasive placenta. In acknowledgement of the high PPH risk, it is recommended that women with suspected placenta accreta should give birth by caesarean section in a specialist centre. Conservative management (when the placenta is left in situ to be absorbed over time) is an option with placenta accreta, though this is associated with a significant incidence of major complications from infection and bleeding, and the woman must be monitored closely for several weeks (sometimes months) following discharge.

Internal iliac artery ligation is occasionally performed but requires a high degree of surgical skill. Radiologically directed arterial embolization is an option in the management of PPH, provided that the woman is stable for transfer to the radiology theatre suite. This procedure is highly specialised and is performed by interventional radiologists. Embolization often enables haemorrhage to be controlled without resorting to hysterectomy.

SECONDARY POSTPARTUM HAEMORRHAGE

This is usually caused by infection of the uterine cavity (endometritis), retained products of conception, or both. Exceptionally, it is due to trophoblastic disease. Pulse rate, blood pressure and temperature are measured and the uterus palpated for tenderness. Endocervical and vaginal swabs are sent for culture. An ultrasound scan is often helpful in ruling out retained tissue.

The management decision is usually between conservative management with antibiotics or arranging for an evacuation of retained products under regional or general anaesthesia. In the first week, the evacuation can often be carried out digitally without the need to instrument the uterus. Clinical judgement is important, often giving broad-spectrum antibiotics in the first instance if the bleeding is not severe and arranging an evacuation if the bleeding does not settle. Care is required to avoid perforating the postpartum uterus. Many clinicians perform the evacuation with real-time ultrasound to ensure that the instrument remains within the uterine cavity.

Key Points

- **Obstetric haemorrhage is one of the leading causes of maternal mortality. While a number of risk factors for obstetric haemorrhage are recognised, APH and PPH are often unpredictable. Maternity care staff should be trained and prepared to deal with this obstetric emergency.**
- **It can be rapidly fatal – it is important to establish adequate IV access, initiate resuscitation and identify the cause of the bleeding.**
- **Early involvement of senior obstetric, anaesthetic and midwifery staff is important.**
- **Providing an explanation to the woman and her birth partner ensures that the anxiety generated by experiencing the haemorrhage is reduced.**

Chapter 27

Fetal Growth and Surveillance

Philip Owen, Katie McBride

Chapter Outline

Introduction

The focus of this chapter is on fetuses who appear to be small for their gestational age. These babies may simply be small—in other words, they are normal unborn babies who just happen to be at the lower end of a normal range (constitutionally or genetically small) or they may be small for a pathological reason. These latter fetuses are referred to as being affected by fetal growth restriction (FGR, previously called 'intrauterine growth restriction'). As a group, small-for-gestational-age (SGA) fetuses are at increased risk of perinatal mortality but most adverse outcomes are within the group affected by FGR.

The key issues are how to screen a low-risk population in order to identify these small fetuses and, once identified, how best to identify those that are risk of developing problems in utero or in labour.

Accuracy of Dating

The reliable diagnosis of SGA and FGR requires knowledge of gestational age. The estimated date of delivery is calculated as 40 weeks after the date of the start of the last menstrual period (LMP), provided that the cycle length is 28 days. A correction may be made for those with regular longer or shorter cycles. For example, if the cycle is 35 days long, then 7 days should be added to the date of the LMP. However, menstrual dating has inherent potential inaccuracies: the dates may be inaccurately recalled, the cycle may be irregular, and bleeding in early pregnancy may be mistaken for a period. Abdominal palpation is an inaccurate way of establishing gestational age, as is the date that fetal movements were first noted. Gestational age is most accurately determined by an ultrasound scan undertaken before 20 weeks' gestation, as it is reasonable to assume that all fetuses of a given gestational age are of a similar size up until this point. The natural variation in size after this stage makes pregnancy dating less accurate. The most reliable fetal measurements for dating are the crown rump length between the 10th and 14th weeks and the head circumference between the 15th and 20th weeks.

The rest of this chapter will assume that gestational age is reliably established.

Small for Gestational Age

SGA describes the fetus or baby whose estimated fetal weight or birth weight is below the 10th centile. As the centile reduces, for example, to the fifth or third, the risk of adverse outcome increases.

Fetal Growth Restriction

The term 'FGR' indicates 'a fetus which fails to reach its genetic growth potential'. FGR presents as a fetus whose growth on serial ultrasound scanning falls below a certain threshold. This threshold is poorly defined and is often implied as the 'crossing of centiles' on a chart of fetal biometry (see later discussion).

Babies with FGR appear thin, as quantified by the ponderal index (the ratio of body weight to length) and their skin-fold thickness, a measure of subcutaneous fat, is reduced. There is clearly an overlap in the categorisation of small and/or growth-restricted fetuses; a proportion of SGA fetuses will be growth restricted, but the majority will be constitutionally small, that is, genetically determined to be small. Some growth-restricted fetuses will not be SGA, that is, their growth is failing but they do not have a size below the 10th centile.

Aetiology

Fetal growth is determined by the baby's intrinsic genetic potential, which is then modified by various fetal, maternal and placental factors (Box 27.1).

FETAL FACTORS AFFECTING FETAL GROWTH

The genetic make-up of the fetus is the main determinant of its growth and is related to a number of factors, including ethnicity. Asian mothers, for example, have smaller babies than their European counterparts.

BOX 27.1 FACTORS AFFECTING FETAL GROWTH

Fetal Factors
- Genetic—Depends on ethnic background and personal characteristics. Maternal genes are more relevant than paternal genes.
- Chromosomal—Decreased growth in association with fetal aneuploidy
- Fetal anomaly

Maternal Factors
- Pre-pregnancy maternal disease, for example, renal disease, essential hypertension
- Drugs/cigarette smoking
- Maternal disease in pregnancy, for example, pre-eclampsia

Placental Factors
- Adequate/inadequate invasion of maternal spiral arteries
- Adequate/inadequate vascular function

This intrinsic genetic drive to grow is more related to the maternal genome than the genome of the father and involves 'genomic imprinting'. It is well recognised that while large women often have correspondingly large babies, the correlation between large men and the size of their babies is poor.

Many developmentally abnormal fetuses are small, presumably as a result of a decreased intrinsic drive. This is particularly seen with chromosomal abnormalities, for instance, trisomies 18, 13, 21 and triploidy. Small babies are also found in association with structural abnormalities of all of the major organ systems, as well as with fetal infection. These infections include toxoplasmosis, cytomegalovirus and rubella. Worldwide, however, the main association is with malaria.

MATERNAL FACTORS AFFECTING FETAL GROWTH

Small variations in diet do not have a measurable effect on fetal growth, but extreme starvation does cause significant growth impairment. This was observed in the Dutch winter famine of 1944. There is no evidence, however, that food supplementation above a normal diet can improve growth in utero.

Oxygen supply is important. Babies born at high altitude are smaller, presumably as a result of the decreased oxygen content found in the rarefied atmosphere. This is also true of babies born to mothers with chronic hypoxia secondary to congenital heart disease. The fetus is able to partly compensate through placental hypertrophy, but this compensation is incomplete.

Drugs such as tobacco, heroin, cocaine and alcohol may decrease fetal growth. It has been estimated that smoking, for example, will decrease neonatal weight by an average of 150 g. Chronic maternal disease also has a potential adverse effect on fetal growth, particularly if there is renal impairment.

PLACENTAL FACTORS AFFECTING FETAL GROWTH

Adequate placental function depends on adequate trophoblastic invasion. In the first trimester, trophoblast cells invade the maternal spiral arteries in the decidua. In the second trimester, a second wave of trophoblast extends this invasion along the spiral arteries and into the myometrium. This results in the conversion of thick-walled muscular vessels with a relatively high vascular resistance to flaccid thin-walled vessels with a low resistance to flow. In certain conditions, such as pre-eclampsia, it would appear that there has been failure of this secondary trophoblastic invasion, the consequences being subsequent placental ischaemia, atheromatous changes and secondary placental insufficiency. Why this failure should occur is unclear, but it may be related to the immunological interface between the fetal and maternal cells. Impaired trophoblast invasion can be inferred from Doppler studies of the maternal uterine arteries; impaired blood flow is associated with an increased risk of delivering an SGA baby and is an indication for serial ultrasound surveillance of fetal growth (see later discussion).

The overall effect of uteroplacental insufficiency, whatever the cause, is a decrease in the nutrient supply to the fetus. Therefore, it is not surprising that these fetuses are often found to be hypoxic, hypoglycaemic and sometimes acidotic. To compensate for this hypoxia, the fetus increases erythropoiesis in order to increase its oxygen-carrying capacity and redistributes blood away from the peripheral circulation, gut, and liver towards the brain, heart and adrenal glands.

The result is a baby with normal growth in length and brain development, but who is thin and has a reduction in subcutaneous fat. Glycogen stores are minimal. As these babies have relatively large heads compared with their bodies, their growth has previously been described as 'asymmetrical', although the terms 'symmetrical' and 'asymmetrical' are no longer used to describe patterns of fetal growth or neonatal nutritional status.

Screening and Diagnosis

A number of risk factors for delivery of an SGA baby have been identified. Some of these are identifiable at the first visit, whereas others feature only during the course of the pregnancy (Box 27.2). The presence of such a risk factor justifies undertaking serial ultrasound fetal biometry from 26 to 28 weeks onwards in order to diagnose poor fetal growth. However, small babies are often identified following routine clinical examination.

CLINICAL EXAMINATION

Estimation of fetal weight from clinical examination is unreliable. The fundus reaches the umbilicus by around 20 to 24 weeks and the xiphisternum by approximately 36 weeks. The height of the uterine fundus should be measured with a tape measure at each antenatal clinic visit from 26 weeks onwards; the height of the uterus in centimetres, measured from the pubic symphysis, is approximately equal to the gestation in weeks. Symphysis fundal height (SFH) charts facilitate the interpretation of these measurements. An SFH less than the 10th centile or serial SFH

BOX 27.2 RISK FACTORS FOR DELIVERY OF A SMALL-FOR-GESTATIONAL-AGE (SGA) BABY

Available From Maternal History
- Age >40 years
- Smoker >10/day
- Cocaine use
- Previous SGA baby
- Previous stillborn baby
- Chronic hypertension
- Diabetes with vascular disease
- Renal impairment
- Antiphospholipid syndrome

Current Pregnancy Complications or Results
- Threatened miscarriage (heavy bleeding = menstruation)
- Pre-eclampsia
- Placental abruption
- Unexplained antepartum haemorrhage (especially if recurrent)
- Abnormal uterine artery Doppler waveform
- Low level of maternal plasma associated placenta protein-A (PAPP-A; a component of Down syndrome screening)
- Hyperechogenic fetal bowel (usually at the time of fetal anomaly scan)

measurements suggestive of poor growth is an indication for ultrasound fetal biometry.

ULTRASOUND EXAMINATION

Ultrasound is used to establish or refute the diagnosis of fetal SGA or FGR. Certain diagnosis of SGA or FGR can only be made postnatally, but this is of little value to the obstetrician and midwife in planning antenatal care/surveillance. Measurements can be made of the fetal head circumference, the abdominal circumference and the femur length, and equations can be used to calculate estimated fetal weight (EFW). For practical purposes, it is reasonable to consider the abdominal circumference alone, as measurements below the 10th centile have an approximately 80% sensitivity in the prediction of SGA neonates in high-risk pregnancies. Estimating fetal weight is attractive since it is more readily conveyed to and understood by parents. However, caution is required since the percentage error of estimating weight is typically ±15%.

SMALL FOR GESTATIONAL AGE OR FETAL GROWTH RESTRICTION?

This is a key question and one that is not always possible to answer. Those fetuses less than the 10th centile include those who are simply constitutionally small (around 50%–70%) and those who have FGR. The increased risks of stillbirth, birth hypoxia, neonatal complications and impaired neurodevelopment are principally in the FGR group, and it would be beneficial to be able to reliably differentiate between the two groups. The diagnosis of SGA is straightforward, but the diagnosis of FGR less so. Consensus criteria defining FGR have recently been published and include a drop of 50 centiles in EFW and increased resistance in the umbilical artery Doppler waveform (see later discussion). FGR is also diagnosed if a single biometric measurement shows the fetus to be below the third centile. Clinical practice is to plot two or more fetal measurements on a chart of EFW (or abdominal circumference) against gestational age. Examples of such measurements and their interpretation from four fetuses are presented in Fig. 27.1.

A similar but subtly different strategy is to employ charts of fetal size which have been customised or individualised to a specific pregnancy. By calculating a 'term optimal fetal weight' based upon a number of

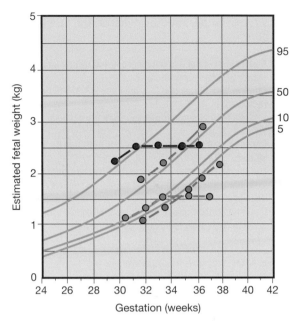

Fig. 27.1 Fetal growth charts. ⊘ The fetus is growing along the 50th centile. ⊘ The fetus is small for gestational age (SGA) but does not have fetal growth restriction (FGR). ◐ The fetus becomes SGA and has FGR. ● The fetus is growth restricted but is not SGA.

easily obtained maternal and pregnancy physiological variables that have an influence upon fetal size—for example, maternal weight, parity and ethnic origin—a customised 'growth' curve with centiles can be produced. This chart will be different for each pregnancy. A fetus with an estimated weight below the 10th centile of a customised chart is more likely to be growth restricted than a fetus that is small based on a population chart.

Once SGA or FGR is diagnosed, it is necessary to evaluate other parameters of fetal well-being, which are considered later. In practice, most fetuses with an abdominal circumference measurement or EFW less than the 10th centile require close observation; whether they have FGR or are SGA (or both) often becomes apparent only in retrospect.

Management

The main principle is to monitor the fetus and deliver at the appropriate time (Box 27.3). No antenatal therapy is of proven benefit. The options for fetal monitoring include fetal movement counting charts, fetal

BOX 27 3 CLINICAL MANAGEMENT OF THE SGA OR FGR FETUS

- Screen with serial ultrasound prompted by risk factors and/or SFH measurements.
- Confirm with ultrasound that the baby is small or growth restricted.
- Exclude fetal abnormality (unless already done at 20-week scan).
- Consider whether the fetus is SGA or FGR. Use Doppler studies.
- Monitor with Doppler studies and CTG as appropriate.
- Consider corticosteroids if <34 weeks and delivery is anticipated.
- Deliver if fetal demise is anticipated; threshold for delivery is strongly influenced by gestation.

CTG, Cardiotocography; *FGR,* fetal growth restriction; *SFH,* symphysis fundal height; *SGA,* small-for-gestational-age.

cardiotocography (CTG), amniotic fluid volume and Doppler blood flow studies. Of these, Doppler flow studies are the most valuable.

FETAL MOVEMENT MONITORING

A poorly nourished fetus will attempt to conserve energy by becoming less active. It is conventional practice to ask the mother about the frequency of perceived fetal movements. Any sudden change in the pattern of movements—reduced fetal movements (RFM)—may be important and should be brought to the attention of the woman's midwife or obstetrician. However, the utility of routine, self-documented formal fetal movement counting is not supported by objective evaluation of its efficacy in reducing perinatal deaths.

CARDIOTOCOGRAPHY (CTG)

The interpretation of CTGs is discussed on page 386. The CTG gives an indication of fetal well-being at a particular moment but has limited longer-term value. CTG interpretation prior to labour is subtly different to interpretation during labour: accelerations of the fetal heart rate and an absence of decelerations are expected in a normal antenatal CTG, whereas they may be absent and/or present, respectively, in a normal intrapartum CTG. Routinely performed CTG recordings are interpreted by obstetric and midwifery staff, whereas computerised CTG involves automated analysis of the CTG pattern and will determine whether the

CTG is normal or abnormal using prespecified criteria (the Dawes Redman criteria, which analyse baseline heart rate, short-term variability long-term variability, accelerations and decelerations). The computerised analysis evaluates the data every 2 minutes until all criteria are met or until 60 minutes is reached, at which point the CTG will be labelled as abnormal. In the context of pre-term FGR, computerised CTG analysis, in combination with fetal arterial Doppler studies, is more effective than visual CTG analysis in preventing fetal death.

The routine use of antenatal CTG is not associated with an improved perinatal outcome; thus, antenatal CTG monitoring should be restricted to specific indications, such as in the presence of RFM.

AMNIOTIC FLUID VOLUME

Redistribution of blood flow within the fetal circulation as a response to hypoxia results in reduced perfusion of the fetal kidneys, a reduction in fetal micturition and reduced amniotic fluid volume (oligohydramnios). In the absence of ruptured membranes, reduced amniotic fluid volume identified by ultrasound is characteristic of FGR.

Using ultrasound, amniotic fluid volume is described by either measuring the maximum vertical pool (MVP) of fluid or by adding together the MVP of each quadrant of the uterus to generate the amniotic fluid index (AFI).

DOPPLER ULTRASOUND

Doppler ultrasound of the umbilical artery is used as an assessment of 'downstream' placental vascular resistance. A normal waveform (described by semi-quantitative pulsatility or resistance indices) indicates that an SGA fetus is constitutionally small rather than growth restricted because of impaired placental function. Reduction or loss of end-diastolic flow identifies a fetus at high risk of hypoxia, and absent end-diastolic flow (AEDF) is a useful discriminator between those growth-restricted fetuses at high risk of perinatal death and those at a lower risk (Fig. 27.2). The use of umbilical artery Doppler to monitor high-risk fetuses reduces perinatal morbidity and mortality.

Doppler studies of the fetal cerebral circulation can also provide additional useful information, particularly in the term fetus (Fig. 27.3). As the

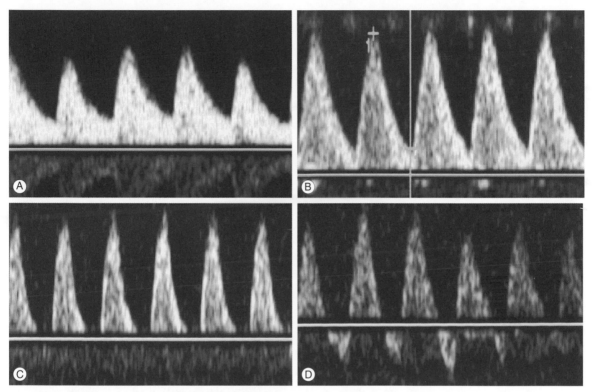

Fig. 27.2 Doppler ultrasound of the umbilical cord demonstrating normal (A), reduced (B), absent (C) and reversed end-diastolic flow (D). Absent and reversed end-diastolic flow are associated with fetal compromise of placental origin.

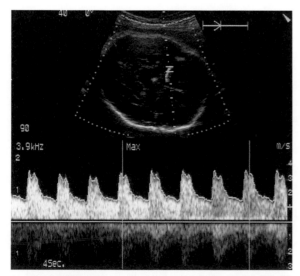

Fig. 27.3 In fetal growth restriction, there is an increased flow in the middle cerebral artery.

growth-restricted fetus redistributes its blood flow away from the less vital organs towards the brain in response to hypoxia, it is reasonable to expect an increased cerebral flow. This is indeed observed to happen, with Doppler studies showing a decreased resistance of the middle cerebral artery. As the hypoxia becomes more severe, this resistance increases again, possibly secondary to cerebral oedema. Doppler examination of the fetal venous circulation provides useful information when considering the timing of delivery. Doppler signals from the ductus venosus (a vein within the fetal liver) can be used to indirectly interpret the function of the right side of the fetal heart. Abnormal ductus venosus waveforms herald fetal demise.

The typical sequence of changes observed with progressive fetal hypoxia is impaired growth, abnormal umbilical artery waveform, increased cerebral blood flow, abnormal ductus venosus flow followed very

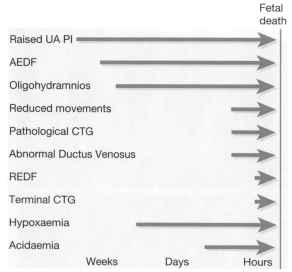

Fig. 27.4 The 'decompensation cascade' of fetal growth restriction. Absent end-diastolic flow (AEDF) is a relatively early sign of hypoxaemia, with reduced fetal movements, cardiotocographic abnormalities and reversed end-diastolic flow (REDF) late features. *UA PI,* Umbilical artery pulsatility index.

closely by an abnormal fetal heart rate pattern, and fetal demise. The rate of deterioration in fetal condition is unpredictable and this sequence of changes is not always observed. However, it does permit the development of a strategy for the management of the SGA/FGR fetus.

OVERALL STRATEGY

Fig. 27.4 illustrates the probable sequence of events in fetal decompensation. As umbilical artery Doppler abnormalities are the first to appear, it is logical to use Doppler as the main screening tool. Thereafter, the optimal surveillance strategy in fetuses with absent or reduced end-diastolic flow involves frequent monitoring with CTG and Doppler studies of fetal vessels. The timing of the delivery will be decided by balancing the risks of keeping the baby in utero against the risks of prematurity, but delivery is appropriate when the CTG becomes pathological, there is AEDF in the umbilical artery with abnormal ductus venosus flow, or there is reversal of end-diastolic flow. If FGR is suspected before 34 weeks and delivery is anticipated, it is appropriate to administer corticosteroids to the mother to enhance fetal lung maturation.

BOX 27.4 CLINICAL SIGNIFICANCE OF FETAL GROWTH RESTRICTION

Increased chance of:
- Perinatal death, including stillbirth
- Perinatal asphyxia
- Operative birth
- Neonatal hypoglycaemia and hypocalcaemia
- Necrotizing enterocolitis
- Long-term handicap
- Type 2 diabetes and coronary artery disease in adult life

One strategy for the outpatient management of women with an SGA pregnancy is presented in Fig. 27.5.

The mode of delivery depends on the individual circumstances, but it must be remembered that the placental reserve of some of these fetuses may be extremely low and careful monitoring in labour is required. Early recourse to caesarean section is appropriate if the monitoring shows signs of fetal compromise. Pre-labour caesarean section may be appropriate if there are significant concerns about fetal well-being, particularly if there is absent or reversed flow in the umbilical artery Doppler waveform.

Long-Term Implications of Fetal Growth Restriction

Babies exposed to FGR are at increased risk of perinatal mortality, including stillbirth (Box 27.4). Antenatal or intrapartum hypoxia may lead to long-term neurological handicap, as may more acute intrapartum hypoxia. Even if there is no overt evidence of handicap, studies of long-term development suggest that growth-restricted fetuses may be more clumsy and that their IQ may be 5 to 10 points lower than a normally grown sibling.

There is also evidence to suggest that FGR predisposes babies to problems much later in life, particularly type 2 diabetes and coronary heart disease. It may be that the fetus alters its metabolism to cope with poor nutrition in utero and is subsequently less able to cope with normal carbohydrate levels in later postnatal life. It is also possible that there are vascular compensatory changes with FGR that predispose to later arterial disease.

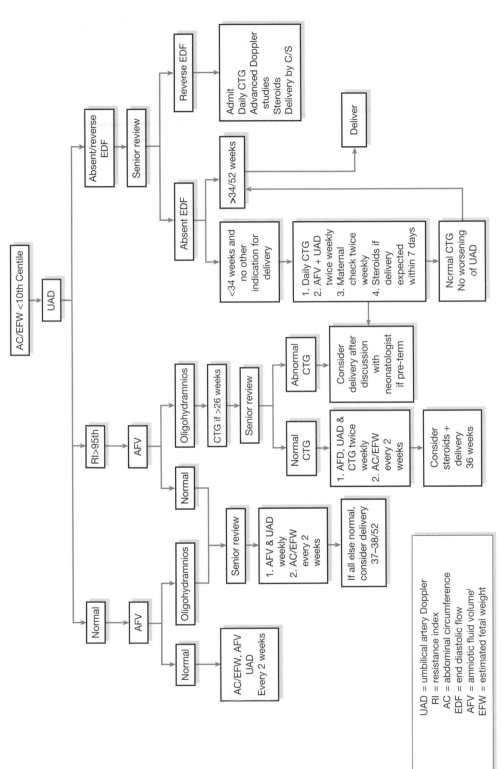

Fig. 27.5 Flowchart for the management of a small-for-gestational-age fetus.

Key Points

- An accurate estimation of gestation is a prerequisite to the accurate diagnosis of fetal growth abnormality.
- SGA refers to those fetuses whose estimated weight is <10th centile for their gestational age. Most SGA fetuses are healthy.
- FGR refers to any fetus failing to achieve its growth potential. Not all SGA fetuses are growth restricted and not all growth-restricted fetuses are SGA. FGR carries an increased risk of intrapartum asphyxia, neonatal hypoglycaemia and possible long-term neurological impairment. There is also an increased risk of perinatal mortality.
- Diagnosis of FGR requires at least two ultrasound scans at least 3 weeks apart. The use of customised or individualised charts of fetal size more reliably differentiates between the SGA and FGR fetus.
- Successful management involves appropriate monitoring, with expedited delivery as necessary.

Chapter 28

Hypertension in Pregnancy

Laura I. Stirrat

Chapter Outline

Hypertensive disorders of pregnancy are responsible for over 60,000 maternal deaths worldwide annually. Both maternal and neonatal morbidity and mortality are increased in pregnancies complicated by hypertension, including chronic hypertension and pre-eclampsia. There is significant personal cost to families affected by the disease and economic implications for the health service.

Women who are hypertensive and pregnant may be subdivided into those with chronic pre-existing hypertension or those with pregnancy-induced hypertension (PIH). Women with PIH (also known as 'gestational hypertension') can be classified further; the majority have non-proteinuric PIH, a condition associated with less maternal or perinatal sequelae if pre-eclampsia does not develop before delivery, whereas a minority have the major pregnancy complication of pre-eclampsia, historically known as 'toxaemia of pregnancy', (PET).

Definitions

HYPERTENSION

Threshold values of ≥140 mmHg systolic or 90 mmHg diastolic blood pressure define hypertension in pregnancy (Fig. 28.1), with blood pressure ≥160 mmHg systolic or ≥110 mmHg diastolic described as severe hypertension.

CHRONIC HYPERTENSION

Chronic hypertension is defined as:
- The presence of hypertension before 20 weeks' gestation (in the absence of a hydatidiform mole) or
- Persistent hypertension beyond 6 weeks postpartum.

Chronic hypertension may be further subclassified into:
1. Chronic hypertension (without proteinuria)
2. Chronic renal disease (proteinuria with or without hypertension)
3. Chronic hypertension with superimposed preeclampsia (new-onset proteinuria)

GESTATIONAL HYPERTENSION

Gestational hypertension may be classified into:
1. Gestational hypertension (without proteinuria)
2. Gestational proteinuria (without hypertension)
3. Gestational proteinuric hypertension (preeclampsia).

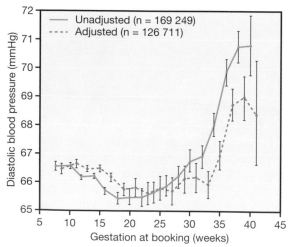

Fig. 28.1 Maternal diastolic blood pressure measurements throughout pregnancy.

PRE-ECLAMPSIA

The definition of pre-eclampsia was revised in 2014 to reflect the multisystem nature of the condition and is defined as hypertension developing after 20 weeks' gestation with one or more of the following: proteinuria, maternal organ dysfunction or fetal growth restriction. This new definition means that proteinuria is no longer essential for diagnosis.

Potential forms of maternal organ dysfunction include:
- Renal insufficiency (creatinine >90 µmol/L)
- Liver involvement (elevated transaminases—at least twice the upper limit of normal ± right upper quadrant or epigastric abdominal pain)
- Neurological complications (examples include eclampsia, altered mental status, blindness, stroke or, more commonly, hyperreflexia when accompanied by clonus, severe headaches when accompanied by hyperreflexia, persistent visual scotomata)
- Haematological complications (thrombocytopenia—platelet count below 150,000/dL, disseminated intravascular coagulation, haemolysis).

ECLAMPSIA

Eclampsia is a complication of severe PET, affecting 5 in 1000 pregnancies, and is characterised by convulsions that cannot be attributed to a primary neurological problem (e.g., epilepsy, cerebral infarction, tumour cerebral infection, or ruptured aneurysm). Forty-four percent of eclamptic seizures occur in the postpartum period. There are significant risks of both maternal and neonatal morbidity and mortality. Neurological complications include focal motor deficits, coma, cortical blindness and cerebral haemorrhage.

Pathophysiology

PHASE 1: ABNORMAL PLACENTATION

Placentation occurs between 6 and 18 weeks' gestation. During normal placental development, major structural alterations of the spiral arteries occur, allowing an increase in blood supply to the placenta. Trophoblast invasion of the maternal spiral arteries causes the diameter of these arteries to increase approximately five-fold, converting a high-resistance, low-flow system to one with a low resistance and high flow. In women who develop pre-eclampsia, there is inadequate trophoblast invasion, resulting in inadequate or deranged placental perfusion.

During early pregnancy, trophoblast invasion is regulated at the maternal decidual barrier by the action of factors expressed within the decidua and on the trophoblast cells. These regulatory factors include cell adhesion molecules and the extracellular matrix, proteinases and their inhibitors, growth factors and cytokines. Underlying genetic and immunological abnormalities may result in abnormalities in any one of these factors.

It has been suggested that the primary factor in the aetiology of pre-eclampsia is immunological in origin. Abnormal placentation may be the result of maternal immune rejection of paternal antigens expressed by the fetus. For example, women who develop pre-eclampsia appear to have an extra-villous trophoblast that does not express human leucocyte antigen G. The predominance of pre-eclampsia in first pregnancies and the protective effect of parity further support an immunological mechanism for the condition.

PHASE 2: ENDOTHELIAL DYSFUNCTION

The second phase of pre-eclampsia is characterised by widespread endothelial damage and dysfunction. This is likely to be mediated through oxidative stress originating from the ischaemic placenta. Women with pre-eclampsia have increased circulating levels of markers of endothelial dysfunction. Endothelial damage promotes platelet adhesion and thrombosis and disturbs the normal physiological modulation of vascular tone, further amplifying the response. This phase of pre-eclampsia is characterised by an exaggerated maternal systemic inflammatory response, with associated activation of leucocytes, platelets and the coagulation system.

There is a relative deficiency of prostacyclin, which is a vasodilator. This occurs either because of reduced prostacyclin synthesis or because of an increased production of thromboxane A_2 (a vasoconstrictor with a tendency to promote platelet aggregation). This imbalance leads to platelet stimulation as well as vasoconstriction and hypertension. Aspirin may reduce risks by redressing this imbalance.

Epidemiology of Hypertensive Disorders in Pregnancy

Hypertension is the most common medical problem encountered in pregnancy, complicating 10% to 15% of pregnancies. Pre-existing or chronic hypertension is one of the most common conditions in women of childbearing age and is becoming more prevalent due to increasing maternal age and increased prevalence of obesity. Chronic hypertension is estimated to affect 1% to 5% of pregnant women and is frequently diagnosed for the first time during antenatal care.

The prevalence of pre-eclampsia varies with the definition used and the population studied; however, pre-eclampsia occurs in less than 5% of an average antenatal population. The incidence of non-proteinuric PIH is approximately three times greater.

The World Health Organization (WHO) reports the prevalence of eclampsia globally to be 0.6%. In the United Kingdom, the incidence of eclampsia has been steadily declining, with a reduction of over 90% observed since the 1920s, related to improved detection and management of hypertensive pregnancies. Risks of serious adverse maternal and perinatal outcomes are high among women with eclampsia. In areas with low maternal mortality, the case-fatality rate is below 1%, but severe maternal complications (such as coma, stroke and acute respiratory distress) occur in 10% to 30% of cases, with 5% to 8% of pregnancies resulting in a perinatal loss.

Chronic Hypertension

The cause of primary hypertension is considered to be multifactorial, with both genetic and environmental contributions. Secondary hypertension is identified in less than 5% of the general population but has been shown to be present in 14% of women of childbearing age. Renal disease is the most common cause of secondary hypertension in pregnancy. Chronic kidney disease affects up to 3% of women aged 20 to 39 years and pregnancy may be the first time it is identified.

HISTORY AND EXAMINATION

The majority of women will be asymptomatic. However, a careful history for end organ damage and potential underlying aetiology should be taken. Questioning about late enuresis and recurrent urinary tract infections in childhood may suggest reflux nephropathy, and a detailed family history may confirm a genetic basis for primary hypertension or identify familial renal disease. Paroxysmal or severe hypertension associated with headache and sweating or palpitations may be indicative of a phaeochromocytoma, which can be fatal in pregnancy if missed.

Examination should include fundoscopy to identify hypertensive retinopathy and assessment for radio-femoral delay (coarctation of the aorta). Other findings may include enlarged kidneys (polycystic kidneys), a renal bruit (renal artery stenosis) and clinical features of endocrine disease (e.g., hyperthyroidism, tachycardia, goitre, proptosis). Some of these conditions may have genetic or endocrine implications for the fetus.

Investigations

Any woman of childbearing age identified to have chronic hypertension should have confirmation with 24-hour ambulatory monitoring and should be investigated for end organ damage, including an echocardiogram to assess for left ventricular hypertrophy and assessment of renal function and proteinuria. Referral for investigation for secondary causes should be made to an appropriate specialist depending on local expertise and interest (e.g., nephrology, clinical pharmacology, cardiology and endocrinology).

Chronic Kidney Disease

The most common causes of renal disease in women of childbearing age are reflux nephropathy, lupus nephritis, immunoglobulin A nephropathy and autosomal-dominant polycystic kidney disease (ADPKD), although hypertensive nephropathy and obesity-related focal segmental glomerulosclerosis are becoming increasingly common. Women with reflux nephropathy and ADPKD may have affected family members but both conditions can also occur spontaneously.

Endocrine

Many endocrine disorders are associated with hypertension. The most common is hyperthyroidism in women of childbearing age. A careful clinical history and examination may identify features of other conditions, including primary hyperparathyroidism, phaeochromocytoma, carcinoid and acromegaly.

MANAGEMENT

Pre-Pregnancy Counselling

Pre-pregnancy counselling is essential for all women with chronic hypertension in order to optimise their hypertensive control, to plan switching from teratogenic medication to alternative agents and inform women about potential complications in the pregnancy. Women should be advised that statin and fibrate treatment should be stopped before or at conception.

In addition, exacerbating factors can be addressed with lifestyle adaptation, such as weight loss, reduced alcohol intake, a low-salt diet and exercise. Smoking cessation should be recommended for all smokers.

Regarding treatment for chronic hypertension, some drugs that are commonly used in the non-pregnant (such as angiotensin-converting enzyme inhibitors) are best avoided as they have adverse fetal effects. The agents commonly used, labetalol and methyldopa, are outlined in Table 28.1. The dose of a single agent should be maximised before introduction of a second agent.

TABLE 28.1	Drug Treatment of Hypertension in Pregnancy		
Drug	**Action**	**Side Effects**	**Comments**
Methyldopa (oral)	Central acting	Initial drowsiness	Safe; slow onset of action. Not suitable if history of depression.
Labetalol (oral/intra-venous [IV])	Alpha- and beta-antagonist	Postural hypotension, tiredness	Widely used in antenatal setting (oral) and hypertensive crisis (IV)
Hydralazine (oral/IV)	Direct-acting vasodilator	Precipitate; precipitates hypotension	Widely used in hypertensive crisis (IV)
Nifedipine (oral/sub-lingual)	Calcium-channel antagonist	Flushing, headaches	Caution—interacts with magnesium sulphate. Watch for precipitous fall in blood pressure

All women with essential hypertension should be advised to take 100 to 150 mg aspirin from 12 weeks until delivery in order to reduce the risk of pre-eclampsia.

Maternal Complications

The incidence of superimposed pre-eclampsia in women with chronic hypertension is approximately 20% but can be higher in women with secondary hypertension. Women with chronic hypertension may have undetectable renal damage that is only revealed by pregnancy. Therefore, a quantitative assessment of proteinuria should be performed at booking for comparison in later pregnancy.

Superimposed pre-eclampsia may be difficult to distinguish from physiological changes, but the following features are suggestive of the condition:

- A rapid rise in hypertension
- New onset or doubling of proteinuria
- Other laboratory parameters, for example, low platelets, or raised liver enzymes or creatinine.

Timing of Delivery

Pre-term delivery, often iatrogenic, is more common in women with chronic hypertension compared with the general population. Timing of delivery should be guided by the severity of hypertension and the presence of proteinuria and fetal compromise, and balanced against the risks of prematurity at lower gestations. UK guidelines suggest that delivery for women with chronic hypertension should be managed as for women with gestational hypertension or, if proteinuria is present, then as for pre-eclampsia.

Neonatal Complications

Neonatal complications are also more commonly reported for women with chronic hypertension than normotensive women, including higher rates of perinatal mortality, fetal growth restriction and admission to neonatal special care units.

Postpartum Management

Peak postpartum blood pressure usually occurs at 3 to 5 days. It is recommended that women with chronic hypertension should continue to have their blood pressure measured postpartum, and treatment titrated to keep blood pressure lower than 140/90 mmHg.

Women with previously diagnosed chronic hypertension can be discharged when their blood pressure is stable and <140/90 mmHg or <150/100 mmHg with treatment. All women with chronic hypertension should be offered a medical review 6 to 8 weeks after delivery for future pre-pregnancy counselling.

It is recommended that estrogen-containing contraceptives be avoided in women with hypertension due to their potential to exacerbate sodium retention and hypertension.

Gestational Hypertension and Pre-Eclampsia

RISK FACTORS

More than a third of pre-eclampsia occurs in women with risk factors – not recognising risk accounts for a considerable amount of substandard care in maternal deaths. Distinguishing at-risk women allows administration of antiplatelet agents (100–150 mg aspirin) prior to 16 weeks' gestation, which appears to reduce the incidence of pre-eclampsia by 15%, particularly reducing earlier presentations of the syndrome. Recognised risk factors for gestational hypertension and pre-eclampsia are shown in Box 28.1.

One of the strongest risk factors for development of pre-eclampsia is a history of the disease in previous

BOX 28.1 PREDISPOSING FACTORS FOR DEVELOPING GESTATIONAL HYPERTENSION/PRE-ECLAMPSIA

- First pregnancy
- Family history—mother/sister
- Extremes of maternal age
- Obesity
- Medical factors:
  - Pre-existing hypertension
  - Renal disease
  - Acquired thrombophilia—antiphospholipid antibodies
  - Inherited thrombophilia
  - Connective tissue disease (e.g., systemic lupus erythematosus)
  - Diabetes mellitus
- Obstetric factors:
  - Multiple pregnancy
  - Previous pre-eclampsia
  - Hydatidiform mole
  - Triploidy
  - Hydrops fetalis (immune and non-immune)
  - Inter-pregnancy interval of >10 years

pregnancies, particularly those requiring delivery before 37 weeks, resulting in a 20% chance of developing pre-eclampsia again. A family history in a first-degree relative increases the risk of pre-eclampsia four- to eight-fold, illustrating the strong genetic influence.

A woman has double the risk of pre-eclampsia if pregnant by a partner who had previously fathered an affected pregnancy. This indicates the immunological element to the disease process, in which there is an effect of exposure to the paternal antigen via either the fetus or the partner. Pre-eclampsia occurs more commonly in first pregnancies; miscarriages or terminations of pregnancy provide some reduction in risk in subsequent pregnancies. A new partner increases risk, whereas non-barrier methods of contraception and increased duration of sexual cohabitation reduce risk. It is sustained exposure to a partner's protective 'foreign' antigens that links these risk factors. Teenage mothers and pregnancies conceived by donor insemination have an increased risk of pre-eclampsia, presumably due to the lack of exposure.

Underlying medical disorders, particularly those involving vascular disease such as chronic hypertension, increase the risk of pre-eclampsia (to >20%). All forms of glucose intolerance, including gestational diabetes, are associated with an increased risk. This may be related to obesity, which is an independent risk factor. Other maternal risk factors include chronic kidney disease and autoimmune disorders. Women with antiphospholipid syndrome and multiple pregnancies are at increased risk. Risk may be related to the size of the placenta; molar pregnancies have been associated with pre-eclampsia, as have pregnancies complicated by hydrops fetalis (mirror syndrome) or trisomy chromosomal complement.

Other moderate risk factors include first pregnancy, age 40 years or more, a pregnancy interval greater than 10 years, body mass index of 35 kg/m² or more, polycystic ovarian syndrome, vitamin D deficiency and multiple pregnancy. Low dietary calcium and low serum calcium concentrations are associated with pre-eclampsia, although the role of calcium in preventing pre-eclampsia remains controversial.

CLINICAL ASSESSMENT

Women may have raised blood pressure during their pregnancy or up to 6 weeks postpartum. Full clinical

---

BOX 28.2 SIGNS AND SYMPTOMS OF PRE-ECLAMPSIA

Symptoms of Pre-Eclampsia

Severe headache	Visual disturbances,
Severe right upper quadrant and epigastric abdominal pain	including blurring, flashing or scotoma
	Vomiting
Sudden swelling of the face, hands or feet	Restlessness or agitation

Signs of Pre-Eclampsia

Hypertension and proteinuria	Clonus
	Haemolytic anaemia
Hyperreflexia	Elevated liver enzymes
Serum creatinine raised	Retinal haemorrhages
Platelet count decreased	and papilloedema

---

assessment is important to differentiate between the hypertensive disorders of pregnancy and determine severity. There are many non-specific symptoms and signs that are important indicators of widespread multisystem involvement. These symptoms may herald the onset of severe pre-eclampsia (Box 28.2).

When women have the presenting symptom of hypertension, both gestational age and previous pregnancy history are important factors in establishing risk of progression to pre-eclampsia. Late-onset hypertension after 37 weeks' gestation rarely results in serious morbidity to mother or baby. However, prophylactic delivery may be justified and induction of labour does not result in an increased risk of caesarean section. In cases of pre-eclampsia, delivery at 37 weeks' gestation is routinely recommended. However, in those who develop early-onset gestational hypertension, particularly before 28 weeks, almost half will develop pre-eclampsia.

1. *Blood Pressure Measurement (Fig. 28.2A)*

Care in assessing blood pressure will prevent misdiagnosis; blood pressure measurement is poorly performed in clinical practice. The antenatal population within the United Kingdom has a significant proportion of obese women. The standard bladder used in sphygmomanometer cuffs (23 × 12 cm) is too small for about a quarter of the antenatal population, resulting in the over-diagnosis of hypertension, usually by more than 10 mmHg. Automated 'oscillometric' devices often under-read the true blood pressure in pre-eclampsia; thus, only those shown to be specifically

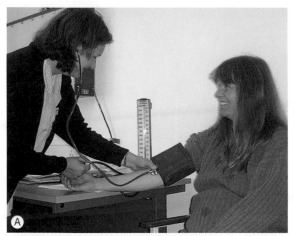

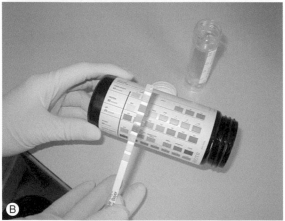

Fig. 28.2 Early detection of pre-eclampsia is important. (A) Measurement of blood pressure. **(B)** Testing for urinary protein.

accurate in pregnancy should be used. Otherwise, Korotkoff sounds by a trained observer should be used for decision-making. Repeating the blood pressure readings or obtaining a series of readings in the day unit will limit the over-diagnosis of hypertension. Uncontrollable blood pressure may indicate need for urgent delivery.

2. Urine Tests (Fig. 28.2B)

Assessing for proteinuria, typically by dipstick of a midstream urine sample, is a routine screening tool that should be performed at each clinical interaction with all pregnant women. Urinary protein excretion is considered abnormal in pregnant women when it exceeds 30 mL/dL, a level that usually correlates with 1+ on a

urine dipstick. However, errors in the interpretation of proteinuria are common with dipstick urine analysis, as false positives may be caused by dehydration, contamination of samples after ruptured membranes or certain medications. False negatives may occur due to dilutional effects of drinking and overhydration. The gold standard confirmation of the diagnosis would be 24-hour collection of urine (with >300 mg proteinuria in 24 hours being considered elevated). However, this is not routinely performed in most cases. Albumin:creatinine ratio (ACR) and protein:creatinine ratio (PCR) are commonly used in clinical practice to quantify urinary protein, with 30 mg/mmol used as a threshold for significant proteinuria.

3. Blood Tests

In addition to blood pressure and proteinuria, pre-eclampsia has significant effects on other organs (Table 28.2).

Uric acid has been used in the past to detect pre-eclampsia but is not reliable. Spuriously high levels of uric acid are associated with acute fatty liver of pregnancy. Aspartate transaminase (AST) and other transaminases indicate hepatocellular damage and should be checked routinely. It should be remembered that the normal range for transaminases is approximately 20% lower than the non-pregnant range.

When liver involvement is associated with haemolysis and low platelets, this is known as HELLP (*h*aemolysis, *e*levated *l*iver enzymes and *l*ow *p*latelets) syndrome, which is a severe variant of pre-eclampsia and will require urgent delivery. If proteinuria excretion is high (usually >3 g/24 h), circulating albumin may fall, increasing the risk of pulmonary oedema. A

TABLE 28.2 **Blood Test Investigations in Pre-Eclampsia**	
Investigation	Finding in pre-eclampsia
Full blood count	Reduced platelets, reduced haemo-globin, haemolysis on blood film
Renal function	Reduced urine output
	Increased urate, increased urea, increased creatinine
Coagulation system	Prolonged coagulation indices
Hepatic system	Elevated alanine transaminase and aspartate transaminase

raised AST can be associated with either haemolysis or liver involvement, lactate dehydrogenase levels are also elevated in the presence of haemolysis.

If delivery or induction of labour is likely to be imminent, or if the platelet count is low, it is also sensible to screen for clotting abnormalities. Pre-eclampsia can cause disseminated intravascular coagulation, and clotting must be adequate for regional anaesthesia.

A low albumin, low platelet count or clotting derangement may indicate urgent need for delivery, as the disease of pre-eclampsia is progressive and the only cure is removing the placenta.

4. Fetal Assessment

Fetal well-being must be carefully considered in all cases, particularly with early-onset disease. A symphysis fundal height should be carefully measured in all women who present with pre-eclampsia in addition to discussing patterns of fetal movements. At early gestations, or in pregnancies with suspected growth restriction, it is usual to confirm fetal growth with ultrasound and to assess the amniotic fluid volume and umbilical artery Doppler waveform. When fetal compromise is detected, urgent delivery is important to prevent fetal demise.

5. Prediction of Pre-Eclampsia

Research focusing on the prediction of pre-eclampsia has identified both ultrasonographic markers and biomarkers that may help identify at-risk women.

Ultrasonographic

Doppler velocimetry to assess impedance of uteroplacental flow in pregnancies complicated by pre-eclampsia was described in the 1980s. A more recent meta-analysis study reported that the uterine artery pulsatility index with notching in the second trimester predicted pre-eclampsia. As the disorder originates in the placenta, blood flow in the uterine artery is abnormal in most women destined to present with the syndrome (Fig. 28.3).

Biomarkers

Angiogenic factors such as placental growth factor (PlGF) levels and soluble fms-like tyrosine kinase 1(sFlt-1) have a role in identifying pre-eclampsia. PlGF promotes placental vascular development and sFlt-1 can cause vasconstriction. Low levels of PlGF and high

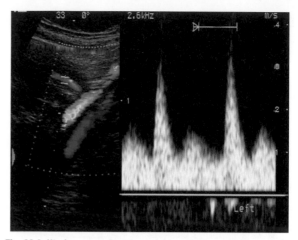

Fig. 28.3 Uterine artery Doppler notching at 24 weeks is predictive of pre-eclampsia and fetal growth restriction in high-risk mothers.

levels of sFlt-1 have been shown to predict PET such that in the United Kingdom, the National Institute for Health and Care Excellence (NICE) recommends use of PlGF and the sFlt-1/PlGF ratio, in conjunction with standard clinical assessment, to help rule out PET in suspected cases between 20 weeks and 34+6 weeks.

PlGF measurements have also been shown to reduce the time to diagnosis from 4.1 days to 1.9 days. This may improve outcomes, particularly at preterm gestations, by allowing more time for administration of steroids to accelerate fetal lung maturation or facilitating in utero transfer to a unit with neonatal intensive care capability if earlier delivery is anticipated.

Further research is required for use of both angiogenic markers and uterine artery Doppler to predict and 'rule-in' PET.

Prophylaxis

Various preventive strategies have been employed in women considered to be at risk of developing pre-eclampsia (Box 28.3).

Aspirin inhibits prostaglandin synthesis via cyclooxygenase, and the dose of aspirin required to inhibit thromboxane synthesis is less than that required for prostacyclin inhibition. Low-dose aspirin should reduce the vascular and prothrombotic effects of thromboxane A_2 in women at risk of developing pre-eclampsia. Taking 100 to 150 mg aspirin daily from 12 weeks' gestation leads to a 15% reduction in the incidence of pre-eclampsia.

BOX 28.3 PREVENTION OF PRE-ECLAMPSIA

Proven to be of Value
- Low-dose aspirin

Possibly of Value
- Calcium supplementation

Not of Value
- Diet with high protein content
- Restriction of salt in diet
- Restriction of weight gain
- Vitamins C and E

Restriction of salt intake and limiting weight gain during pregnancy are not useful.

Clinical Management of Hypertension in Pregnancy Without Proteinuria

If the maternal blood pressure is found to be elevated, measurement should be repeated after 10 to 20 minutes. If it settles, and there are no other signs or symptoms of pre-eclampsia, no further action is needed. If still elevated, further assessment is required, ideally at an antenatal daycare unit.

In the absence of severe hypertension (blood pressure ≥160/110 mmHg), significant proteinuria or symptoms of pre-eclampsia, and with normal biochemistry and haematology results, the woman can usually be managed as an outpatient. She should be seen at least twice weekly for blood pressure and urinalysis checks. Serum biochemistry and haematology should also be repeated at least once a week. The woman should be advised to return to hospital if she feels unwell or if there is any headache, visual disturbance or epigastric pain.

Treatment of the woman with antihypertensive drugs controls the hypertension but does not alter the course of pre-eclampsia. Treatment of hypertension may allow prolongation of the pregnancy and thereby may indirectly improve fetal outcome. Antihypertensive treatment should be commenced with consistent blood pressure recordings of ≥140/90 mmHg.

CLINICAL MANAGEMENT OF PRE-ECLAMPSIA

In a woman with pre-eclampsia, it is important to consider the overall picture rather than make decisions on the basis of a single parameter. Progression of the disease is not consistent; thus, further management should be tailored to the individual woman.

All women with pre-eclampsia should be admitted at initial diagnosis for assessment, as the condition may progress aggressively or follow a longer time course.

The aim should be to prolong the pregnancy in order to reduce the risk to the baby, but this must be balanced against the risks to the mother. The only true 'cure' for pre-eclampsia is delivery of the fetus and placenta.

The decision to deliver and the method of delivery are dependent on many factors. There are usually fetal advantages to conservative management before 34 weeks if the blood pressure, laboratory values and fetal condition are stable.

The principles of management of pre-eclampsia follow.
- *Control the maternal blood pressure.* Reduce the diastolic blood pressure to <100 mmHg using labetalol, nifedipine, hydralazine or methyldopa (Table 28.2). Effective control of hypertension is essential to prevent cerebrovascular accidents. As intracerebral haemorrhage contributes to a significant proportion of deaths, systolic blood pressure should always be <150 mmHg and treated aggressively if not. Labetalol is now recommended as first-line treatment. Regimens vary, but NICE guidelines now recommend a standard approach to hypertensive management.
- *Assess maternal fluid balance.* Pre-eclampsia is associated with an increased vascular permeability and a reduced intravascular compartment. In women with pre-eclampsia, administering too little fluid risks maternal renal failure and giving too much fluid may cause pulmonary oedema. Therefore, fluid input and urine output should be monitored. In severe pre-eclampsia, the maternal oxygen saturation (SaO_2) should also be monitored, along with serum urea and electrolytes, liver function tests, haemoglobin, haematocrit, platelets and coagulation. If there is marked oliguria, central venous pressure monitoring may be helpful to differentiate intravascular volume depletion from renal impairment.
- *Prevent seizures (eclampsia).* The use of magnesium sulphate ($MgSO_4$) in severe pre-eclampsia halves the risk of subsequent eclampsia and may reduce the risk of maternal death. $MgSO_4$ given to those who have had an eclamptic seizure prevents further seizures.

- *Consider delivery.* The timing of this depends on the maternal condition, fetal condition and gestational age. Maternal indications for delivery include gestation ≥37 weeks, an inability to control hypertension, deteriorating liver or renal function, progressive fall in platelets or neurological complications. Fetal indications include abnormal fetal heart rate monitoring or a fetal condition that is clearly deteriorating. If pre-term delivery is being considered at <34 weeks' gestation, corticosteroids should be administered to the mother to reduce the risks associated with prematurity unless there is acute compromise requiring immediate delivery.
- *To optimise postnatal care.* Women with pre-eclampsia who remain hypertensive in the initial postpartum period are still at risk of pre-eclampsia-related complications, particularly for the initial 72 hours following delivery when the blood pressure often peaks. Continued vigilance is advisable during this period, as an inpatient if necessary.

COMPLICATIONS

Complications of pre-eclampsia involve several organs and the clotting system (Box 28.4), with the most common complication being compromised placental blood supply leading to fetal growth restriction (Fig. 28.4), fetal hypoxia or intrauterine death. Additionally, since the successful management of pre-eclampsia revolves

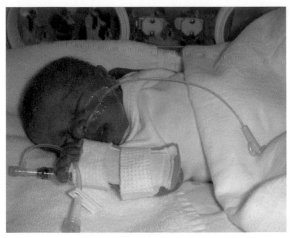

Fig. 28.4 This baby, born at 36 weeks to a mother with severe pre-eclampsia, weighed 1.6 kg. The usual weight at 36 weeks is 2.2 to 3.3 kg.

around delivery, prematurity and its related problems are more common among babies born to mothers with pre-eclampsia.

HELLP syndrome (which affects 10%–20% of eclamptic pregnancies) is defined by the presence of haemolysis, elevated liver enzymes and a low platelet count. Associated morbidity commonly includes disseminated intravascular coagulation, placental abruption and acute renal failure. It is also associated with maternal mortality in between 1.1% and 25% of cases (with the most common causes of mortality being haemorrhage and stroke).

Eclampsia is a less common complication, considered to complicate approximately 1% of pregnancies with pre-eclampsia, although this rate is higher in low-resource settings. It occurs when tonic-clonic seizures (not attributable to other causes) complicate pre-existing hypertensive disease of pregnancy. The management of eclampsia is outlined in Box 28.5.

A diagnosis of pre-eclampsia usually has no long-term serious sequelae. However, it rarely may result in a range of complications with significant long-term implications on the mother, such as liver rupture, stroke, pulmonary oedema or kidney failure. Furthermore, the diagnosis may have future implications on the management of the health of the mother, as a history of pre-eclampsia is a risk factor for future cardiac disease and stroke.

BOX 28.4 COMPLICATIONS OF PRE-ECLAMPSIA

Maternal

Placental rupture	Eclampsia
Disseminated intravascular coagulation	Liver failure or haemorrhage
	Stroke
	Death
HELLP syndrome	Long-term cardiovascular morbidity
Pulmonary oedema	
Aspiration	

Neonatal

Pre-term delivery	Perinatal death
Intrauterine growth restriction	Long-term cardiovascular morbidity (associated with low birth weight)
Hypoxia-neurological injury	

HELLP, Haemolysis, elevated liver enzymes and low platelets.

BOX 28.5 TREATMENT OF ECLAMPSIA

- The woman should be turned onto her left side to avoid aortocaval compression. The airway should be secured and high-flow oxygen should be administered.
- Magnesium sulphate ($MgSO_4$) should be administered intravenously to terminate the seizure and then by intravenous (IV) infusion to reduce the chance of further convulsions. In settings where IV infusion pumps are not available, $MgSO_4$ can be administered intramuscularly (IM) to reduce the risk of over- or under-dosing. The infusion should be continued for at least 24 hours following delivery or after the last seizure. $MgSO_4$ can depress neuromuscular transmission and the woman should be monitored for signs of toxicity. The respiratory rate and patellar reflexes should be monitored (reduced patellar reflexes usually precede respiratory depression). If there is significant respiratory depression, calcium gluconate can be used to reverse the effects of $MgSO_4$ and consideration given to ventilation.
- Urgent delivery is necessary if the seizure has occurred antenatally or intrapartum.
- Paralysis and ventilation should be considered if the seizures are prolonged or recurrent.

Global Challenges

The most serious of all complications of pre-eclampsia is maternal death. It is a triumph of modern obstetric care that maternal death rate in the United Kingdom from hypertensive disorders is at the lowest ever, with less than one maternal death per million births, which equates to less than one death per year.

The low rate of maternal deaths from pre-eclampsia in the United Kingdom is in stark contrast with the global setting, where an estimated 60,000 women die each year from this condition, which equates to about five deaths every hour. Eighty-five percent of this burden lies with sub-Saharan Africa and Southern Asia, where restricted or understaffed maternity services, particularly in rural areas with poor transport systems, mean that women may present late or infrequently to antenatal care (see Chapter 39).

Long-Term Implications of Hypertension in Pregnancy

Pregnancy has been described as a cardiometabolic 'stress test' such that the physiological changes of pregnancy unmask subclinical conditions, including diabetes and hypertension. While gestational hypertensive disorders resolve after pregnancy, affected women remain at increased risk of cardiovascular disease later in life.

Following a pregnancy complicated by PET, women have a three-fold increased risk of developing hypertension, a two-fold increased risk of developing ischaemic heart disease and a two- to three-fold increased risk of developing type 2 diabetes mellitus. Women with recurrent PET have a six-fold increased risk of developing hypertension in later life. It is not clear whether pre-eclampsia is a causative factor or whether there are simply shared risk factors (e.g., obesity, age and diabetes).

Pregnancy presents an opportunity to promote health and prevent disease in this at-risk population. The role of the obstetrician extends beyond providing pregnancy care to educating women about the future implications of their pregnancy complications and highlighting these women to their primary care providers. Women who have had a gestational hypertensive disorder should be advised that they are at increased risk of hypertension and explain the complications that may arise later in life. However, further evidence is needed for specific screening and management strategies.

Key Points

- **Pre-eclampsia is an important complication of pregnancy, resulting in effects on multiple organ systems with severe consequences if not detected and managed adequately.**
- **Clinical assessment involves determining a woman's symptoms, examination, accurate blood pressure assessment, testing for proteinuria, checking liver and renal function, assessing platelet count and monitoring of the fetus.**
- **Complications include maternal stroke, liver failure, pulmonary oedema, seizures and ultimately death, along with fetal effects, including growth restriction and stillbirth.**
- **Appropriate management involves prompt detection of the condition, blood pressure management with antihypertensives,**

monitoring fluid balance, $MgSO_4$ to reduce seizure risk and timely delivery of the baby.

- In the United Kingdom, this has resulted in low maternal death rates. However, many global challenges exist which must be overcome to continue the promising improvements that have been made in reducing the mortality from pre-eclampsia and eclampsia over recent years.

- Women who have had a pregnancy complicated by pre-eclampsia are at increased risk of hypertension, cardiovascular disease and type 2 diabetes mellitus in later life.

Chapter 29

Pre-Term Birth

Sarah Stock, Anna King

Chapter Outline

Introduction

Pre-term birth is defined as birth before 37 weeks' completed gestation. It occurs in around 10% of births and affects 15 million pregnancies worldwide annually. Almost one-third of pre-term births in the United Kingdom are iatrogenic (following deliberate medical intervention) when the risks of continuing the pregnancy, for either the mother or the baby, outweigh the risks of prematurity.

Prematurity is the leading cause of perinatal morbidity and mortality; pre-term birth is responsible for over a quarter of all neonatal deaths. Prematurity is associated with significant early neonatal morbidity, including ischaemic brain injuries, necrotising enterocolitis, retinopathy and respiratory distress syndrome. Later pre-term births are associated with neurodevelopmental delay in the infant and in adulthood with metabolic conditions, including diabetes and hypertension. The resultant short- and longer-term medical needs of these individuals have huge economic implications for health systems worldwide. While there is substantial morbidity with early pre-term births, there are far greater numbers of moderate to late pre-term births, which contribute a greater overall burden to health care systems. Prematurity is a global issue. However, there is stark contrast in mortality between countries, with 90% of extremely pre-term infants dying in low-resource settings versus 90% survival in high-resource settings, where advanced neonatal care is available.

Research into the definitive mechanisms involved in pre-term labour and its prevention has proven to be a difficult task. As a result, prematurity is one of the most challenging problems facing obstetricians and neonatologists.

Definitions

Pre-term: Birth at gestation of less than 37 completed weeks

Late pre-term: Birth at gestation between 34^{+0} and 36^{+6} completed weeks

Moderately pre-term: Birth at gestation between 32^{+0} and 33^{+6} completed weeks

Very pre-term: Birth at gestation between 28^{+0} and 31^{+6} completed weeks

Extremely pre-term: Birth at gestation of less than 28 completed weeks

Pre-term labour: Regular uterine contractions accompanied by effacement and dilatation of the cervix before 37 completed weeks' gestation

Pre-term pre-labour rupture of the membranes (PPROM): Rupture of the fetal membranes before 37 completed weeks' gestation, at least 1 hour before the onset of labour

Aetiology and Predisposing Factors

Around two-thirds of pre-term births are following spontaneous pre-term labour, with the remainder physician indicated. However, many of the conditions triggering decision to perform iatrogenic pre-term birth overlap with those causing spontaneous pre-term labour. The observed precursors to pre-term birth are heterogenous, as listed in Box 29.1, and are likely multifactorial.

Inflammation has emerged as a potential unifying feature, with localised release of cytokines and proteases potentially triggering cervical ripening, rupture of amniotic membranes, and initiation of uterine activity. Progesterone acts as an endogenous tocolytic and is functionally suppressed by cytokines. Bacterial infection – and, thus, inflammation, both intra- and

---

BOX 29.1 RISK FACTORS FOR PRE-TERM BIRTH

Maternal
- Previous pre-term birth (2–5 times risk; dependent on previous gestation at birth)
- Uterine malformation
- Previous cervical surgery
- Previous full dilatation caesarean birth
- Maternal disease (particularly pre-eclampsia and eclampsia)
- Smoking
- Mental health disorders, including depression and stress
- Domestic violence
- Extremes of maternal age (particularly age over 40 years)
- Black ethnicity
- Short interpregnancy interval (conception less than 12 months since previous birth)

Fetal/Pregnancy Related
- Multiple pregnancy
- Polyhydramnios
- Growth restriction
- Congenital anomaly
- Chorioamnionitis
- Extrauterine infection
- Antepartum haemorrhage
- Assisted reproduction

---

extrauterine – carries a significant risk of pre-term birth, whilst non-infective inflammatory conditions such as uterine stretch (polyhydramnios, multiple pregnancy) and antepartum haemorrhage are also associated with pre-term birth. Fetal and maternal stressors, including fetal growth restriction and maternal depression, are known to be associated with pre-term birth.

Identifying Women at Increased Risk of Pre-Term Birth

A number of strategies have been proposed to identify women who have an increased risk of pre-term birth. These include clinical risk scoring, cervical assessment and the measurement of fetal fibronectin (fFN). The available strategies, as outlined later, are moderately useful in identifying at-risk women and targeting interventions but better at helping to avoid unnecessary intervention in low-risk women.

Whilst a number of risk-scoring systems have been devised based on the recognised risk factors, none has been shown to be reliably effective in the prediction of pre-term birth. The strongest association is a history of previous pre-term birth, increasing this risk of recurrent pre-term birth by up to 5 times. Across the United Kingdom, there has been an increase in the provision of specialist antenatal care for women with risks for pre-term birth, which can help provide tailored antenatal care and surveillance.

Cervical insufficiency affects around 1% of pregnancies, and is associated with almost 10% of midtrimester losses. Cervical length measurement is a useful tool in risk stratification. A normal cervical length in pregnancy, when measured by transvaginal ultrasound, is between 34 and 40 mm and with no funnelling at the internal os (Fig. 29.1). Women with a cervix less than 25 mm in length can be considered at risk. The predictive value is best when applied to an already at-risk population rather than a mixed population; therefore, screening is advocated only in women with other significant risk factors for pre-term birth. Up to half of women with a cervical length under 25 m will remain pregnant beyond 34 weeks.

fFN is an adhesion molecule involved in maintaining the integrity of the choriodecidual extracellular matrix. It is usually not detectable on a high vaginal swab of cervicovaginal secretions after 20 weeks until term or membrane rupture; thus, if it is found to be present, it implies disruption of the matrix. Whilst most useful in stratifying women with symptoms of threatened pre-term labour, fFN has potential to be useful in asymptomatic women. A positive fFN in an asymptomatic woman confers a 14 times relative risk of birth before 32 weeks' gestation. The sensitivity is optimal when used in a high-risk population (e.g., women with previous pre-term birth). However, good-quality data on effectiveness in clinical practice are lacking. Other biomarkers are also available; however, fFN is the best characterised and most widely used in the United Kingdom.

Screening for vaginal infection has been considered to be a method to identify those at high risk of pre-term labour but is not routinely done in the low-risk, asymptomatic population. Bacterial vaginosis, which is present in 10% to 20% of pregnant women, is associated with a doubling of the odds of pre-term birth if identified in the third trimester. Unfortunately, clinical trials have demonstrated that the risk of pre-term labour is unchanged after treating bacterial vaginosis.

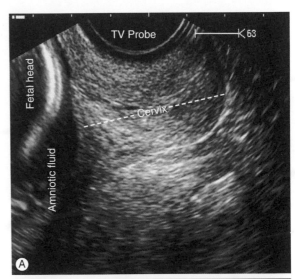

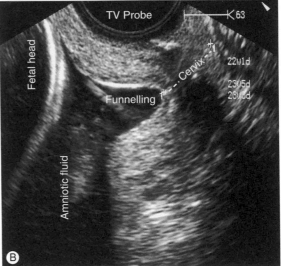

Fig. 29.1 Transvaginal ultrasound images of a cervix. The probe is seen at the top of the imaging, looking laterally through the cervical canal with the fetal head to the left of the screen. **(A)** A cervix without evidence of loss of integrity at the internal os. **(B)** Evidence of cervical shortening and funnelling of the internal os.

In those considered to have other risk factors for pre-term labour, it is reasonable to treat bacterial vaginosis if identified, rather than screen asymptomatic women.

Prevention of Pre-Term Labour

The aim of the following interventions is to improve the perinatal morbidity and mortality associated with pre-term birth. Research is ongoing to see whether women treated with these interventions to prolong gestation have corresponding improvements in long-term outcomes for their children.

SMOKING CESSATION

Smoking is associated, in a dose-dependent manner, with a third of pre-term births in industrialised nations as well as conferring many other pregnancy and neonatal risks. Smoking cessation clearly has wide-reaching benefits for the mother but, in particular, cessation prior to and during early pregnancy has been shown to mitigate risk of pre-term birth. A range of psychological interventions, including monetary incentives, have been shown to be effective in achieving smoking cessation in the pregnant population.

ASPIRIN

Aspirin is used widely in antenatal care to limit risk of pre-eclampsia and fetal growth restriction, both of which are significant risk factors for pre-term birth. There is also evidence to suggest that high-dose aspirin (150 mg at night) confers a benefit directly to preventing pre-term birth, potentially via anti-inflammatory pathways.

ANTIBIOTICS

Over 50% of very pre-term births are associated with infection. Evidence suggests that screening for, and treating, asymptomatic bacteriuria can reduce the risk of pre-term labour. There is a lack of evidence to suggest that screening and treating asymptomatic women for vaginal infections is an effective reduction strategy for pre-term birth prevention.

Aggressively treating extra-uterine infections with antibiotics – for example, cholecystitis or appendicitis – initially serves to minimise the risk of maternal sepsis and, therefore, minimise the risk of pre-term birth. In some scenarios, operative management of infections may be required with a careful risk-benefit analysis for each case.

CERVICAL CERCLAGE

There is evidence that cervical cerclage (with a Shirodkar or McDonald suture) performed in early second trimester is of benefit in women with a short cervix (<25 mm). As previously discussed, a short cervix has low predictive value in a mixed population. Therefore, this intervention is only routinely offered to women with other risk factors, including a personal history of pre-term labour, mid-trimester miscarriage or significant cervical surgery. In this high-risk group of women, cerclage can reduce the chance of pre-term birth prior to 28, 34 and 37 weeks' gestation.

Under anaesthesia (usually regional), with a vaginal approach, a non-absorbable high-strength suture (Mersilene or similar) is placed through the tissue of the cervix in a purse-string fashion. It is removed between 36 and 37 weeks' gestation or as an emergency if labour commences or fetal membranes rupture beforehand. Anaesthesia is not required for removal.

Abdominal cerclage is a specialist procedure reserved for those with a poor pregnancy outcome despite previous standard cervical cerclage. It can be performed pre-conception by laparotomy or laparoscopy. Subsequent birth has to be by caesarean section and the suture is usually left in place for the benefit of any future pregnancies.

'Rescue' cerclage refers to the emergency insertion of a cervical suture in women with exposed membranes before or around the limit of viability. Careful selection criteria are employed, since cerclage in the presence of infection can result in significant maternal morbidity without advantage to the baby.

PROGESTERONE

Progesterone supplementation is offered as an alternative to cervical cerclage. Potential mechanisms are oxytocin antagonism (leading to relaxation of smooth muscle), maintenance of cervical integrity and anti-inflammatory effects. Progesterone is administered vaginally or rectally, and is usually commenced around 16 weeks. Studies into the effects of progesterone have been conflicting regarding outcome; however, meta-analyses have suggested that vaginal progesterone may be effective at reducing the rates of pre-term birth before 36 weeks by 20% to 40% amongst women with singleton pregnancies and a short cervix, both with or without previous pre-term birth. However, other large trials have shown no benefit in reducing pre-term birth or improving newborn or longer-term outcome. There is no evidence that progesterone has any significant fetal or maternal side effects, but there is a lack of long-term safety data.

Neither progesterone nor cerclage have been shown to be of benefit to women with twin pregnancies.

IMMEDIATE POSTPARTUM CONTRACEPTION

A short inter-pregnancy interval (less than 12 months) is associated with subsequent pre-term birth; encouraging comprehensive provision of post-natal contraception can help to reduce this risk.

Inhibition of Pre-Term Labour

There is a lack of robust evidence to suggest a substantial benefit with use of tocolytics (drugs which suppress uterine contractions) once pre-term labour appears to have begun.

In view of the high morbidity and mortality associated with prematurity, an attempt may be made to delay labour to allow a course of corticosteroids to be administered (the benefits of which are discussed later) or an in-utero transfer to take place should adequate neonatal care facilities not be available in the current location. Whether this delay in itself translates into an improvement for the baby in the long term remains unproven. As no tocolytic drug has been shown to reduce perinatal mortality or neonatal morbidity, it is also reasonable to use no tocolysis. Contraindications to tocolysis include chorioamnionitis, significant bleeding, fetal distress, and severe maternal condition, in which case prompt birth would be indicated.

The most commonly used tocolytics are discussed next. If the decision is made to use a tocolytic drug, nifedipine and atosiban appear to have comparable effectiveness in delaying birth, with fewer maternal adverse effects. It is not recommended that any tocolytics be used in combination with one another. There is little information about the long-term growth and development of babies exposed to any of these medications.

NIFEDIPINE

This calcium-channel blocker inhibits inward calcium flow across cell membranes. The side effects of dizziness, hypotension (sometimes profound), flushing and headache are all related to peripheral dilatation, and serious adverse effects are rare. There seem to be no obvious adverse fetal effects provided that there is no precipitous fall in maternal blood pressure resulting in under-perfusion of the uterus.

OXYTOCIN ANTAGONIST

Atosiban is a synthetic competitive inhibitor of oxytocin, resulting in uterine smooth muscle relaxation. It is given as a continuous intravenous infusion, has been shown to be as effective as nifedipine, and has minimal maternal or fetal side effects.

CYCLO-OXYGENASE INHIBITORS

Indomethacin is the most commonly used tocolytic agent of this class of drug. It works via inhibition of prostaglandin production. Side effects include maternal gastrointestinal irritation, headaches and dizziness. The main risks are to the baby. The ongoing patency of the ductus arteriosus in the fetus is prostaglandin dependent, and ductal constriction has been demonstrated in human fetuses in response to these drugs. Significant adverse neonatal effects have not been convincingly demonstrated; caution is advised, nonetheless.

BETA AGONISTS

Terbutaline and salbutamol, beta-2 agonists, are used in the emergency treatment of uterine hyperstimulation, in which cessation of contractions is required to relieve fetal distress. The use of these drugs for inhibition of pre-term labour is not routinely recommended due to the risk of severe maternal side effects, including cardiac arrhythmias, pulmonary oedema and myocardial ischemia.

Pre-Term Pre-Labour Rupture of the Membranes

PPROM complicates 2% to 3% of all pregnancies and occurs in 20% to 40% of all spontaneous pre-term deliveries. It is more likely with polyhydramnios, twin pregnancy and vaginal infection. If the mother does not establish in labour, the problem is balancing the increased risk of developing ascending chorioamnionitis, leading to maternal and fetal morbidity, against the risks of prematurity. The neonatal prognosis is poorer the earlier the membrane rupture occurs on account of secondary pulmonary hypoplasia (lung development occurs between 18 and 28 weeks' gestation) and skeletal deformities resulting from the absence of amniotic fluid. The amniotic fluid normally allows fetal movement and it circulates into the fetal lungs (Box 29.2).

BOX 29.2 RISKS ASSOCIATED WITH SPONTANEOUS PRE-TERM PRE-LABOUR RUPTURE OF MEMBRANES

- Chorioamnionitis
- Pre-term labour
- Cord prolapse or cord compression
- Fetal lung hypoplasia
- Skeletal

After 37 weeks' gestation, 85% of babies are born within 48 hours following rupture of membranes. There is a longer interval at pre-term gestations; with PPROM, 50% of babies are born within 48 hours.

Diagnosis of PPROM is largely clinical, by taking a history and confirming pooling of liquor in the vagina by sterile speculum examination. In the absence of visible amniotic fluid, biochemical markers can be detected on vaginal swabs, most commonly insulin-like growth factor binding protein-1 or placental alpha microglobulin-1, lending further confidence to a diagnosis of PPROM. There is no clear evidence to suggest that any of the biochemical tools currently available are superior to another. The use of ultrasonographic assessment of liquor volume for diagnosis of PPROM is not recommended, as oligohydramnios may be the result of growth restriction or fetal renal problems.

Chorioamnionitis is potentially extremely serious for both mother and baby, as both may develop rapid and overwhelming sepsis, which can be fatal. The diagnosis of chorioamnionitis is suggested by maternal pyrexia, maternal and fetal tachycardia, abdominal pain, uterine tenderness, drainage of offensive liquor and raised serum inflammatory markers. Infection is more likely if vaginal examinations have been performed. Thus, examinations are contraindicated unless there is high suspicion of pre-term labour. The membrane rupture may be a secondary process resulting from an already established infection. Therefore, screening for infection with high vaginal swab and urine culture is recommended. Expediting birth is beneficial for mother and baby in the presence of chorioamnionitis.

MANAGEMENT OF PRE-TERM PRE-LABOUR RUPTURE OF THE MEMBRANES

Prophylactic antibiotics will reduce the risk of chorioamnionitis in women with confirmed PPROM; 10 days oral erythromycin (250 mg QID) is the current UK recommendation. Antibiotic prophylaxis improves some immediate neonatal outcomes when compared with placebo and can increase the time between membrane rupture and birth. However, there is no evidence to show long-term benefit to the child. Some antibiotics, including co-amoxiclav (amoxicillin and clavulanic acid), have been shown to have adverse effects on the neonate. Given the high risk of pre-term labour, corticosteroids can be considered for women under 34 weeks' gestation due to the benefits outlined later.

It is considered acceptable practice to manage these women on an outpatient basis following an initial inpatient stay. Aiming for birth around 36 to 37 weeks' gestation is appropriate when the risk of ascending infection and prematurity is felt to be in balance. In the presence of group B streptococcal colonisation, the risk of prematurity outweighs that of ascending infection until around 34 weeks. Therefore, birth may be planned earlier in this group.

Close monitoring is recommended, with routine weekly hospital follow-up that includes measurement of maternal temperature, C-reactive protein and cardiotocography (CTG). Regular growth scanning of the fetus is also routinely performed. Women should be advised to attend for urgent assessment in hospital if they develop symptoms of infection or pre-term labour. Tocolytics for the prevention of pre-term labour are not recommended with PPROM, as there is a tendency towards increased maternal infection rates with no evidence of benefit to the baby.

Diagnosis and Management of Pre-Term Labour

The diagnosis of pre-term labour is similar to the diagnosis of labour at term: regular painful contractions associated with progressive cervical effacement and dilatation. Diagnosis may be difficult in the early stages because, in many cases, regular painful contractions with normal abdominal and speculum examination may not progress to established labour. Labour may be insidious, or heralded by a 'show', bleeding or abruption.

Objective assessment may be helpful in the presence of normal examination findings. With a good sensitivity but low specificity, fFN has a low positive predictive value in women with symptoms of pre-term labour, but a threshold of less than 50 ng/mL as a negative result has high negative predictive value. A negative fFN result means that less than 5% of symptomatic women will deliver in the week following the test, and 91% will remain pregnant at 34 weeks. Similarly, a cervical length of >15 mm is reassuring, with a negative predicative value of 96%, and a high threshold for intervention can then be set.

Fetal well-being can be assessed with CTG and then ideally with ultrasound to evaluate liquor volume, presentation and estimated fetal weight. The neonatal team should be alerted and consideration given to in utero transfer if local facilities for neonatal care are insufficient for the current gestational stage.

CORTICOSTEROIDS

Corticosteroids are generally recommended if pre-term birth before 34 weeks' gestation is considered likely within 7 days. They are most effective if administered within 48 hours of birth. Among their many effects, they cross the placenta and increase the amount of pulmonary surfactant produced by type II fetal pneumocytes, reducing the incidence of respiratory distress syndrome (hyaline membrane disease). Betamethasone or dexamethasone given by intramuscular injection in divided doses over 24 hours provides many neonatal benefits. Antenatal corticosteroids confer a 31% reduction in perinatal death, with 46% reduced incidence of intraventricular cerebral haemorrhage and a 44% reduction in neonatal respiratory distress. There is no identifiable increase in the incidence of maternal or fetal infection, but steroids are contraindicated if there is active maternal sepsis.

Corticosteroids are potent drugs with multisystem effects. Animal studies have shown impact upon the developing brain, and they are associated with a small increase in subsequent behavioural problems in children. Multiple courses of corticosteroids are associated with poorer outcomes for babies. Thus, the aim is to give the first, and only, course to women 48 hours to a week before pre-term birth. Corticosteroids can be used in pregnant women with diabetes; however, as they can precipitate ketoacidosis, additional measures to control blood glucose are recommended, with an insulin sliding scale if necessary.

The use of antenatal corticosteroids in low-resource settings is largely extrapolated from trial data from countries where accurate gestation stage is known and pre-term babies are cared for in high-resource settings with specialist neonatal facilities. Despite this, antenatal corticosteroids are recommended in low-resource settings, as there is a high burden of pre-term birth. Thus, even small reductions in neonatal morbidity are likely to be important. The use of dexamethasone in these settings was shown to reduce neonatal morbidity when there was less certainty about gestational age, without any increase in maternal morbidity.

MAGNESIUM SULPHATE

Magnesium sulphate ($MgSO_4$) was identified as a neuroprotective agent incidentally in the 1990s when infants of mothers treated with $MgSO_4$ for severe pre-eclampsia were found to be at 80% reduced risk of cerebral palsy. This finding has been subsequently corroborated and infants of mothers treated with $MgSO_4$ shown to have better gross motor function in early childhood. This neuroprotective effect is more pronounced at earlier gestations, with babies less than 30 weeks' gestation likely to benefit most, but $MgSO_4$ can be considered up to 34 weeks' gestation. $MgSO_4$ is beneficial to the pre-term baby regardless of mode of birth (vaginal or caesarean). A regime of 4 g intravenous bolus of $MgSO_4$ over 15 to 20 minutes, followed by an intravenous infusion of 1 g per hour until the birth or for 24 hours (whichever is sooner), is routinely used in settings where intravenous infusion pumps are available for administration. The infusion should ideally be started more than 4 hours before birth to ensure the optimal effect, although even a short exposure to magnesium prior to birth is likely to be of benefit. Vigilance is required to assess the mother for magnesium toxicity. Once birth has occurred, the magnesium can be stopped unless also being given to prevent maternal eclampsia, in which case it should be continued until 24 hours postpartum (see Chapter 28).

PREVENTION OF INFECTION

In women known to be colonized with group B *Streptococcus* (*Streptococcus agalactiae*), antibiotic prophylaxis (benzylpenicillin or clindamycin) is offered at all gestational stages, when the woman is in labour, to reduce the risk of severe infection of the neonate. This is also recommended in women in established pre-term labour without evidence of group B streptococcal colonisation.

Should a woman with PPROM develop clinical signs of chorioamnionitis, broad-spectrum antibiotics should be administered and birth expedited in both the maternal and fetal interests: the mother to remove the source of infection and the baby to minimize the risk of sepsis and subsequent risk of cerebral palsy.

INTRAPARTUM MONITORING

In the event of pre-term labour, close monitoring is important as a pre-term baby is more susceptible to intrapartum hypoxia and acidosis than a baby at term. Women in pre-term labour are best cared for on a specialist-led labour ward with monitoring, usually in the form of a continuous CTG if the fetus is over 26 weeks' gestation, although intermittent auscultation may also be appropriate. The use of fetal scalp electrodes is generally avoided, and expediting birth by forceps or caesarean is preferred to fetal blood sampling in this scenario.

Mode of Birth

How the baby is born needs to be considered, but there is a lack of high-quality evidence to guide decisions. Caesarean section may be indicated for an apparently compromised fetus. Pre-term birth by caesarean section at very early gestations often requires a vertical uterine incision (as the lower uterine segment may be poorly formed), which can have significant implications for future pregnancies. Vaginal birth is preferred, on the whole, for those with cephalic presentation; there is no routine recommendation for epidural, forceps or episiotomy. Transverse or oblique lie, however, is more likely in the pre-term baby than at term and makes safe vaginal birth impossible. There is uncertainty about the most appropriate route of birth in those with breech presentation. However, most babies in breech presentation before 26 weeks are born vaginally and many of those above this gestational stage by caesarean section.

In the event that an assisted vaginal birth is required, forceps are safer than vacuum devices for a baby less than 34 weeks' gestation to avoid the increased risks of cephalohaematoma, subgaleal haematoma, and intraventricular haemorrhage.

If the condition of the baby and mother permit, optimal cord clamping (>60 seconds and <3 minutes) after the baby is born will improve fetal circulating blood volume and, hence, organ perfusion. Very pre-term babies are particularly susceptible to hypothermia (see Chapter 38). It is often helpful to place these babies promptly into a plastic bag to minimise heat loss (Fig. 29.2).

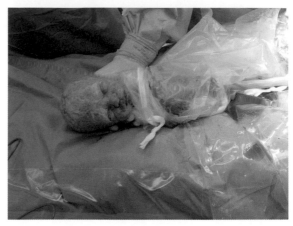

Fig. 29.2 A plastic bag minimises heat loss in very pre-term babies.

In settings where advanced neonatal care is available to babies born pre-term, the survival of babies born at 34 weeks' gestation or beyond is equivalent to babies born at term. The survival at 27 and 31 weeks' gestation is 89% and 95%, respectively.

Key Points

- **Pre-term birth affects 10% of pregnancies and has significant associated morbidity and mortality.**
- **There is no universal screening tool to predict pre-term birth. However, identifying risk factors and applying tools such as serial cervical length measurement and biomarkers in risk groups may be useful.**
- **Cervical cerclage may reduce risk of pre-term birth in carefully selected pregnancies.**
- **Corticosteroids significantly decrease the neonatal morbidity associated with pre-term labour under 34 weeks' gestation.**
- **Magnesium sulphate can improve neurological outcomes in babies born under 30 weeks' gestation.**
- **Prophylactic antibiotics for women with pre-term rupture of membranes reduce risk of chorioamnionitis and early-onset neonatal infection.**
- **Tocolytics are not routinely recommended but may be considered to allow for corticosteroid administration or in utero transfer to a location with appropriate neonatal facilities.**

Chapter 30

Multiple Pregnancy

Janice Gibson, Mark D. Kilby

Chapter Outline

Introduction

The natural incidence of twinning has a large geographical variation, ranging from 54 in 1000 in Nigeria, 12 in 1000 in the United Kingdom, to 4 in 1000 in Japan. This difference is almost entirely due to variations in the rate of non-identical twins, while the incidence of identical twins remains remarkably constant at around 3 in 1000. However, immigration of ethnic groups with higher rates of multiple pregnancy has contributed to the increasing rates overall in countries which previously had lower rates. In the United Kingdom, the actual incidence of twin pregnancies is significantly greater than the natural incidence due to the widespread use of in vitro fertilization and ovulation induction techniques. Around 25% of twin pregnancies, 50% to 60% of triplet pregnancies and 75% of quadruplet pregnancies are a result of assisted-reproduction techniques. One in 64 (15.6/1000) pregnancies in the United Kingdom is now a twin pregnancy.

Twins babies have a nearly two-fold risk of stillbirth and over a three-fold risk of neonatal death compared with singletons. This reflects an increased risk of pathological conditions, such as pre-term birth, fetal growth restriction (one or both fetuses), twin-to-twin transfusion syndrome (TTTS), and an increased

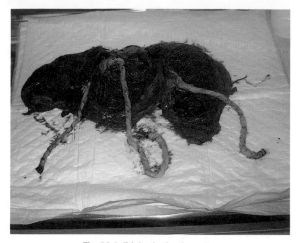

Fig. 30.1 Trichorionic placenta.

incidence of congenital malformations (mostly discordant). Perinatal mortality rates rise exponentially with fetal number in higher-order pregnancies. The outcome of any multiple pregnancy is also significantly affected by its chorionicity (whether each fetus has its own or shares a placenta; Fig. 30.1).

The Nature of Twinning and Chorionicity

'Zygosity' refers to whether the twins have developed from a single ovum or from different ova – in other words, whether they are identical or non-identical, respectively (this cannot be identified clinically). 'Chorionicity' refers to the number of placentae (Fig. 30.2).

DIZYGOTIC TWINNING (NON-IDENTICAL)

Dizygotic twins account for approximately 70% of twins. This process occurs when two ova are fertilized and implant separately into the decidua. Each developing embryo will form its own outer chorion (chorionic membrane and placenta) and its own inner amniotic membrane. Dizygotic twin pregnancies are described as dichorionic and diamniotic.

MONOZYGOTIC TWINNING (IDENTICAL)

Monozygotic twins (30% of twins) are derived from the splitting of a single embryo and the configuration of placentation depends on the age of the embryo when the split occurred (see Fig. 30.2). Division that occurs at or before the eight-cell stage (3 days

post-fertilization) will occur before the outer chorion has differentiated and, therefore, will give rise to two separate embryos that will each proceed to form its own chorion. Therefore, these twin pregnancies, like dizygotic twins, will be dichorionic and diamniotic. Embryo division at the blastocyst stage (4–8 days post-fertilization) will occur after the chorion has started to differentiate; therefore, the fetuses will share an outer chorion (placenta and outer chorionic membrane). These twins will be monochorionic diamniotic and are the most common form of monozygotic twins. Division of the embryo between 8 and 14 days will result in the inner amniotic cavity and membrane being shared (monochorionic monoamniotic twins). Splitting beyond 14 days following fertilization is extremely rare, giving rise to conjoined twins (Fig. 30.3 and Table 30.1). The later the time before division of the embryo, the higher the risk of complications affecting the twin pregnancy.

In monochorionic twins, the shared placental mass inevitably contains several types of vascular anastomoses between the two fetal-placental circulations. The very presence of a shared vascular system dictates that the well-being of each twin is directly dependent on the well-being of the other. The number and nature of these placental vascular connections places monochorionic twins at risk of specific complications and an increased perinatal loss and morbidity rate. Therefore, determining chorionicity is essential to allow risk stratification (Table 30.2). Chorionicity has key implications for prenatal diagnosis and antenatal monitoring. It is most easily determined before 14 weeks' gestation by ultrasound:

- Widely separated first-trimester sacs or separate placentae are dichorionic.
- Those with a 'lambda' or 'twin-peak' sign at the membrane insertion are dichorionic (Fig. 30.4A).
- Those with a 'T' sign at the membrane insertion are monochorionic (Fig. 30.4B).
- Those with no dividing membrane are monochorionic monoamniotic.

After 14 weeks' gestation, these ultrasound signs may become less obvious. Discordant fetal sex is helpful to assume dizygosity and, therefore, dichorionicity. If chorionicity cannot be accurately determined, the pregnancy should be managed as if it is monochorionic.

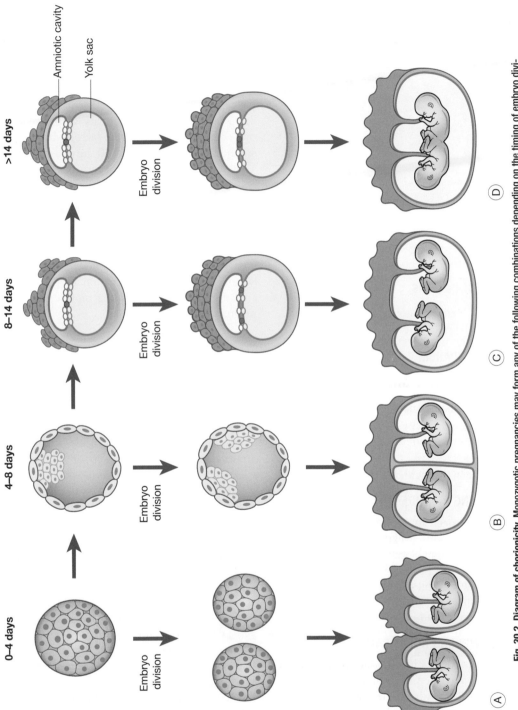

Fig. 30.2 Diagram of chorionicity. Monozygotic pregnancies may form any of the following combinations depending on the timing of embryo division: (**A**) dichorionic diamniotic; (**B**) monochorionic diamniotic; (**C**) monochorionic monoamniotic; (**D**) conjoined twins.

0–4 days

4–8 days

8–14 days

>14 days

Amniotic cavity

Yolk sac

Embryo division

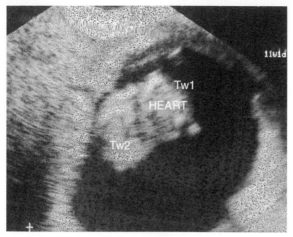

Fig. 30.3 Conjoined twins. Diagnosed at 12 weeks' gestation. This is a cross-sectional view through the thoraces of both twins. In view of the shared cardiac structures, management includes the option of termination of pregnancy.

Maternal Complications

The incidence of many maternal complications is increased in multiple pregnancy.

HYPEREMESIS GRAVIDARUM

The increased placental mass and, therefore, increased maternal circulating human chorionic gonadotrophin concentration is associated with an increased incidence and earlier onset of hyperemesis gravidarum.

ANAEMIA

There is an increase in the incidence of anaemia associated with multiple pregnancy, which is not completely explained by a haemodilutional effect of the increased plasma volume. The need for iron and folate supplementation should be assessed early in the pregnancy with a full blood count performed at 20 to 24 weeks' gestation in addition to the usual antenatal anaemia screen performed at 28 weeks in all pregnancies.

PRE-ECLAMPSIA

The incidence of pre-eclampsia in twin pregnancy is three to four times greater than that in singleton pregnancies. It tends to develop earlier and may be more severe. Women carrying a multiple pregnancy should be assessed for any additional risk factor for pre-eclampsia (first pregnancy; age ≥40 years; pregnancy interval of more than 10 years; body mass index of ≥35 kg/m² or family history of pre-eclampsia). If one or more additional risk factors exist, the woman should be advised to take 150 mg of aspirin daily from 12 weeks until birth as a measure aimed to reduce her overall risk of this complication (see Chapter 28).

ANTEPARTUM HAEMORRHAGE

Placenta praevia is more common with multiple gestations because of the larger placental surface. The management of this condition in multiple pregnancy is similar to that of a singleton pregnancy. Placental abruption also appears to be more common in twin pregnancies.

THROMBOEMBOLIC DISEASE

Multiple pregnancy is a risk factor for venous thromboembolic disease. This may be due to the adverse effects of the increased size of the pregnant uterus on venous blood flow. Women with multiple pregnancy are also more likely to have other independent risk factors for venous thrombosis, such as advanced maternal age, assisted conception, high parity, pre-eclampsia and immobility. Assessment of risk factors for thromboembolic disease should be performed throughout pregnancy. Antenatal thromboprophylaxis may be indicated throughout pregnancy or from 28 weeks' gestation dependent on the number and nature of concurrent risk factors. Risk assessment should be repeated postpartum. Operative birth is an additional significant risk factor for thromboembolic disease.

TABLE 30.1	Chorionicity in Monozygous Twins		
Timing of Embryonic Separation After Fertilization (Days)	Number of Chorions	Number of Amniotic Sacs	Percentage of Monozygous Twins (%)
<4	Dichorionic	Diamniotic	30
4–8	Monochorionic	Diamniotic	66
8–14	Monochorionic	Monoamniotic	3
>14	Monochorionic (conjoined)	Monoamniotic	<1

TABLE 30.2	Fetal Loss by Chorionicity	
	Dichorionic (%)	Monochorionic (%)
Fetal loss before 24 weeks	1.8	12.2
Fetal loss after 24 weeks	1.6	2.8
Delivery before 32 weeks	5.5	9.2

The high early fetal mortality in monochorionic pregnancy before 24 weeks is probably largely the result of severe early-onset twin-to-twin transfusion syndrome.

OTHER MATERNAL COMPLICATIONS

Women with multiple pregnancies are at increased risk of gestational diabetes, general discomfort, varicose veins and dependent oedema, delivery trauma, caesarean section, postpartum haemorrhage, psychological disorders and breastfeeding and parenting challenges.

Fetal Complications

CHROMOSOMAL ABNORMALITIES

These are usually confined to one twin (i.e., non-concordant) in dizygotic twins and almost always concordant in monozygotic twins. Therefore, the maternal age-related risk for carrying at least one fetus with trisomy 21 (Down syndrome) is approximately doubled in dichorionic twin pregnancies (most of which are dizygotic, i.e., the woman carries two individuals each with a risk) but remains unaltered in monochorionic (monozygotic) twins. Maternal serum screening for trisomy 21 performs poorly in twin pregnancy (and only gives a pregnancy-related risk). Nuchal translucency measurement (with or without biochemistry) is a more useful screening test and gives a fetal-specific risk. Analysis of cell-free fetal DNA in the maternal blood (non-invasive prenatal screening) is likely to be the most sensitive and specific screening test for fetal chromosomal anomalies in twin pregnancies (albeit as a pregnancy-related risk). In the United Kingdom, it is anticipated that this test will be incorporated into the routine care of women with twins in the very near future.

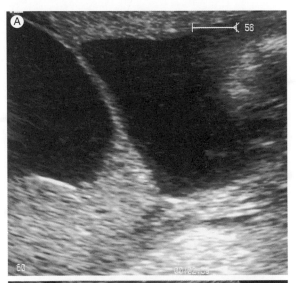

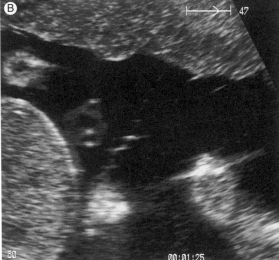

Fig. 30.4 (A) Dichorionic twins – lambda sign. (B) Monochorionic twins – no lambda sign. The two amniotic membranes form a 'T' sign as they join the placenta.

If a screening test suggests an increased risk of a chromosomal anomaly in any twin, diagnostic testing should be offered. Amniocentesis of each amniotic sac is required in dichorionic pregnancies; care must be taken to document which sample has come from which sac. Monochorionic (identical twins) only exceptionally have different karyotypes (i.e., rarely there may be post-division loss of some chromosome material in one twin). Sampling of one sac is acceptable unless one has an obvious structural abnormality.

Chorionic villous sampling is not usually appropriate for twin pregnancies, as it may be difficult to be sure that both placentae have been sampled, particularly if they are lying close together.

Before any screening or invasive diagnostic test is undertaken, the parents should be comprehensively counselled about the psychological difficulties they may face if a risk or diagnosis of an anomaly is confined to a single fetus along with the physical and psychological risks associated with selective termination of one twin.

STRUCTURAL DEFECTS

The incidence of structural fetal abnormality in dichorionic twins is similar to that seen in singleton pregnancies, but it is two- to three-fold greater in monochorionic twins. It is thought to be the process of embryo division which is inherently teratogenic, particularly if this occurs late. Characteristic abnormalities include cardiac defects, neural tube and other central nervous system defects and gastrointestinal atresia. Therefore, in a twin pregnancy, the woman will have a two- to six-fold increased risk of carrying a fetus with a structural abnormality. It is appropriate to offer all women with multiple pregnancies a detailed mid-trimester ultrasound scan. Women with monochorionic twin pregnancies should be offered an extended ultrasound assessment of fetal heart structure. The abnormalities are usually confined to one twin; for example, if there is a neural tube defect in one twin, the other twin is normal in 85% to 90% of cases. Selective termination with intracardiac potassium chloride (KCl) is possible only in dichorionic pregnancies. However, the procedure carries a 5% risk of miscarriage of the healthy co-twin. In monochorionic twins, due to the shared fetoplacental vascular system, specialized cord vessel occlusive techniques are required but carry an increased (10%–20%) risk of loss to the other twin due to the invasiveness of this procedure. Technical and ethical challenges, and the complication risks of selective reduction, in both dichorionic and monochorionic twins increase with gestational age.

PRE-TERM BIRTH

Approximately 60% of twin pregnancies result in spontaneous pre-term birth before 37^{+0} weeks' gestation and approximately 10% deliver before 32 weeks' gestation. Triplet pregnancies (75%) typically result in spontaneous pre-term birth before 35^{+0} weeks'

gestation. Twins account for 25% of all pre-term births, despite accounting for only 3% of births per year. Pre-term birth is higher in monochorionic compared with dichorionic twins (see Table 30.2). Increased uterine distension, early myometrial contractility and TTTS may be causative factors in pre-term labour in multiple pregnancy. At present, there is no known effective treatment to prevent pre-term labour in twin pregnancies. As spontaneous labour may occur at extreme pre-term gestation (22–26 weeks' gestation) women should be counselled as to the risks of pre-term labour early (ideally at 16 weeks' gestation) in their pregnancy. Women should be encouraged to seek assistance early with any symptoms of suspected pre-term labour so that they and their babies may be optimally prepared for pre-term birth. Therapies such as maternally administered corticosteroids to accelerate fetal lung maturation and magnesium sulphate (in very pre-term babies) as a potential fetal neuroprotective agent benefit from time to be considered, discussed with the parents, and optimally administered.

In addition to spontaneous pre-term birth, multiple pregnancies are at increased risk of medically indicated planned pre-term birth (iatrogenic pre-term birth). This may be required due to the development of maternal or fetal complications of pregnancy, especially pre-eclampsia, fetal growth restriction and the complications of monochorionicity.

FETAL GROWTH RESTRICTION

Abdominal palpation is not a reliable method for monitoring fetal growth in multiple pregnancy. Serial ultrasound should be performed to obtain an estimated fetal weight (EFW). EFW is derived from combinations of fetal biometry, including abdominal circumference, head circumference and femur length measurements, which should be plotted on a chart serially throughout pregnancy (see Chapter 27). Twins typically reflect singleton size charts until 28 to 30 weeks' gestation and then growth naturally slows. Approximately 30% of twins are small for gestational age by singleton standards and a significant difference in the growth of one twin compared with the other is seen in 12% of pregnancies. This is defined by a discordance in EFW of 20% to 25% (the difference in EFW of the twins divided by the EFW of the larger twin) and the smaller twin is <10th centile for EFW and predicts perinatal morbidity. Placental dysfunction underlies fetal growth restriction in twin pregnancies, as it does in singleton pregnancies. In monochorionic twins, unequal sharing of the placental mass is an additional pathological risk.

If diagnosed, growth restriction requires increased surveillance of fetal well-being with umbilical artery Doppler (and other fetal Doppler velocimetry assessments) and cardiotocography (CTG) monitoring, so that birth of the twins can be optimally timed. Monochorionic twins are at increased risk of growth restriction and require a lower threshold for birth owing to the specific adverse consequences to the co-twin in the event of a single intrauterine death in these twins (see later discussion).

TWINS WITH ONE FETAL DEATH

First-trimester intrauterine death in a twin has not been shown to have adverse consequences for the survivor. This probably also holds true for the early second trimester in dichorionic twins, but loss in the late second or third trimester commonly precipitates labour. Most affected pregnancies will deliver both fetuses before 34 weeks' gestation, often within 3 weeks of the loss. Therefore, prognosis for a surviving dichorionic fetus is influenced primarily by its gestational stage. When one monochorionic twin dies in utero, however, there are additional complicating risks of co-twin death in 20% of cases and in single twin survivors at least a 25% risk of cerebral damage because of the shared fetal circulations through placental anastomoses. As these are probably related to acute hypoperfusion/hypotension in the co-twin at the time of the other's death, early delivery of the surviving twin is unlikely to improve its outcome and may compound morbidity if performed at a premature gestation.

Antenatal Problems Specific to Monochorionic Twin Pregnancies

TWIN-TO-TWIN TRANSFUSION SYNDROME

This complicates 10% to 15% of monochorionic multiple pregnancies and accounts for a significant proportion of perinatal mortality in twins. In this condition, there is a net blood flow from one twin to the other through arterial to venous anastomoses in the shared placenta. The circulation of the recipient twin becomes hyperdynamic, with the risk of high-output

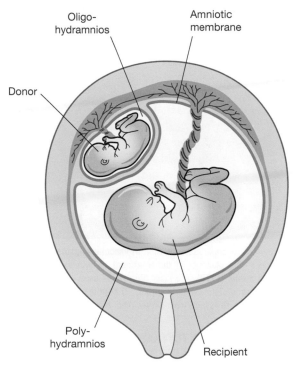

Fig. 30.5 Monochorionic twins demonstrating twin-to-twin transfusion syndrome (TTTS). Oligohydramnios-polyhydramnios sequence.

cardiac failure. Activation of the renal renin-angiotensin pathway and excessive fetal urine production results in polyhydramnios within the recipient twin's sac. Conversely, the donor twin develops oliguria and oligohydramnios, and often suffers growth restriction (Fig. 30.5). The ultrasound finding of the oligohydramnios-polyhydramnios sequence is the key to establishing an antenatal diagnosis. The severity of TTTS can be staged by the degree of fetal cardiovascular compromise (known as Quintero staging).

Without treatment, TTTS is associated with a >80% pregnancy loss rate. Two interventions have proven useful: serial amniodrainage and laser ablation of the causative placental vascular anastomoses (Fig. 30.6). Evidence has emerged that laser ablation is the most effective intervention (76% survival of at least one twin vs 51% survival of at least one twin with amnioreduction). Therefore, it is the treatment of choice in all but the mildest form of TTTS. Laser therapy is also associated with a lower rate of significant neurological morbidity in surviving twins compared with amnioreduction (6% vs 14%).

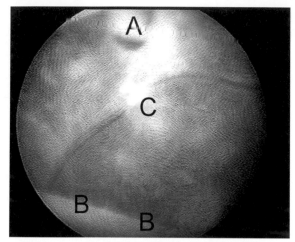

Fig. 30.6 Fetoscopic laser ablation of vascular anastomoses on the surface of the placenta in the treatment of twin-to-twin transfusion syndrome (TTTS). The laser fibre (A) is used to ablate vessels (C) crossing the inter-twin membrane (B) from the donor twin as they anastomose with vessels from the recipient twin.

TWIN ANAEMIA POLYCYTHAEMIA SEQUENCE

In this condition, there is a slow, low-volume transfer of blood from one fetus to the other through exceedingly small-calibre placental anastomoses. This causes one fetus to become anaemic and the other polycythaemic (Fig. 30.7), without the large haemodynamic fluid shifts seen in TTTS. Therefore, the liquor volumes are not altered as in TTTS. The anaemic twin may develop cardiac failure and hydrops. Intervention is difficult with all potential therapies (intrauterine transfusion, laser therapy and early delivery), having a significant risk of not being effective or of fetal and neonatal morbidity. Screening for the anaemia which occurs in this condition can be performed by fetal middle cerebral artery (MCA) Doppler. In the absence of an ideal therapy, this may be cost-effective only following laser therapy for TTTS, in which the incidence (up to 13%) is higher than is seen in other monochorionic twins (1%–2%).

SEVERE SELECTIVE INTRAUTERINE GROWTH RESTRICTION (sIUGR)

If severe sIUGR of one monochorionic twin occurs before viability, selective termination by cord-occlusion techniques may be considered in the interests of the co-twin. sIUGR is associated with an increased risk of in utero demise.

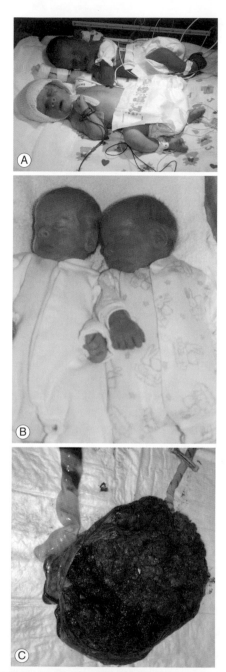

Fig. 30.7 Twin anaemia polycythaemia sequence. These monochorionic twins were born at 37 weeks' gestation. Although their weights were almost identical, there was significant difference in haemoglobin concentrations at birth. This is a recently described (chronic) form of fetal-to-fetal transfusion. (A) At delivery. (B) Post corrective blood transfusion to the anaemic twin (with permission). (C) The monochorionic placenta demonstrating the features of Twin Anemia Polycythemia Sequence (TAPS).

MONOAMNIOTIC TWINS

Twins who occupy a single amniotic sac are at risk of demise due to cord entanglement in utero. Frequent CTG monitoring is required once they reach viability. Birth is usually electively planned for between 32 and 33 weeks' gestation but is indicated earlier if cord compression is suggested by abnormal fetal heart rate patterns on CTG analysis. Birth should be by caesarean section, as the risk of a cord accident is particularly high during labour.

TWIN REVERSED ARTERIAL PERFUSION SEQUENCE

If the heart of one monochorionic twin stops or does not form, the body of this acardiac twin may continue to be partially perfused by the surviving twin via a large fetal arterial-to-arterial anastomosis within the shared placenta. The dead twin undergoes atrophy of its upper body and heart due to the especially poor oxygenation of these tissues and becomes what has been described as an 'acardiac monster'. The condition is rare, affecting <1% of monochorionic twins. There is a high incidence of mortality in the normal ('pump') twin due to intrauterine cardiac failure and prematurity. This risk increases with the relative size of the acardiac twin. Cord vessel–occlusive techniques, when performed on large acardiac twins (>50% size of the normal twin), appear to improve survival rates of the normal twin.

Care of Women With Multiple Pregnancy

INITIAL VISIT

It is important to ensure that chorionicity has been established on scan. Ideally, this should be performed between 11 and 13+6 weeks' gestation, as it becomes increasingly difficult to do so with advancing gestation.

The parents are often excited and shocked. Thus, initial counselling should be focused and include positive aspects. The parents should be counselled regarding their options for antenatal screening for fetal anomalies and should understand the potential dilemmas that may arise if one normal and one abnormal twin is diagnosed. It should be explained that more frequent antenatal visits will be required than in a singleton pregnancy to monitor both the maternal and fetal well-being and that ultrasound will play the key role in fetal assessments. Risk assessment for pre-eclampsia should be undertaken and low-dose aspirin initiated as indicated.

SUBSEQUENT VISITS

Women should be cared for in a dedicated multiple pregnancy clinic by a multidisciplinary team, including a specialist obstetrician and midwife. Detailed counselling about specific risks of each woman's pregnancy ideally should be performed by her specialist obstetrician at 16 weeks. The risks, symptoms and management of pre-term labour, fetal growth disorders and the specific complications of monochorionicity (if appropriate) should be discussed. Subsequent multidisciplinary antenatal care within the specialist clinic should be timed to coincide with the ultrasound assessments, the schedule of which will depend on chorionicity.

Monochorionic twins:
- Every 2 weeks from 16 weeks until birth to survey for TTTS and fetal growth restriction
- Detailed structural survey at 18 to 20 weeks' gestation
- Detailed fetal cardiac scan at 22 weeks' gestation.

Dichorionic twins:
- Detailed structural survey at 18 to 20 weeks' gestation
- Every 2 to 4 weeks from 24 weeks until birth for fetal growth assessment.

The woman should be monitored for complications such as pre-eclampsia and anaemia. Risk assessment for thromboembolic disease should be performed at each visit or if admitted to hospital. Discussion around mode of birth and management of twin labour is useful from 24 weeks' gestation and should be revisited throughout ongoing care. Tailored parentcraft advice or classes should be offered and include dietary, breastfeeding and perinatal mental health advice. Contact details of support groups for parents with multiple pregnancies should be offered.

Management of Twin Birth

In uncomplicated twin pregnancies, birth is planned for 37 weeks' gestation in dichorionic twin pregnancies and for 36 weeks' gestation in monochorionic pregnancies. This guidance is based on the increased risk of stillbirth in these populations after these gestational periods.

Presentations at term are typically:
- Cephalic/cephalic (40%)
- Cephalic/breech (40%)

- Breech/cephalic (10%)
- Other, for example, transverse (10%).

In general, provided that the presentation of the first twin is cephalic and the pregnancy has progressed beyond 32 weeks, the balance of current evidence would suggest that planned vaginal birth and planned caesarean birth are both safe choices. Significant growth discordance or any other concern of fetal well-being may be a reason to consider caesarean birth. If the labour is significantly pre-term (26–32 weeks' gestation) or if the mother has had a previous caesarean section, many clinicians would also consider birth by caesarean section. Extreme pre-term labour (<26 weeks) requires an individualized assessment regarding the risks of different modes of birth.

If labour is induced or spontaneous, the first stage is managed as for singleton pregnancies. Care should be taken to ensure that both twins are being monitored with CTG rather than one twin being monitored twice. This is best achieved by monitoring twin I with a fetal scalp electrode and twin II with an abdominal transducer.

An experienced obstetrician, an anaesthetist, two paediatricians and two midwives should be present for the birth. If not already required, an oxytocin infusion should be ready in case uterine activity decreases after the birth of the first twin. After the first twin is born, it is often helpful to have someone 'stabilise' the lie of second twin to longitudinal by abdominal palpation while a vaginal examination is performed to assess the station of the presenting part. A portable ultrasound machine is helpful to confirm the lie and presentation of the second twin. The membranes of twin II should not be broken until the presenting part has descended into the pelvis. If twin II lies transversely after the delivery of twin I, external cephalic or breech version is appropriate. If the lie is still transverse, the choice is between performing an internal podalic version (ideally keeping the membranes intact while the obstetrician's hand enters the uterus to identify, grasp and bring down a fetal foot) followed by subsequent breech extraction, or performing a caesarean section. The CTG of twin II should be carefully monitored throughout and birth expedited if fetal heart rate abnormalities are observed. The second twin has the highest risk of adverse outcome in labour.

A maternal epidural is useful in the management of twin labour owing to the increased risks of obstetric intervention, particularly assisted birth of twin II.

Owing to the enlarged uterine size, there is an increased risk of atonic postpartum haemorrhage. This should be anticipated. Management of the third stage should be active with the administration of oxytocin or ergometrine. Rapid escalation to a postpartum haemorrhage protocol should follow if indicated by ongoing blood loss. Risk assessment for thromboembolic disease should continue postnatally.

Triplets and Higher-Order Multiples

In these pregnancies, the perinatal mortality and morbidity is high, mostly because of the high risk of pre-term labour. It may be appropriate to discuss reducing the number of fetuses to twins at 12 to 14 weeks' gestation. With quadruplets or higher-order pregnancies, there is likely to be a greater chance of at least one or two survivors if fetal reduction is carried out, despite the miscarriage risk associated with the procedure itself. Reduction of any monochorionic twin pairs will have the greatest positive effect on outcomes. For triplets, the situation is less clear. The emotional and ethical problems associated with these decisions are considerable.

Triplets and higher-order multiple pregnancies require intensive antenatal care. These pregnancies are best delivered by caesarean section due to the inability to effectively monitor all fetuses in labour and the higher risk of fetal malpresentation.

Key Points

- It is essential to establish chorionicity by 11^{+0} to 13^{+6} weeks' gestation in multiple pregnancies to plan and deliver appropriate antenatal care.
- Increasing fetal number and monochorionicity are associated with increased risks of adverse outcomes.
- The shared fetal circulations within a monochorionic placenta can cause specific complications, such as TTTS, but also make the care of other generic twin complications, such as selective fetal growth restriction or anomaly of one twin, more complex.
- Pre-term labour is the most common cause of neonatal morbidity and mortality in multiple pregnancies.

Chapter 31

Labour and Analgesia

Marie-Anne Ledingham

Chapter Outline

Introduction

Labour is a challenging time for mothers and their babies. The success of labour and the ability of the fetus to negotiate a journey through the maternal pelvis depends upon the successful interaction of three variables – the 'power' (contractions), 'passenger' (fetus) and 'pelvis' (bony pelvis and pelvic soft tissues). For women, this is often a life-changing event, with the experience that a woman has at this time potentially having both short- and long-term physical and emotional effects. For most women, this is a positive, joyous life event, but the challenges faced during labour can potentially result in adverse outcomes for mother and baby. Midwives and obstetricians are intimately involved in the care of women in normal labour, in trying to ensure normality, in recognising at an early stage when obstetric intervention may be required in the maternal or fetal interest, and in ensuring that the woman's choices and opinions are respected. The majority of women in the United Kingdom will have a normal delivery in pregnancy after 37 weeks' gestation after a healthy uncomplicated pregnancy, with almost two-thirds of women going into labour spontaneously. Of these women, 40% will be in their first pregnancy. Good communication with women is essential at this time to help them feel supported and in control, with the aim of making birth a positive experience for all concerned.

Evolution and Human Labour

Labour is defined as the onset of regular uterine activity associated with effacement and dilatation of the cervix and descent of the presenting part through the cervix. The control and timing of delivery is crucial to the survival of any species and, in most, the interval between conception and parturition varies little. This is not the case in human pregnancy, in which delivery can occur many weeks before or after the expected due date.

Labour in humans is surprisingly hazardous. Evolution ought to have favoured those mothers who deliver without problems. Yet, for those without access to good medical care, the lifetime risk of dying from labour and postnatal complications may be as high as 10%.

Apes are able to give birth with little problem. Their pelvises are relatively large, the fetal head is relatively small, and the fetus is born facing anteriorly. When the Australopithecines adopted an upright posture around 4 million years ago, the pelvic shape became narrower in the anteroposterior plane to allow more efficient weight transfer from the trunk to the femurs. As the fetal head was still relatively small, the Australopithecines were also able to deliver without much problem, although this time the head was in the transverse position.

With further evolution 1.5 million years ago to *Homo erectus* and then *Homo sapiens*, the volume of the brain increased from around 500 mL to 1000 to 2000 mL. This increased the chance of the head being bigger than the pelvis (cephalopelvic disproportion), and to deliver successfully it became necessary for the head to rotate during birth. The head entered the pelvic brim in the transverse position as the inlet is widest in the transverse plane, but rotated at the pelvic floor to the anteroposterior plane, which is the widest diameter of the pelvic outlet.

This process requires efficient uterine activity and is aided by 'moulding' of the fetal head. Moulding is possible because the individual skull bones are unfused – therefore, they can move or even override each other to form the most efficient shape for delivery. The pelvic ligaments, particularly the cartilaginous joint of the symphysis pubis, relax antenatally under the influence of relaxin to maximise the pelvic diameters. Successful delivery also requires the fetus to enter the pelvis in the appropriate position. When these criteria are not met, problems may occur, which are discussed further in Chapter 34. The difficulty with human delivery is related to the balance between our need to run (and, therefore, have a narrow pelvis) and our need to think (and, therefore, have a big head).

Primigravid Compared With Multigravid Labour

There is a considerable difference between the labour of a primigravida (a woman having her first labour) and that of a parous woman who has had a previous vaginal birth (Table 31.1). A successful vaginal birth first time around usually leads to subsequent births being relatively uneventful. Conversely, a caesarean section or other complications in a first labour can lead to subsequent obstetric problems.

The Uterus During Pregnancy

The uterus is a thick-walled hollow organ, normally located entirely within the lesser pelvis (Table 31.2) in the non-pregnant state. The smooth muscle fibres interdigitate to form a single functional muscle that increases markedly during pregnancy, mainly by hypertrophy (an increase in size of cells) and to a lesser extent by hyperplasia (an increase in the number of smooth muscle cells).

From early pregnancy onwards, the uterus contracts intermittently; the frequency and amplitude of these contractions increase as labour approaches. These 'Braxton Hicks' contractions are irregular, low frequency and high amplitude in character, and are only occasionally painful. They are thought to begin at

TABLE 31.1 The Differences Between a Normal Primigravid and Multigravid Labour

Primigravida	Multigravida
Unique psychological experience	
Inefficient uterine action is common; therefore, labour is often longer.	Uterine action is efficient and the genital tract stretches more easily; therefore, labour is usually shorter.
The functional capacity of the pelvis is not known – cephalopelvic disproportion is a possibility.	Cephalopelvic disproportion is rare. If it occurs, it is usually secondary to a serious problem.
Serious injury to the child is relatively more common. The incidence of instrumental birth is higher.	Serious injury to the child is rare. Risk of birth injury is less when the baby is born by propulsion rather than traction.
The uterus is virtually immune to rupture.	Small risk of uterine rupture, particularly if there is a pre-existing caesarean section scar.

TABLE 31.2 Changes in the Uterus and Cervix During Pregnancy

	Non-Pregnant Uterus	Term Uterus
Weight (g)	50	950
Length (cm)	7.5	30
Depth (cm)	2.5	20
Shape	Flattened pear	Ovoid and erect
Position	Anteverted and anteflexed in pelvic cavity	Rotated to right in the abdominal cavity
	Non-Pregnant Cervix	**Cervix At Term**
Length (cm)	2.5	2.5
Colour	Pink	Blue and vascular

Modified from Harrison JM. The initiation of labour: physiological mechanisms. *Br J Midwifery.* 2000;8:281–285.

a 'pacemaker point' close to the junction of the uterus and the fallopian tube (although this has never been confirmed anatomically) and spread from this point downwards. The intensity of contractions is maximal at the fundus (where the muscle is thickest), intermediate at the mid-zone and least at the lower segment.

The Initiation of Labour

In humans, despite major advances in molecular biology and the science of reproduction, there is still much that is not known about the physiological processes involved in the initiation of labour. Some of the information we have about this process is derived from animal studies in which our understanding is more complete. In some mammals, changing levels of estrogen and progesterone regulate the timing of onset of labour. In other animals – for example, sheep – there is some evidence that the fetal adrenal secretion of corticosteroids is the trigger. In humans, however, the process appears to be more complicated, involving the coordinated inhibition and activation of a variety of factors. Our limited understanding of this process means that any proposed mechanism is hypothetical and open to constant change as our knowledge advances.

There is increasing evidence that human parturition involves activation of inflammatory pathways finally leading to cervical ripening, the onset of uterine activity, and membrane rupture. This process appears to be controlled in some way by a complex interaction of various mediators. Therefore, the onset of labour appears to occur when there is the coordinated 'release' of the uterus and cervix from the inhibitory effects of various pro-pregnancy factors and the simultaneous activation of various pro-labour factors (Box 31.1). How these factors interact and why labour occurs at a specific time (whether pre-term or at term) is unclear and still the subject of much ongoing research.

BOX 31.1 PRO-PREGNANCY FACTORS AND PRO-LABOUR FACTORS

Pro-Pregnancy Factors
- Progesterone
- Nitric oxide
- Catecholamines
- Relaxin

Pro-Labour Factors
- Estrogens
- Oxytocin
- Prostaglandins
- Corticotrophin-releasing hormone
- Prostaglandin dehydrogenase
- Inflammatory mediators

Pro-Pregnancy Factors

Progesterone is derived from the corpus luteum for the first 8 weeks or so of pregnancy and thereafter from the placenta. It has the direct effect of decreasing uterine oxytocin receptor sensitivity and, therefore, promotes uterine smooth muscle relaxation. In addition, progesterone seems to have an anti-inflammatory role. It also decreases cytokine production and the influx of immune cells into the myometrium and cervix occurring in normal labour. Its role in maintenance of uterine quiescence during pregnancy is illustrated by the fact that the progesterone antagonist mifepristone increases myometrial contractility and has been successfully used to induce labour. Progesterone withdrawal has been shown in animal studies in sheep and goats to trigger labour. However, human parturition is not associated with a fall in serum progesterone levels, suggesting instead that there may be a 'functional' progesterone withdrawal, perhaps caused by changes in the progesterone receptor. This may lead, in turn, to a decrease in the transcription of genes which cause uterine relaxation and an increase in the transcription of genes which increase the sensitivity of the myometrium to uterotonic agents and also cause activation of inflammatory pathways within the cervix and myometrium.

Nitric oxide, a highly reactive free radical, is also a pro-pregnancy factor. Some studies have observed a fall in uterine nitric oxide synthetase activity as pregnancy advances, but these findings are not confirmed in other studies. Nitric oxide may be involved in the process of cervical ripening, which involves remodelling of the extracellular matrix and collagen. Catecholamines act directly on the myometrial cell membrane to alter contractility and beta-sympathomimetics have been used as tocolytics to suppress pre-term labour. The specific roles of catecholamines in physiological terms and the role of the hormone relaxin are unclear, although they may indirectly cause uterine muscle relaxation by stimulating prostacyclin production.

Pro-Labour Factors

Oxytocin, a nonapeptide from the posterior pituitary, is a potent stimulator of uterine contractility. However, circulating levels do not change as term approaches. The rise in oxytocin receptor levels explains the increase in sensitivity of the uterus to circulating levels of oxytocin as pregnancy advances. It is unlikely that the onset of labour in humans is triggered by oxytocin release. However, it is clear that oxytocin release during labour increases the frequency and force of uterine contractions.

Changes in oxytocin receptor concentration are mediated in part by activation of the fetal hypothalamic–pituitary axis with release of fetal adrenocorticotrophic hormone. Prostaglandin levels also increase prior to the onset of labour. These are synthesised from arachidonic acid by cyclo-oxygenase (COX); COX-2 enzyme expression in the fetal membranes has been observed to double by the time labour begins. Prostaglandins promote cervical ripening and stimulate uterine contractility both directly and by upregulation of oxytocin receptors. There is some evidence that the increased levels may be mediated by maternal corticotrophin-releasing hormone secretion. Inflammatory cells are recruited into the fetal membranes, uterus and cervix at the onset of labour, perhaps as a result of distension of the uterus and/or endocrine hormone signaling from the fetus itself. A number of cytokines are produced – such as interleukin (IL)-8, tumour necrosis factor (TNF)-alpha, IL-6, and IL-1β) – which, in turn, set up activation of pro-inflammatory transcription factors. This inflammatory response is thought to contribute to cervical ripening and membrane rupture via an increase in collagenase activity. It may also contribute to an increase in uterine activity by inhibition of progesterone and activation of contractile genes (COX-2, oxytocin receptor).

The Mechanism of Normal Labour and Birth (See Also Chapter 1)

The mechanism of labour involves effacement and then dilatation of the cervix, followed by expulsion of the fetus by uterine contractions. The lower part of the uterus is anchored to the pelvis by the transverse cervical (or cardinal) ligaments and uterosacral ligaments, allowing the shortening uterine muscle to drive the fetus downwards (Box 31.2).

BOX 31.2 SUMMARY OF THE MECHANISM OF LABOUR

- Head at pelvic brim in left or right occipitolateral position.
- Neck flexes so that the presenting diameter is suboccipitobregmatic.
- Head descends and engages.
- Head reaches the pelvic floor and occiput rotates to occipitoanterior.
- Head delivers by extension.
- Descent continues and shoulders rotate into the anteroposterior diameter of the pelvis.
- Head restitutes (comes into line with the shoulders).
- Anterior shoulder delivered by lateral flexion from downward pressure on the baby's head; posterior shoulder delivered by lateral flexion upwards.

CERVICAL RIPENING

The cervix is composed of a network of collagen fibres embedded in ground substance made of extracellular matrix. During the later stages of pregnancy, it softens and begins to efface so that birth can occur. Prostaglandins increase cervical ripening by inhibiting collagen synthesis and stimulating collagenase activity to break down the collagen. This collagenase activity comes, in part, not only from fibroblast cells but also from an influx of inflammatory cells, supporting the theory that labour is, in part, like an inflammatory process. Dermatan sulphate (a proteoglycan molecule) is replaced with hyaluronic acid, which is more hydrophilic, and the water content of the cervix increases. As a result of these changes, the concentration of collagen fibres decreases and the cervix becomes softer and ready to dilate. In clinical practice, cervical ripening is assessed using the Bishop score (Table 31.3). The parameters of this score include cervical length, cervical dilatation, consistency and position and station of the presenting part (relative to the ischial spines in the woman's pelvis).

ACTIVATION OF THE MYOMETRIUM

Contractions in the uterus, like any other smooth muscle, involve adenosine triphosphonate (ATP)-dependent binding of myosin to actin. The process involves phosphorylation of the enzyme myosin light chain kinase, which is dependent on calcium and calmodulin for its activity. Hence, calcium-channel blockers and beta agonists inhibit uterine activity by decreasing intracellular free calcium levels, and prostaglandins and oxytocin increase uterine activity by bringing about an increase in free calcium.

The uterine smooth muscle cells are embedded in a supporting framework of collagen fibres and extracellular matrix. The myometrial fibres communicate with each other by means of gap junctions between cells. These gap junctions facilitate cell signalling and allow the smooth muscle to act as a syncytium, with contractions spreading from one cell to another. During pregnancy, gap junctions are few in number. However, as pregnancy advances, they increase in concentration and size within the uterus. One of the actions of estrogen and prostaglandin is to increase gap junction formation, while human chorionic gonadotrophin may decrease their formation.

DESCENT AND BIRTH OF THE BABY

As the cervix dilates and the uterus contracts, the fetus needs to descend into the pelvis. The widest two points of the fetus are the head in the anteroposterior plane (Fig. 31.1) and the shoulders laterally, from one shoulder tip to the other (bisacromial diameter). The head rotates from a lateral position at the pelvic brim to the anteroposterior position at the outlet (Figs 31.2–31.4). This rotation has the advantage that by the time the head is delivering through the outlet, the shoulders will be entering the inlet in the transverse position, maximising the chance of successful birth.

The position of the head as it traverses the canal is described according to the position of the occiput in relation to the mother's pelvis. The head usually enters the pelvic brim in either the right or left occipitotransverse position (Fig. 31.5A). The contracting uterus above causes the head to flex so that the smallest diameter is presented for birth.

As the head descends it reaches the V-shaped pelvic floor at the level of the ischial spines (see Fig. 31.5B–D). The shape of the pelvic floor encourages the fundamentally important head rotation. Fig. 31.6 illustrates the tendency for the longest part of the head to fit into the lowest part of the V-shaped gutter, achievable only by

TABLE 31.3	Bishop Score			
Parameter	0	1	2	3
Dilatation (cm)	<1	1–2	2–4	>4
Length (cm)	>4	2–4	1–2	<1
Consistency	Firm	Average	Soft	
Position	Posterior	Mid	Anterior	
Station	–3	–2	–1, 0	+1, +2

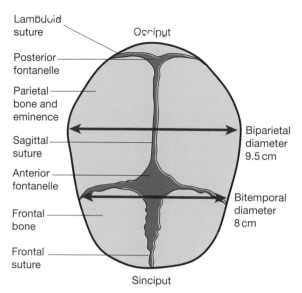

Fig. 31.1 **The fetal skull.** The widest diameter is anteroposterior.

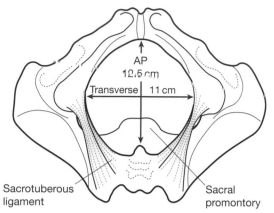

Fig. 31.3 **The maternal pelvic outlet.** The widest diameter is antero-posterior (AP).

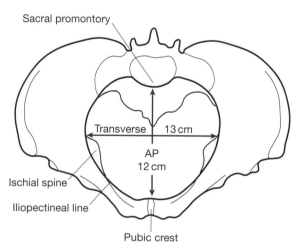

Fig. 31.2 **The maternal pelvic inlet.** The widest diameter is from one side laterally to the other. *AP,* Anteroposterior.

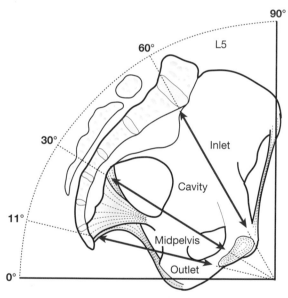

Fig. 31.4 **Lateral view of the pelvis.**

a 90-degree rotation to either the occipitoanterior (OA) or occipitoposterior position. In most cases, the head rotates anteriorly. The consequences of posterior rotation are discussed on page 415. The head, now OA, descends beyond the ischial spines and extends, distending the vulva until it is eventually delivered (see Fig. 31.5E, F).

Meanwhile, at the pelvic inlet, the shoulders are now presenting in the transverse position. They, too,

descend to the pelvic floor and rotate to the antero-posterior position in the V of the pelvic floor (see Fig. 31.5G). By this time, the head has been completely delivered and it is free to rotate back to the transverse position along with the shoulders. The anterior shoulder can then be delivered by downward traction of the head so that the lateral traction on the fetal trunk allows the shoulder to be freed from under the pubic arch (see Fig. 31.5G). The posterior shoulder is delivered with

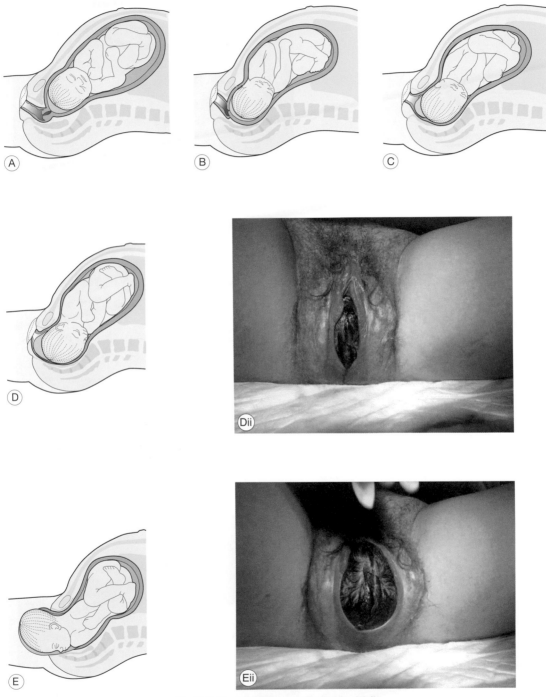

Fig. 31.5 Normal labour; A–I. See text for details.

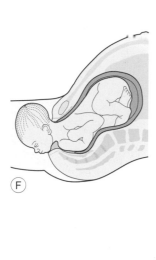

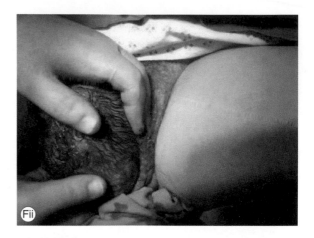

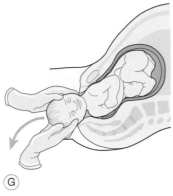

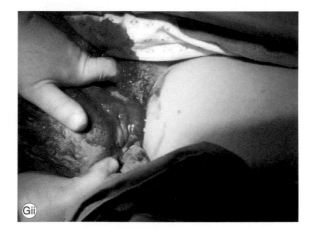

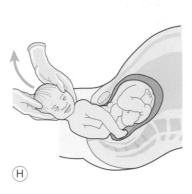

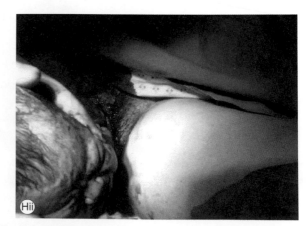

Fig. 31.5, cont'd

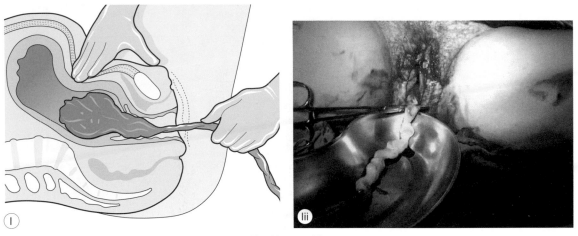

Fig. 31.5, cont'd

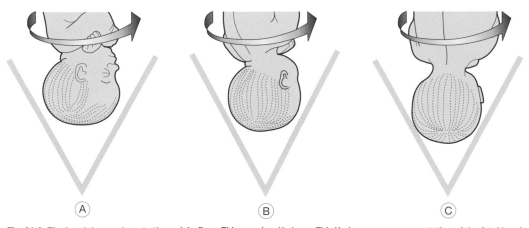

Fig. 31.6 The head descends onto the pelvic floor. This runs in a V-shape. This V-shape encourages rotation of the fetal head.

upward lateral traction and the rest of the baby usually follows without difficulty (see Fig. 31.5H).

The third stage of labour is from birth of the baby until delivery of the placenta. The uterus contracts, shearing the placenta from the uterine wall. This separation is often indicated by a small rush of dark blood and a 'lengthening' of the cord. The placenta can then be delivered by gentle cord traction (see Fig. 31.5I). However, caution is required to avoid uterine inversion.

DIAGNOSIS OF LABOUR

The diagnosis of 'labour' is important but often surprisingly difficult. The presence of palpable contractions does not necessarily mean that a woman is in labour, as Braxton Hicks contractions are common antenatally. For a diagnosis of labour, there needs to be 'uterine contraction' together with 'effacement (thinning) and dilatation of the cervix'.

Effacement has occurred when the entire length of the cervical canal has been 'taken up' into the lower segment of the uterus, a process that begins at the internal os and proceeds downwards to the external os until the cervical tissue becomes continuous with the uterine walls (Figs 31.7A–C). This is analogous to pulling a polo-necked sweater over your head. It is of note that 'dilatation' refers only to the dilatation of the external os. Again, there is an important difference between primigravid and multigravid labours, as

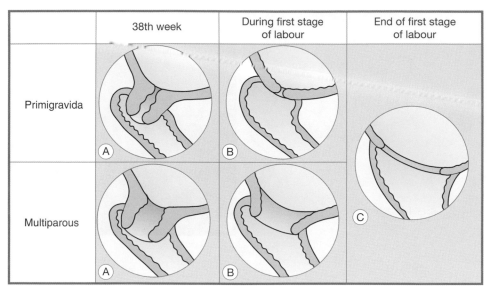

	38th week	During first stage of labour	End of first stage of labour
Primigravida	A	B	
Multiparous	A	B	C

Fig. 31.7 Cervical dilatation – primigravida versus multigravida. Note that in a multigravida, the cervix may dilate before effacement is complete.

dilatation will not begin in a primigravida until effacement has occurred, whereas both may occur simultaneously in a parous woman (see Fig. 31.7).

If there are regular contractions and a fully effaced cervix, the woman can be said to be in labour. If, however, there are contractions with only a partially effaced cervix, further objective evidence must be sought in the form of either a 'show' or spontaneous membrane rupture. A 'show', or bloodstained mucous discharge, has occurred in approximately two-thirds of women by the time of presentation and supports the diagnosis in those with regular contractions. Spontaneous membrane rupture in the presence of regular contractions also confirms the diagnosis.

RUPTURE OF THE MEMBRANES

Rupture of the fetal membranes is a vital part of normal labour. In 6% to 12% of labour, the membranes will rupture prior to the onset of uterine contractions or cervical dilatation, 'pre-labour rupture of the membranes'. The mother will usually describe the feeling of 'water' leaking vaginally, and if a speculum examination is carried out, a pool of liquor is typically seen in the posterior vaginal fornix. A digital vaginal examination is not routinely indicated, as this increases the risk of introducing infection. If managed conservatively, 60% of mothers will establish in labour spontaneously by 24 hours and 90% by 48 hours. However, this conservative management carries a small risk of ascending infection, which may lead to chorioamnionitis. Rarely, chorioamnionitis may progress to rapid overwhelming fetal and maternal sepsis.

Nonetheless, in view of the high chance of spontaneous labour over the first 24 hours, a conservative approach may be appropriate. This is provided that the mother is apyrexial, the baby is in cephalic presentation, the liquor is clear and fetal monitoring is normal. In women presenting with rupture of the membranes prior to the onset of labour, the risk of serious neonatal infection is 1% compared with 0.5% for women with intact membranes. Induction of labour may be offered after 24 hours if there are no signs that labour is becoming established. Women who present with pre-labour rupture of the membranes may also be offered induction of labour on admission, as this may reduce the incidence of neonatal infection with no increase in the rate of caesarean birth. Women with pre-labour rupture of membranes should be counselled about their options, and they and their partners should be involved in the decision-making process. Women who opt for conservative management should be made aware of signs and symptoms of infection and advised to attend hospital if there is any change in the colour or smell of their discharge or any decrease in fetal movements. If there is clinical suspicion of chorioamnionitis, with pyrexia or passage of meconium (see later discussion), the birth should be expedited. Pain and discharge are late features of intrauterine infection.

Clinical Progress in Labour

Labour is divided into three stages of unequal length (Table 31.4). There is no 'normal' time for the length of labour. However, the mean length of established labour (i.e., from 4 cm dilated, with regular painful contractions) is 8 hours for primigravid women but can be up to 18 hours. The mean length for second and subsequent labours is 5.5 hours but can be up to 12 hours. Even after a labour of 40 hours, the chance of a vaginal birth is still around 50%. Fetal distress (hypoxia) is only partly related to the length of labour. The highest incidence of caesarean birth for distress is in the first hour of labour, probably related to babies already compromised

antenatally with some pre-existing problem. Even after 24 hours, however, the chance of fetal distress remains low. It is recognised that markedly prolonged labour is associated with subsequent maternal pelvic floor dysfunction and fistulae. Therefore, there is no 'optimal' length of labour – each mother should be assessed on an individual basis with her views being taken into account when making decisions about her ongoing care.

FIRST STAGE

The onset of labour is often gradual, with changes occurring in the cervix and myometrium during pregnancy in preparation for this process. The first stage of labour is timed from the onset of regular uterine activity associated with progressive effacement and dilatation of the cervix. The first stage is complete when the cervix becomes fully dilated (10 cm). Progress in the first stage of labour is measured in terms of dilatation of the cervix and descent of the fetal head.

There are two phases of the first stage. The latent phase describes the time interval between the onset of labour and the completion of effacement. The cervix will be 3 to 4 cm dilated at the end of this stage. The length of the latent phase is particularly variable, especially for women having their first pregnancy. For some women, this stage of labour can be prolonged and potentially unsettling due to the uncertainty associated with the length of time it will take. Women should be supported at this time and encouraged to mobilise if possible. Simple analgesia can be advised. Some women may choose to use breathing exercises, massage and immersion in water to help with pain relief. Women can often remain at home in the latent phase; they should be informed that there is no reason to restrict eating and drinking at this time.

The active phase describes the time interval between the end of the latent phase and full dilatation (10 cm). When a woman presents in labour, a risk assessment will be performed to identify whether it is appropriate for her to continue with midwifery-led care. Initial assessment will include a review of her past obstetric history to identify potential complications. This may prompt referral to an obstetric-led rather than a midwifery-led unit. Baseline recordings of her pulse, blood pressure, temperature and urinalysis should be made along with an assessment of the length, strength and

TABLE 31.4	The Three Stages of Labour	
	Stage	**Phases**
First stage	From the onset of labour until the cervix is fully dilated; further subdivided into two phases.	Latent – onset of contractions until the cervix is fully effaced and 3–4 cm dilated
		Active – cervical dilatation
Second stage	From full cervical dilatation until the head has delivered. It also has two phases.	Propulsive – from full dilatation until head has descended onto the pelvic floor
		Expulsive – from the time the mother has an irresistible desire to bear down and push until the baby is born
Third stage	From birth of the baby until expulsion of the placenta and membranes.	

frequency of contractions. Women should be asked if their membranes have ruptured and about the colour and amount of amniotic fluid lost. Notes should also be made of any discharge or bleeding and whether the fetal movements are normal. A vaginal examination is often performed to confirm whether active labour has commenced. An abdominal examination is performed to assess fundal height, lie, presentation and engagement of the presenting part prior to this. The midwife makes an assessment of the contractions by palpation of the woman's abdomen and auscultation of the fetal heart is performed with either a handheld Doppler device or a Pinard stethoscope. Some hospitals will perform a cardiotocography (CTG) on low-risk women at first presentation in labour. This is controversial, as the benefit of CTG monitoring in low-risk women has not been proven. However, some women may request a CTG on admission. Their wishes should be respected following a discussion about the possible limitations of its use.

During labour, information about maternal observations (blood pressure, temperature, pulse), fetal heart rate, progressive cervical dilatation, descent of the presenting part in fifths palpable, the strength and frequency of contractions and the colour of the amniotic fluid draining are plotted on the partogram. This should be commenced when a woman is established in labour (Fig. 31.8). It forms a graphic record of clinical findings and any relevant events. The purpose is to help early recognition of abnormal labour, to ensure appropriate transfer of care where indicated, and to aid continuity of care.

Although there is no research on the ideal frequency of vaginal examinations in labour, the World Health Organization recommends that 4-hourly vaginal examinations are adequate. These should ideally be performed by the same professional to minimise interobserver variation (Table 31.5). Vaginal examinations should not be regarded as routine; they are unpleasant, may be painful and are associated with a risk of infection even when performed in a 'sterile' manner. The average rate of cervical dilatation in primigravidae is around 1 cm/h, although it is accepted that 0.5 cm/h can be normal.

Descent of the fetal head is measured in labour by abdominal examination, when the amount of the fetal head palpable above the pelvic brim (in fifths) is

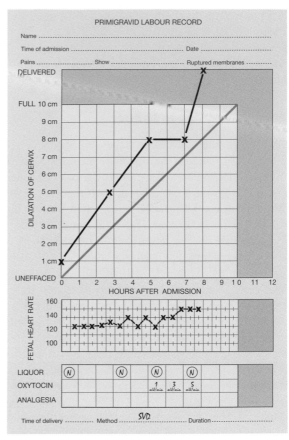

Fig. 31.8 Partogram suitable for recording a primigravid labour.

TABLE 31.5 Vaginal Examinations	
Findings on Vaginal Examination	**Details**
Presence or absence of meconium	Meconium staining might suggest fetal distress.
Dilatation of the cervix	In centimetres from 0 to 10 cm
Station of the presenting part	In centimetres above or below the ischial spines
Position of the head	With reference to the occiput if cephalic, or sacrum if breech. A note should be made of whether the head is flexed or deflexed.
Presence of caput and/or moulding	If excessive, might suggest obstructed labour.

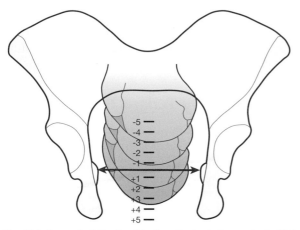

Fig. 31.9 Descent of the head is described relative to the ischial spines.

documented on the partogram. If only two-fifths or less of the fetal head is palpable abdominally, then the head is determined to be 'engaged' (Fig. 31.9).

On vaginal examination, the 'station' of the fetal head with respect to the ischial spines is recorded. Sometimes, it can be difficult to ascertain this accurately, as increasing caput succedaneum (see later discussion) can make the head seem artificially lower in the pelvis on vaginal examination. The ischial spines are designated 'station zero'. When the head is above the spines, it is said to be at –1, –2, –3 or –4 cm. If the head is below the spines, the notation is +1, +2, +3 or +4 cm. If the head is at the level of the ischial spines, it must be engaged.

It is important to note that the 'position' of the head on vaginal examination (VE) is with reference to the occiput, for example, OA, right occipitotransverse (ROT) or left occipitoposterior (LOP).

'Caput' (succedaneum) is oedema of the scalp owing to pressure of the head against the rim of the cervix and is classified somewhat arbitrarily as '+', '++' or '+++'. 'Moulding' describes the change in head shape, which occurs during labour, made possible by movement of the individual scalp bones. It is arbitrarily termed '+' if the bones are opposed, '++' if they overlap but can be reduced by digital pressure and '+++' if they overlap but cannot be reduced.

Uterine activity is routinely monitored in labour by palpation – measuring length, strength and frequency of contractions. Uterine activity over a 10-minute

period is plotted on the partogram. Women often report increasing regular uterine activity at the onset of labour.

In the first stage, an assessment of the fetal heart rate is made every 15 minutes by intermittent auscultation. If any abnormalities are detected by this method, CTG monitoring is advised in the first instance. For some women, this may mean transfer to hospital from home or a low-risk midwifery-led setting.

Passage of meconium in itself is not concerning. A healthy term baby will often pass meconium during labour; under these circumstances, it will be thin and green/brown in colour. However, passage of thick meconium, which is often more greenish in colour (pea soup), can be a sign of fetal hypoxia or acidosis.

SECOND STAGE

This begins when the cervix is fully dilated and ends with birth of the baby. In a similar way to the first stage of labour, the duration of the second stage of labour is different for nulliparous and parous women. It is generally recommended that for nulliparous women, birth would be expected to take place within 3 hours of the start of the active second stage of labour. For parous women, birth would be expected to take place within 2 hours of the start of the active second stage of labour. Progress is measured in terms of descent and rotation of the fetal head on vaginal examination. There are two distinct phases:

1. The propulsive/passive phase. This is from full dilatation until the head reaches the pelvic floor. During this time, the head is relatively high in the pelvis, the position is typically occipitotransverse, the lower vagina is not stretched, and the mother has no or little urge to push. In many respects, it is a natural extension of the first stage of labour.
2. The expulsive/active phase. This begins when the fetal head reaches the pelvic floor, the head becomes visible, and the mother usually has a strong involuntary desire to push.

With pushing, the head usually delivers. Normally, it does so in the OA position. After delivery it restitutes, returning to an occipitolateral position by rotating with the shoulders as they descend into the pelvis. The birth attendant then applies lateral traction to the head, moving it in the direction of the mother's back to allow the birth of the anterior fetal shoulder (see earlier discussion). At this point, an oxytocic is injected intramuscularly into the mother's thigh to encourage a prolonged uterine contraction and minimise the chance of postpartum haemorrhage. The head is then lifted anteriorly to allow delivery of the posterior shoulder, after which the rest of the baby is delivered with lateral flexion of the fetal body. The umbilical cord is clamped and cut. If the baby does not require resuscitation, cord clamping should be delayed and the baby may be placed on the mother's abdomen and skin-to-skin contact encouraged. If this is not the woman's preference, the baby should be wrapped in a warm towel and handed to the parents.

THIRD STAGE

This is the time from birth of the baby to delivery of the placenta and membranes. The third stage of labour can be managed physiologically or actively. Active management of the third stage of labour has been shown to decrease the risk of postpartum haemorrhage and the need for blood transfusion. It involves the use of an oxytocic (as mentioned earlier), deferred clamping and cutting of the cord, and gentle controlled cord traction using the Brandt-Andrews method after separation of the placenta has been diagnosed (see Fig. 31.5I). Placental separation is recognised by apparent lengthening of the cord and a gush of dark blood per vaginam. The operator exerts traction on the cord while the other hand maintains pressure upwards on the fundus. The main risk of cord traction is uterine inversion; the fundus is continually 'guarded' to prevent this (see p. 431). Once the placenta passes the vulva, it may be gently twisted to allow the membranes to peel off completely and the uterine fundus is rubbed up to ensure that the uterus is well contracted. Some women may choose to have a physiological third stage of labour. This involves no routine use of uterotonic drugs, no clamping of the cord until pulsation has ceased, and delivery of the placenta by maternal effort only. The third stage is prolonged if it is not completed within 30 minutes after birth of the baby with active management and within 60 minutes of birth of the baby with physiological management.

The labia, vagina and perineum are inspected for tears and sutured if bleeding. Finally, the placenta is examined to ensure that it is complete.

The normal blood loss at delivery is about 300 mL. The routine use of an oxytocic following delivery of the anterior shoulder reduces the risk of postpartum haemorrhage by about 60%.

Episiotomies and Perineal Tears

Episiotomy should not routinely be performed at the time of a normal vaginal birth, as there is no clear evidence that this reduces the incidence of third- or fourth-degree tears. Midline episiotomy in particular does not protect the perineum or sphincters during childbirth and may impair anal continence. If an episiotomy is to be performed, a right (or, less commonly, left) mediolateral episiotomy is preferred (Fig. 31.10).

Restricting the use of episiotomy to specific fetal and maternal indications leads to lower rates of posterior perineal trauma, less need for suturing, and fewer long-term complications. A spontaneous tear may be

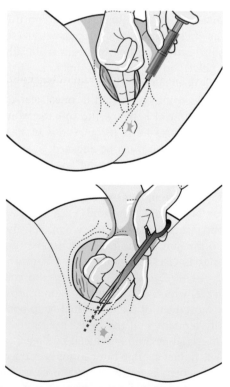

Fig. 31.10 If required, an episiotomy is usually carried out after infiltration of the perineum with local anaesthesia.

less painful than an episiotomy and may also heal better.

Possible indications for an episiotomy are as follows:

- A rigid perineum which is preventing birth
- If it is judged that a large tear is imminent
- Most instrumental deliveries (forceps or ventouse)
- Suspected fetal compromise
- Shoulder dystocia (to permit access to the birth canal).

Prior to an episiotomy, local anaesthetic is injected into the subcutaneous tissues of the perineum and vagina (unless there is an effective regional block). A right mediolateral cut is made and pressure on the fetal head is maintained so that the delivery is slow and the head remains flexed, minimising the possibility of the incision extending. The cut should begin at the vaginal fourchette and be at angle of between 45 and 60 degrees to the vertical axis.

Spontaneous tears are categorised into four degrees (Table 31.6). An episiotomy is an iatrogenic second-degree tear. Anterior perineal trauma is classified as any injury to the labia, anterior vagina, urethra or clitoris, and is described as such.

REPAIR OF EPISIOTOMIES AND PERINEAL TEARS

Before performing repair of a perineal tear or episiotomy, it is important to ensure that the woman has been offered analgesia and that she is in a comfortable position so that the genital area can be adequately examined. Good lighting is essential and the examination should be done gently and with sensitivity. A rectal examination should be performed as part of the

TABLE 31.6	Classification of Spontaneous Perineal Tears
	Tear Involves
First degree	Injury to the vaginal epithelium and vulval skin only
Second degree	Injury to the perineal muscles, but not the anal sphincter
Third degree	Injury to the perineum involving the anal sphincter complex
Fourth degree	Injury to the perineum involving the anal sphincter complex and anal/rectal mucosa

procedure to ensure that there is no damage to the anal sphincter or to the perineal muscles.

Repair should be with a rapidly absorbable synthetic material, using a continuous subcuticular (non-locking) technique to minimise short- and long-term problems (Fig. 31.11). These newer suture materials result in less short-term pain and less analgesic requirements than do older materials, such as catgut and non-absorbable sutures. Good perineal hygiene after delivery is likely to aid healing, and the use of ice packs and analgesia may be useful to alleviate discomfort. The use of rectal non-steroidal analgesia may be helpful provided that there is no contraindication to its use.

REPAIR OF EPISIOTOMY AND FIRST- OR SECOND-DEGREE TEARS

The perineum is infiltrated with local anaesthetic (Fig. 31.11A; unless an epidural is in place or there has been a pudendal block or perineal infiltration prior to birth). The apex of the vaginal incision or tear

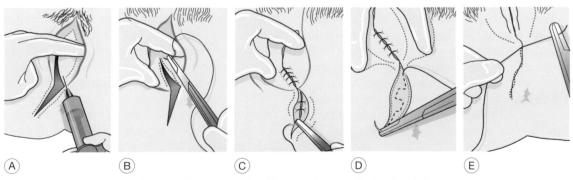

(A)   (B)   (C)   (D)   (E)

Fig. 31.11 Repair of a perineal tear or episiotomy. See text for details.

is identified and the first suture placed just above this level (Fig. 31.11B; care is needed because the rectum is just posterior to the vaginal wall).

The use of a loose, continuous non-locking method for vaginal mucosa and perineal muscles and a continuous subcuticular technique for perineal skin is recommended (Fig. 31.11C–E).

REPAIR OF THIRD- OR FOURTH-DEGREE TEARS

This should be by an experienced clinician, in theatre, with good analgesia, good light, the appropriate instruments and an assistant. The anal mucosa (if involved) is repaired using interrupted dissolving sutures, with the knot of each suture placed in the anal canal. The internal anal sphincter is then identified and its ends approximated and sutured with a monofilament suture, such as polydioxanone. Next, the ends of the external anal sphincter are identified and either approximated or overlapped – again, with the monofilament suture. The rest is as described earlier for first- and second-degree tears. Antibiotics, laxatives, and physiotherapy are important to facilitate healing.

Analgesia in Labour

Although there is an acceptance, to a degree, that labour is a painful experience, we must guard against the inevitability that labour should be painful. Pregnant women, especially primigravidae, find it difficult to conceptualise the amount of pain they may experience or their ability to cope with it until they are in established labour. They may choose to suffer some pain, but the extent to which women should experience pain should ideally be agreed upon, mainly by the woman but in consultation with a midwife and/or obstetrician and/or anaesthetist.

The pain of labour can be severe. It is a complex mix of physiological, psychological and emotional factors and can be difficult to treat. Many different forms of analgesia have been suggested; each has varying efficacies, risk profiles and potential complications.

Pain is unpleasant for the woman, although there is often some amnesia, which can positively influence its perception in retrospect. It is also recognised that the childbirth experience is influenced by maternal expectations and preparation, and by the severity of pain in labour.

FACTORS INFLUENCING PAIN

The severity of labour pain can vary depending on obstetric, psychological and emotional factors. Pain scores have been shown to be higher in primigravid women than in multiparous women, especially if they have not had any antenatal preparation. Reports have also shown that primigravid women generally experience more sensory pain during early labour compared with multiparous women, who experience more intense pain much later in labour as a result of rapid descent of the fetus.

Long labours are perceived as being more painful. Labour is also reported to be more painful with fetal malposition. In particular, a woman whose baby is occipitoposterior may experience continuous backache and a prolonged labour.

PHYSIOLOGY OF LABOUR PAIN

There are two components to the pain of labour: visceral (relating to an organ, i.e., the uterus) and somatic (relating to other tissues).

Visceral labour pain occurs during the first stage of childbirth. It is due to progressive mechanical dilatation of the cervix, distension of the lower uterine segment and contraction of the uterine muscles. Labour pain may also be a result of the myometrial and cervical ischaemia that occurs during contractions. Severity of this pain mirrors the duration and intensity of contractions. Visceral pain is transmitted by small unmyelinated 'C' fibres, which travel with sympathetic fibres and pass through the uterine, cervical and hypogastric nerve plexuses into the main sympathetic chain. The pain fibres from the sympathetic chain then enter the white rami communicantes associated with the T10 to L1 spinal nerves and pass via their posterior nerve roots to synapse in the dorsal horn of the spinal cord. Chemical mediators involved in this pain transmission include bradykinin, leucotrienes, prostaglandins, serotonin, substance P and lactic acid. This pain is dull in character and is sensitive to opioid drugs.

Somatic labour pain occurs during the late first stage and second stage of labour. It is due to stretching and distension of the pelvic floor, perineum and vagina. It occurs as a result of descent of the fetus; during this stage of labour, the uterus contracts more intensely in a rhythmic and regular manner. Somatic pain is transmitted by fine, myelinated, rapidly transmitting

'A delta' fibres. Transmission occurs via the pudendal nerves and perineal branches of the posterior cutaneous nerve of the thigh to the S2 to S4 nerve roots. Somatic fibres from the cutaneous branches of the ilio-inguinal and genitofemoral nerves also carry afferent fibres to L1 and, to some degree, L2.

All resulting nerve impulses (visceral and somatic) pass to dorsal horn cells and, finally, to the brain via the spinothalamic tract. Direct pressure of the fetus on the lumbosacral plexus also results in neuropathic pain during labour.

PSYCHOLOGY OF LABOUR PAIN

Maternal control makes labour a more positive experience. Attitudes towards pain and pain relief in labour depend on personal aspirations, expectations, cultural factors, learned behaviours, peer group influences, desirability of the pregnancy, previous experiences of pain, pre-existing anxiety or depression and preparation, education and communication.

Methods of Pain Relief

NON-PHARMACOLOGICAL METHODS

Maternal Support

Psychological support is extremely valuable and allows pharmacological intervention to be minimised. With continuous 1 : 1 support in labour, women need less analgesia, are more likely to have a vaginal birth, and are more satisfied with their labour. The supporting person does not need to be the woman's partner or a midwife. Indeed, it may be more useful if the supporting person is not part of the woman's social network at all.

Environment

Women may choose to have music played in labour and may opt to have a light diet as long as her labour is uncomplicated. Women are encouraged to be mobile, to walk and to try to achieve comfortable positions; it is recognised that pain is increased by being flat on the back. Positions such as squatting, all fours, or a birthing chair or birthing ball may reduce the need for pharmacological pain relief.

Birthing Pools

The use of warm baths and birthing pools (Fig. 31.12) has been shown to reduce pain and the need for

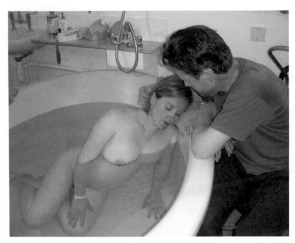

Fig. 31.12 A birthing pool. The environment for labour and birth is important in reducing the need for pharmacological intervention.

regional analgesia. These should not be used within 2 hours of the administration of opioids or if the woman is drowsy.

Education

Maternal education has some effect in engendering calm and making expectations realistic. This thereby improves control and reduces pain and distress in labour.

Breathing and relaxation techniques, the playing of music, massage, acupuncture, acupressure and hypnosis are used by many women, but have limited evidence to support their effectiveness. There is no evidence that transcutaneous electrical nerve stimulation (TENS) has any benefit.

PHARMACOLOGICAL METHODS

Inhaled Analgesics

Entonox (a 50 : 50 mixture of oxygen and nitrous oxide) is commonly used by labouring women. Despite its widespread use, studies have shown that it is not a potent analgesic in labour. Reassuringly, however, there is good evidence for its safety. That said, any pain relief it offers is limited, and it can lead to nausea, vomiting, drowsiness and light-headedness.

The anaesthetic gases isoflurane, desflurane and sevoflurane can be used safely at sub-anaesthetic concentrations with or without nitrous oxide to improve analgesic efficacy during labour. Although studies have shown that sevoflurane is superior to Entonox in providing pain relief, these gases are not widely available for use in the labour setting.

Systemic Opioid Analgesia

Systemic opioids have a limited effect, irrespective of the drug, the route or the method of administration. There is some limited evidence that intramuscular diamorphine gives more effective analgesia than other opioids, and it may have fewer side effects. There is the potential for maternal nausea, vomiting and drowsiness, and short-term respiratory depression and drowsiness in the neonate. Opiates should be avoided if delivery is thought to be likely to occur within 4 hours of administration. Antiemetics should be administered when parenteral opioids are used. Women should be aware that the use of opioids during labour may interfere with breastfeeding and bonding after delivery.

Opioids can be given as a subcutaneous or continuous intravenous infusion which is controlled by the woman – patient-controlled analgesia (PCA) – rather than as intramuscular injections. Remifentanil is often used under these circumstances, as it is short acting and women can control dose administration to coincide with contractions.

Pudendal Analgesia

The pudendal nerve, derived from the second, third and fourth sacral nerve roots, supplies the vulva and perineum. It crosses the sacrospinous ligament behind the ischial spine along with the pudendal artery (Fig. 31.13). Local infiltration at this point may provide useful perineal analgesia for a low-outlet forceps or ventouse delivery. A pudendal needle is inserted through the sacrospinous ligament. After aspirating to ensure that the injection is not intravascular, a local anaesthetic is injected behind the ligament on that side. The injection is repeated on the other side; it is usual to infiltrate the perineum directly at the same time.

Regional Analgesia

This refers to the delivery of analgesic drugs into the intrathecal (subarachnoid) space or into the epidural space (Fig. 31.14). In obstetric anaesthesia, the introduction of a drug to the intrathecal space tends to be

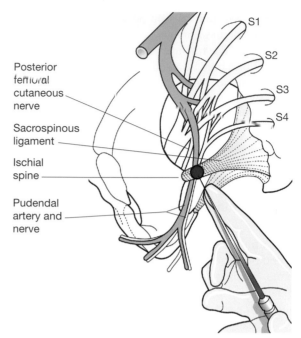

Fig. 31.13 The pudendal nerve runs behind the sacrospinous ligament.

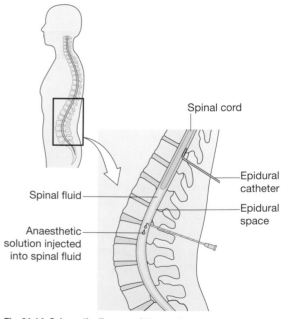

Fig. 31.14 Schematic diagram of the meninges.

known as 'a spinal' and the introduction of drug to the epidural space, as 'an epidural'.

In general, epidurals are used for analgesia in labour and spinals as a form of anaesthesia for caesarean section and other operative procedures (Table 31.7). The use of regional techniques for anaesthesia has resulted in a reduction in the use of general anaesthesia for caesarean section and other operative procedures. This, in turn, has had an impact on maternal morbidity and mortality from anaesthetic causes.

Epidural Analgesia for Labour

There is good evidence that epidurals provide more effective pain relief than parenteral opioids. The main indication for epidural analgesia is maternal request, but there may be obstetric indications, for example, in twin delivery to allow manipulation of the second twin if necessary. Continuous electronic fetal monitoring is recommended. Epidurals do not cause a prolonged first stage, do not lead to an increased rate of caesarean section, and are not associated with long-term backache. However, they have been associated with a prolonged second stage and a higher rate of instrumental birth, but this may be less of an issue with some lower-dose regimens. The addition of opioid to the epidural solution allows less local anaesthetic use and, therefore, greater mobility. Epidural analgesia should be continued until after the third stage and for perineal repair if necessary.

Where labour proceeds to a trial of instrumental vaginal birth or caesarean section, or if complications requiring operative intervention are encountered, the epidural can be topped up or a spinal can be used instead.

Side effects of epidurals (Table 31.8) can arise from the mechanical nature of the technique or from the drugs themselves. Neurological complications from mechanical insertion are rare. However, inadvertent dural puncture may occur and subsequent

TABLE 31.7 Differences Between Epidural and Spinal Analgesia

Epidural	Spinal
Extradural catheter placement	Subarachnoid injection
Cannula allows top up for prolonged use	One-off injection lasting 2–4 hours
Analgesic effect may be patchy	Dense and relatively reliable anaesthetic blockade

TABLE 31.8 Complications of Regional Analgesia

Complication	Details
Dural puncture headache	Occurs due to cerebrospinal fluid leak from subarachnoid space. Headache when sitting upright and relieved when lying flat. Blood patch may be necessary to treat.
Hypotension	Fall in blood pressure due to blockage of sympathetic tone to peripheral blood vessels, resulting in vasodilatation.
Local anaesthetic toxicity	Systemic toxicity occurs when local anaesthetic is injected into blood vessel. Affects central nervous system and cardiovascular systems, ultimately progressing to cardiovascular collapse and death.
Accidental total spinal block	Occurs with accidental injection of epidural doses of local anaesthetic into the subarachnoid space. Implies anaesthesia has spread to brainstem, resulting in loss of consciousness, respiratory arrest, and profound hypotension. Treatment involves intubation, ventilation, and circulatory support.
Neurological complications	Peripheral nerve injury can occur secondary to direct needle trauma, intraneural injection of local anaesthetic, compression from haematoma or abscess formation, stretch injury, or nerve ischaemia. Majority of injuries are transient; 95% resolve in 4–6 weeks and 99% resolve in 1 year.
Effects on labour	Epidural analgesia increases assisted vaginal birth rates unless second stage is actively managed.
Bladder dysfunction	Loss of sensation can predispose to bladder overdistension. This can lead to long-term voiding dysfunction. Bladder care in labour is important and catheterization should be performed in women having difficulty voiding.

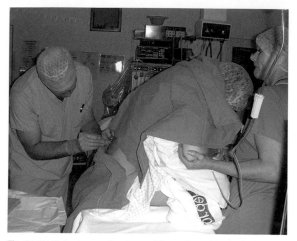

Fig. 31.15 Spinal anaesthesia provides a dense block, which is particularly useful for caesarean birth and some instrumental births.

ongoing cerebrospinal fluid leakage can lead to a 'spinal headache'. This leakage can be sealed using a technique known as a 'blood patch'. Side effects from the local anaesthetic and opioid are hypotension, urinary retention, pyrexia, pruritus, maternal respiratory depression and neonatal respiratory depression. The hypotension results from sympathetic blockade and peripheral vasodilatation. It should be managed by lying the woman in the left lateral position, giving oxygen, and treating with either intravenous fluids or vasopressors.

Spinal Anaesthesia

Spinals can be used primarily for analgesia, but are more commonly used for anaesthesia before caesarean birth, instrumental birth or the surgical management of postpartum complications, such as a retained placenta or the repair of third- and fourth-degree tears (Fig. 31.15). In obstetric anaesthesia, spinals are invariably carried out as a single shot, which provides a dense block for 2 to 4 hours. As with epidurals, the addition of an opioid allows some sparing of the local anaesthetic volume (and, therefore, dose). This, in turn, allows some sparing of the side effects of sympathetic block.

Complications of spinal anaesthesia can again be considered as related to the procedure and to the drugs. The mechanical complications are similar to those of the epidural. Hypotension also often occurs and is managed as described earlier. A high block

(which blocks fibres above T4), however, can lead to bradycardia, which, in turn, compounds any hypotension. A total spinal is a rare complication in which local anaesthetic affects the brain directly and leads to unconsciousness.

Combined spinal–epidural (CSE) is a technique whereby the epidural space is accessed using an epidural needle and then a spinal needle is passed down the epidural needle and advanced to the intrathecal space. 'Spinal doses' of drugs are given down the spinal needle; this needle is then removed and an epidural catheter introduced down the epidural needle to the epidural space. The epidural catheter can then be 'topped up' as necessary. CSE is used when rapid-onset analgesia is needed. However, the procedure may be prolonged such that epidural top-ups also may be needed or when the woman's condition cannot risk the potential sympathetic block, which might occur with a full spinal (cardiac disease) or a high motor block (respiratory disease). A smaller-dose spinal can then be used, with the facility to top this up epidurally.

General Anaesthesia

General anaesthesia in pregnancy carries more risk than in the non-pregnant patient. As there is reduced gastro-oesophageal tone, increased intra-abdominal mass and reduced gastric emptying, regurgitation of gastric contents and their aspiration to the lungs is more likely. In addition, as the gastric contents are more acidic in pregnancy, any aspiration is more likely to lead to pneumonitis. Difficult and failed intubation is more likely than in non-pregnant patients because of pregnancy-related obesity. Therefore, regional anaesthesia is to be preferred if possible.

Key Points

- **The correct diagnosis of 'labour' is central to good care.**
- **Labour is considered in three stages: the first from the onset of labour until the cervix is fully dilated, the second from then until birth of the baby, and the third from that point until delivery of the placenta and membranes.**
- **Compared with a multigravida, the labour of a primigravida is likely to be longer and more likely to result in both instrumental delivery and neonatal injury.**

- The choice of analgesia should be a balanced, well-informed decision based upon maternal preference following discussion about the efficacy, risks, and side effects of the analgesic methods available.
- Non-pharmacological options include psychological support from a birthing partner, a positive attitude from professionals, remaining mobile and finding comfortable positions, the use of warm baths and birthing pools, and other techniques of the woman's choice.
- Entonox is not a potent analgesic but there is good evidence for its efficacy and safety. Systemic opioid analgesia also has limited effect.
- There is good evidence for the analgesic benefits of epidural analgesia compared with systemic opioids. A 'low-dose' local anaesthetic and opioid mixture may be optimal.

Monitoring of the Fetus in Labour

Philip Owen

Introduction

The purpose of monitoring the fetus in labour is to identify those who might be at increased risk of death or hypoxic injury so that delivery can be expedited and harm prevented. Fetal monitoring involves fetal heart rate (FHR) assessment, either by intermittent auscultation or by continuous electronic measurement (cardiotocography (CTG): 'cardio' meaning heart, 'toco' meaning labour). Intermittent auscultation of the fetal heart is appropriate for monitoring fetal condition in labours at 'low risk' of fetal hypoxia, with electronic fetal monitoring being advised in labours at increased risk ('high risk') of hypoxia or if concern is raised by preceding intermittent auscultation. A 'normal' CTG reliably identifies the nonhypoxic fetus, but the converse is not true regarding an 'abnormal' CTG; there is a high false-positive rate and many fetuses suspected to be hypoxic are not. As a consequence, the use of the CTG increases the rate of obstetric intervention in return for limited neonatal benefit.

The term 'fetal distress' is widely used to describe a clinical scenario in which there is concern regarding fetal well-being. Unfortunately, the term lacks a precise definition and its use is not encouraged. A standardised categorisation of the CTG enables a more meaningful way of communicating the magnitude of concern. Analysis of the electrocardiogram (ECG) waveform in association with the CTG can improve its ability to correctly identify hypoxia.

Fetal Physiology

Fetal oxygenation depends on a number of factors.

MATERNAL BLOOD SUPPLY TO THE PLACENTA

During a contraction, the intramural vessels supplying the placenta are constricted by the smooth muscle fibres of the uterus. Provided that the contractions are not too long or too frequent, the placental blood supply has time to recover before the next contraction begins. In hyperstimulation, when the uterus is contracting too frequently, placental oxygenation may be impaired. In other circumstances, there may be placental hypoperfusion – for example, following the distal sympathetic blockade and associated hypotension – which can occur with spinal or epidural anaesthesia.

FUNCTIONAL CAPACITY OF THE PLACENTA

A small or poorly functioning placenta is less capable of adequate oxygen transfer than a larger or normally functioning placenta. In this situation, the fetus may already be growth restricted prior to the onset of labour and, therefore, more susceptible to hypoxic stress. In cases of placental abruption, partial placental separation leaves a reduced surface area for vascular communication. This results in less efficient oxygen exchange.

FETAL CIRCULATION

The fetus responds to hypoxia with peripheral vasoconstriction and redistribution of the blood to the heart and brain. Prolonged vasoconstriction may lead to damage in other organs manifesting in the neonatal period, such as the gastrointestinal tract (resulting in necrotising enterocolitis) and kidneys (renal impairment). Regardless of the protective effect of such redistribution, in the absence of intervention, prolonged or severe hypoxia and acidosis results in hypoxic brain damage or death.

Persistent or severe hypoxia leads to anaerobic metabolism and acidosis. The acid–base balance within the fetal circulation reflects the degree of oxygenation, which forms the basis of intrapartum fetal blood sampling (FBS).

Risk Assessment

FHR monitoring is recommended to all labouring women. The use of continuous electronic monitoring in 'low-risk' labours may increase the rate of intervention for little or no demonstrable benefit in terms of improved neonatal outcomes. It is important to consider which labours are at increased risk of hypoxia (so-called 'high-risk' labours) and which are 'low risk'. Some of these factors are outlined in Box 32.1

MECONIUM STAINING OF THE AMNIOTIC FLUID

Meconium (fetal stool) staining of the amniotic fluid is present in 15% of all deliveries at term and in about 40% at 42 weeks. The mechanism is considered to be stimulation of the vagus (parasympathetic) nerves in

---

BOX 32.1 PREGNANCIES AT INCREASED CHANCE ('HIGH RISK') OF FETAL HYPOXIA AND ACIDOSIS IN LABOUR

Fetal Factors
- Fetal growth restriction or small for gestational age (see p. 325)

Placental Factors
- Hypertension (see p. 333)
- Antepartum haemorrhage (see p. 315)

Obstetric Factors
- Precipitate labour (see p. 402)
- Pre-term labour (see p. 345)
- Prolonged labour (see p. 403)
- Induced labours or those augmented with oxytocin (see p. 395)
- Epidural analgesia
- Previous caesarean section
- Meconium (fetal stool) stained amniotic fluid (see later discussion)

---

utero, causing the fetal bowel to contract and the anal sphincter to relax. This often happens for no particular reason, but it also may occur as a response to fetal hypoxia. While often not of clinical significance, the presence of meconium staining increases the likelihood that there is underlying fetal hypoxia. A 'normal' CTG provides reassurance. An 'abnormal' CTG is more likely to truly represent fetal hypoxia in the presence of meconium staining.

Meconium staining may give rise to the 'meconium aspiration syndrome'. This is a form of neonatal pneumonitis. Clinical features range from mild neonatal tachypnoea to severe respiratory compromise. The incidence is probably unrelated to the presence or absence of fetal hypoxia; however, the syndrome is more likely to be severe if there is associated hypoxia or acidosis. It is also more severe when the meconium is thick.

Meconium can be graded as follows:
- Grade 1: Good volume of liquor stained lightly with meconium
- Grade 2: Reasonable volume of liquor with heavy suspension of meconium
- Grade 3: Thick undiluted meconium of 'pea soup' consistency.

The grading of meconium is subjective and correlates relatively poorly with fetal condition and neonatal outcome. Generally, the higher the grade, the more likely it is to be associated with metabolic acidosis and the meconium aspiration syndrome. It is appropriate to consider continuous electronic FHR recording if meconium staining is identified.

Fetal Heart Rate Recording

INTERMITTENT MONITORING (INTERMITTENT AUSCULTATION)

Assessment of the FHR is used to provide information about fetal well-being. In low-risk labours, it is recommended to auscultate the fetal heart every 15 minutes before and after a contraction during the first stage of labour and every 5 minutes between contractions in the second stage of labour. A baseline tachycardia or bradycardia and the presence of decelerations are indications for further evaluation with continuous CTG monitoring. The heartbeat can be auscultated using either a Pinard stethoscope or an electronic Doppler device.

CONTINUOUS MONITORING

A CTG provides a continuous printed or electronic record of the FHR and uterine contractions. The contractions are registered by a pressure monitor held on to the mother's abdomen by an elastic belt and the FHR is measured using either:

- an abdominal ultrasonic transmitter–receiver Doppler probe, which detects fetal cardiac movements; or
- a metal clip known as a fetal scalp electrode (FSE) which is attached to the baby's scalp and detects the R–R wave of the fetal ECG. It is usually used if transabdominal monitoring is technically unsatisfactory or if fetal ECG monitoring is employed.

Analysis of the CTG is undertaken in a systematic fashion, whereby each of the three features are categorised as 'reassuring', 'non-reassuring' or 'abnormal' (Table 32.1). Such an analysis is subsequently distilled in order to provide an overall categorisation of the CTG as 'normal', 'suspicious' or 'pathological' (Table 32.2).

The mnemonic DR C BRaVADO is widely used to facilitate systematic analysis of the CTG. DR is 'define risk' (low or high risk), C is 'contractions' (frequency, strength), BRa is 'baseline rate', V is 'variability', A is 'accelerations', D is 'decelerations' and O is 'overall category'.

The baseline FHR is normally between 110 and 160 beats per minute (bpm). This rate represents a balance between the sympathetic and parasympathetic systems. Sustained tachycardia may be associated with prematurity; the rate slows physiologically with advancing gestation. Tachycardia may also be associated with fetal acidosis (probably as a response to increased sympathetic stimulation) or maternal pyrexia (fetal temperature closely reflects maternal temperature). Fetal cardiac tachydysrhythmias are rare but can cause extremely high heart rates.

TABLE 32.1	Categorisation of the Individual Features of the Intrapartum Cardiotocography		
Feature	**Reassuring**	**Non-Reassuring**	**Abnormal**
Baseline fetal heart rate (beats per minute)	110–160	100–109 or 161–180	<100 or >180
Variability	5–25	<5 for 30–50 minutes	<5 for >50 minutes
Decelerations	None or early. Variable with no concerning features for <90 minutes	Variable with no concerning features for >90 minutes OR Variable with concerning features over 50% of contractions for <30 minutes OR Late in >50% of contractions for <30 minutes	Variable with concerning features in >50% contractions for 30 minutes OR Late decelerations for >30 minutes OR Acute bradycardia lasting 3 minutes or more

Note: The presence of accelerations makes acidosis unlikely but the absence of accelerations in the intrapartum period does not in itself indicate hypoxia or acidosis.
Modified from Intrapartum care for healthy women and babies (CG190) National Institute for Health and Care Excellence (NICE) 2017.

TABLE 32.2	Categorisation of the Cardiotocograph in Labour
Normal	**All Features Reassuring**
Suspicious	One non-reassuring and two reassuring features
Pathological	One abnormal feature or two non-reassuring features

Modified from Intrapartum care for healthy women and babies (CG190) NICE 2017.

A baseline bradycardia is associated with severe fetal acidosis (e.g., following placental abruption, uterine rupture or cord prolapse), but it is more commonly found in the presence of maternal hypotension, typically following epidural analgesia. Fetal congenital heart block is rare but can occur especially in association with maternal systemic lupus erythematosus.

Baseline variability describes the fluctuations in the FHR and is due to the balance between the parasympathetic and the sympathetic nervous systems. Since the nervous system of the fetus develops as pregnancy advances, the baseline variability is relatively reduced at earlier gestations. Baseline variability is described as normal or reduced and it gives a relatively good indication of fetal oxygenation. Normal variability is 5 to 25 bpm; the most common reason for loss of baseline variability is the 'sleep' phase of the fetal behavioural cycle, which may last up to 50 minutes. Loss of variability is also associated with prematurity, fetal acidosis and some drugs administered to the mother (e.g., opiates or benzodiazepines).

Accelerations of the FHR are a sign of a healthy fetus (accelerations indicate that the fetus is moving). However, their absence in labour is not unusual. Prior to labour, there should be at least two accelerations per 20 minutes, each with an amplitude >15 bpm and lasting for at least 15 seconds.

The presence of decelerations increases the likelihood of fetal hypoxia. Accurate categorisation of decelerations is important, but there is often a difference of opinion between clinicians regarding the classification of decelerations. Most decelerations in labour are 'variable' in nature (Fig. 32.1). Decelerations represent a reduction in FHR from baseline of at least 15 bpm and last for more than 15 seconds. Early decelerations occur with contractions; the trough of the deceleration coincides with the peak of the contraction. Early decelerations reflect increased vagal tone (intracranial pressure rises during a contraction) and are probably physiological. As

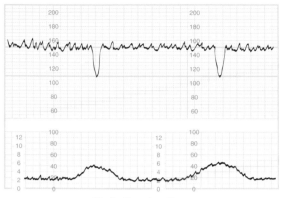

Early Decelerations

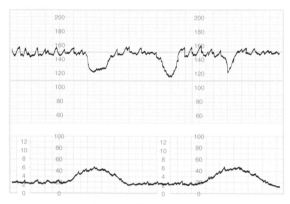

Variable Decelerations

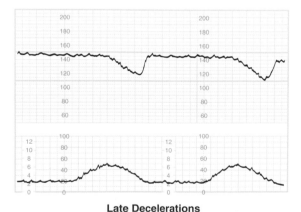

Late Decelerations

Fig. 32.1 Characteristic appearances of cardiotocography (CTG) decelerations.

the name suggests, 'variable' decelerations vary in both timing and shape. Variable decelerations probably represent intermittent cord compression and are subcategorised into 'typical' and 'with concerning features'. A small increase in FHR at the beginning and end of a variable deceleration (shouldering) suggests that the fetus is coping physiologically with the hypoxic stress of the intermittent compressions; absence of 'shouldering' is a concerning feature. Other concerning features include a deceleration lasting >60 seconds and a biphasic (W) shape. Variable decelerations may resolve if the mother's position is changed. Late decelerations occur more than 15 seconds after the contraction, where the trough of the deceleration typically falls outwith the duration of the contraction. Late decelerations suggest reduced placental perfusion and hypoxia during that period. The recommended actions following categorisation of the CTG are summarised in Table 32.3. It is essential to explain to women in labour your findings and proposed actions.

Computerised analysis of the intrapartum CTG has been developed as an aid to interpretation and clinical decision-making. Unfortunately, such analysis has been demonstrated not to improve clinical outcomes for mothers or babies.

TABLE 32.3 Actions to be Followed When the Cardiotocography Is Categorised as 'Suspicious' or 'Pathological'	
Category	**Action**
Suspicious	Correct any underlying cause, for example, maternal hypotension, uterine hyperstimulation.
	Adopt one or more conservative measures, for example, change maternal position, adjust oxytocin infusion.
	Inform obstetrician or senior midwife.
	Talk to the woman and birth partner regarding their preferences.
Pathological	Exclude an acute event, for example, placental abruption, cord prolapse.
	Correct hyperstimulation, that is, stop oxytocin, consider tocolysis.
	Adopt conservative measures, for example, change of maternal position, correct maternal hypotension.
	Consider fetal blood sampling or expedite delivery.
	Inform obstetrician and senior midwife.
	Take the views/preferences of the woman into account.

Modified from Intrapartum care for healthy women and babies (CG190) NICE 2017.

FETAL ELECTROCARDIOGRAM

Analysis of the fetal ECG in labour, particularly the ST segment, can improve the specificity (i.e., reduce the number of false positives) of the CTG. An FSE is required to obtain the ECG, the signal from which is a reflection of the electrical activity in the myocardium.

Myocardial hypoxia leads to changes in the ECG waveform. Used in conjunction with the CTG, fetal ECG analysis results in a reduction in the number of FBS procedures and a reduction in instrumental deliveries; the rate of caesarean sections and infants born with encephalopathy is unaffected. The fetal ECG is used in some maternity units.

Fetal Blood Sampling

Also known as fetal scalp sampling, this is a diagnostic test for fetal acidosis. The CTG is used as a screening test to identify the fetus who is experiencing hypoxia and acidosis. The CTG is highly sensitive (good at detecting true positives) but poorly specific (there are many false positives). CTG use leads to an approximately four-fold increase in caesarean section rates for presumed fetal hypoxia, a figure much reduced if FBS is used to identify a normal pH in the false positives.

The principal indication for undertaking an FBS is the presence of a 'pathological' CTG, in which case knowledge of the fetal pH is likely to influence the management of labour. FBS is contraindicated when there is a risk of infection transmitted from the mother (e.g., human immunodeficiency virus, hepatitis B, herpes), a fetal bleeding diathesis (e.g., von Willebrand disease), and before 34 weeks' gestation. FBS is not appropriate in the presence of an acute event necessitating immediate delivery, for example, cord prolapse or placental abruption. Consideration of the whole clinical picture is crucial to good decision-making.

TECHNIQUE OF FETAL BLOOD SAMPLING

Explanation is given to the mother and her verbal consent to proceed is obtained. The mother is placed in the lithotomy position with a 15-degree lateral tilt or in the left lateral position.

Immediately prior to undertaking an FBS, the fetal scalp is digitally stimulated. If this prompts an acceleration of the FHR, then the likelihood of fetal acidosis is very low and the indication for an FBS can be reconsidered. An amnioscope appropriate for the dilatation of the cervix is inserted and the scalp is dried with a swab on sponge holders. The scalp is then sprayed with ethyl chloride to induce hyperaemia and the area is covered with a thin layer of paraffin jelly (so that the blood will form a blob). A blade is used to make a small incision in the scalp and the blob of fetal blood is touched with the capillary tube. When **possible, three samples are taken to ensure consistency of** results. The pH of the sample is determined on a near-patient analyser. Serum lactate measurement may be employed as an alternative to determining pH.

INTERPRETATION OF RESULTS

The scalp blood pH reflects the acid–base status of the fetus at the time of the sample. Correlation between the CTG and scalp pH is not precise. However, as a general rule, the greater the number of non-reassuring or abnormal features contained in the CTG, the higher the chance of acidosis. It is usual practice to deliver the baby if the pH is 7.20 or below (Table 32.4).

Fetal Monitoring Scenarios

See Figs 32.2–32.9.

TABLE 32.4 Categorisation of pH Results Following Fetal Blood Sampling

pH		
>7.25	Normal	No action
7.21–7.24	Borderline	Repeat in 30–60 minutes if not delivered.
7.20 or below	Abnormal	Instrumental vaginal delivery or caesarean section
		Consider tocolysis with a beta-2 agonist.

Long-Term Prognosis Following Delivery

There are two key issues to be considered here:

1. Whether a particular infant, born with apparent compromise, will later turn out to be neurologically normal, that is, prospective prediction
2. Whether an infant, later discovered to be affected by cerebral abnormality, sustained its injury prior to the onset of labour or as the result of an intrapartum insult, that is, retrospective evaluation.

Before considering these two overlapping issues, it should be noted that the term 'birth asphyxia' is best avoided unless there is evidence of a pale baby with no tone and not breathing, with evidence of metabolic acidosis on umbilical cord arterial blood.

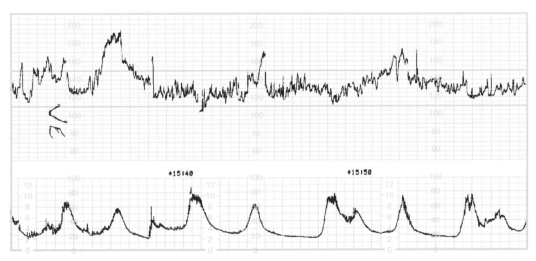

Fig. 32.2 A 29-year-old para 2, with a history of two previous normal deliveries admitted in labour at 38 weeks. The cervix was 3 cm dilated and fully effaced, but there was thick meconium staining. The cardiotocography (CTG) was reassuring, with a baseline of 130 bpm, good baseline variability and presence of accelerations. She was given diamorphine for pain relief.

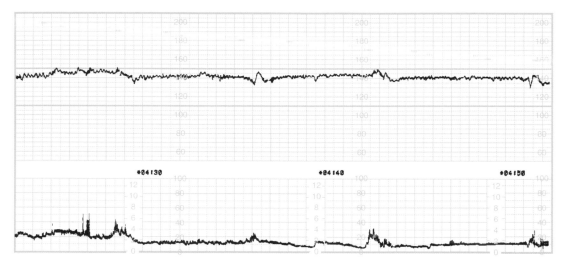

Fig. 32.3 After a further 2 hours, baseline variability was reduced. Although there were no decelerations, it was recognised that meconium staining increases the risk of fetal hypoxia and fetal blood sampling (FBS) was performed. The pH was 7.31 (normal) and she went on to have a normal delivery 3 hours later. The baby was born in good condition.

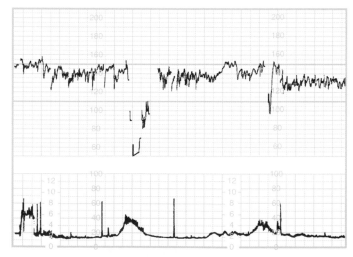

Fig. 32.4 A 40-year-old primigravida was admitted after spontaneous rupture of membranes at 39 weeks. The amniotic fluid was clear and she was having mild contractions every 8 minutes. The cardiotocography (CTG) baseline was 130 to 140 bpm with normal variability but there were variable decelerations. These are not uncommon after membrane rupture, as amniotic fluid cushions the cord. The decelerations resolved with change of maternal position.

PROSPECTIVE PREDICTION

The actual length of time and degree of hypoxia required to produce cerebral palsy in a previously healthy fetus are unknown, but there are specific mechanisms which protect the fetus for considerably longer than an adult with similar blood gas concentrations. Nonetheless, hypoxia, whether of antenatal or intrapartum origin, can cause cerebral injury. Attempts have been made to correlate status at delivery with long-term neurological outcome. CTG abnormalities, Apgar scores, neonatal behaviour and neonatal brain imaging have all been evaluated.

The CTG and Apgar scores are of very limited value in assessing long-term prognosis. There is a high incidence of 'abnormal' CTGs in what later become normal infants. The same is true for Apgar scores, which are

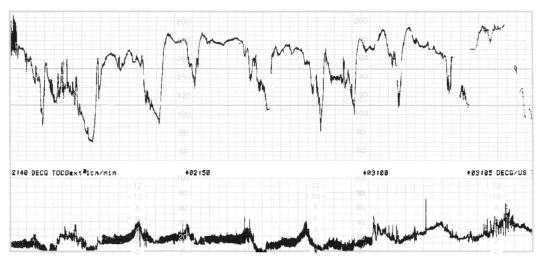

Fig. 32.5 A 27-year-old primigravida was induced at 40 weeks +12 days, as she was 'post-dates'. After prostaglandin gel was administered vaginally, the cervix was suitable for membrane rupture and the induction was continued with an oxytocin infusion. This cardiotocography (CTG) was seen at 6 cm dilatation. It shows a baseline around 180 bpm (tachycardia) with reduced variability and variable decelerations, some with concerning features; the CTG was 'pathological'. fetal blood sampling (FBS) revealed a pH of 7.28, but on repetition 30 minutes later, the pH was 7.19. By this time, the cervix was fully dilated and the baby was born by ventouse extraction in good condition.

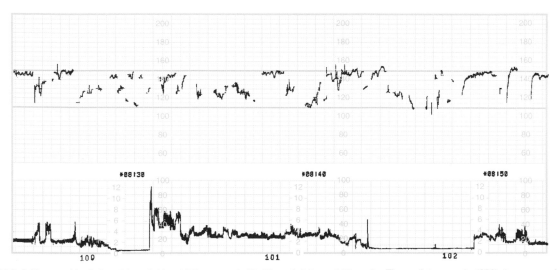

Fig. 32.6 A 19-year-old primigravida weighing 115 kg was admitted in early labour at 38 weeks. The cardiotocography (CTG) shows poor pick-up from the abdominal transducer; after the membranes were ruptured, a scalp clip was applied. The subsequent CTG recording was technically good and categorised as normal. She proceeded to a normal birth of a baby in good condition.

intended as a guide to the need for resuscitation rather than a reflection of the degree of hypoxic injury. Low Apgar scores do not indicate the cause of the baby's poor condition and are a reflection of its immediate status.

Abnormal neonatal behaviour, referred to as 'neonatal encephalopathy', is more useful. This is a clinically defined syndrome of disturbed neurological function occurring during the first week after birth. It is characterised by difficulty with initiating and maintaining respiration, depression of tone and reflexes, altered level of consciousness, and seizures. There are three grades:

1. Hyperalert and jittery, with reduced tone and dilated pupils. This usually resolves within 24 hours without long-term sequelae.

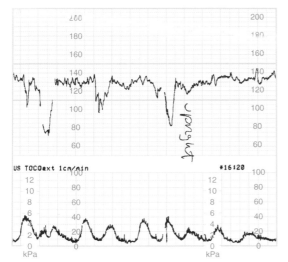

Fig. 32.7 A 26-year-old primigravida was induced at 33 weeks for worsening pre-eclampsia. The fetus was small for gestational age, but the amniotic fluid volume was normal and the antenatal cardiotocography (CTG) was normal. Eight hours after vaginal administration of prostaglandin gel, with the cervix still closed, there were three variable decelerations. The baseline FHR and variability were both normal, which might have warranted more conservative management in a normally grown, term fetus in labour, but the underlying risk factors for fetal hypoxia in this case were sufficient to warrant delivery by caesarean section. The baby, weighing 1.6 kg (1st centile) was awarded Apgar scores of 9 and 10 at 1 and 5 minutes, respectively and made uneventful progress. It is essential to consider the whole clinical picture when interpreting the CTG.

2. Lethargic, with seizures and a weak suck. There is an approximately 20% chance of severe sequelae.
3. Flaccid, no suck, no Moro reflex and prolonged seizures. The chance of severe sequelae is 70% to 80%.

The prognosis is generally good if the baby does not develop Grade 3 neonatal encephalopathy or if Grade 2 neonatal encephalopathy lasts less than 5 days.

Radiological assessment is also of value in assessing long-term neurological function. The prognosis is good if a magnetic resonance imaging scan appears normal but is not as good if there is evidence of cerebral damage. At term, partial but prolonged hypoxia (as indicated by repeated decelerations with loss of variability over a prolonged period) may give rise to motor cortical atrophy and quadriplegia. If the hypoxia is sudden and profound (as with a prolonged bradycardia), it is more likely to result in injury to the thalamus, giving rise to an athetoid or dyskinetic type of cerebral palsy.

Early cerebral oedema suggests a recent event, as oedema usually appears within 6 to 12 hours of an insult and clears by 4 days afterwards. Further clinical evaluation may be available from an electroencephalograph (EEG). The incidence of death or handicap is low if the EEG is normal. However, despite these

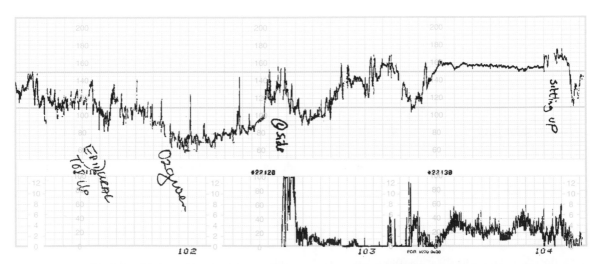

Fig. 32.8 A 34-year-old primigravida in spontaneous labour at 39 weeks had an epidural sited when 4 cm dilated. After epidural top-up there was a fetal bradycardia, which evolved into a tachycardia before finally returning to normal. It is recognised that the maternal hypotension associated with regional anaesthesia leads to placental hypoperfusion and fetal bradycardia. The bradycardia usually resolves spontaneously or following maternal fluid volume expansion.

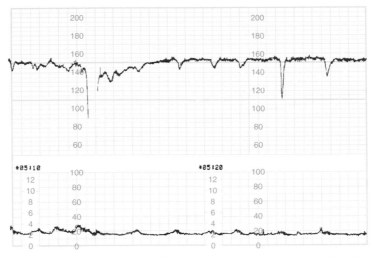

Fig. 32.9 A primigravida at 40 weeks who was admitted from home in spontaneous labour at 8 cm dilatation. The cardiotocography (CTG) demonstrated reduced variability and there were shallow late decelerations. A fetal blood sample showed a pH of 7.09 and an emergency caesarean section was performed. The baby had Apgar scores of 3 at 1 minute and 7 at 5 minutes, and weighed 2.23 kg (1st centile). The baby's subsequent progress was normal. Although seemingly 'low risk', this pregnancy was affected by unrecognised fetal growth restriction.

measures, the prognosis often cannot be defined with accuracy and only long-term follow-up will reveal the true clinical picture.

RETROSPECTIVE EVALUATION

Cerebral palsy, which is characterised by non-progressive abnormal control of movement or posture, is usually not diagnosed until months or years after birth. It is often at this point that questions are asked about whether the cause lay in some difficulty with the delivery. In many instances, it is impossible to say whether the cerebral insult was antenatal in origin (usually of an unspecified nature) or whether it occurred during labour, but this seemingly academic point has two important implications. First, if most cases of cerebral palsy are antenatal in origin, then intrapartum monitoring and subsequent intervention will have little impact upon eventual outcomes. Second, there may be medicolegal ramifications. If a cerebral insult is found to have occurred as the result of substandard care during labour, a substantial sum of money may be paid in compensation.

Epidemiological studies suggest that in about 90% of cases, the cerebral injury is antenatal in origin and that in the remaining 10%, the problems may have been the result of intrapartum difficulties. In particular, there is a strong association between cerebral palsy and prematurity, fetal growth restriction, intrauterine infection, fetal coagulation disorders, antepartum haemorrhage and chromosomal or congenital anomalies.

There are sometimes conflicting views about the criteria required to implicate intrapartum events as the cause of cerebral palsy. One set of views is expressed in Box 32.2.

BOX 32.2 CRITERIA OFTEN USED TO DEFINE AN ACUTE INTRAPARTUM HYPOXIC EVENT AS THE CAUSE OF LATER CEREBRAL INJURY

- Evidence is required of a metabolic acidosis in an intrapartum fetal blood sample, umbilical arterial cord blood, or in very early neonatal blood. Metabolic acidosis at birth is not rare (2% of all births) and the large majority of these infants do not develop cerebral palsy. An appropriate cut-off point that correlates with an increased risk of neurological deficit is often considered to be a pH of <7.00 and a base deficit of >16 mmol/L.
- There should be moderate or severe (Grade 2 or 3) neonatal encephalopathy.
- Cerebral palsy should be of the spastic quadriplegic or dyskinetic type. Spastic quadriplegia and, less commonly, dyskinetic cerebral palsy are the only subtypes of cerebral palsy associated with hypoxic intrapartum events at term.

The large majority of neurological pathologies causing cerebral palsy occur as a result of multifactorial and mostly unpreventable events during either fetal development or the neonatal period. However, this is not an excuse for substandard intrapartum care. Every effort should be made to identify and act upon identifiable causes of potential cerebral injury.

Key Points

- The purpose of monitoring the fetus in labour is to identify those who might be at risk of hypoxic injury so that delivery can then be expedited prior to irreversible harm. This monitoring involves FHR assessment, either with intermittent auscultation or by continuous electronic measurement.

- Meconium (fetal stool) staining of the liquor increases the chance that fetal hypoxia is present.
- Misinterpretation of the CTG is a relatively common cause of substandard care and subsequent litigation. A systematic approach to analysing the CTG maximises the likelihood of correct interpretation.
- FBS is used to reduce the incidence of false-positive diagnosis of fetal acidosis.
- Interpretation of the CTG must take account of the whole clinical situation rather than the CTG in isolation.
- Cerebral palsy is usually the result of antenatal factors rather than intrapartum hypoxia and acidosis.

Chapter 33

Induction of Labour

Katharine Rankin

Chapter Outline

Introduction

Induction of labour is one of the most common obstetric interventions, occurring in approximately 20% of pregnancies in the United Kingdom. It is indicated in women for whom vaginal birth is planned when the risks of continuing the pregnancy are felt to be greater than the risks of induction of labour. Balancing these risks is often difficult, particularly at pre-term gestations; both fetal and maternal factors must be considered. There should be a careful discussion about the risks and benefits with the mother, especially as the process may have an impact on the pregnancy outcome, the woman's experience of labour, and future pregnancies. It should be noted that 'induction' is different from 'augmentation'. Induction refers to the process of starting labour in someone who is not labouring. Augmentation describes the process of accelerating labour which is already underway (see Chapter 34).

Indications

PROLONGED PREGNANCY

The most common reason for induction of labour is prolonged pregnancy. For 5% to 10% of women, their pregnancy continues beyond 42 weeks' gestation. The chance of perinatal death increases as the pregnancy continues, rising from 1 in 1000 at 37 weeks to 6 in 1000 at 43 weeks' gestation. Although absolute numbers of stillbirths are small, it is reasonable to advocate induction of labour, when the gestational age is reliably established, for otherwise uncomplicated pregnancies between 41 and 42 weeks' gestation. The risk of stillbirth increases with maternal age, with a rate of 0.75/1000 for mothers over 40 years old. These women may be offered induction earlier – at 40 weeks' gestation.

OTHER POTENTIAL REASONS FOR INDUCTION OF LABOUR

- Maternal diabetes, including gestational diabetes
- Twin pregnancy

- Fetal growth restriction and suspected fetal compromise
- Hypertensive disorders of pregnancy, including pre-eclampsia
- Deteriorating maternal medical conditions (e.g., cardiac or renal disease)
- Maternal request

Contraindications

Induction is not appropriate in situations in which a vaginal delivery would be very risky or impossible, such as placenta praevia or transverse fetal lie. In general, induction of labour is not recommended for breech presentations. There is an increased risk of uterine hyperstimulation with induction of labour in those who have had a previous history of precipitate labour.

Caution is required in women who have had a previous caesarean section or uterine surgery. In women with a previous caesarean section, induction of labour carries a higher risk of uterine scar rupture than if the woman labours spontaneously. A greater proportion of the cases in which scar dehiscence or rupture occurred were associated with induction using prostaglandins. In these circumstances, many clinicians prefer mechanical methods to start the induction process. Oxytocin infusions can be used with due caution if required.

Methods

Before induction, gestation should be confirmed again, the fetal presentation confirmed to be cephalic, and any contraindications excluded. Various induction methods are available (Fig. 33.1), including mechanical (balloon catheter insertion or amniotomy) and pharmacological (oxytocin and prostaglandins). Deciding on the most appropriate technique depends on the favourability of the cervix, as assessed by the Bishop scoring system (Table 33.1 and Box 33.1).

Unfavourable Cervix

PROSTAGLANDINS

Prostaglandins promote cervical ripening and stimulate uterine contractility. They are administered orally or vaginally. The main side effect is gastrointestinal upset with nausea, vomiting and diarrhoea, which

TABLE 33.1 Bishop Scoring System for Cervical Assessment

Score	0	1	2
Cervical dilatation (cm)	<1	1–2	3–4
Length of cervix (cm)	>2	1–2	<1
Station of presenting part (cm)	Spines −3	Spines −2	Spines −1
Consistency	Firm	Medium	Soft
Position	Posterior	Central	Anterior

BOX 33.1 OVERVIEW OF INDUCTION

- If Bishop score is ≤6 ('unfavourable'), the cervix should be ripened with prostaglandins (e.g., gel or pessary) or using a mechanical method.
- If Bishop score is >6 ('favourable'), prostaglandins, artificial rupture of the membranes (ARM, or amniotomy) ± intravenous oxytocin may be considered.

may occur in up to 50% of women depending on the route of administration. Vaginal preparations have the fewest side effects.

Prostaglandin E2 (PGE2) is used in clinical practice. A gel or tablet is inserted into the posterior fornix and the cervix is reassessed after 6 hours if labour has not started. If the Bishop score is >6, an amniotomy may be performed, reassessment made 2 hours later, and intravenous oxytocin started if there is no change. Prostaglandins are not required if there is regular uterine activity, to minimise the risk of hyperstimulation. Misoprostol (a methyl ester of prostaglandin E1) can also be used either orally or vaginally but carries a higher incidence of hyperstimulation than PGE2 preparations, which is also less likely to resolve with tocolysis.

Sustained-release preparations containing PGE2 are also available as a polymer-based vaginal insert. This is placed in the posterior fornix for 24 hours. This is removed with its attached string when the Bishop score is reassessed. This preparation has the advantage that the insert can be removed if hyperstimulation develops, and there is evidence that it is associated with a reduced likelihood of operative vaginal birth compared with other prostaglandin formulations. Sustained-release preparations of misoprostol are used in some countries.

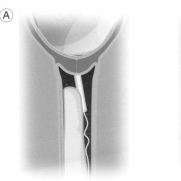
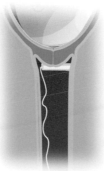

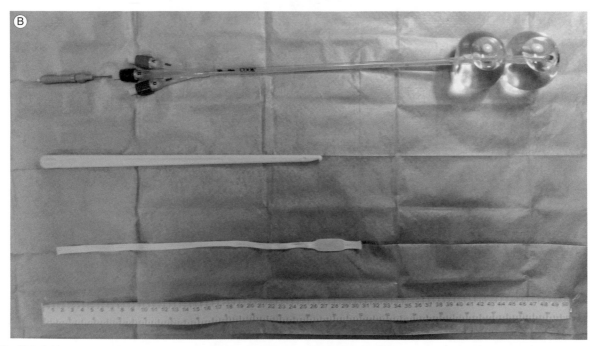

Fig. 33.1 A. The vaginal sustained-release prostaglandin pessary is placed behind the cervix to release prostaglandins adjacent to the cervix. **B.** Upper: The cervical ripening balloon is shown with both balloons filled; Middle: Amniotomy hook; Bottom: Sustained release PGE2 vaginal insert, with 25cm tail to aid removal.

MECHANICAL METHODS OF INDUCTION

Mechanical induction methods include intracervical insertion of balloon devices. These devices aim to ripen and dilate the cervix and promote onset of labour by applying pressure to the internal cervical os. A standard urinary catheter has been commonly used, with the balloon inflated in the extra-amniotic space. Increasingly, double-balloon catheters are being used (Fig. 33.2). The double balloon aims to stimulate local prostaglandin release by squeezing the cervix between the upper and lower balloon, thereby leading to cervical ripening.

Procedure

The balloon catheter is usually inserted with the woman in a lithotomy position. A sterile speculum

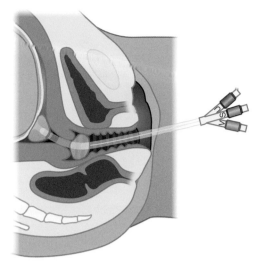

Fig. 33.2 The cervical ripening balloon is used to mechanically shorten and widen the cervix. It can be used in most women and is particularly useful in women with previous caesarean section, as prostaglandins have a higher incidence of uterine scar dehiscence.

is inserted to gain access to the cervix. The cervix is then prepared by cleaning with an antiseptic solution. A double-balloon catheter (with a uterine balloon and vaginal balloon) is inserted through the cervical canal and into the uterus so that the tip of the catheter lies in the uterus. The uterine balloon is then inflated with saline and the catheter is gently pulled back until the uterine balloon lies against the internal cervical os. The vaginal balloon is also inflated with saline so that it lies against the external cervical os. Both balloons are inflated alternately and incrementally with small amounts of saline. When the balloons are fully inflated and in place on each side of the cervix, the speculum is removed. The external end of the device can be loosely taped to the woman's thigh. Following the insertion of the double balloon, the mother and fetus are monitored and the device is left in place for up to 24 hours or until it falls out spontaneously.

The device is removed if labour begins, membrane rupture occurs or fetal distress is suspected. If the balloon is removed because labour has not started, then an amniotomy can usually be performed, followed by an intravenous oxytocin infusion if required.

Efficacy and Safety

Increasing evidence suggests that mechanical methods of induction of labour are as effective as prostaglandins for achieving vaginal birth within 24 hours, particularly for women in their first pregnancy.

Mechanical methods have lower rates of hyperstimulation compared with vaginal prostaglandins. Both methods are associated with similar rates of caesarean section and postpartum haemorrhage.

Favourable Cervix

If the cervix is favourable (Bishop Score over 6), the choice is between:
- Prostaglandins
- Artificial rupture of membranes (ARM; amniotomy)
- ARM and intravenous oxytocin

It remains unclear which of these methods is best, but there is some evidence that maternal satisfaction and likelihood of achieving vaginal birth within 24 hours is greater with prostaglandins. The requirement for analgesia and rates of postpartum haemorrhage may also be lower with prostaglandins. Pharmacological preparations all cause uterine contractions. They also have the potential to reduce uterine blood flow and cause fetal distress. Therefore, cardiotocography (CTG) monitoring is indicated.

ARTIFICIAL RUPTURE OF THE MEMBRANES

ARM may be used for induction in those with a sufficiently favourable cervix and is used for augmentation as well. It also allows assessment of the colour of the liquor (see meconium staining of the liquor, p. 385). Although ARM is effective in the case of a favourable cervix, it is associated with more frequent need for oxytocin augmentation compared with vaginal prostaglandins.

Before ARM, an abdominal and vaginal examination is performed to ensure that the baby is in a cephalic presentation, with the fetal head engaged in the pelvis. The fetal head should be well applied to the cervix to minimise the risk of cord prolapse. With asepsis, the tips of the index and middle fingers of one hand should be placed through the cervix onto the membranes (Fig. 33.3). The amniotomy hook should be allowed to slide along the groove between these fingers (hook pointing towards the fingers) until it reaches the cervix. The point is then turned upwards, breaking the membrane sac. Liquor is usually seen but may be absent in oligohydramnios or with a well-engaged fetal head. Cord prolapse should be excluded before removing the fingers; then, the fetal heart should be auscultated. Absent liquor following ARM should be treated in the same way as meconium-stained liquor – by carefully monitoring fetal well-being until birth.

OXYTOCIN

Intravenous oxytocin (Syntocinon) is a synthetic version of the naturally occurring hormone produced by the pituitary gland in labour, which stimulates uterine contractions. This may be used for induction after ARM with a favourable cervix or for augmentation of a slow non-obstructed labour (see Chapter 34). Oxytocin should be started only after membrane rupture, and continuous CTG monitoring is mandatory. The dose should be titrated against the contractions, aiming for 3 to 4 contractions every 10 minutes.

Other Methods of Induction of Labour

MEMBRANE SWEEP

This involves performing a vaginal examination and inserting a finger through the internal cervical os to separate the membranes from the uterine wall, thus releasing endogenous prostaglandins (Fig. 33.4). Carrying out one membrane sweep after 40 weeks' gestation doubles the spontaneous labour rate especially in those with low Bishop scores. The risk of infection is considered minimal, but it can often be uncomfortable for the mother.

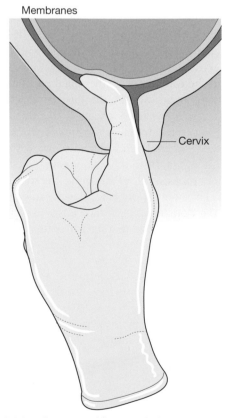

Fig. 33.4 A 'membrane sweep' increases the incidence of spontaneous labour.

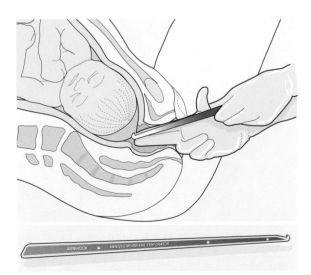

Fig. 33.3 Artificial rupture of membranes can be used to induce or augment labour. (Redrawn from Greer IA, Cameron IT, Magowan BA, et al. *Problem-Based Obstetrics and Gynaecology.* Churchill Livingstone; 2003.)

Complications

Induction of labour risks are largely related to the use of medicines that are used to stimulate uterine activity. The most concerning side effect is uterine hyperstimulation, carrying the risk of fetal distress. Hyperstimulation occurs in 1% to 5% of prostaglandin-induced labours and is defined as >5 contractions in 10 minutes for >20 minutes, associated with fetal heart rate abnormalities. It necessitates removal of the prostaglandin (if possible), consideration of tocolysis with a beta-agonist (such as subcutaneous terbutaline) and potentially immediate emergency birth if the abnormal fetal heart rate persists. Induction may also be associated with increased obstetric intervention (including operative vaginal birth), but large population studies suggest no increase in caesarean section rates when induction is performed at 41 weeks.

Unsuccessful Induction

Despite these techniques, induction is sometimes unsuccessful. The plan then depends on the reason for the induction. If it was for a significant fetal or maternal indication, there is probably little choice but to consider caesarean section as the alternative. If the reason was less pressing, it may be worth considering a more conservative approach with a repeat attempt at induction of labour. This would depend on an informed discussion with the woman and revisiting the central question of whether the risks of induction of labour still outweigh the risks of continuing the pregnancy.

Key Points

- **The risks of induction of labour need to be balanced against the risks of awaiting spontaneous labour.**
- **The use of oxytocics and prostaglandins carry an increased risk of uterine hyperstimulation. Close fetal monitoring is important.**
- **If the cervix is unfavourable, prostaglandins or a mechanical method should be used for ripening before moving to amniotomy and intravenous oxytocin as required.**

Chapter 34

Malpresentation and Slow Labour

Lorna Hutchison

Chapter Outline

Introduction

Labour is defined as the onset of regular uterine activity, cervical effacement and dilatation with descent of the presenting part. The duration of labour is variable and is influenced by factors including parity, gestation or whether the labour was spontaneous or induced. First labours on average last 8 hours and are unlikely to last over 18 hours. Second and subsequent labours last on average 5 hours and are unlikely to last over 12 hours. In order to determine whether labour is progressing adequately, it is important to assess cervical dilatation and rate of change, uterine activity, and the position and station of the presenting part. The parity of the woman should always be considered for reasons just outlined. National clinical guidelines advise offering vaginal examination every 4 hours in labour in addition to abdominal palpation and assessment of vaginal loss.

Abdominal palpation should aim to define the lie, presentation, and position of the fetus. The lie refers to the long axis of the fetus in relation to the long axis of the uterus. The lie may be longitudinal, transverse or oblique. The presentation is that part of the fetus that is at the pelvic brim, in other words, the part of the fetus presenting to the pelvic inlet. 'Normal' presentation refers to the vertex of the fetal head, which is the area bounded by the anterior fontanelle (bregma), posterior fontanelle and biparietal eminences. 'Malpresentation' describes any non-vertex presentation. This may be of the face, brow, breech or some other part of the body if the lie is oblique or transverse.

The position of the fetus refers to the way in which the presenting part is positioned in relation to the maternal pelvis. This refers to any presenting part. However, it will be considered here in relation to those fetuses presenting head first (cephalic). As discussed in Chapter 31, the head is usually occipitotransverse at the pelvic brim and rotates to occipitoanterior (OA) at the pelvic floor. 'Malposition' is when the head, coming vertex first, does not rotate to OA, presenting instead as persistent occipitotransverse or occipitoposterior (OP). Vaginal examination should be performed to assess cervical dilatation and effacement in addition to station and position of the fetal head.

Uterine activity is monitored by measuring the strength, duration and frequency of contractions. This activity is recorded on the partogram in addition to the vaginal examination. During active labour, effective uterine activity is considered to be four to five contractions over a 10-minute period, lasting 40 seconds or more. Uterine overactivity presents as rapid, painful contractions, which are often associated with fetal distress. This can happen spontaneously but is more commonly associated with the use of oxytocics. Inadequate uterine activity is often associated with absent or slow cervical dilatation. Slow labour may result from inadequate uterine activity, cephalopelvic disproportion (CPD) or, more commonly, a combination of the two.

CPD refers to how well the fetal head fits through the pelvis and may occur if the fetal head is too big or the pelvis too small. It is subdivided into 'true' CPD if the head is in the correct position and 'relative' CPD if the obstruction is caused by malposition.

Precipitate Labour

Precipitate labour has been defined as rapid birth of the fetus (a combined first stage and second stage of labour duration) within less than 2 to 3 hours of the onset of contractions, and may result from uterine overactivity.

Excessive uterine activity is commonly termed 'uterine tachysystole' or 'hyperstimulation'. It is defined as more than five uterine contractions per 10 minutes in at least two consecutive intervals. There may be signs of fetal distress on the cardiotocograph due to interference with the placental blood supply.

Spontaneous hypercontractility, excessive uterine activity not resulting from the administration of medications,

is rare. Spontaneous uterine hypercontractility may be associated with placental abruption (see p. 316).

Uterine hyperstimulation occurs much more commonly. By definition, it is caused by the use of oxytocics. Both oxytocin and prostaglandins may be implicated. The choice of dosage regimens for each represents a compromise between efficacy and the risk of hyperstimulation. The appropriate dose of oxytocin remains controversial, but there is good evidence for starting at a low dose, around 0.5 to 4 mU/min, and increasing incrementally to 12 mU/min. The dose should be increased no more frequently than every 30 minutes until there are 4 to 5 contractions in 10 minutes. While the licenced maximum dose in the United Kingdom is currently 20 mU/min, some clinicians support the use of regimens up to 32 or even 40 mU/min.

With prostaglandins, hyperstimulation is also a significant risk but is less likely if their administration is intravaginal rather than oral, intracervical or directly extra-amniotic.

Precipitate labour resulting from either spontaneous hypercontractility or uterine hyperstimulation may lead to fetal distress. Normal labour, with sufficient physiological relaxation time, allows the oxygenation level of an uncompromised baby to be restored between contractions. However, strong contractions and a shortened relaxation time does not allow the blood supply to the placenta to return to baseline levels before the next contraction, which can result in fetal acidosis (Fig. 34.1). Precipitate labour may also predispose to uterine rupture in parous women, particularly if there is a pre-existing caesarean section scar.

Management of precipitate labour is largely dependent on the fetal condition. If an oxytocin infusion is running, it should be stopped and the woman turned to the left lateral position. A tocolytic agent (a drug to relax the uterine muscle, for example, a bolus of subcutaneous terbutaline or sublingual glyceryl trinitrate spray) may be administered. If severe fetal distress is apparent, it may be necessary to expedite the birth of the baby, either instrumentally or by caesarean section, depending on the dilatation of the cervix. If a caesarean section is arranged, a vaginal examination prior to starting the operation should be considered, as the cervix may dilate rapidly during the time taken to transfer to theatre, especially in a parous woman.

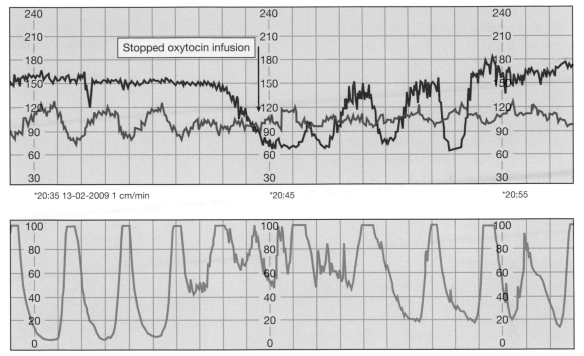

Fig. 34.1 Cardiotocograph trace in precipitate labour. There is hyperstimulation secondary to oxytocin administration. When the oxyocin infusion is stopped, the contractions become less frequent and the cardiotocograph improves.

Precipitate labour is associated with an increased risk of complications for the woman, including cervical and perineal tears, retained placenta, postpartum haemorrhage and the need for a blood transfusion.

Frequent uterine contractions are also a feature of placental abruption (see Chapter 26). Contractions with a frequency of more than one every 2 minutes are highly suggestive of this and these frequent contractions may increase the distress of a fetus already compromised by partial placental separation. The diagnosis of placental abruption is even more likely if there is associated lower abdominal pain, backache or vaginal bleeding. As a general rule, tocolytic drugs should not be used to manage the uterine hypercontractility associated with placental abruption, as uterine relaxation may exacerbate the bleeding and precipitate further placental separation.

Slow Labour

Slow progress in the first stage of labour is diagnosed by assessing the rate of cervical dilatation. As discussed on pages 374 and 404, progress can be monitored on a partogram, and alert lines can be used to identify women who are progressing slowly. Early identification and intervention makes it more likely that the woman will have a vaginal birth. The definition of slow labour is controversial; traditional obstetric practice suggested that any nulliparous woman with a rate of cervical dilatation less than 1 cm/h required treatment for slow progress. More recently, a rate of cervical dilatation of less than 0.5 cm/h has been adopted as the threshold. UK national clinical guidance suggests that a diagnosis of delay in labour should be made when there is dilatation of less than 2 cm in 4 hours.

The second stage of labour is defined as between full dilatation of the cervix to birth of the baby, and is divided into passive and active stages. Active second stage is commenced when the woman develops expulsive contractions with the urge to push or when active pushing is commenced and usually follows 1 to 2 hours of passive second stage. Delay in the second stage should be diagnosed if birth is not imminent despite 2 hours of active second stage in a primigravida or 1 hour in a parous woman.

Slow labour is associated with:

- Eventual fetal 'distress' and risk of fetal hypoxic injury
- Increased risk of intrauterine infection, leading to fetal and maternal morbidity
- Increased risk of postpartum haemorrhage
- Maternal anxiety and longer-term psychological morbidity
- A loss of confidence in those providing maternity care.

These, in turn, are associated with a greater chance of the woman giving birth by caesarean section or requiring an instrument vaginal birth. The causes of slow labour are summarised in Table 34.1 and the outcomes in Table 34.2.

PROLONGED LATENT PHASE

Chapter 31 describes how the first stage of labour is divided into two parts: the latent phase (from the onset of contractions until the cervix is fully effaced) and the active phase (when the cervix begins to dilate). The normal duration of the latent phase of labour in primigravidae ranges from 1.7 hours up to 15.0 hours. The latent phase is most likely to be prolonged in those whose cervix

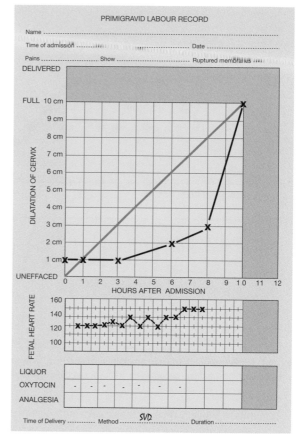

Fig. 34.2 Partogram with prolonged latent phase.

is unfavourable. Therefore, a prolonged latent phase is much more common in primigravidae (Fig. 34.2).

There is rarely any serious cause for a prolonged latent phase. CPD is usually evident at more advanced stages of cervical dilatation. With a prolonged latent phase, the woman often becomes weary, exhausted and demoralised from what can sometimes be discomfort over a number of days. A prolonged latent phase of labour is associated with more obstetric intervention (e.g., caesarean birth) and poor fetal outcomes

TABLE 34.1 Clinical Classification of Slow Labour	
Clinical Features	**Caused by**
Prolonged latent phase	Idiopathic
Prolonged active phase and secondary arrest	Inadequate uterine activity: • Hypoactive • Incoordinate Obstruction (CPD): • True CPD (head too big or pelvis too small) • Relative CPD (malposition of the head increases the diameter of the presenting part)

CPD, Cephalopelvic disproportion.

TABLE 34.2 Birth Outcomes Based on Pattern of Labour (%)				
	Cases	Spontaneous Vertex Birth	Instrumental Birth	Caesarean Birth
Normal pattern	65–70	80	18	2
Prolonged latent phase	2–5	75	10	15
Prolonged active phase	20–30	55	30	15
Secondary arrest	5–10	40	35	25

(e.g., admission to the neonatal unit). Within reason, it is important to resist the temptation to actively intervene by artificially rupturing the membranes or administering oxytocics, at least until the cervix is 2 or 3 cm dilated and fully effaced with a well-applied presenting part. Intervention may actually increase the risk of further obstetric intervention in what might, with patience, have been an uneventful labour. Reassurance, encouragement, hydration and appropriate analgesia over this time are extremely important.

PROLONGED ACTIVE PHASE AND SECONDARY ARREST

The active phase may be prolonged because of inadequate uterine activity or CPD (Fig. 34.3).

Inadequate Uterine Activity

The uterus may be hypoactive or incoordinate. A hypoactive uterus is one with low resting tone and only weakly propagated contractions. There is often a

longer interval between contractions and the contractions are not particularly painful.

Incoordinate uterine activity may occur because of inadequate 'fundal dominance'. Normal uterine contraction begins at a pacemaker point close to the junction of the uterus and the fallopian tube. It spreads from this point downwards, with its intensity maximal at the fundus (where the muscle is thickest), intermediate at the mid-zone, and least at the lower segment. Uterine contractions can be described in terms of baseline tone, amplitude, frequency, and duration. With incoordinate uterine activity, the intensity profile appears to be reversed, with the maximal intensity in the lower segment (where the muscle is thinnest) and weakest at the fundus. This is much less efficient. The resting tone is increased throughout and, therefore, the threshold for pain is reached earlier in the contraction. Incoordinate uterine activity is common, especially in women in their first labour. Contractions may be incoordinate in terms of frequency, duration or strength, or a combination.

Inadequate uterine activity has no specific cause— it may simply be a developmental feature of the uterine muscle. There is evidence that many will resolve spontaneously given sufficient time. There is also some evidence that inadequate uterine activity is associated with CPD. This is because cervical dilatation itself may improve uterine activity, but it is less likely to occur if the presenting part is pressing less firmly on the cervix.

If progress is satisfactory, there is no need to consider treatment of incoordinate uterine activity. Most will respond well to oxytocics, usually given by a stepwise intravenous oxytocin infusion, as described earlier. As labour is likely to be prolonged, care should be taken to make sure that the woman does not become dehydrated or ketotic, as this will further exacerbate the uterine problem.

Cephalopelvic Disproportion

This may occur because of the following:

1. The baby's head is presenting in the optimal way but is too large relative to the pelvis ('true' CPD). It is diagnosed only if the head does not become engaged despite adequate uterine activity. It is not possible to predict CPD antenatally, and even using the strictest antenatal criteria,

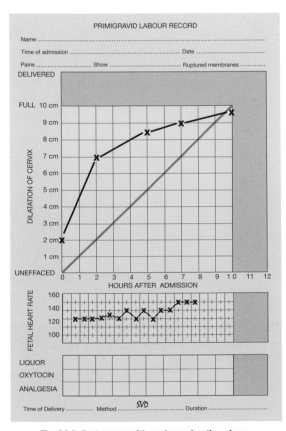

Fig. 34.3 Partogram with prolonged active phase.

many of those considered to be at risk by clinical pelvic assessment will go on to have a vaginal birth. More complicated attempts to predict CPD using ultrasound measurements of the fetal head together with X-ray or computed tomography pelvimetry measurements have also proved to be unreliable and only lead to unnecessary surgical intervention. Short maternal stature or small shoe size are not predictive of CPD. The only true test is labour itself.

2. There is a malpresentation or malposition of the baby's head so that a wider part of the head is being presented to the pelvis. This is 'relative' CPD. It may occur with deflexed malpresentations (particularly of the brow and face; see p. 409), but the most common cause of relative CPD occurs when the head rotates to the OP (see p. 417) rather than the OA position. The first stage and second stage progress more slowly, although spontaneous delivery is quite possible with the head coming out 'face to pubis', secondary arrest is not uncommon.

3. There is some form of pelvic abnormality. Major abnormalities are uncommon, particularly in well-resourced settings, and are usually associated with disease, injury or severe nutritional problems. The obstetric classification is based on the shape of the pelvic brim, as it is the pelvic inlet, which seems to be the major determinant of vaginal birth (Fig. 34.4).

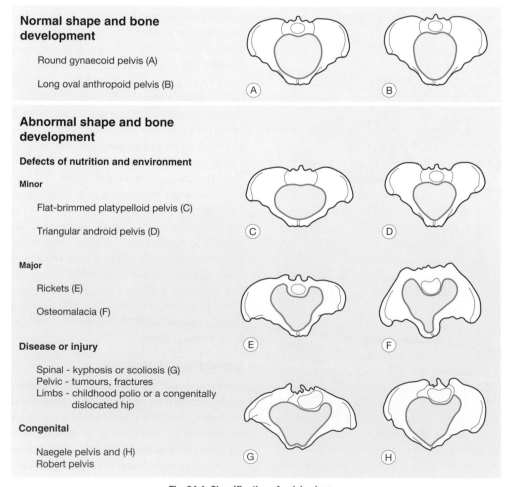

Normal shape and bone development

Round gynaecoid pelvis (A)

Long oval anthropoid pelvis (B)

Abnormal shape and bone development

Defects of nutrition and environment

Minor

Flat-brimmed platypelloid pelvis (C)

Triangular android pelvis (D)

Major

Rickets (E)

Osteomalacia (F)

Disease or injury

Spinal - kyphosis or scoliosis (G)
Pelvic - tumours, fractures
Limbs - childhood polio or a congenitally dislocated hip

Congenital

Naegele pelvis and (H)
Robert pelvis

Fig. 34.4 Classification of pelvic shapes.

PELVES WITH NORMAL SHAPE AND BONE DEVELOPMENT

The round 'gynaecoid' pelvis is the most common and, as would be teleologically predicted by the theory of natural selection, it is obstetrically ideal. The long oval 'anthropoid' pelvis is also relatively common but is associated with OP presentation.

PELVES WITH ABNORMAL SHAPE AND BONE DEVELOPMENT

Defects of Nutrition and Environment

Minor

The flat-brimmed 'platypelloid' pelvis and the triangular 'android' pelvis are considered to be minor variations associated with adverse nutrition in infancy and childhood. The flat-brimmed pelvis is found relatively more commonly in African women and the triangular pelvis in those from southern Europe.

Major

Rickets is caused by prolonged vitamin D deficiency in early life, leading to poorly mineralised bones containing large areas of soft, uncalcified osteoid. Weight bearing produces bony deformities by pushing the sacral promontory forward and pivoting the sacrum backwards. The result is a marked reduction in the anteroposterior measurement of the pelvic brim, with possible further mid-cavity narrowing in severe cases as the acetabula are also forced inwards. Low vitamin D concentrations are present in a large proportion of the UK population. Therefore, it is recommended that women who are pregnant or breast-feeding should have vitamin D supplementation (10 µg a day).

Disease or Injury

Abnormal pressure on the pelvis from kyphosis or scoliosis gradually moulds the pelvis into funnelled or asymmetrical shapes. Asymmetrical weight bearing from polio or a congenitally dislocated hip may also mould the pelvis to less favourable proportions. Pelvic fractures may leave the pelvis asymmetrical. Excessive bone formation at the fracture site may further narrow the passage.

Congenital Malformations

Congenital absence of one or both sacral masses (Naegele pelvis and Robert pelvis, respectively) is very uncommon. It results in direct fusion of the sacrum to the ilium and marked narrowing.

Management of Slow Labour

When progress is slow or when there is secondary arrest, it is important to distinguish whether the cause is inadequate uterine activity or CPD.

The strength of contractions is difficult to assess reliably and cannot be done from a cardiotocograph recording. Direct intrauterine pressure monitoring using a pressure catheter is essentially only a research tool and is rarely, if ever, used in clinical practice. Some idea of the strength can be gained by observing the woman and abdominal palpation of contractions. The examining hand is placed between the umbilicus and the uterine fundus, and the duration and frequency of the uterine contractions are assessed over a 10-minute period. With an experienced observer, this can provide useful clinical information. In the presence of CPD, there will be caput (a diffuse swelling of the scalp) and moulding (an alteration in the relation of the fetal cranial bones). Malposition or malpresentation may be identified by careful vaginal examination. If delay in labour is suspected or confirmed, amniotomy should be offered with a view to repeat examination in 2 hours to ensure adequate progress in labour.

In practice, the clinical decision is usually whether or not to start an oxytocin infusion. The main risks of starting oxytocin are:

- Hyperstimulation of the uterus and subsequent fetal distress
- Rupture of the uterus (this applies almost exclusively to multiparous women and is more likely in those with a previous caesarean section scar).

In primigravidae with slow progress or secondary arrest who do not have a prohibitive malpresentation (e.g., brow presentation) it is reasonable to offer and commence oxytocin. This is not appropriate if there is suspected fetal distress and should only be after the membranes have been ruptured or have ruptured spontaneously. The aim is to titrate the infusion to the point at which the contractions are coming at a frequency of 4 to 5 every 10 minutes. Vaginal examinations should be offered and repeated every 3 to

4 hours after the infusion has started to ensure adequate progress. If progress is still inadequate (cervical dilatation has increased by less than 2 cm in 4 hours), then operative delivery will be required.

In parous women, the decision is more difficult, mainly because of the risk of uterine rupture (see p. 433). Rupture can occur suddenly and leads to expulsion of the fetus into the peritoneal cavity. In this situation, fetal hypoxia and death is not uncommon. If the woman has had a previous vaginal birth, true CPD is extremely unlikely, but if the only previous birth was an elective caesarean section (e.g., for breech presentation), there is no guide to the likelihood of true obstruction. Therefore, an oxytocin infusion should be used with caution and only in those women thought to have inadequate uterine activity with no evidence of obstruction. Following discussion with the woman, vaginal examinations should again be repeated every 3 to 4 hours to ensure adequate progress, with a lower threshold for caesarean birth in those thought to have some degree of CPD.

Malpresentation

As described earlier, 'malpresentation' is a term used to describe any non-vertex presentation. Over 95% of fetuses are in cephalic presentation at term. Malpresentations include face presentation, brow presentation and breech presentation. When the fetus has a cephalic presentation, the presenting diameter is dependent on the degree of flexion or extension of the fetal head—deflexed and brow presentations offer a wide diameter to the pelvic inlet (Table 34.3 and Fig. 34.5).

As the fetal skull is made up of individual bony plates (the occipital, sphenoid, temporal and ethmoid bones), which are joined by cartilaginous sutures (the frontal, sagittal, lambdoid and coronal sutures), it has the potential to be 'moulded' during labour. This allows the head to fit the birth canal more closely (Fig. 34.6). Moulding should be distinguished from caput succedaneum, which refers to oedema of the presenting part of the scalp. Both moulding and caput can occur in any cephalic presentation, but are more likely to occur in malpresentation. The presence or absence of moulding and caput should be documented during each vaginal

TABLE 34.3	Presenting Diameters of the Fetal Head	
Presentation	**Presenting Diameter**	
Vertex	Suboccipitobregmatic	9.5 cm
Deflexed OP	Occipitofrontal	11.5 cm
Brow	Mentovertical	14 cm
Face	Submentobregmatic	9.5 cm

OP, Occipitoposterior.

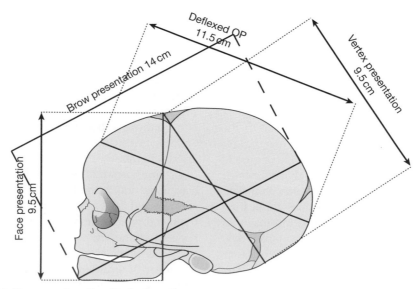

Fig. 34.5 The presenting diameter is dependent on the degree of flexion or extension of the fetal head
OP, Occipitoposterior.

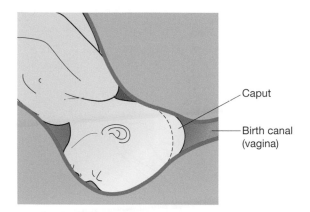

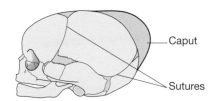

Fig. 34.6 'Moulding' refers to the change in shape of the fetal skull during labour as it 'moulds' to the birth canal. Caput refers to oedema of the presenting part of the scalp.

examination in labour; excessive moulding and caput are suggestive of an obstructed labour due to CPD.

FACE PRESENTATION

This occurs in about 1:500 births and occurs when the fetal head extends right back (hyperextended so that the occiput touches the fetal back; Fig. 34.7A). It is associated with prematurity, tumours of the fetal neck, loops of cord around the fetal neck, fetal macrosomia and anencephaly. Face presentation is usually recognised only after the onset of labour and, if the face is swollen (see Fig. 34.7D), it is easy to confuse this presentation with that of a breech. The position of the face is described with reference to the chin, using the prefix 'mento'. The presenting diameter is submentobregmatic (9.5 cm; see Fig. 34.5).

The face usually enters the pelvis with the chin in the transverse position (mentotransverse) and 90% rotates to mentoanterior so that the head is born with flexion (see Fig. 34.7B). If mentoposterior, the extending head presents an increasingly wider diameter to the pelvis, leading to worsening relative CPD and impacted obstruction (see Fig. 34.7C). A caesarean birth is usually required.

BROW PRESENTATION

This occurs in only approximately 1:700 and 1:1500 births and is the least favourable for delivery (Fig. 34.8). The presenting diameter is mentovertical, measuring 14 cm. The supraorbital ridges and the bridge of the nose will be palpable on vaginal examination. The head may flex to become a vertex presentation or extend to a face presentation in early labour. If the brow presentation persists, a caesarean birth will be required.

BREECH PRESENTATION

Breech presentation describes a fetus presenting bottom first. The incidence is around 40% at 20 weeks, 25% at 32 weeks and only 3% to 4% at term. The chance of a breech presentation turning spontaneously after 38 weeks is less than 4%. Breech presentation is associated with multiple pregnancy, bicornuate uterus, fibroids, placenta praevia, polyhydramnios and oligohydramnios. It may also rarely be associated with fetal anomaly, particularly neural tube defects, neuromuscular disorders and autosomal trisomies. At term, 65% of breech presentations are frank (extended), with the remainder being flexed or footling (Fig. 34.9). Footling breech carries a 5% to 20% risk of cord prolapse (see p. 425).

Mode of Delivery

There has been extensive debate about the safest route of delivery—whether it should be a vaginal or caesarean birth. The risks of vaginal birth are small, but include intracranial injury, widespread bruising, damage to internal organs, spinal cord transection, umbilical cord prolapse and hypoxia following obstruction of the after-coming head. The risks of caesarean birth are largely maternal and related to surgical morbidity and mortality. A planned caesarean birth is associated with less perinatal mortality and less serious neonatal morbidity than planned vaginal birth at term. The risks of serious maternal complications are much the same, partly because planned vaginal birth often ends with an intrapartum caesarean section, which carries

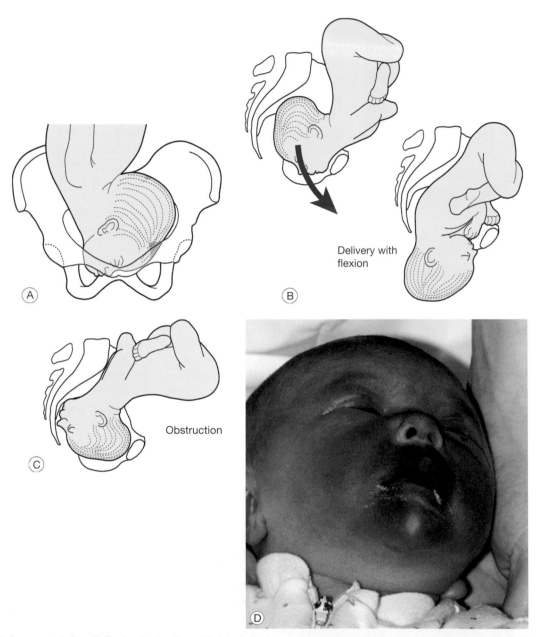

Fig. 34.7 Face presentation. (A) The head enters the pelvic brim in the transverse position. **(B)** Most rotate to the mentoanterior position and are born without problems. **(C)** Those that rotate to mentoposterior will obstruct. **(D)** Face presentation is often associated with oedema and bruising. This baby recovered without problems.

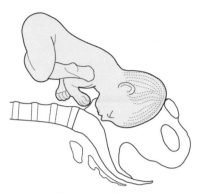

Fig. 34.8 Brow presentation.

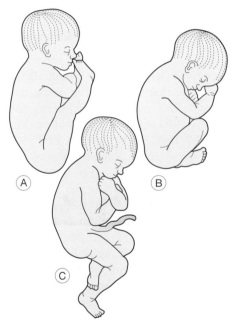

Fig. 34.9 Breech presentation. Those presenting by the breech may be **(A)** extended (or frank), **(B)** flexed, or **(C)** footling.

greater risks than a planned elective section. The problem of vaginal breech delivery can be removed if it is possible to turn the baby prior to the onset of labour. This process is called external cephalic version (ECV).

External Cephalic Version

All women with a breech presentation at term should be offered ECV unless there is an absolute contraindication (outlined in Box 34.1). It is good practice to offer ECV from 36 weeks in nulliparous women and from 37 weeks in multiparous women. The success rate is approximately 50%.

BOX 34.1 CONTRAINDICATIONS TO EXTERNAL CEPHALIC VERSION (ECV)

Absolute Contraindications
- When caesarean delivery is required regardless of presentation (e.g., placenta praevia)
- Antepartum haemorrhage within the last 7 days
- Abnormal cardiotocograph
- Major uterine anomaly
- Ruptured membranes
- Multiple pregnancy (except delivery of second twin)
- Absence of maternal consent

Relative Contraindications Where ECV Might be More Complicated
- Nuchal cord
- Fetal growth restriction
- Proteinuric pre-eclampsia
- Oligohydramnios
- Major fetal anomalies
- Hyperextended fetal head
- Morbid maternal obesity

Note: ECV after one caesarean birth appears to have no greater risk than with an unscarred uterus.

Procedure

A cardiotocograph and ultrasound scan should be performed. Some obstetricians prefer the woman to be fasted and prepared for theatre since there is a very small risk of fetal distress during the procedure. Although this is usually not necessary, it is reasonable to have access to theatre close at hand. ECV is most likely to be successful in parous women when the presenting part is free, the liquor volume is normal, the head is easy to palpate, and the uterus feels soft. A flexed breech is more likely to turn than an extended (frank) breech.

The woman is asked to lie flat with a 30-degree lateral tilt. The use of tocolysis, such as a betamimetic drug, to soften the uterus is associated with an increased success rate. Applying scanning gel to the abdomen allows easier manipulation and permits scanning during the procedure if required. The breech is disengaged if necessary, with the scan probe or hands. Then, attempts are made to rotate in the direction in which the baby is facing (i.e., 'forward roll'). The fetal heart rate should be checked throughout the procedure. If a forward roll is unsuccessful, a backward 'somersault' can be tried. If the procedure is only partially successful (i.e., the fetus is converted to a transverse lie), the fetus should be returned to breech rather than leave it transverse. A cardiotocograph should be performed after the procedure is completed. Women who are rhesus D negative should undergo testing for fetomaternal haemorrhage and anti-D immunoglobulin should be offered.

Caesarean Section for Breech Presentation

Planned caesarean section at term for breech presentation is associated with a small reduction in perinatal mortality compared with a planned vaginal birth. However, the decision to perform a caesarean section has important implications for future pregnancies, such as the risks of opting for vaginal birth after caesarean section, increased risk of complications in future caesarean sections and the risk of an abnormally invasive placenta.

Pre-Term Breech

For those in pre-term labour with breech presentation, the mode of delivery should be individualised. The decision should be based on the stage of labour, type of breech, fetal well-being, and the availability of a clinician experienced in vaginal breech birth.

Vaginal Birth for Breech Presentation

Women should be assessed and counselled in the antenatal period regarding the risks associated with vaginal breech birth. A planned vaginal breech birth is expected to be more complicated in the following circumstances: hyperextended neck on ultrasound, high/low estimated fetal weight, footling presentation, and evidence of fetal compromise. If a woman presents in labour with a breech presentation, her intrapartum care will depend on her preferences, the stage of labour, and the availability of clinical expertise. Induction of labour is not usually recommended.

In women aiming for a vaginal birth with a breech presentation, the role of epidural analgesia is controversial—its use may facilitate manipulation of the fetus, but its presence may inhibit the desire to push, which is particularly important in breech delivery. Augmentation of slow progress should be considered only in the event of inadequate uterine activity in the presence of an epidural. There is no contraindication to a fetal 'scalp' electrode being applied to the breech provided that care is taken to avoid genital injury. A

standing or semi-recumbent position in an 'all fours' position has been recommended.

At full dilatation, the woman can be encouraged to push when she experiences an urge. The temptation to pull must be resisted. Ideally, the baby should be left alone to birth by itself ('hands off'), taking care to ensure that the back remains uppermost when advancing. If there is undue delay, or there are concerns about fetal well-being (e.g., movements stopping, baby becoming floppy, no response to stimuli), assisted delivery can be used to encourage a more rapid birth. The techniques of 'hands off' and 'assisted breech' are illustrated in Figs 34.10 and 34.11. Breech extraction may be considered when delivering the second twin (see p. 362).

One of the key risks of breech delivery is that pulling may lead the head to extend and become stuck at the pelvic brim. 'The importance of maternal effort at this stage, rather than traction from below, cannot be overemphasised—it allows the head to flex and minimises the risk of it becoming stuck at the pelvic brim'.

Should the head of a pre-term breech become entrapped behind an incompletely dilated cervix, it should first be flexed as far as is possible to narrow the presenting diameter. Failing this, the options are then to incise the cervix at the 4 and 8 o'clock positions (risking massive, potentially fatal maternal haemorrhage) or to push the fetus back up and perform a caesarean section (a very difficult manoeuvre). Because such interventions are hazardous to the woman, it may be preferable to await spontaneous birth even if this compromises the well-being of the baby.

All babies presenting by the breech should be examined for developmental dysplasia of the hip and Klumpke paralysis.

TRANSVERSE LIE AND OBLIQUE LIE

These are uncommon, occurring in less than 1% of pregnancies at term (Fig. 34.12). There is usually no specific cause, but abnormal lie is more common in multiparous women, multiple pregnancies, pre-term labour and polyhydramnios. It may also be associated with placenta praevia, congenital abnormalities of the uterus, lower uterine fibroids and other pelvic masses, such as an ovarian cyst.

If transverse lie is identified antenatally, a scan should be undertaken to exclude placenta praevia,

As the breech descends with pushing, it rotates to the anteroposterior and advances over the perineum. It then rotates with the back uppermost. Any movement of the back posteriorly should be corrected.

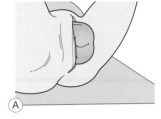
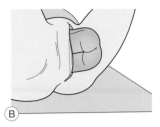

The legs will free themselves as the baby advances, and will hang down

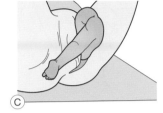
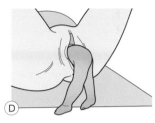

With pushing, the arms will deliver

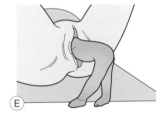
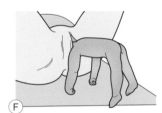

The breech should be allowed to hang in order for the head to flex, waiting for the nape of the neck to become visible

After delivery of the other arm, flexion of the baby's head is encouraged by placing the second and third fingers of the lower hand over the malar bones on the face, pulling them towards you....

....while the second and third fingers of the other hand are used to push the occiput (back) of the head away from you. With maximum flexion, the head can then be delivered. An episiotomy can be used if necessary

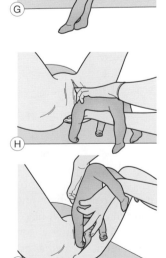

Fig. 34.10 'Hands off' vaginal breech delivery.

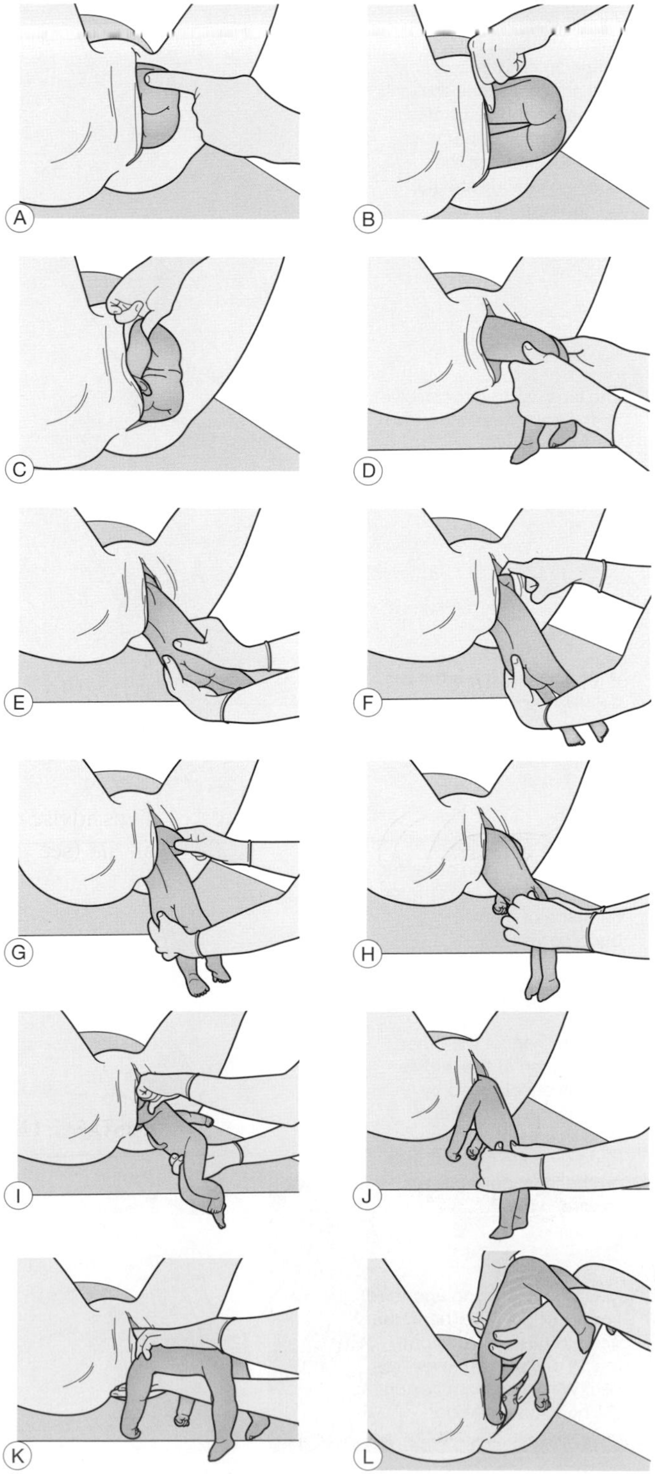
The knees can be flexed to deliver the legs
A
B
Once the legs are delivered, it is important to wait for the body to advance further, before holding the bony pelvis firmly as shown
C
D
Rotation allows one arm to be freed, flexed and brought down....
E
F
....while rotation the other way allows the other arm to be similarily delivered
G
H
After delivery of the other arm, flexion of the baby's head is again encouraged by allowing the breech to hang down....
I
J
....and the head is delivered as for the 'hands off' vaginal breech delivery
K
L

Fig. 34.11 Assisted vaginal breech birth.

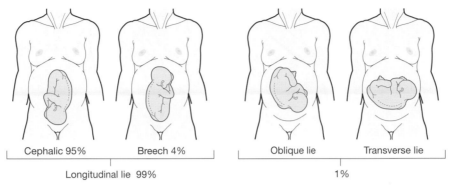

Cephalic 95%   Breech 4%   Oblique lie   Transverse lie

Longitudinal lie 99%   1%

Fig. 34.12 Fetal lie at term.

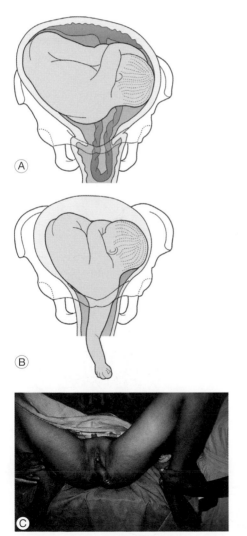

Fig. 34.13 Transverse lie is associated with (A) cord prolapse and (B,C) arm prolapse.

polyhydramnios, lower uterine fibroids and a pathologically enlarged fetal head. ECV is usually possible (see earlier discussion), and the woman should be reviewed a few days later to ensure that the lie is still cephalic. She should be advised to come to hospital if there is any suspicion of early labour, as it may still be possible to carry out an ECV at that stage, provided that the membranes are still intact. She should also be advised to go to the hospital immediately if there is any suspicion of membrane rupture, as there is a risk of cord prolapse or prolapse of a limb (Fig. 34.13A–C). In view of the small risk of cord prolapse, some clinicians advise that women with a transverse lie or unstable lie (see later discussion) are admitted to hospital from 38 weeks to await birth or until a longitudinal lie is maintained.

If the lie is transverse in established labour, particularly after membrane rupture, a caesarean section will usually be required. These caesarean sections can be technically very difficult, and a vertical uterine incision may be necessary to allow adequate access for delivery.

UNSTABLE LIE

An unstable lie is one that varies from examination to examination. The options are:

- Manage conservatively, with repeated ECVs as required, and await the spontaneous onset of labour. Should the membranes rupture with the fetus in a non-cephalic presentation, there may be a risk of cord prolapse. As described earlier, inpatient care is considered appropriate by some.
- Arrange to turn the baby to cephalic presentation and then induce labour. This is sometimes referred to as a 'stabilising induction'. The disadvantage is

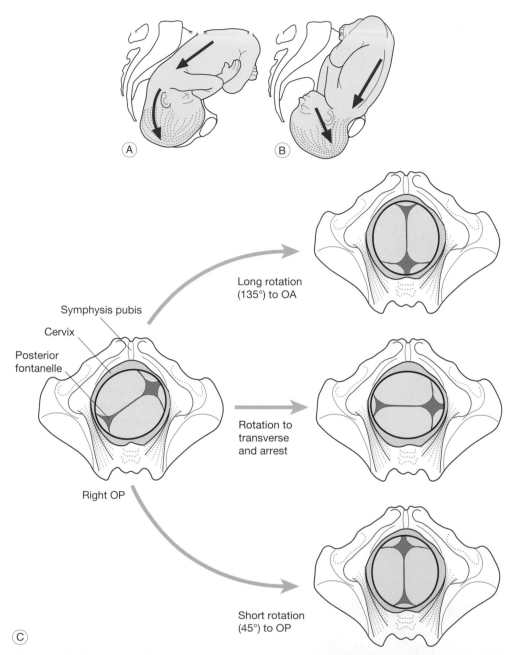

Symphysis pubis

Cervix

Posterior
fontanelle

Right OP

Long rotation
(135°) to OA

Rotation to
transverse
and arrest

Short rotation
(45°) to OP

Fig. 34.14 Occipitoposterior (OP) position (A) compared with an occipitoanterior (OA) position (B). (C) Occiput rotation.

that the induction itself is not without risks, and the lie may become unstable again even after the membranes have been ruptured.

- Carry out a caesarean section.

MALPOSITION

The fetal head normally engages at the pelvic brim in the occipitotransverse position, flexing as it descends into the pelvic cavity and rotating to OA at the level of the ischial spines. The head then extends as it descends, distending the vulva until it is delivered. In about 10% of pregnancies, the fetal head enters the pelvis in a more OP position than transverse or anterior, either by chance or in association with an unfavourably shaped pelvis, particularly the long oval 'anthropoid' pelvis. The baby is then in a direct OP position or with the occiput to the right or left of the midline, referred to as right or left OP.

There are then three main possibilities (Fig. 34.14C):

- The occiput will rotate anteriorly (through approximately 135 degrees) to OA, and then (usually) deliver normally (65%).
- The occiput will partially rotate to occipitotransverse and not deliver (20%).
- The occiput will rotate more posteriorly to OP (15%).

Those that remain OP have greater difficulty negotiating the birth canal and are less likely to birth spontaneously. The normal mechanism of birth involves extension of the head to OA, but extension is not possible in the OP position and a wider diameter is presented to the outlet (occipitofrontal 11.5 cm; see Table 34.3 and Fig. 34.14A,B). With malposition, the first and second stages of labour are usually longer, partly because of the greater presenting diameter (relative CPD) and partly because the head is less well applied to the cervix and, therefore, less able to facilitate its dilatation. Back pain in labour appears to be more common with the OP position. The woman is more likely to request an epidural, is more likely to experience secondary arrest due to relative CPD, and is more likely to require augmentation with an oxytocin infusion.

If the cervix does not reach full dilatation despite oxytocin augmentation, a caesarean section will be required. If full dilatation is reached, it is quite possible for a baby to be born in the OP position (with the head coming out 'face to pubis'). Not uncommonly, manual rotation, rotational ventouse, or a Kielland rotational forceps birth will be required (see p. 437). Third- and fourth-degree perineal tears are more likely to occur when a baby is born in an OP position.

Key Points

- **Progress in labour requires adequate uterine activity and an appropriately proportioned fetal head compared with the size of the maternal pelvis.**
- **Precipitate labour is most commonly iatrogenic following oxytocin administration.**
- **Slow progress is often corrected with the use of an oxytocin infusion, whether due to inadequate uterine activity or a small degree of CPD. Care must be taken to exclude a significant malpresentation before the infusion is started. An oxytocin infusion carries a risk of uterine rupture, especially in parous women.**
- **Normal presentation is with the vertex of the fetal head; the word 'malpresentation' describes any non-vertex presentation. It may be of the face, brow, breech or some other part of the body if the lie is oblique or transverse.**
- **Those who are presenting by the brow usually become obstructed, and those who are lying transversely always become obstructed.**
- **Babies presenting by the breech can often birth vaginally, but there is a small risk of intrapartum injury. Women whose baby is presenting by the breech at term should be offered ECV if there is no contraindication.**
- **Babies with a face presentation are usually born without significant problems.**

Chapter 35

Obstetric Emergencies

Tim Draycott, Sophie Renwick, Emily Hotton, Cameron Hinton, Katie Cornthwaite

Chapter Outline

Introduction

Across the world, one woman dies every minute of every day from a complication of pregnancy. In high-resource settings, maternal death is rare, but the UK maternal death audit programme (MBRRACE-UK) identifies substandard care in around two-thirds of cases. Many obstetric emergencies are uncommon and can deteriorate quickly. There is an evidence base for multi-professional training that appears to be one of the most promising strategies to improve maternal and perinatal outcomes after obstetric emergencies. In particular, a structured approach with integrated teamwork training and communication is associated with better outcomes.

This chapter will discuss the obstetric emergencies listed here:

- Shoulder dystocia (SD)
- Cord prolapse
- Impacted fetal head (IFH) at caesarean section
- Maternal collapse and cardiac arrest
- Amniotic fluid embolism (AFE)
- Sepsis
- Uterine inversion
- Uterine rupture

See also obstetric haemorrhage (Chapter 26), eclampsia (Chapter 28), pulmonary embolism (pp. 277) and practical obstetrics and gynaecology (Chapter 44).

General Principles

TEAMWORK AND TRAINING

A team-based approach to obstetric emergencies is required, as multiple actions are often required simultaneously within a short time frame.

Simulation training can help prepare staff to manage rare, life-threatening emergencies. However, not all training is equal or effective. Local, multi-professional training in the clinical area (within the maternity unit) appears to be most effective and is more realistic than delivering training outside of the settings where care is delivered. Simulated scenarios enable teams to rehearse technical skills while testing the environment and systems in place in the maternity unit – for example, making sure that equipment is available and functional as well as ensuring that interactions with supporting systems (porters, laboratories and so on) are efficient.

COMMUNICATION

Non-technical skills (communication, leadership and teamwork) in obstetric emergencies have consistently been identified as contributors to outcomes for mothers and babies. There is good evidence that training as a team improves these non-technical skills in real emergencies. Additional tools, such as checklists, may support effective communication. Emergency boxes or trolleys (e.g., for postpartum haemorrhage, eclampsia or sepsis), which contain all of the essential equipment required to manage an emergency in one place, enable teams to provide the correct care reliably and rapidly (Fig. 35.1).

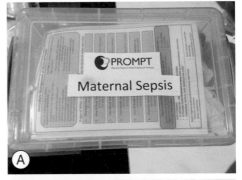

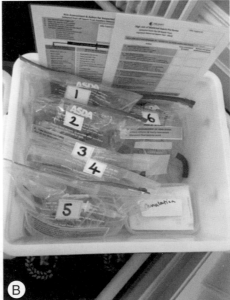

Fig. 35.1 Example of an emergency box for maternal sepsis, containing all of the equipment to commence 'Sepsis 6'.

BOX 35.1 EXAMPLE OF AN SBAR HANDOVER IN AN EMERGENCY

BOX 35.1 EXAMPLE OF AN SBAR HANDOVER IN AN EMERGENCY

> **Situation:** This is a suspected uterine rupture.
> **Background:** Catherine is a Para 1. She had a previous caesarean section 12 months ago and has presented in spontaneous labour.
> **Assessment:** She has constant pain over her caesarean section scar, new fresh vaginal bleeding, and the cardiotocography is pathological. Catherine is 6 cm dilated on vaginal examination.
> **Recommendation:** I would like a senior obstetrician, midwife and anaesthetist to attend immediately.

Team members should be aware that communication is often impaired under stress. It is important to declare the emergency to incoming colleagues to initiate the required actions, for example, 'This is a shoulder dystocia'. Handing over of information in a succinct manner can be achieved using a structured format, such as SBAR (**S**ituation, **B**ackground, **A**ssessment, **R**ecommendation), an example of which is shown in Box 35.1.

General communication, such as the delegation of a task, should be clear, addressed to specific individuals, and acknowledged by the individual receiving the information – for example, 'Jane, please fetch the postpartum hemorrhage (PPH) trolley'. When a team member completes a task, the individual should report back to the team leader so that the leader can maintain a 'helicopter view' of the emergency. Another useful tool can be '20 seconds to plan next 20 minutes', in which the team members pause for 20 seconds to recap care and plan for the next 20 minutes of care.

Effective communication with the mother and her partner is essential. The psychological trauma of obstetric emergencies may lead to long-term psychiatric problems, including postnatal depression and post-traumatic stress disorder. Women are more likely to report a traumatic birth experience when they feel communication has been poor. Therefore, explanation of events as they are happening, appropriate consent, and debriefing after such experiences is vital. It may be appropriate for one of the team to be allocated the role of keeping the woman and her family up-to-date with events during the emergency; women want information similar to that shared amongst the team about their baby, their own safety and next steps. It may also be appropriate to offer an appointment for follow-up to the woman and her family some weeks after the event to discuss the events and answer any questions they may have (debriefing).

RISK ASSESSMENT AND PREPARATION

Although many emergencies are difficult to predict, an appreciation of risk factors and continual risk assessment, both antenatally and intrapartum, can help with anticipation, preparation and prevention (if not of the emergency, then at least some of the consequences). For example, if a woman has had a previous SD, or other risk factors for SD such as diabetes, it is important to ensure that she has been offered an opportunity to discuss antenatally the risks, benefits and available options, including place or mode of birth. Furthermore, SD can complicate any vaginal birth; therefore, teams should be ready and able to manage it when it arises.

In obstetric emergencies, there are often two lives at stake. However, only the mother can be resuscitated directly. 'Resuscitate the mother and you will resuscitate the fetus' is a useful principle. A structured approach can be applied generically to the initial management of all obstetric emergencies associated with maternal compromise (e.g., maternal collapse, postpartum haemorrhage, sepsis), which is outlined in Box 35.2.

BOX 35.2 INITIAL STEPS IN MANAGEMENT OF AN OBSTETRIC EMERGENCY

1. **Call for help:** Pull the emergency buzzer or emergency bleep the obstetric emergency team. This should include senior obstetricians, anaesthetists and midwives. It may also include theatre staff, someone skilled in neonatal resuscitation, and porters.
2. **Declare the emergency** to the incoming team – for example, 'this is a uterine inversion'.
3. **Request emergency equipment** – for example, postpartum haemorrhage emergency box.
4. **Allocate team roles**, including a scribe to clearly document actions.
5. Ensure that the environment is safe for you and **perform an ABC assessment** (if appropriate).
   - **Airway:** Have woman lie flat, assess airway.
   - **Breathing:** Assess respiratory rate and oxygen saturations, and consider administering high-flow oxygen (15 L/min).
   - **Circulation:** Assess pulse and blood pressure. Insert two wide-bore cannulae, take urgent bloods and administer intravenous fluids.
6. Continue with **specific emergency management**, which may be aided by an emergency algorithm or checklist.

Shoulder Dystocia

SD is an unpredictable and time-critical obstetric emergency. Efficient and effective management is required to prevent fetal mortality or long-term fetal and maternal morbidity.

DEFINITION

SD is an impaction of the fetal shoulders at the maternal pelvis, occurring after the birth of the head. It is defined by the need for additional obstetric manoeuvres to assist the birth of the infant, when routine axial traction has failed to deliver the anterior shoulder. Routine axial traction is used to deliver an infant without SD. Most commonly, SD is caused by the anterior shoulder impacting behind the maternal symphysis pubis. However, it may also be caused by the posterior shoulder impacting on the sacral promontory. The incidence is in the range of 0.1% to 3% of vaginal births and is increasing.

RISK FACTORS AND PREVENTION

A number of antenatal and intrapartum risk factors have been identified (Box 35.3). However, these offer limited predictive value; 50% of SD occurs in normal-sized fetuses and 98% of large babies do not have SD. The most significant risk factor is SD with a previous birth, which increases the incidence to 12% to 17%. Therefore, all women with a previous SD should receive counselling about their birth options in the antenatal period, with discussion between caesarean or vaginal birth with the relevant risks and benefits; a Cochrane decision tool is available to guide the discussion. Induction of labour between 37 and 39 weeks for

BOX 35.3 RISK FACTORS FOR SHOULDER DYSTOCIA

Antepartum
Previous shoulder dystocia
Macrosomia
Maternal diabetes mellitus
Advanced gestational age
Maternal obesity
Intrapartum
Prolonged first stage
Prolonged second stage
Augmentation of labour
Instrumental birth (forceps or vacuum)

babies with an estimated fetal weight of >4 kg at term has been demonstrated to reduce the risk of SD by 40%, but with no improvement in clinical outcomes and a three-fold increase in severe perineal injury.

RECOGNITION

There are a number of clinical signs that may precede an SD, which include:
- Slow or difficult birth of the face and chin
- Tight retraction of the head against the vulva
- Chin retraction ('turtle-neck sign')
- Lack of restitution of the fetal head.

However, a diagnosis cannot be made until there is failure of delivery of the anterior shoulder with routine axial traction.

CARE OF WOMEN WITH SHOULDER DYSTOCIA

A timely and systematic team approach is required to deliver the impacted fetal shoulder whilst also minimising the likelihood of fetal injury. Current international guidelines all recommend four basic manoeuvres, most commonly attempted in the following order, with the least invasive first:
- McRoberts position
- Suprapubic pressure
- Delivery of the posterior arm
- Internal rotation manoeuvres

These are outlined in more detail in Fig. 35.2.

The first step is to call for help and clearly state the emergency of 'shoulder dystocia' to the team. It is important to document the time of delivery of the head and of subsequent management. Communicate what is happening to the parents and ask the mother to stop pushing, as further pushing increases the impaction. Lie the bed flat and bring the mother to the edge of the bed. After each manoeuvre, diagnostic traction (an attempt to deliver the shoulders) should be applied to the fetal head to see if the manoeuvres have successfully released the impaction. All traction should be in an axial direction (in line with the axis of the fetal spine) with the same amount of traction as for a routine vaginal birth without SD, to prevent brachial plexus injury (Fig. 35.3).

The **McRoberts position** optimises the diameter of the pelvic inlet. It is the least invasive manoeuvre, with success rates of up to 50%. Therefore, it should routinely be attempted first. With the mother lying flat, an assistant on each side should hyperflex the mother's

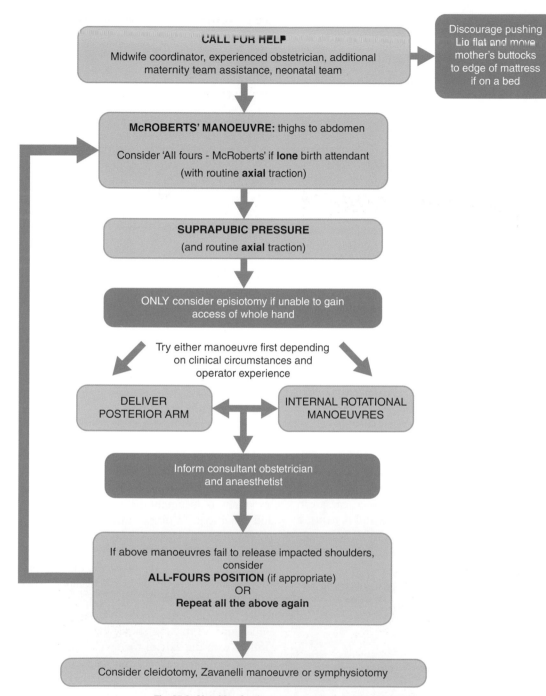

Fig. 35.2 Algorithm for the management of shoulder dystocia.

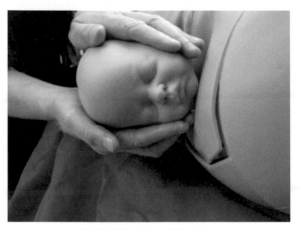

Fig. 35.3 Routine axial traction.

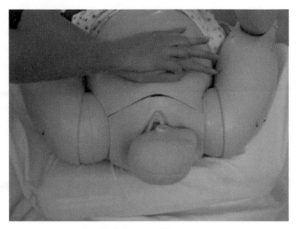

Fig. 35.5 Suprapubic pressure.

legs against her abdomen. When the manoeuvre is executed correctly, the maternal buttocks should lift off the bed (Fig. 35.4). **All-fours McRoberts**, positioning the mother in a flexed all-fours position with thighs against the abdomen, can also be attempted.

Suprapubic pressure (SPP) (1) can be applied with McRoberts and reduces the fetal shoulder-to-shoulder diameter with (2) rotation of the shoulders away from the narrowest, anteroposterior pelvic diameter. An additional assistant should apply pressure suprapubically, with outstretched arms and inter-clasped hands in a 'CPR' (cardiopulmonary resuscitation) position (Fig. 35.5), ideally applied from the side of the fetal back. There is limited evidence as to whether rocking or continuous pressure is more effective.

Episiotomy will not relieve the bony obstruction of SD and can be difficult to perform after delivery of

the head. Therefore, perform or extend an episiotomy only if there is not enough space to perform internal manoeuvres.

Internal manoeuvres include (1) **delivery of the posterior arm** to reduce the diameter of the shoulders and (2) **internal rotation** to move the shoulders away from the narrow anteroposterior pelvic diameter. Both are performed with the insertion of the accoucheur's hand posteriorly into the sacral hollow at 6 o'clock, including the thumb, with the hand in the position of putting on a bangle (Fig. 35.6). Once access has been gained, the most appropriate manoeuvre can be attempted first, depending on whether the fetal hand and forearm can be felt. If the forearm of the posterior fetal arm can be grasped, deliver the posterior arm. If not, move on to attempt internal rotation by applying pressure on the anterior aspect of the posterior

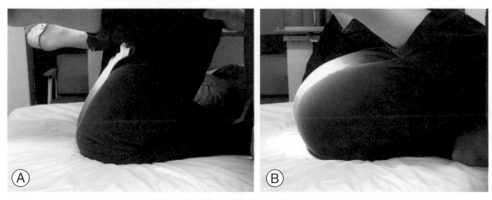

Fig. 35.4 A: Lithotomy position. B: McRoberts position.

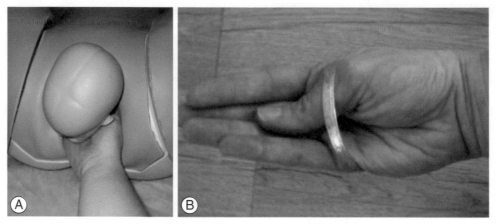

Fig. 35.6 (A) Correct vaginal access to perform internal manoeuvres for shoulder dystocia. (B) The hand position is the same as for putting on a bangle.

shoulder, with SPP in the same rotational direction; internal rotation applies pressure to the front of the posterior shoulder and enhances the effect of SPP in rotating the anterior shoulder away from the antero-posterior pelvic diameter. If the initial round of manoeuvres fail to release the impacted shoulder, repeat the sequence.

Other manoeuvres – including (1) Symphysiotomy, division of the symphysial joint with scalpel to increase the pelvic diameter (Fig. 35.7), and (2) the Zavanelli manoeuvre, replacing the fetal head in the uterus and then birth by caesarean – are 'last-resort' measures, associated with poor outcomes, and should be used only in extremis.

COMPLICATIONS

The umbilical cord can be occluded between the fetal trunk and the maternal pelvis, leading to rapid fetal hypoxia that may lead to brain injury and death. Studies have demonstrated low rates of hypoxic ischaemic encephalopathy (HIE; see Chapter 43) when the head-to-body interval is less than 5 minutes. However, it is not possible to recommend an absolute time limit for the management of SD. There are new data from the United States that neonatal fluid resuscitation may be useful for infants who are difficult to resuscitate post-SD, probably due to hypovolaemia post–cord occlusion.

Excessive traction, downward traction, and rapid application of force (jerking) are all associated with

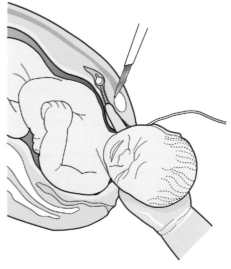

Fig. 35.7 Symphysiotomy. The left forefinger is shown displacing the urethra to the maternal left. A scalpel is positioned above the pubic symphysis and the joint divided anterior to posterior.

neonatal injury, particularly permanent injury to the anterior brachial plexus. Brachial plexus injury occurs in 2.3% to 16.0% of SD cases (Fig. 35.8). Most are temporary, but 10% of will be permanent (>12 months), leading to life-long disability of the upper limb. Neonatal fractures of the humerus and clavicle may also occur as well as maternal complications, such as genital tract trauma and postpartum haemorrhage.

Complications relating to SD are one of the biggest areas of litigation in obstetrics. Training, accurate

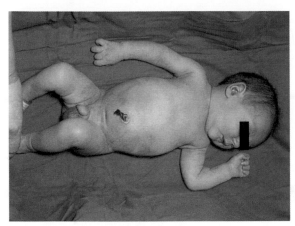

Fig. 35.8 A baby with a right-sided Erb's palsy following a shoulder dystocia. The baby was otherwise well. (From Rymer J. *Picture Tests Obstetrics and Gynaecology.* Churchill Livingstone; 1995, Fig. 168, p. 85.)

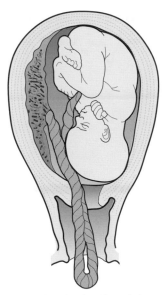

Fig. 35.9 Umbilical cord prolapsing through incompletely dilated cervix. This is due partially to a high presenting part.

documentation, a systematic approach to the manoeuvres and avoidance of excessive traction have been associated with significant reduction of fetal injury, particularly permanent brachial plexus injury.

Cord Prolapse

DEFINITION

'Cord presentation' is defined as the presence of the cord between the presenting part of the baby and the membranes prior to membrane rupture. 'Cord prolapse' refers to the same situation after membrane rupture, in which the cord descends through the cervix. The cord can remain alongside the presenting part (occult prolapse) or can pass the presenting part (overt prolapse), when it will be palpable in the vagina or visible at the introitus (Fig. 35.9). Cord prolapse is a time-critical obstetric emergency due to the high chance of complete occlusion of blood flow to the baby before birth.

EPIDEMIOLOGY

The incidence is related to fetal presentation (Table 35.1). Antenatal risk factors include high presenting part, multiparity, breech presentation, unstable lie, polyhydramnios, fetal congenital abnormalities, external cephalic version and a small (e.g., small-for-gestational-age or pre-term) fetus. Intrapartum risk factors include amniotomy, internal podalic version and disimpaction of the fetal head during rotational assisted vaginal birth.

TABLE 35.1 Incidence of Cord Prolapse in Relation to Presentation	
Presentation	**Incidence (%)**
Vertex	0.4
Frank breech	0.5
Flexed breech	4–6
Footling breech	15–18

CLINICAL FEATURES/INVESTIGATION

Early diagnosis is crucial. There are two potential insults during a cord prolapse, both of which may lead to cessation of fetal blood flow and fetal death. First, there is direct cord compression by the fetal head or body against the maternal pelvis. Second, there can be cord vasospasm from exposure to the cool external atmosphere and/or excessive handling of the cord.

Cardiotocography (CTG) usually indicates fetal compromise in the form of deep variable decelerations or a fetal bradycardia (Fig. 35.10).

The cord may be clearly visible, protruding through the vagina ('overt' cord prolapse), or may be identified at a vaginal examination carried out in response to a CTG abnormality ('occult' cord prolapse). It is important to routinely exclude cord prolapse during every vaginal examination but especially following artificial

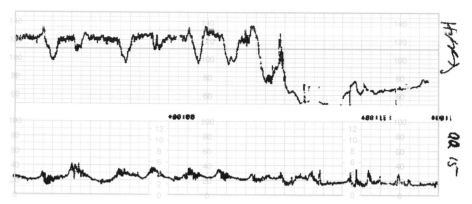

Fig. 35.10 In an occult umbilical cord prolapse, the only indication may be cardiotocography abnormalities, which should mandate a vaginal examination.

rupture of the membranes or when there is a sudden change in fetal heart rate, for example, bradycardia.

CARE OF WOMEN WITH CORD PROLAPSE

Duration is critical; there is significant correlation between bradycardia-to-delivery interval and cord arterial pH in umbilical cord prolapse with fetal bradycardia. Structured management and training have been associated with improved neonatal outcomes by reducing the duration of the hypoxic insult of the cord prolapse.

First, declare the emergency and call for help. Then, relieve pressure on the cord by manually elevating the presenting part. This can be done by:

- Digital elevation of the presenting part
- Maternal positioning through exaggerated lateral recumbent or the knee–chest position (Fig. 35.11)
- Bladder filling with a catheter

Bladder filling is a useful approach when transferring a woman from a setting where immediate birth is not possible, for example, from a primary birthing

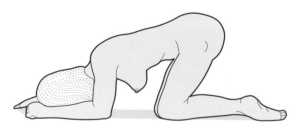

Fig. 35.11 The knee–chest position should be adopted on the way to theatre. Gravity ± an assistant's hand displaces the presenting part away from the umbilical cord.

centre to a hospital with facilities for operative birth. Bladder filling can be achieved by inserting a Foley catheter and filling the maternal bladder with 500 mL of fluid – tubing from a 'blood-giving set' can be used for this. The catheter can be clamped, which can relieve the pressure on the cord, with the filled bladder displacing the fetal presenting part upwards. If loops of cord are outside the vagina, a gentle attempt can be made to replace them within the vagina to reduce vasospasm. A dry pad can be used to keep the cord inside the vagina, without further handling the cord.

It is important to plan for immediate birth or transfer. Continuous monitoring of the fetal heart rate should be undertaken if in hospital and intravenous (IV) access should be secured. A tocolytic (e.g., terbutaline 250 µg subcutaneously) can be considered to minimise uterine contractions and related pressure on the cord.

Birth should be achieved by the quickest safe means, dependent on the fetal heart rate and gestational age. If the cervix is fully dilated, preparation can be made to expedite the birth by forceps or ventouse; if not fully dilated, preparation should be made for immediate (i.e., 'category 1') caesarean section. Regional anaesthesia can be considered depending on the fetal and maternal condition. A neonatologist should be called to attend. Post-birth, it is important to take paired umbilical cord gases, ensure clear documentation and debrief the mother and birth partner.

When declaring a cord prolapse, it is important to establish the fetal heart rate. The absence of palpable cord pulsation does not necessarily indicate fetal death, particularly if the prolapse is acute. Where there is doubt, particularly after a transfer, the fetal heart rate should be visualized directly by ultrasound before proceeding to caesarean. If fetal death has occurred, sadly there is no longer an urgent need to expedite birth, and aiming for a vaginal birth can be considered.

OUTCOMES

Despite increased access to operative birth and improvement in neonatal intensive care, the fetal mortality related to cord prolapse remains around 10%.

Impacted Fetal Head at Caesarean Section

DEFINITION

There is currently no consensus on the definition for IFH at caesarean section. However, there is agreement that these are technically difficult births where the fetal head is low and fixed in the mother's pelvis. Usually, additional techniques are required to disimpact the fetal head to allow the baby to be born.

EPIDEMIOLOGY

There is little data on incidence.

CLINICAL FEATURES/INVESTIGATION

IFH is more common during caesarean section at full dilatation. However, it may also occur during the first stage of labour. It is diagnosed when the clinician performing the caesarean section is unable to disimpact the fetal head using routine manoeuvres (flexion of the fetal head and then steady upward pressure by the accoucheur with a cupped hand below the fetal head).

APPROACHES TO AN IMPACTED FETAL HEAD AT CAESAREAN SECTION

A number of strategies have been reported to deliver an IFH. However, there is no consensus on an optimal approach or sequence of manoeuvres.

Techniques include a push up (which involves an assistant inserting the entire hand into the vagina to cradle and flex the baby's head to elevate it), reverse breech extraction (in which the baby's feet are delivered first), and a modification of reverse breech extraction in which the shoulders are delivered first (Patwardhan method). A 'T' or 'J' incision may be performed to extend the uterine incision and improve

access for a reverse breech extraction. Tocolytics such as sublingual glyceryl trinitrate or subcutaneous terbutaline are widely used but with no evidence of effect. Novel devices have been developed to equalise the pressure gradient between the abdomen and the vagina and assist with atraumatic elevation of the fetal head. However, there is as yet insufficient evidence to support their widespread use.

OUTCOMES

Difficulties delivering an IFH can delay the birth of a (potentially already compromised) fetus and may result in significant complications for mother and baby. Potential maternal complications include uterine injury postpartum haemorrhage, urinary tract injury, and hysterectomy. Potential neonatal complications include skull fracture, HIE, intraventricular haemorrhage and neonatal death.

Maternal collapse

Maternal collapse is characterised by cardiorespiratory compromise and altered consciousness. It is rare in pregnancy, and there are a broad range of obstetric and non-obstetric causes (Table 35.2). However, the initial management is the same regardless of cause.

Prevention and/or preparation should be the primary objective, which starts with risk stratification. A thorough antenatal assessment should be performed to identify women at risk and then strategies for mitigation should be implemented – for example, centralising care for women with congenital heart disease to a specialist tertiary centre or ensuring that crossmatched blood is available at a caesarean section for placenta praevia. Obstetric-specific early warning charts for recording systemic observations facilitate early identification of deterioration and promote communication and escalation, which may result in interventions that prevent deterioration to the point of collapse.

The care of women with maternal collapse must account for the anatomical and physiological changes of pregnancy. It is important to remember that there may be two lives to care for. While fetal distress may be evident in maternal collapse, resuscitation of the mother is always the priority and will usually improve the condition of the baby.

TABLE 35.2 Causes of Maternal Collapse (the 6 Hs)	
Head	Eclampsia
	Epilepsy
	Cerebrovascular event
	Intracranial haemorrhage
	Vasovagal response
Heart	Myocardial infarction
	Arrhythmias
	Peripartum cardiomyopathy
	Congenital heart disease
	Dissection of thoracic aorta
Hypoxia	Asthma
	Pulmonary embolism
	Pulmonary oedema
	Anaphylaxis
Haemorrhage	Abruption
	Uterine atony
	Genital tract trauma
	Uterine rupture
	Uterine inversion
	Ruptured aneurysm
wHole body and Hazards	Hypoglycaemia
	Amniotic fluid embolism
	Septicaemia
	Trauma
	Complications of anaesthesia
	Anaphylaxis

PREGNANCY-SPECIFIC CONSIDERATIONS IN MATERNAL COLLAPSE

- After 20 weeks' gestation, the gravid uterus may compress the aorta and vena cava in the supine woman, limiting venous return and resulting in reduced cardiac output.
- Progesterone causes relaxation of the oesophageal-gastric junction, increasing the risk of aspiration of acidic stomach contents and chemical pneumonitis (Mendelson syndrome).
- Difficult endotracheal intubation is more common in pregnancy.
- Changes in lung function, including diaphragmatic splinting and increased oxygen consumption, mean that pregnant women may become hypoxic more readily and can be more difficult to oxygenate.
- The fetus and placenta take a share of the circulating blood volume from the mother and increase oxygen demand.

CARE OF WOMEN WITH MATERNAL COLLAPSE

Initial management of maternal collapse should follow resuscitation guidelines, such as those from the Resuscitation Council (UK), using the standard 'ABCDE' approach, with modifications for pregnancy physiology.

CALL FOR HELP!

The obstetric emergency team should be called. At a minimum, this should include a senior obstetrician and anaesthetist, neonatologist, junior medical staff and senior midwife.

ASSESS FOR SIGNS OF LIFE

If signs of life are not present, commence basic life support.

ADOPT AN ABCDE APPROACH

A – Airway
- Open the airway if compromised (chin lift or jaw thrust).
- In cases of cardiac arrest, intubation should be undertaken as soon as possible by an experienced anaesthetist.
- Use of cricoid pressure during intubation may reduce the risk of aspiration.

B – Breathing
- Apply high-flow oxygen 15 L/min.
- A pulse oximeter should be applied for monitoring oxygen saturations.

C – Circulation
- Assess heart rate, blood pressure, and capillary refill.
- Secure large-bore IV access.
- An initial blood screen should include a full blood count, urea and electrolytes, liver function test, clotting, blood group and screen, and venous blood gas.
- Fluid resuscitation – initial stat 500-mL bolus of crystalloids, for example, 0.9% sodium chloride, except when the suspected diagnosis is fluid overload.
- Manual displacement of the uterus to the left should be performed (if >20 weeks' gestation) to reduce aortocaval compression.

D – Disability
- Assess responsiveness with the AVPU method (**A**lert, responds to **V**oice, responds to **P**ain, **U**nresponsive).
- Check capillary blood glucose.
- Check whether pupils are equal and responsive to light.

E – Exposure
- Check temperature.
- Inspect for evidence of bleeding, including suspecting occult bleeding.
- Examine the abdomen, palpate the uterus and perform a speculum or vaginal examination when there is evidence of vaginal bleeding.

Conduct a Detailed Survey

Once an initial ABCDE approach has been undertaken, a more thorough appraisal of the clinical situation, or 'primary survey', should take place. This should comprise history, examination, investigation, continued monitoring and consideration of any additional specialist tests or multidisciplinary input. Under certain conditions, such as significant antepartum haemorrhage, it may be necessary to urgently stabilise the maternal condition in order to expedite the birth of the baby.

Maternal cardiac arrest

Maternal cardiac arrest is exceptionally rare, complicating approximately 1 in 30,000 pregnancies in the United Kingdom. Standard cardiac arrest drugs and doses should

---

BOX 35.4 CAUSES OF MATERNAL CARDIAC ARREST

Four Hs
Hypoxia
Hypovolaemia
Hypo- and hyperkalaemia
Hypothermia

Four Ts
Thromboembolism
Toxins (including local anaesthesia)
Tamponade (cardiac)
Tension pneumothorax

Also consider
Eclampsia (including magnesium toxicity)
Amniotic fluid embolus

---

be used for pregnant women, with early defibrillation with standard energies for shockable cardiac rhythms.

The 'four Hs and four Ts' describe reversible causes of collapse that should be considered for maternal cardiac arrest (Box 35.4). To reduce aortocaval compression by the gravid uterus, left manual uterine displacement should be performed during CPR, with the woman lying flat (Fig. 35.12).

A peri-mortem caesarean section should be performed if there is no response to correctly performed CPR within 4 minutes of cardiac arrest and immediate assisted vaginal birth is not possible. Peri-mortem caesarean sections are primarily performed to improve maternal resuscitation efforts and increase the woman's chance of survival by:
- Improving venous return by relieving aortocaval compression by emptying the gravid uterus

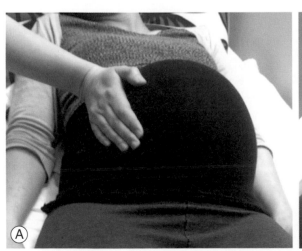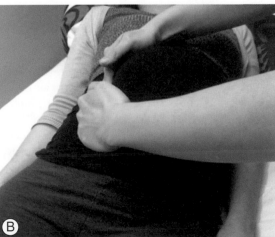

Fig. 35.12 Left manual uterine displacement using one-handed (A) and two-handed (B) techniques.

- Improving ease of ventilation by reducing upward displacement of the lungs by the gravid uterus
- Reducing oxygen requirement, as fetal oxygenation is no longer required.

There are also improvements to neonatal survival rates when birth is expedited in this time frame. As the peri-mortem caesarean section should be performed within 4 minutes, preparation to do so should take place alongside the primary survey.

Amniotic Fluid Embolism

AFE, sometimes referred to as 'anaphylactoid syndrome of pregnancy', is characterised by respiratory distress, sudden cardiovascular collapse and disseminated intravascular coagulation in a pregnant (usually intrapartum) or recently postpartum woman in the absence of another cause. The incidence is reported to be much higher in North America (around 1 in 15,000) than in the United Kingdom (1 in 50,000). Risk factors for AFE include maternal age over 35 years, black ethnicity, multiple pregnancy, placenta praevia, induction of labour and operative birth.

AFE may present with one or a combination of the following features:
- Acute fetal compromise
- Cardiac arrhythmias or arrest
- Coagulopathy
- Seizures
- Hypotension
- Maternal haemorrhage
- Premonitory symptoms, for example, restlessness, numbness, agitation, tingling
- Shortness of breath

PRESENTATION

AFE characteristically presents with acute hypoxia, hypotension and respiratory distress. Other causes for symptoms should be considered and excluded. Pulmonary hypertension develops either secondary to cellular debris or vasoconstriction. Left ventricular impairment and disseminated intravascular coagulopathy ensue, with massive postpartum haemorrhage (Box 35.5).

CARE OF WOMEN WITH AFE

The management of AFE is supportive and directed towards the maintenance of oxygenation, cardiac output

BOX 35.5 SYMPTOMS AND SIGNS OF AMNIOTIC FLUID EMBOLUS

Symptoms
Chills
Shivering
Sweating
Anxiety
Coughing
Signs
Cyanosis
Hypotension
Bronchospasm
Tachypnoea
Tachycardia
Arrhythmias
Myocardial infarction
Seizures
Disseminated intravascular coagulopathy

and blood pressure, and correction of coagulopathy. The pathophysiology of the condition is probably inflammatory, as in anaphylaxis or severe sepsis, but there is no specific treatment. Intensive care is almost always required.

OUTCOMES

Case fatality for women with AFE has improved from 80% to around 20% but long-term neurological sequelae have been reported in surviving women. Outcomes for the fetus (if AFE occurs prior to birth) are similarly poor, with a reported 60% perinatal mortality.

Sepsis

DEFINITION

Maternal sepsis is a life-threatening syndrome in which organ dysfunction arises as a consequence of infection during pregnancy, birth or the postpartum period. Some infections are more common in pregnancy and the postnatal period, including urinary tract infection, chorioamnionitis, endometritis and mastitis. Sepsis may be caused by bacterial, viral or fungal pathogens. Pregnant and postpartum women appear to be particularly vulnerable to Group A *Streptococcus*, a bacterium commonly carried on the skin and nasal passages. It initially may present with localized upper respiratory tract infections (such as a sore throat) or skin infections but may lead to very rapid deterioration and sepsis with circulatory shock.

The term 'sepsis' should not be used interchangeably with infection. They are clearly related but separate: the immune dysfunction caused by sepsis leads to haemodynamic instability and tissue damage. Severe sepsis may lead to septic shock, with hypotension that is resistant to fluid resuscitation, necessitating vasopressor support. The physiological and immunological changes of pregnancy make pregnant women more susceptible to sepsis. Worldwide, sepsis is thought to contribute to 25% to 40% of maternal deaths. In the United Kingdom, 10% of maternal deaths are directly related to sepsis.

PREVENTION

Primary prevention using aseptic technique and appropriate antibiotic prophylaxis is a keystone of modern obstetric care, particularly at caesarean and instrumental birth.

DIAGNOSIS

Plotting maternal observations on a modified early warning score (MEWS) chart may improve early detection of sepsis. Red flag symptoms for sepsis include:

- Confusion
- Systolic blood pressure <90 mmHg
- Heart rate >130 beats per minute
- Respiratory rate >25 breaths per minute
- Oxygen saturations <92% on air
- Non-blanching rash/mottled/ashen/cyanotic
- Lactate >2 mmol/L
- Oliguria (not passed urine in 18 hours)

CARE OF WOMEN WITH SEPSIS

When there is concern over evolving sepsis, prompt intervention is required. A serum lactate >2 mmol/L is a helpful tool to determine when care should be escalated.

The "Sepsis Six" bundle comprises six actions that must be performed as quickly as possible (ideally within 1 hour) for suspected sepsis:

1. Administer high-flow oxygen.
2. Take blood cultures.
3. Give broad-spectrum antibiotics.
4. Give IV crystalloid fluids.
5. Check serum lactate (serum lactate >4 mmol/L indicates severe tissue hypoperfusion and septic shock, but lactate >2 mmol/L may be abnormal).
6. Monitor urine output.

CARE OF WOMEN WITH SEVERE SEPSIS/SEPTIC SHOCK

Senior obstetricians, anaesthetists and intensive care specialists should be involved in the care of women with severe sepsis. In some circumstances, such as sepsis secondary to chorioamnionitis, it may also be necessary to expedite birth. In women with severe sepsis or septic shock, treatment in an intensive care or high dependency unit reduces mortality rates. Fetal risks include miscarriage, stillbirth and pre-term delivery.

Uterine Inversion

DEFINITION

Uterine inversion is a rare complication of the third stage of labour, in which there is descent of the uterine fundus through the genital tract. There are reported rates between 1 in 1,500 to 1 in 20,000 births and, although it is uncommon, awareness of the complication with prompt recognition and intervention improves outcomes.

The uterus may undergo varying degrees of inversion. In its extreme form, the fundus may pass through the cervix such that the whole uterus is turned completely inside out. As there is a rich vagal nerve supply to the cervix, inversion can lead to profound neurogenic (vasovagal) shock.

PATHOLOGY

Inversion is most often iatrogenic and related to umbilical cord traction prior to placental separation as part of active management of the third stage of labour (Fig. 35.13). Additional risk factors are listed in Box 35.6.

CLINICAL PRESENTATION

Uterine inversion may be difficult to diagnose, especially if the fundus is not visible at the introitus. The first symptom may be sudden maternal shock or collapse disproportionate to any blood loss. Vaginal examination should be performed with abdominal examination to identify whether there is a non-palpable or abnormally shaped uterine fundus. With complete inversion, the uterus will appear as a mass protruding from the vagina, which may be purple or blue in colour. In extreme cases, there can also be vaginal eversion. In approximately 50% of cases, the placenta remains attached.

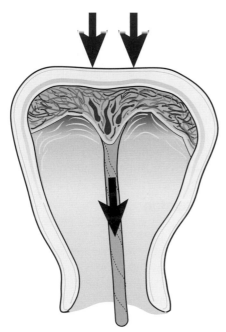

Fig. 35.13 Undue traction on a fundally sited placenta without guarding the uterus may result in uterine inversion.

Sudden death following neurogenic shock (bradycardia and hypotension) has been reported. However, more commonly, there is hypovolaemic shock (tachycardia and hypotension) associated with accompanying haemorrhage.

CARE OF WOMEN WITH UTERINE INVERSION

Immediate resuscitation is required (see ABCDE approach in earlier 'Maternal Collapse' section) and should involve the most senior available obstetric and anaesthetic team members. Uterine inversion is associated with severe atonic postpartum haemorrhage in 90% of cases, often occurring after the uterus has been replaced and placenta removed. Attempts to replace the uterus should occur simultaneously with resuscitation, as restitution of the uterus is the quickest way to treat neurogenic shock and minimise haemorrhage. Furthermore, the earlier the uterus is replaced, the more likely it is to be successful as oedema can rapidly occur, making replacement more difficult. No attempt should be made to separate the placenta before replacing the uterus, as this will exacerbate haemorrhage.

If the woman is stable and does not have analgesia, rapid transfer to theatre for pain relief or anaesthesia

before replacing the uterus should be considered. The uterus should be manually replaced by following the umbilical cord to the fundus and applying pressure on the fundus towards the umbilicus (Fig. 35.14).

Should this fail, the O'Sullivan hydrostatic technique can be employed. A silastic ventouse cup, if available, can be used to create a seal at the introitus, followed by 2 L of warmed saline passed through the cup (using a wide-bore giving set) into the vagina. The resulting vaginal distension and hydrostatic pressure promotes pushing the uterus back to its anatomical position.

Once replacement has been successful, by whichever method, the uterus should be stabilised until oxytocics have been given, to prevent recurrence. Subsequent removal of an adherent placenta should be performed in theatre.

Should all of these attempts fail, a laparotomy should be considered for direct replacement of the inversion (Fig. 35.15) or to perform a hysterectomy.

Uterine Rupture

DEFINITION

Uterine rupture is an important complication of labour that can be a life-threatening obstetric emergency, particularly for complete rupture, in which the baby may be displaced into the abdominal cavity and the placenta may start to separate, causing fetal distress or demise. Uterine ruptures can extend laterally into the uterine arteries or the broad ligament plexus of veins, and there may be severe intra-abdominal haemorrhage.

In caesarean section scar dehiscence, the fetal membranes remain intact, there is usually minimal bleeding, and the rupture does not usually involve the

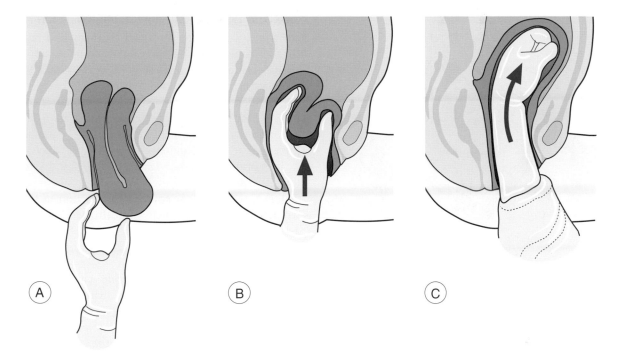

Fig. 35.14 Replacing an inverted uterus. (A) Recognition of uterine inversion. **(B)** Replacement of the uterus through the cervix. **(C)** Restitution of the uterus.

entire scar length. Occasionally, dehiscence is an incidental finding at a pre-labour caesarean section.

RISK FACTORS

The risk factors for uterine rupture are summarized in Box 35.7. Any previous breach of the uterine muscle wall creates a potential weak point that predisposes to rupture, particularly with contractions. Previous uterine perforation or myomectomy increases the risk of uterine rupture. However, the most common risk factor is previous caesarean section. Attempting a vaginal birth after caesarean (VBAC; also known as trial of labour after caesarean (TOLAC)), carries a 0.5% (5 per 1000) risk of rupture. Medical induction or augmentation in VBAC further increases the risk; up to 3 times with oxytocin and 14 times with prostaglandin use.

The risk of uterine rupture is higher with increasing numbers of previous caesarean sections and when the previous caesarean section was 'classical' rather than 'lower segment' (i.e., midline, extending into the upper segment of the uterus, rather than a lower uterine segment transverse incision). Spontaneous rupture of an unscarred uterus is rare (2 per 10,000 births)

> **BOX 35.7 RISK FACTORS ASSOCIATED WITH UTERINE RUPTURE**
>
> **Spontaneous Rupture of Unscarred Uterus (Rare)**
> Grand multiparity
> Oxytocin administration
> Obstructed labour
> Macrosomia
> Malpresentation
> Cephalopelvic disproportion
> Abnormally invasive placenta
> Uterine abnormalities
> Iatrogenic, for example, during internal obstetric manipulations and forceps delivery
> **Previous Uterine Scarring**
> Caesarean section
> Myomectomy
> Previous uterine perforation, e.g. at hysteroscopy

and extremely rare in primigravidae with no other risk factors.

CLINICAL FEATURES

The most common sentinel sign of uterine rupture is fetal compromise, particularly an acute fetal

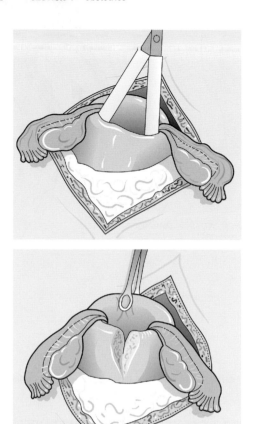

Fig. 35.15 It may be possible to reduce the inversion with division of the involuted rim at laparotomy.

bradycardia, which occurs in 70% of cases of uterine rupture. Other features may include vaginal bleeding, abdominal pain, haematuria and sudden cessation of uterine contractions.

There can be maternal shock (tachycardia and hypotension), which may be disproportionate to the degree of vaginal bleeding, reflecting concealed intra-abdominal haemorrhage. The abdomen may change shape, with easily palpable fetal parts and the presenting part may be higher in the pelvis or not palpable at all at vaginal examination.

CARE OF WOMEN WITH UTERINE RUPTURE

Summon immediate senior obstetric and anaesthetic help. A standard maternal resuscitation (ABCDE approach) should be commenced, followed by urgent emergency laparotomy to deliver the baby and repair the uterus. Uterine repair may be uncomplicated if the rupture or dehiscence has followed a caesarean scar. If there are extensions or involvement of the bladder or large vessels, a hysterectomy may be required. If complete uterine rupture is suspected, early activation of the major obstetric haemorrhage protocol may be useful to pre-empt the likely requirement for blood products.

It is important to be vigilant for signs and symptoms of rupture in high-risk women in labour, and consider early recourse to caesarean section in these women when there are signs of obstructed labour, to avoid uterine rupture.

ANTENATAL COUNSELLING

Any women with a history of uterine scarring (caesarean or otherwise), should have an individual risk assessment and a discussion of birth options in the antenatal period. 'VBAC calculators' have been developed for personalised risk calculations, such as the one published by the Maternal and Fetal Medicine Unit Network.

Women who have had a previous uterine rupture should be advised to have a pre-labour caesarean section in subsequent pregnancies at 37 to 38 weeks' gestation.

Key Points

- Obstetric emergencies can unfold rapidly and require a team approach to manage them effectively.
- Simulation training can provide a useful opportunity to practice the management of emergencies as well as the opportunities to test the systems in the maternity unit and improve teamwork and communication.
- Assessment of risks and preparation for emergencies are vital.
- It is important to remember that communication can be impaired in obstetric emergencies.
- Remember to communicate clearly with the woman and her partner and debrief with them after the emergency.

Chapter 36

Operative Birth

Deirdre J. Murphy

Chapter Outline

Introduction

The term 'operative birth' is used to describe both instrumental vaginal delivery (also known as 'operative vaginal delivery' or 'assisted vaginal birth') and caesarean section. Operative deliveries are usually performed by obstetricians and account for a third or more of all births in most high-resource settings. Caesarean sections can be performed before the onset of labour as either elective (or scheduled) when planned, or pre-labour emergency caesarean sections when unplanned. All caesarean sections in labour are considered emergency procedures and occur in either the first or second stages of labour. Emergency caesarean sections occasionally occur after an unsuccessful attempt at instrumental delivery.

Instrumental vaginal delivery using a ventouse (also known as vacuum device) or forceps can be performed only in the second stage of labour. It is preferable that instrumental delivery is completed with the first choice of instrument. However, in circumstances in which the ventouse dislodges and the baby's head is close to the perineum, the delivery may be completed with forceps, a situation known as 'sequential' instrumental delivery. The indications for operative delivery can be classified as 'fetal' or 'maternal', with a high degree of overlap. The majority of instrumental vaginal deliveries occur in women labouring for the first time. The majority of caesarean sections occur in either women labouring for the first time or women who have had a previous caesarean section.

Instrumental Vaginal Delivery

The most common indications for instrumental vaginal delivery are suspected fetal compromise (e.g., fetal heart rate abnormalities on cardiotocography) and second-stage delay. Second-stage delay may occur as a result of maternal exhaustion, fetal malposition (occipitoposterior (OP) or occipitotransverse (OT)) or cephalopelvic disproportion (relative mismatch between the size of the fetus and the birth canal). In practice, the indication for assistance frequently includes both fetal and maternal elements; for example, a prolonged second stage of labour is often associated with fetal heart rate abnormalities. The safety criteria in Box 36.1 must

BOX 36.1 CRITERIA FOR INSTRUMENTAL VAGINAL DELIVERY

- Consent from the mother obtained
- The cervix fully dilated and the membranes ruptured
- The head fully engaged, at the level of the ischial spines or below, with no more than one-fifth of the head palpable abdominally
- The position of the head known
- The bladder empty
- Analgesia satisfactory (perineal infiltration and pudendal block usually suffice for mid-cavity forceps and ventouse deliveries, but regional anaesthesia is required for Kielland rotational forceps)
- Neonatal resuscitation available
- Contingency planning in case delivery is unsuccessful and an emergency caesarean section is required

be fulfilled before an instrumental vaginal delivery can be attempted.

A careful assessment is required prior to instrumental delivery, including abdominal palpation, vaginal examination, assessment of the fetal heart rate pattern, analgesia requirements and the preferences of the labouring woman. There should be no fetal head palpable above the symphysis pubis on abdominal examination (0/5ths), although occasionally one-fifth is palpable in an OP position. One of the most difficult parts of assessment is being certain of the fetal head position prior to applying the forceps or ventouse. A systematic vaginal examination should determine the orientation of both the anterior and posterior fontanelles, as the most common mistake is diagnosing an occipitoanterior (OA) position when, in fact, it is OP. If there is a suspicion from palpation of the sutures that the fetal head is OT, it may be helpful to feel for an ear anteriorly under the symphysis pubis. The station of the fetal head should be determined relative to the ischial spines of the maternal pelvis. This is important because instrumental delivery should not be attempted when the fetal head is above the ischial spine's 'high station'. The degree of flexion (ideally well flexed with the fetal chin on its chest), caput (scalp swelling) and moulding (overlap of fetal skull bones), and the dimensions of the pelvis should be assessed.

Where uncertainty exists regarding the position of the fetal head, some obstetricians use transabdominal ultrasound to confirm the position; others will seek a second opinion or re-examine the woman in an operating theatre with good anaesthesia. Incorrect assessment

of the fetal head position or the station of the presenting part results in a higher incidence of failed instrumental delivery and traumatic injury to the mother and baby.

Instrumental vaginal delivery requires a multidisciplinary approach to maximise the likelihood of success and minimise maternal and fetal trauma. In addition to the attending midwife, a practitioner experienced in neonatal resuscitation should be present and an anaesthetist should be available to provide adequate anaesthesia. Umbilical artery and vein acid–base status should be routinely tested and recorded immediately after delivery. This is a reflection of the oxygenation of the baby immediately prior to birth. The Apgar scores at 1 and 5 minutes reflect the early condition of the neonate and the response to resuscitation, if required. A midwife will write a contemporaneous record of the birth events and timings, and the obstetrician will complete a detailed record immediately following the procedure.

COMPLICATIONS

Complications include failure with the chosen instrument, resulting in either caesarean section or use of sequential instruments. Perinatal complications include low Apgar scores, fetal acidosis (on cord blood testing), cerebral trauma (haemorrhage/haematoma or skull fracture) and brachial plexus injury or skeletal fractures (clavicle or humerus) if shoulder dystocia is encountered. Maternal complications include perineal tearing that may involve obstetric anal sphincter injury (OASI, classified as third- or fourth-degree tears), postpartum haemorrhage (PPH), subsequent perineal infection, urinary or bowel incontinence, dyspareunia or subsequent fear of childbirth (tokophobia). In appropriately selected cases, the incidence of complications is low. When considering potential complications, the morbidity associated with instrumental vaginal delivery should be compared with the morbidity associated with a caesarean section in the second stage of labour, which is itself a potentially complex procedure associated with maternal and perinatal complications.

FORCEPS DELIVERY

There are three main types of obstetric forceps (Fig. 36.1):

1. Low-cavity outlet forceps (e.g., Wrigley's), which are short and light and are used when the head is on the perineum (these forceps can also be used to assist delivery of the fetal head at caesarean section)

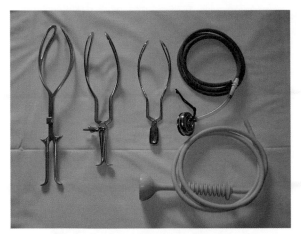

Fig. 36.1 Selected types of forceps and ventouse cups. The forceps, from left to right, are Kielland, Haig Ferguson, and Wrigley. The orange tubing is attached to an O'Neill occipitoanterior metal cup, and the blue ventouse is a silastic cup.

2. Mid-cavity forceps (e.g., Haig Ferguson, Neville-Barnes, Simpson), for use when direct traction is required and the sagittal suture is in the antero-posterior plane (preferably OA)
3. Kielland forceps for rotational delivery to an OA position from OP or OT. The reduced pelvic curve of the forceps allows rotation about the axis of the handle.

Low- or Mid-Cavity Non-Rotational Forceps

The procedure is explained to the woman and her verbal consent to proceed is obtained. The woman is placed in the lithotomy position with her bottom just over the edge of the bed (the bottom half of the bed usually lifts away) and her legs supported in stirrups. Using an aseptic technique, the perineum is cleaned and draped, the bladder is emptied, and the vaginal examination findings are rechecked. A pudendal block and perineal infiltration (local anaesthesia) are provided if required or the epidural anaesthesia is tested to ensure that it is effective. The forceps are assembled discreetly before application, care being taken to ensure that the pelvic curve of each blade will be sitting over the malar aspect of the baby's head, convex towards the baby's cheeks. Traction is applied in conjunction with the uterine contractions and maternal effort is encouraged by the attending midwife. The rest of the technique is shown in Fig. 36.2.

Rotational Forceps

These forceps, known as Kielland forceps (Fig. 36.3), lack the pelvic curve of direct traction (mid-cavity) forceps and can be applied directly to the baby's head, if OP, to allow gentle rotation to OA. After rotation, delivery is the same as for the mid-cavity forceps. If the baby's head is OT, the blades may be applied directly or the anterior blade applied initially posteriorly before being 'wandered' past the baby's face to the anterior position (Fig. 36.4). These forceps require considerable skill and may be associated with greater maternal injury than rotational ventouse or manual rotation. Hence, they should be used only by experienced obstetricians.

MANUAL ROTATION

'Manual rotation' of the head followed by direct traction forceps is an alternative approach to rotational forceps. It is usual to use the right hand for left occipitotransverse or left occipitoposterior (LOT/LOP) positions (Fig. 36.5) and the left hand for right occipitotransverse or right occipitoposterior (ROT/ROP) positions. The fingertips are applied to the lambdoid suture and the fetal head is gently rotated or dragged with a pronation movement. Some operators prefer to rotate during a contraction to minimise the risk of disengaging the head up out of the pelvis. If rotation is successful, it may be necessary to stabilise the new position with one hand while applying non-rotational forceps with the other to prevent the fetal head rotating back again. Delivery with mid-cavity forceps is then completed in the usual way.

VENTOUSE

Whether to use ventouse or forceps remains an area of debate. The decision depends to a large degree on the operator's experience and preference for the clinical circumstances. The aim should be to deliver safely with one instrument. Ventouse has the theoretical advantage that less pelvic space is required – with forceps, the diameter of the presenting part includes both the fetal head and the width of the forceps, whereas with the ventouse it is only the diameter of the head that needs to be delivered. The disadvantages are that the mother needs to push well, which may be a limiting factor with maternal fatigue or dense regional analgesia, and that where there is marked fetal scalp swelling (caput), the cup may dislodge easily with traction (termed a 'pop-off').

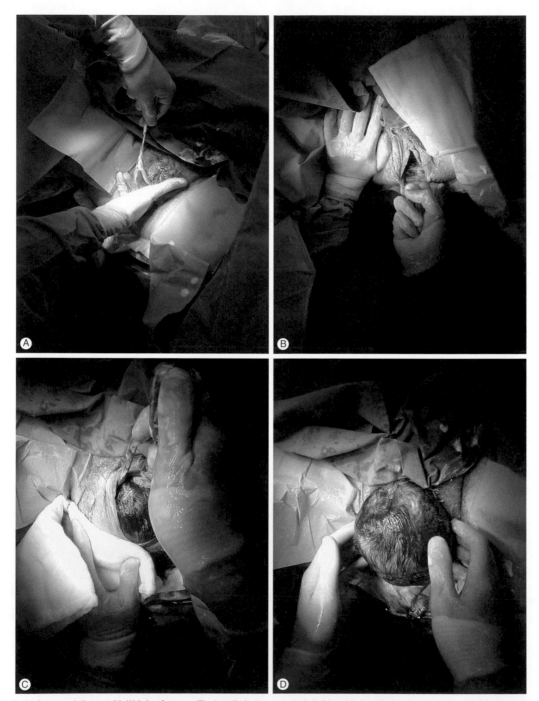

Fig. 36.2 Outlet forceps delivery with Wrigley forceps. The handle in the operator's left hand is inserted to the mother's left side by placing the right hand into the vagina to prevent injury and slipping the blade between the hand and baby's head between contractions **(A)**. Opposite hands are used to insert the right blade; the blades are locked into position by lowering the handles and allowing articulation to occur gently. Traction is applied by pulling initially downwards at an angle of ~60 degrees – maternal pelvis to obstetrician's pelvis if the obstetrician is sitting **(B)** – with the direction of traction becoming horizontal and then upwards as the baby's head advances over the perineum **(C)**. It is usual to perform an episiotomy as the vulva stretches. However, occasionally, as here, this may not be necessary, especially in a parous woman. The forceps are removed after delivery of the baby's head and the remainder of the baby delivered as normal **(D)**.

A systematic review of randomised controlled trials demonstrated that, compared with forceps, the use of ventouse is associated with a higher risk of failure, a higher incidence of neonatal cephalohaematoma and retinal haemorrhage, but less anaesthesia requirements and less maternal perineal or vaginal trauma. No differences in morbidity between ventouse and forceps deliveries were found in the one randomised trial that followed up mothers and children for 5 years.

The use of a soft silastic cup rather than a metal vacuum extractor cup is associated with more failures but fewer neonatal scalp injuries. Therefore, silastic cups are often used for OA deliveries and a metal OP cup or disposable 'Kiwi' cup for transverse and posterior malpositions. Disposable cups (rotational and non-rotational) produce a vacuum using a hand-powered pump and are suitable for single use. The same criteria for safe use apply to ventouse-assisted delivery as to forceps (see Box 36.1).

The cup should be placed in the midline overlying the 'flexion point', just anterior to the posterior

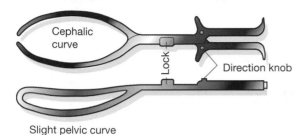

Fig. 36.3 Kielland forceps for rotational delivery.

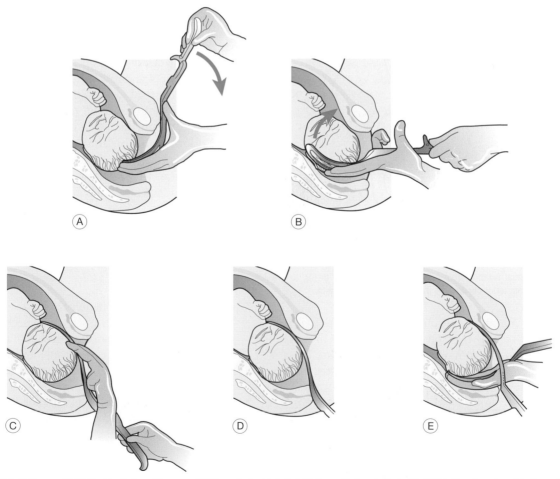

Fig. 36.4 Delivery with Kielland rotational forceps. (A) The anterior blade is initially applied posteriorly. **(B–D)** It is then 'wandered' to the anterior position across the baby's face. **(E)** The posterior blade can then be applied and the baby's head rotated to the occipitoanterior position.

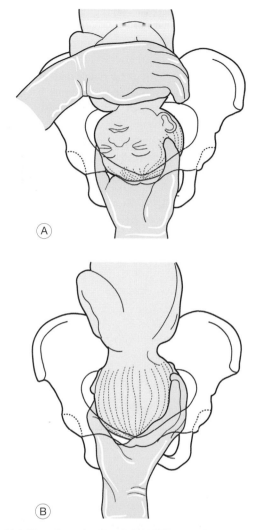

Fig. 36.5 Manual rotation from left occipitoposterior, as in (A), to direct occipitoanterior position, as in (B), using the right hand.

fontanelle, in order to encourage flexion of the head. Failure to correctly position the cup over the flexion point is the most common reason for ventouse failure. Suction is applied, care being taken to ensure that vaginal skin is not included under the cup. Traction is then applied in the axis of the pelvis as for forceps, but delivery is much more likely to be successful if traction is timed with contractions and maternal effort (Fig. 36.6). The risk of significant fetal injury (e.g., subgaleal haemorrhage) is increased with the duration of application, suboptimal application and 'pop-offs' where the cup dislodges abruptly.

Although it has been suggested that ventouse should not be used at gestations of less than 36 weeks because of the risk of cephalohaematoma and intracranial haemorrhage, a case control study suggested that this restriction may be unnecessary. Nonetheless, caution is still required and the ventouse should not be used at less than 34 weeks' gestation. There is minimal increased risk of fetal haemorrhage if the extractor is applied after fetal blood sampling or application of a fetal scalp electrode. The ventouse is contraindicated with a face presentation or if there is a possibility of a fetal bleeding disorder.

ODÓN DEVICE

The Odón device (named after the Argentinian inventor) is a new low-cost device that consists of a plastic sleeve that is inflated around the baby's head and is used to gently pull and ease the head of the fetus through the birth canal (Fig. 36.7). The use of an air chamber to act as the traction point on the fetal head (rather than the metal blades of the forceps) is proposed to reduce adverse events associated with the greater pressures applied to the fetal head during use of forceps. The lack of negative pressure on the fetal head, the mechanism of action of the ventouse, is proposed to reduce the risk of haematoma and haemorrhage associated with the ventouse. The device is currently being evaluated in clinical trials. Its low cost and reported ease of use would facilitate its uptake in low-resource settings if it proved to be safe and effective.

Caesarean Section

Caesarean section may be:
- Pre-labour
    - Elective (planned/scheduled), for example, for previous caesarean section, breech presentation or asymptomatic placenta praevia
    - Emergency (immediate/urgent), for example, following a placental abruption or severe pre-eclampsia
- In labour (i.e., emergency), usually for the reasons listed under 'forceps'. However, the cervix is not fully dilated or the cervix is fully dilated but circumstances are unsuitable for instrumental vaginal delivery.

Maternal mortality is higher for emergency than for elective caesarean section. There is also greater

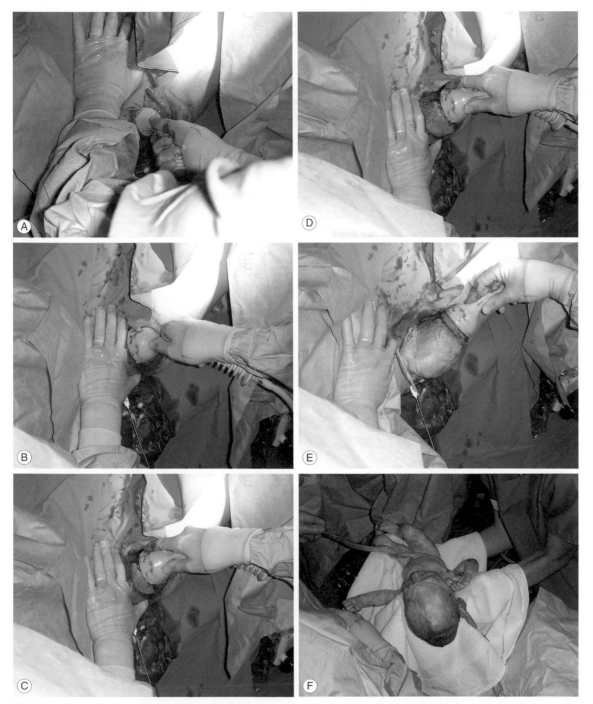

Fig. 36.6 Ventouse delivery. The ventouse cup is applied in the midline overlying, or just anterior to, the posterior fontanelle (the 'flexion point'), care being taken to ensure that the vaginal skin is not included under the cup. Traction is then applied to coincide with maternal effort.

How the BD Odon Device™ works

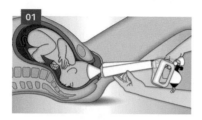

The user places the soft plastic cup on the head of the baby. The cup is designed to help facilitate the proper placement of the device.

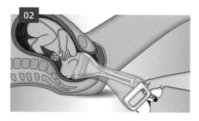

The user pushes on the handle of the inserter to progressively position the BD Odon Device around the head of the baby. The inserter consists of four spatula, which gently slide the sleeve along the birth canal and around the baby's head.

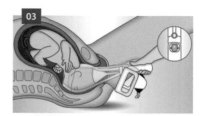

The BD Odon Device is properly positioned when the aircuff sits at the baby's jawline. Once in position, a marker on the handle of the inserter becomes clearly visible in the reading window.

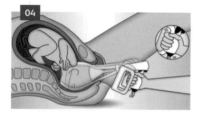

The user then pumps a minimal and self-limited amount of air into the air cuff.

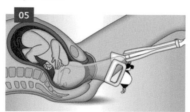

Once inflated, the air cuff produces a secure grasp around the head of the baby and allows for traction. The user now removes the inserter.

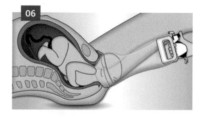

The user pulls on the handles of the sleeve, leveraging the traction created by the air cuff and lubrication of the sleeve, to deliver the baby's head.

Fig. 36.7 The Odón device. (Courtesy and copyright of Becton, Dickinson and Company).

morbidity from haemorrhage, infection and thromboembolic disease. Deaths from thromboembolism have been dramatically reduced by the widespread use of appropriate thromboprophylaxis (low-molecular-weight heparin, early mobilisation, hydration).

Lower uterine segment caesarean section is by far the most commonly used technique and has a lower rate of subsequent uterine rupture, together with better healing and fewer postoperative complications. A 'classical' caesarean section (vertical uterine incision involving the upper segment of the uterus) will provide better access for a transverse lie, in the presence of a vascular anterior placenta praevia, very pre-term fetuses (particularly after spontaneous rupture of the membranes), or where the lower uterine segment is obscured by fibroids. Following a vertical uterine incision, the risk of uterine scar rupture in subsequent pregnancies is much greater than with a transverse incision. Women are advised to have an elective repeat caesarean section (ERCS) following a classical caesarean section.

Preparation for caesarean section includes obtaining written maternal consent, intravenous access, group and save (cross-match when increased blood loss is anticipated), sodium citrate ± ranitidine or a proton pump inhibitor (to reduce the incidence of aspiration of stomach contents into the lungs – Mendelson syndrome), antibiotic prophylaxis, anaesthesia (spinal, epidural or general) and bladder catheterisation. Thromboprophylaxis with low-molecular-weight heparin is typically administered 6 hours following the surgery. The details of the operation are outlined in Fig. 36.8.

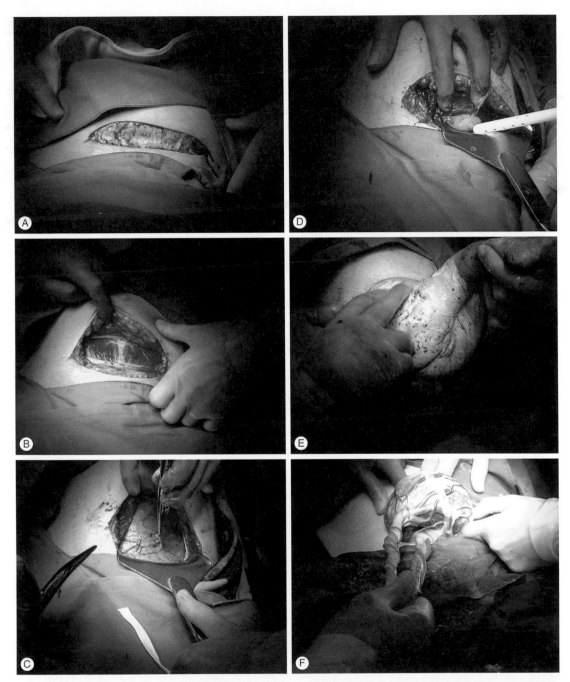

Fig. 36.8 Delivery by caesarean section. The table should be tilted 15 degrees to the left side (to reduce aortocaval compression and hypotension) and a lower abdominal transverse incision made, cutting through the fat **(A)** and the rectus sheath **(B)** to open the peritoneum. The bladder is freed **(C)** and pushed down, and a transverse lower segment incision is made in the uterus **(D)**. If the presentation is cephalic, the head is then encouraged through the incision with firm fundal pressure from the assistant. Wrigley forceps are occasionally required. If the baby is presenting by the breech (as here), traction is applied to the baby's pelvis by placing a finger behind each flexed hip to deliver the bottom first **(E)**. If the lie is transverse, a leg should be identified and pulled through the uterine incision to help deliver the baby (i.e., internal podalic version). After delivery, oxytocin is given intravenously and, after uterine contraction, the placenta is delivered **(F)**.

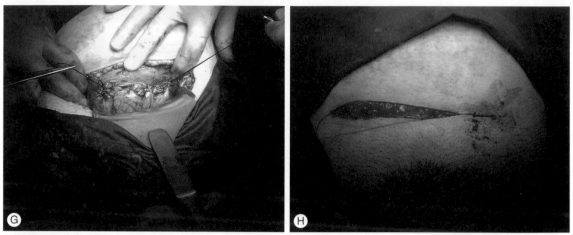

Fig. 36.8, cont'd Haemostasis is secured with clamps and a check is made to ensure that the uterus is empty and that there are no ovarian cysts. The incision is closed, usually with two layers of dissolving sutures to the uterus **(G)**, one layer to the rectus sheath and one layer to the skin **(H)**.

COMPLICATIONS

Complications of caesarean section include infection (wound, urinary, uterine), PPH (which may occur during the course of surgery or afterwards), and, less commonly, thromboembolism or bowel or bladder injury. For the fetus, there is an increased risk of transient tachypnoea of the newborn (TTN) and transfer to the neonatal unit, although this is more likely with pre-labour procedures and at earlier gestational ages. Following a caesarean section, there are implications for any subsequent deliveries, as there is a scar on the uterus with an increased risk of uterine rupture during labour.

SUBSEQUENT BIRTHS

In general, women with a previous caesarean section for a non-recurrent indication – for example, breech presentation, 'fetal distress', or fetal malposition – should be offered a vaginal birth after caesarean section (VBAC), but ERCS should also be discussed. Women with a previous caesarean section are counselled by a senior obstetrician, ideally at the first antenatal visit and again at about 36 weeks' gestation when a care plan can be finalised. Women who attempt VBAC have a vaginal delivery rate of approximately 60% to 70%. The risk of uterine rupture with attempted VBAC of spontaneous onset is estimated to be approximately 1 in 200 to 500, being higher if the labour is induced or contractions are stimulated with an oxytocin infusion. It is possible to attempt labour after two previous

caesareans, although most women opt for an ERCS. Women who have had more than two previous lower uterine segment caesarean sections or a classical caesarean section are advised to have an ERCS.

CAESAREAN SECTION ON MATERNAL REQUEST

Women who have had a previous difficult birth or an adverse birth-related outcome may request an elective caesarean section in their next pregnancy. This may be influenced by both psychological and physical factors. Although a more straightforward delivery can reasonably be anticipated in most cases in which vaginal birth occurred, careful consideration of the advantages and disadvantages of an elective delivery by caesarean section is required.

Some women request an elective caesarean section for a first birth when there is no obstetric indication. The advantages and disadvantages need careful consideration before an informed decision can be reached.

INFORMED CONSENT

Informed consent is an essential part of any intervention in labour, which can be challenging for time-sensitive indications such as the development of a fetal bradycardia. Therefore, it is important that women are informed during the antenatal period about interventions, procedures and potential complications that may occur in labour and that clear, documented explanations are provided at subsequent assessments during labour. The General Medical Council guidance indicates that the consenting process is not a snapshot but a continuing process. Planning for labour emergencies is essential so that the doctor and woman can discuss her wishes if an emergency should arise.

The UK Montgomery v Lanarkshire case of March 2015 brought fresh attention to the importance of informed consent for childbirth. Ms Montgomery, a woman with diabetes and of small stature, had a vaginal birth complicated by shoulder dystocia, resulting in a hypoxic insult to her son and consequent development of cerebral palsy. Ms Montgomery sued for negligence, arguing that if she had known of the increased risks associated with a vaginal birth in her circumstances, she would have requested a caesarean section. Initially, the case was successfully defended but the law on informed consent was eventually changed following a UK Supreme Court judgement that found in her favour. Doctors must now ensure that women are aware of any 'material risks' involved in a proposed treatment and of all the reasonable alternatives, including no intervention.

AUDIT AND RISK MANAGEMENT

Clinical audit is a means of systematically recording rates of operative delivery and associated complications which can be reviewed against explicit audit criteria or standards. Data can be compared within a unit over time and externally with other centres, regions or countries. Monitoring variation in intervention rates or adverse outcomes provides a means of evaluating the quality of care provided within a unit.

When adverse birth-related outcomes occur, this can be very distressing for the mother, her partner and family and for the staff involved in her care. The first priority is to provide supportive care to the woman and her family. However, at the earliest opportunity, a clinical incident form should be completed to initiate a review process. This is an important part of risk management – the aim is to learn from adverse events as an organisation and mitigate against future risks. As with all health professionals, obstetricians have the duty to be candid – the professional responsibility to be open and honest with women when things go wrong.

Key Points

- Operative delivery includes instrumental vaginal delivery by either forceps or ventouse, and caesarean section either pre-labour or during the first or second stages of labour.
- Operative delivery accounts for a third or more of all births in high-income countries.
- The indications for operative delivery may be fetal, maternal or a combination of both.
- Forceps may be low-cavity (outlet), mid-cavity or rotational (Kielland), and should be used only when eligibility criteria have been met.
- Ventouse can be non-rotational or rotational – using a silastic, metal or disposable device – and should be used only when eligibility criteria have been met.
- Compared with forceps, the ventouse is associated with less maternal perineal trauma but more neonatal trauma and more instrumental delivery failures.
- The Odón device is being evaluated as an alternative to vacuum or forceps, with the potential for ease of use and low cost.
- Maternal morbidity is higher for emergency than for elective caesarean section.
- Counselling for birth following a previous caesarean section needs to address the risks and benefits of VBAC versus ERCS.
- Operative delivery can result in physical and psychological complications that should be addressed following the birth and again when planning subsequent births.
- Rates of instrumental vaginal delivery and caesarean section should be audited on a continuing basis and risk management procedures must be in place to address and learn from adverse outcomes.

Chapter 37

Stillbirth and Neonatal Mortality

Alastair McKelvey, Paul Timmons

Chapter Outline

Introduction

The death of a baby and the loss of all the potential of a human life can be a devastating event for women, their partners, families and society. The grief and anguish is often life-changing. The human reactions to grief of disbelief, denial, negotiation and anger can all be seen by those caring for affected women and families. Care of women suffering such loss should be compassionate and professional. The burden on those providing such care, especially on a regular basis, should not be underestimated.

Whilst major improvements in medical care in well-resourced countries have seen reductions in perinatal mortality of around 10-fold in the last 150 years, the incidence in under-resourced countries remains as high as 5%. Despite major efforts in the last 2 decades, the rate of fall in the incidence of perinatal mortality has slowed since the mid 1990s, and the incidence in the United Kingdom remains higher than many other well-resourced countries (Fig. 37.1).

Definitions

The following definitions are used in the United Kingdom.

- **Stillbirth**: This is a legal definition, confirmed in UK legislation by the Still-Birth (Definition) Act (1992) as the death of a fetus in utero after 24 weeks of gestation.

  This is a baby born with no signs of life, when death is known (or believed) to have occurred after 24 weeks. The timing of the death is important – for example, in an originally twin pregnancy in which there had been a fetal reduction at 12 weeks to a singleton, it would not be appropriate to describe the delivery as a stillbirth. Where death occurs in utero before 24 weeks, the term 'miscarriage' or 'late fetal loss' can be used. Death after 20 weeks is sometimes classed as a late fetal loss, but there is no accepted specific definition of such a situation.

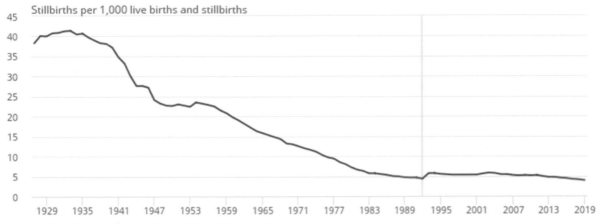

Fig. 37.1 Stillbirths in England and Wales, 1927 to 2019. (From Office for National Statistics, licensed under the Open Government Licence v.3.0.)

Stillbirth can be subclassified as those occurring before labour (antepartum) and during labour (intrapartum), in which the fetus was known to be alive at the onset of labour.

- **Neonatal death**: A baby born alive (at any gestation) who subsequently dies within 28 days of the birth. If the death is within the first week, it is termed 'early'. After the first week, it can be termed 'late'.
- **Perinatal mortality:** This is the combination of stillbirth and early neonatal deaths. The perinatal mortality rate is defined as stillbirth and early neonatal deaths per 1000 births.

Other definitions are used in different countries. The World Health Organization (WHO) continues to use 28 weeks rather than 24 weeks (this was also the UK definition before 1992) as its gestational cut-off or a birthweight less than 1 kg. This reflects the limited availability of advanced neonatal care globally. Adopting this later gestation lowers the apparent incidence of stillbirth. Despite this, the WHO reported 2.6 million stillbirths globally per year or one every 16 seconds. The large majority of these deaths are in low-resource countries, where around half of all stillbirths occur in the intrapartum period, representing the greatest time of risk. The estimated proportion of stillbirths that are intrapartum varies from 10% in well-resourced countries to 60% in under-resourced countries.

Historically, the rate of stillbirths fell dramatically through the second half of the 20th century, from over 40 in 1000 births before the Second World War to around 10 in 1000 by the mid-1970s. This was

believed to be largely a result of improved antenatal care and better nutrition, which mirrored reductions in infant mortality and increased life expectancy generally. The change in definition from 28 to 24 should be taken into account when comparing data before and after 1992. The fall in the stillbirth rate since the mid-1990s has been much slower than the reduction in neonatal mortality during the same period.

In 2019, there were 2346 stillbirths in England, generating a stillbirth rate of 3.6 per 1000 births (a record low). This was a significant fall from a rate of 5.1 in 2010. While this compares relatively well with some global regions (e.g., in sub-Saharan Africa where, even using the narrower WHO definition, the rate was 29 per 1000 births in 2015), the UK government has set a target of continuing to lower this rate. In 2014, the target of halving the number of stillbirths in England by 2025 was announced. This would require a continued reduction to approximately 1600 by 2025, which represents a further decrease of around 750 stillbirths. A recent national review of stillbirths in the United Kingdom concluded that the majority of stillbirths are preventable, particularly by addressing improvements in health care.

Stillbirth

CAUSES

Whilst some stillbirths can be clearly ascribed to a specific cause (such as placental abruption) – even following extensive investigations, including autopsy – a cause is not identifiable in up to 50% of cases. There are a number of classifications of causes. One useful nomenclature is to divide causes into: maternal, fetal, placental, structural, and intrapartum. There may be an overlap of contributory causes. When no specific cause can be established, factors associated with an increased chance of stillbirth – such as maternal obesity, smoking, or advanced age – may be considered to be contributory, though the precise cause of death may remain unclear. The presence of maternal characteristics associated with stillbirth has changed over the last few decades, with an incidence of maternal obesity being 10% in the 1970s, rising to around 30% today. Maternal age has also increased over the same time frame. The principal causes of stillbirth appear in Table 37.1.

TABLE 37.1   Principal Associations With and Causes of Stillbirth
Maternal associations
Smoking – dose dependent
Obesity
Diabetes
Age over 40 years
Black ethnicity
Illicit drug use – especially cocaine
Pre-eclampsia/hypertension
Poor maternal mental health or low educational attainment
Previous stillbirth
Hypovolaemia – hypotension and underperfusion
Antiphospholipid syndrome
Antibody production e.g. haemolytic disease
Placental causes of stillbirth
Placental insufficiency – failure of adequate trophoblastic invasion
Fetal growth restriction
Placental thrombosis/infarction
Placental abruption
Vasa praevia – fetal haemorrhage
Chorioamnionitis – membrane rupture
Fetal causes of stillbirth
Fetal abnormality – aneuploidies
Multiple pregnancy, including twin-to-twin transfusion
Infection, for example, parvovirus B19
Fetomaternal haemorrhage
Cord compression

CARE OF WOMEN WITH A STILLBIRTH

In some cases, the immediate well-being of the mother is the principal concern. Where a woman is haemodynamically unstable (e.g., massive haemorrhage, trauma, or severe pre-eclampsia), the priorities of resuscitation and life support must be addressed without delay. However, in many cases, there is no immediate maternal physical compromise. In that situation, obstetric and midwifery staff will be able to focus on emotional support and sensitive care.

The diagnosis of stillbirth should be made by the most senior clinician available. It is best practice for real-time ultrasound by a trained operator to be performed for at least 1 minute to confirm asystole. Whenever possible, the diagnosis should be confirmed by a second trained operator. In addition to asystole, there may be other features which can give some indication of the duration of death, such as alteration in the brain tissue leading to overlap of the cranial bones (Spalding sign).

The manner in which the fact of death is communicated to the woman and partner is important and must be done sensitively but unambiguously. Terms such as 'sleeping' or 'passed away' should be avoided and a clear but tactful use of the words 'death' or 'has died' will avoid ambiguity. Staff required to communicate such information should have training in how to break bad news. Reiterating the message may also be important in some circumstances. Sometimes, another ultrasound examination will be requested if the woman or her family remain in any doubt about what has happened.

In some cases, the woman will have no suspicion of the baby's death, and it may be a chance finding on a scheduled ultrasound scan. In other scenarios, the woman will be worried about her baby's welfare (often, a lack of fetal movements) and will have attended hospital for an antenatal assessment. Typically, one or more midwives will have attempted unsuccessfully to auscultate the fetal heart before calling for medical assistance. In such cases, there will already be anxiety and fear before the bad news is broken.

This news causes emotional numbness and shock to the woman, in which case further detailed information may not be readily absorbed. A period of privacy and comfort from a partner, family member, or friend is important and should be offered. The reaction will vary from one person to another; staff should accommodate each individual woman's needs as much as possible. It is important to perform basic clinical observations to exclude undiagnosed pre-eclampsia. If it is likely that the fetus died more than 48 hours ago, blood samples taken from the mother to exclude coagulopathy should be considered. An estimation of any fetomaternal haemorrhage by the Kleihauer test is appropriate, especially if the woman is rhesus negative.

After a period of contemplating the bad news, there will come a time when a woman is ready to discuss and plan what happens next. Unless there is maternal physical compromise, this should be avoided until the woman is ready. The fundamental need to deliver the baby should be discussed sensitively with the woman and her family. In most cases, vaginal birth by induction of labour is safer than caesarean birth, though each case will be different and there may be a relative contraindication to induction of labour (such as multiple previous caesareans) or an urgent need to deliver, which cannot wait for birth by induction of labour (e.g., haemorrhage or uncontrolled pre-eclampsia). For some women, when there is no medical indication for caesarean birth, this can seem initially preferable. A careful discussion of the pros and cons of induction versus caesarean should be conducted by a senior clinician.

When there is no maternal physical compromise, many women will choose to leave the hospital to spend some time with family and loved ones at home. Whilst generally a day or two will make little difference, women should be advised that longer prolongation of the pregnancy may lead to additional complications, such as coagulopathy, and can result in deterioration of the baby's physical appearance and a reduction of information available at autopsy. The possibility of passive fetal movements should be discussed – this is the sensation of movement caused by the baby moving inertly within the amniotic sac because of maternal movements.

Whilst standard induction agents and techniques can be used, mifepristone followed by misoprostol (although unlicensed in the United Kingdom for this indication) is effective and safe as an induction technique. The combination of mifepristone and misoprostol gives an average duration of labour of 8 hours (the addition of mifepristone reduces the time interval by about 7 hours over using misoprostol alone). The dose of misoprostol should be tailored to the gestation. Lower doses of misoprostol are used at more advanced gestations, and caution is required when there is a history of caesarean section. Women should be offered as wide a range of analgesia as is safely possible, including epidural anaesthesia (unless there is evidence of coagulopathy or another specific contraindication). There is no indication for the routine use of antibiotics. Women undergoing vaginal birth after caesarean (VBAC) should be monitored for features of scar rupture, such as persistent suprapubic pain and vaginal bleeding.

Many UK obstetric units have a dedicated facility to care for women who are experiencing a stillbirth. Furnishings may be more evocative of home and a television or radio is typically provided. Facilities may include a bathroom and simple kitchen to allow self-contained consumption of meals and hot drinks. Ideally, this will have a separate entrance to the main delivery area to minimise contact with other women and partners. Care should be led by a consultant obstetrician and one-to-one care provided by an experienced midwife. Many units have midwives specially trained in bereavement care in order to provide continuity of contact and support for women and their partner. Many women will already know the gender of the baby and may already have chosen a name. If the gender cannot be determined with certainty at birth, genetic analysis will determine gender within a few working days.

INVESTIGATION

With the agreement of the mother, it is important to try to discover why the baby died. Whilst relatively uncommon, identifying causes which might have a bearing on future maternal physical well-being (such as diabetes mellitus) or which might recur in future pregnancies (such as red cell isoimmunisation) is relevant.

When there is no immediately apparent cause for the stillbirth, women should be offered a full range of investigations to try to find a reason for the fetal death. Even if a cause is strongly suspected, confirmatory evidence from such tests may still be useful. An adapted list of investigations based on recommendations of the Royal College of Obstetricians and Gynaecologists appears in Table 37.2. It is important to explain that

TABLE 37.2   Investigations to Be Considered Following a Stillbirth

Investigation	Rationale
Haematology and bio-chemistry, including C-reactive protein, liver function test, and bile acid	Pre-eclampsia, sepsis, obstetric cholestasis.
Coagulation	Disseminated coagulopathy
Kleihauer test	Identification and quantification of fetomaternal haemorrhage and assessment of requirement for additional anti-D immunoglobulin for unsensitised Rh-negative women.
Red cell antibodies	Red cell isoimmunisation, haemolytic disease
Serology	Cytomegalovirus, toxoplasmosis, syphilis, and specific history-indicated infectious diseases, for example, Zika
Random blood glucose and HbA1c	Diabetes
Thyroid function	Thyroid dysfunction
Thrombophilia screen	Associated with abruption, severe growth restriction
Autoantibodies	Anti Ro + La antibodies can cause fetal heart block
Parental karyotype/ DNA microarray	In the presence of an unbalanced fetal translocation
Maternal urine/hair	If illicit drug use suspected
Placental testing	Histopathology, microbiology
Fetal samples	Skin swabs for microbiology
	Autopsy – full or external only with explicit maternal consent
	Karyotyping of skin or amnion – only with explicit maternal consent

an abnormal result does not necessarily mean that this was the causative factor. A full history should be taken, which may guide additional laboratory testing. For example, overseas travel to an endemic area for certain infections might indicate the need for targeted testing.

Signed consent is required for a perinatal post-mortem examination (autopsy). The woman should be counselled and guided through the consent process by a clinician trained in taking consent for autopsy. For a variety of reasons, women may decide not to have an autopsy and, in some cases, may decide to have a more limited examination, such as an external post-mortem. Under these circumstances, women should be made aware that this is likely to provide more limited information than a full autopsy. The placenta and membranes should be retained and sent for pathological examination. Clear follow-up plans should be in place before hospital discharge of how the information from any tests will be disclosed to the woman and partner.

AUTOPSY

A complete examination by a pathologist with specialised training in fetal and child pathology is likely to yield the greatest amount of information. This will include measurements, photographs, and X-rays. Depending on the parental wishes, small tissue samples on slides can also be retained. Macroscopic and microscopic examination is undertaken. Retention of whole organs requires specific written consent. There is increasing interest in non-invasive autopsy by MRI; where available, this may be acceptable to some women for whom a conventional autopsy is not acceptable. When requesting any form of post-mortem examination, the maximum relevant information should be provided for the pathologist so that laboratory findings can be interpreted within the relevant clinical context.

POST-NATAL NEEDS

All women should be risk assessed for venous thromboembolism (VTE), as stillbirth is in itself a risk factor for VTE and prophylactic low-molecular-weight heparin may be indicated. Women should also be offered lactation suppression, preferably before lactation commences. Cabergoline is safe and effective as a single dose, but care should be taken in the presence of hypertension. A tactful discussion of family planning needs should also be offered before discharge. Hospital chaplains or the patient's own clergy can make contact to help plan funeral arrangements or for blessings or other rights according to religious beliefs the woman may hold. Alternatively, some women prefer the funeral to be organised by the hospital; the chaplaincy department is often responsible for coordinating this. The offer of psychological support should be made. Clinical psychologists provide a valuable service to bereaved women and their partner.

Mementos such as handprints and footprints, a lock of the baby's hair, and photographs should be offered. Specific religious and cultural traditions should be respected and taken into account in helping the woman and her family during their bereavement.

Any appointments for antenatal care should be cancelled. The general practitioner, community midwives, and other relevant community health services should be informed of the stillbirth. Contact details for specific support groups can be provided, such as Sands, the stillbirth and neonatal death society, or other local groups.

The experience of stillbirth will be different for each woman, but talking to others who have been through similar experiences is helpful to many. Continued contact with a bereavement midwife is useful for many women; a meeting with her named consultant should be offered, the timing typically coinciding with the availability of the results of investigations.

In the United Kingdom, a certificate of stillbirth should be issued. The woman can register the birth with the local authority accordingly. Stillbirth must be medically certified by a fully registered doctor or midwife; the doctor or midwife must have been present at the birth or examined the baby subsequently. There is no requirement to inform the coroner or similar authority unless there is a suspicion of criminal intent.

INSTITUTIONAL INVESTIGATIONS

It is good practice for a hospital to look carefully at every stillbirth to identify any individual or systemic problems with care with a view to learning from the event. A structured perinatal review process should be completed by the clinical risk team, a multidisciplinary group principally consisting of clinicians. The woman (and partner when appropriate) should be offered an opportunity to be involved – including specific questions that she may have. The conclusions should be shared with the family. A good example of a structured investigation is the Perinatal Mortality Review Tool developed by the National Perinatal Epidemiology Unit. The identification of specific themes or an unexpectedly high rate of stillbirth in a department may prompt the need for external review and changes in practice as necessary.

POSTNATAL MEETING

The woman and her partner or other supporter should be invited to meet with her consultant obstetrician around 8 weeks following the stillbirth. The lead clinician should prepare for the meeting by reviewing all available results. While the pathologist will usually have issued a report within 6 weeks of the examination, on occasion, a final autopsy report may not be ready. If the report is not ready, then the meeting should be delayed until the pathologist has issued it. It is important to be sensitive to specific dates in order to avoid them, such as the original estimated date of delivery.

The meeting forms an opportunity for the clinician to assess the woman's physical and mental well-being, summarise all of the available information, answer any questions the woman and her supporter may have, and discuss future reproductive plans. When another pregnancy is desired, then a specific antenatal care plan can be made. The plan should be composed of an appropriate enhanced frequency of antenatal visits and fetal surveillance, including ultrasound scans and timing and mode of delivery. Other health issues should be sensitively addressed, including minimising risk factors for stillbirth such as obesity and smoking when relevant. Care should be taken not to imply blame or fault. A letter detailing the discussions should be sent to the woman's general practitioner and a copy or summary should also offered to the woman.

Neonatal Death

EPIDEMIOLOGY

Alongside the fall in the UK stillbirth rate in recent years, a similar gradual reduction in neonatal deaths has been observed – from 3.9 per 1000 total births in England and Wales in the year 2000 to 2.8 in 2019.

As with rates of stillbirth, while these figures compare favourably with an international average of 17 in 1000 births – with the highest rates of up to 40 to 1000 observed in parts of sub-Saharan Africa and central Asia – they nevertheless represent considerably higher death rates when compared with other well-resourced countries. (Fig 37.2).

Epidemiological risk factors for neonatal death are well-described and follow a regrettably predictable trend. Higher rates are seen in infants born to younger (<20 years) and older (>40 years) mothers and women from black, Asian, and minority ethnic backgrounds. Rates of death have an inverse relationship with socioeconomic status.

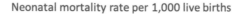

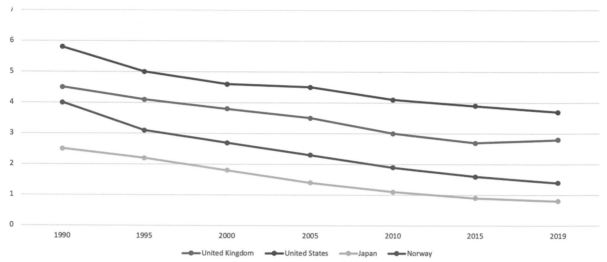

Fig. 37.2 Neonatal mortality rate in the United Kingdom, Japan, Norway, and the United States, 1990 to 2019. (Data from The World Bank: Databank: World Development Indicators.)

Any infant considered to have shown signs of life at birth (Table 37.3), irrespective of gestational age, is considered to be a live birth and registered as such. This leads to a slight disparity of reported rates between Office of National Statistics data, which includes all such live births, and that published by MBRRACE-UK (Mothers and Babies: Reducing Risk through Audits and Confidential Enquiries across the UK), which considers only those occurring at 22 completed weeks of gestation and beyond. The threshold of 22 weeks' gestation reflects current guidance from the British Association of Perinatal Medicine, which advises that resuscitation should be considered only for infants born from 22+0 onwards. The threshold of 24 completed weeks of gestation for stillbirths reflects similar guidance from the time the relevant legislation

was passed (Still-Birth [Definition] Act 1992) on so-called 'thresholds of infant viability' – the suggestion being that survival at gestations earlier than 24 weeks was not possible. On this basis, many clinicians and lay campaigners advocate that a revision of this definition, in light of developments in neonatal care and survival, is now necessary.

CAUSES

The principal causes of neonatal death are presented in table 37.4. Causes are often not mutually exclusive, e.g. an infant with a congenital abnormality is often born prematurely.

Pre-Term Birth

Over 90% of infants who die during the first 28 days of life in the United Kingdom are born prematurely, that is, before 37 completed weeks of gestation. This is in the context of premature births accounting for only 8% of births overall. While prematurity itself is not necessarily the specific cause of death in many of these infants, the ability of a premature infant to successfully make the adaptations necessary to survive outside the womb and respond to the stress of infection, respiratory disease, and more is less than that of an infant born at term.

The majority of premature births arise as a consequence of spontaneous labour. That, in turn, could be caused by a wide range of underlying processes, including

TABLE 37.3	Signs of Live Birth
Live birth is determined by one or more persistent visible signs of life	The following do not warrant classification as signs of life
Easily visible heartbeat	Fleeting reflex activity
Definite movement of arms and legs	Transient gasps
Visible umbilical cord pulsation	Brief visible chest wall pulsations
Breathing, crying, or sustained gasps	Involuntary muscle movement

infection (principally chorioamnionitis), bleeding (principally, abruption), and cervical incompetence or over-distension of the uterus (from polyhydramnios or multiple pregnancies). A substantial proportion of premature births have no identifiable cause.

A smaller number of premature births are iatrogenic – in which the infant is intentionally delivered pre-term either due to a risk to the mother's health (such as pre-eclampsia) should the pregnancy continue or when concerns exist regarding fetal well-being (principally, fetal growth restriction) and it is considered that the risk of intrauterine fetal death outweighs the risks associated with being born prematurely.

While there is wide variation in the potential direct causes of death amongst infants born pre-term, the majority are secondary to respiratory complications (respiratory distress syndrome as a consequence of insufficient surfactant production), sepsis, and neurological complications (most often as a result of intraventricular haemorrhage).

Prevention of Pre-Term Birth and Its Consequences

Given both the individual and societal burdens associated with prematurity, measures aimed at identifying women at increased risk of pre-term birth and its subsequent prevention have long been a focus of research and clinical activity. Nevertheless, there persists a paucity of evidence to support any specific universal screening tools. Thus, the majority of screening and preventive measures are targeted at either the small cohort of women who have identifiable risk factors for pre-term birth or those who present with symptoms of pre-term labour. The majority of infants delivered pre-term in the United Kingdom continue to be born to mothers who have no identifiable risk factors for pre-term birth at the onset of their pregnancy.

There is some research evidence to support a programme of cervical length screening by ultrasound in women who have risk factors for cervical incompetence – those with either a history of spontaneous (typically painless) pre-term birth or second trimester miscarriage or those who have previously undergone cervical surgery (e.g., repeated large loop excision of the transformation zone procedures). Where cervical shortening (defined as less than 25 mm distance between the external and internal cervical os) is present, or the cervix appears 'funnel-shaped' rather than tubular, there may be a role for either cervical cerclage (a stitch inserted to keep the cervix closed, subsequently removed prior to labour) or daily

intravaginal progesterone supplementation. Each of these interventions is associated with only a small improvement in outcomes which must be balanced against the acceptability of the treatment to the woman (see Chapter 29).

When pre-term delivery can be anticipated (spontaneous or iatrogenic), there is evidence of benefit for the administration of magnesium sulphate and/or corticosteroids to the mother, as these reduce the incidence of neurological injury (cerebral palsy) and respiratory distress syndrome, respectively. Antibiotic prophylaxis during pre-term labour should be offered to all women, as this reduces the risk of early-onset Group B Streptococcus infection – a principal source of infective morbidity and mortality in both pre-term and term infants.

Improvements in neonatal care for pre-term infants in recent decades – including improved techniques for respiratory support, the administration of exogenous surfactant, and development of optimal feeding schedules – have led to improved rates of survival at the limits of viability. Survival and serious disability rates in extreme pre-term (<27 completed weeks' gestation) infants by gestation in the United Kingdom are presented in Table 37.5. In settings where advanced neonatal care is available to babies born pre-term, the

TABLE 37.4 Causes of Neonatal Death in the United Kingdom

Causes (MBRRACE-UK 2020)	Percentage
Congenital anomaly	36%
Complications after birth	28%
Extreme prematurity	13%
Infection	7%
Fetal/placental factors	7%
Intrapartum factors	2%
Unspecified/other	7%

TABLE 37.5 Outcomes Amongst Neonates Born Extremely Premature in the United Kingdom

Gestation (Weeks)	Survival	Severe Disability Amongst Survivors
22	30%	33%
23	40%	25%
24	60%	14%
25	70%	14%
26	80%	10%

survival of babies born at 34 weeks' gestation or beyond is equivalent to babies born at term. The survival at 27 and 31 weeks' gestation is 89% and 95%, respectively.

As the rates of both survival and severe disability amongst infants born at very early gestations demonstrate, even small gains in gestational age can make a large difference to eventual outcome. However, caution should be exercised in any attempt to prolong the pregnancy in which the woman is labouring and delivery appears inevitable. The only intervention to delay birth advised in this instance is considering administration of tocolytic drugs such as nifedipine for a maximum duration of 24 hours in order to administer corticosteroids and magnesium sulphate.

REPORTING

All neonatal deaths in the UK beyond 22 completed weeks' gestation are reportable to MBRRACE-UK – a national audit project which examines all maternal deaths, stillbirths and neonatal deaths in the United Kingdom and reports every 3 years on each with a view to identifying trends and making recommendations with broad, national applicability.

All early neonatal deaths (i.e., in the first week of life) of term infants should be reported to the Healthcare Safety Investigation Branch (HSIB), which will, in turn, conduct a thorough independent investigation and root-cause analysis. The HSIB also conducts such investigations into all cases of term intrapartum stillbirth, in which the baby was considered to be alive at the start of labour.

Any case of neonatal death in which the cause of death is unknown, suspicious or related to suboptimal care should be reported to Her Majesty's Coroner (England, Northern Ireland and Wales) or the Procurator Fiscal (Scotland) and, potentially, the police.

Global Perspective

The aetiology of stillbirth and neonatal death in under-resourced nations varies considerably from that seen in well-resourced countries (Fig 37.3). Access to safe intrapartum care remains a major limiting factor in improving rates; across the world, almost half of all stillbirths occur during labour (compared with less than 10% in the United Kingdom).

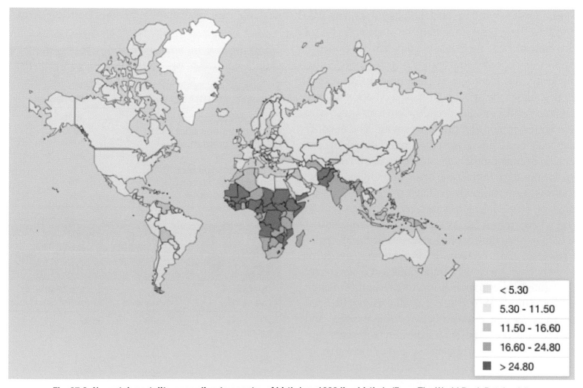

Fig. 37.3 Neonatal mortality according to country of birth (per 1000 live births). (From The World Bank Databank.)

Determining the precise cause of death in low-resource settings is limited by a combination of cultural trends around death and access to adequate investigation. It is estimated that intrapartum hypoxia/birth trauma and infection are each estimated to account for a quarter of all neonatal deaths worldwide, with prematurity accounting for a further third. The WHO estimates that two-thirds of such deaths are preventable with the introduction of simple, evidence-based health measures at birth and in the first week of life (see Chapter 39).

Key Points

- Stillbirth is a unique form of bereavement, which can have devastating consequences.
- The physical health of the woman is the primary initial consideration. For physically well women, psychological support will be the focus.
- A holistic plan of compassionate professional care is needed.
- The incidence of stillbirth is falling in well-resourced countries. Government focus is on further reducing preventable stillbirth.
- Perinatal mortality remains common in under-resourced countries.
- Following a diagnosis of intrauterine death, a vaginal birth is usually recommended. However, cases should be managed individually.
- Induction of labour with mifepristone followed by low-dose misoprostol is safe.
- Pre-term birth at the limit of viability may pose ethical and practical challenges; the use of corticosteroids and magnesium sulphate reduces morbidity and mortality.
- In well-resourced countries, pre-term birth is the principal cause of neonatal mortality.
- In under-resourced countries, infection and birth trauma are common causes of perinatal mortality.

Chapter 38

Neonatal Resuscitation

Nancy O'Hanrahan

Chapter Outline

Physiology

The fetus needs the umbilical cord and placenta for respiration. Within the first minute of life, the newborn infant has to adapt to breathing air. Various stimuli – such as hypoxia, cold air and physical contact – will encourage respiratory effort. Most newborn 'resuscitation' is assisting this normal transition process. The 'healthy' fetus will tolerate well brief periods of hypoxia (part of the normal birthing process). Pathological processes – such as chronic placental insufficiency, acute cord obstruction and infection – interfere with the transition and reduce the ability of the fetus to cope. Being aware of antecedent events or concerns can help predict which babies might need assistance after delivery.

PHYSIOLOGY OF ACUTE HYPOXIA

Significant hypoxia can occur in utero or during or after delivery. This hypoxia will stimulate respiratory effort. If the baby fails to start breathing and oxygen concentration falls further, the baby loses consciousness and enters 'primary apnoea'. The heart rate initially rises and then rapidly falls to around half the normal fetal heart rate (~60 beats per minute [bpm]). Heart rate changes are driven by vagal stimulation and then anaerobic respiration.

After 5 to 10 minutes of primary apnoea, spinal centres, which are normally suppressed by higher centres, begin to cause shuddering gasps at a rate of approximately 12 per minute (agonal gasps). Once gasping stops, the baby enters 'secondary' (or 'terminal') apnoea. Anaerobic metabolism continues and lactic acidosis causes a further drop in the blood pH. The heart rate will gradually fall; without intervention, the outcome will be death. The only way to tell whether a non-breathing newborn infant is in primary or secondary apnoea is by assessment of its response to resuscitation. In primary apnoea, nearly all infants will start breathing within a few breaths. In secondary apnoea, the baby will usually gasp for some time before starting regular respiration. In reality, however, both are initially managed in the same way. Circulation does not fail until late in the process; therefore, very few infants require circulatory support as part of resuscitation. It is this awareness of the normal response to hypoxia in the infant that guides the newborn resuscitation algorithm order, which places a heavy emphasis on airway and breathing support.

Practical Aspects of Neonatal Resuscitation

BEFORE THE BABY ARRIVES

Team briefing and preparation before the baby is born can help communication and readiness for the likely scenario. Before the baby arrives, think about the following things:

- What are the concerns? (e.g., Gestation? Meconium? Fetal monitoring? Suspected or known congenital anomalies? Risk factors for infection?)
- Can we deal with those concerns? Do we need help?
- Do we have the right equipment and is it working? (e.g., dry towels, hat, heat source, masks, self-inflating bag or T-piece resuscitator, suction, resuscitation trolley). Prepare the area by closing windows and doors to reduce draughts.
- Are all team members aware of their role?
- If things do not go according to plan A, what are plans B and C?

By outlining the concerns or the expected situation and allocating roles, the team can work more efficiently. Clear communication is a key part of working well in a resuscitation team – that process starts before the baby is born.

DRY, WRAP, KEEP THE BABY WARM AND ASSESS

Start a timer on the resuscitaire or note the time when the baby is delivered. Dry the baby and then wrap in a warm, dry towel. A naked, wet baby can become hypothermic despite a warm room, especially if there is a draught. A cold baby has increased oxygen consumption and is more likely to become hypoglycaemic and acidotic. Babies also have a large surface area-to-weight ratio; therefore, heat can be lost very quickly. Most of the heat loss is by evaporation; thus, outcome is improved by drying (Fig. 38.1).

Use this 30- to 60-second period of drying and stimulating to assess the baby. Assessment consists of tone, colour, breathing and heart rate. For uncompromised infants, delayed cord clamping for a minimum 1 minute from the complete delivery of the baby is recommended. If intervention is required, the baby should be moved to the area for resuscitation without delay.

APGAR SCORE

The Apgar score is used to evaluate a baby's condition at birth and response to resuscitation. Scores are recorded at 1 and 5 minutes (Table 38.1). Acute clinical assessment will categorise the baby into one of the following three colour groups:

- Pink – regular respirations, heart rate fast (>100 bpm). These are healthy babies, who should be kept warm and given to their mothers.
- Blue – irregular or inadequate respirations, heart rate slow (<100 bpm). If gentle stimulation does not induce effective breathing, the airway should be opened. If the baby responds, no further resuscitation is needed. If not, progress to lung inflation.
- Blue/white – apnoeic, heart rate slow (<60 bpm). Whether an apnoeic baby is in primary or secondary apnoea, the initial management is the same.

AIRWAY

Before a baby can breathe, the airway needs to be open. The baby's head should be in the neutral position. The typically prominent occiput of a newborn may cause flexion and pharyngeal collapse. A folded towel placed under the neck and shoulders may help to maintain the airway in a neutral position, taking care not to overextend the neck (Fig. 38.2). A jaw thrust may be needed to bring the tongue forward and open the airway, especially if the baby is floppy.

Suction should be reserved for infants who have airway obstruction due to visible material (e.g., blood, mucous, meconium or vernix) that cannot be resolved by positioning. Material should be gently suctioned from the oropharynx under direct visualization.

If tracheal obstruction is suspected, inspection using a laryngoscope may be performed. If seen, obstructing material may be removed by intubating and suctioning on withdrawal of the endotracheal tube. Prolonged attempts to suction should be avoided. The priority should be providing ventilation, especially if bradycardia is ongoing.

BREATHING

If the baby is not breathing or breathing ineffectively (e.g., gasping), artificial ventilation should be commenced within the first minute of life. The first five breaths should be inflation breaths, preferably using

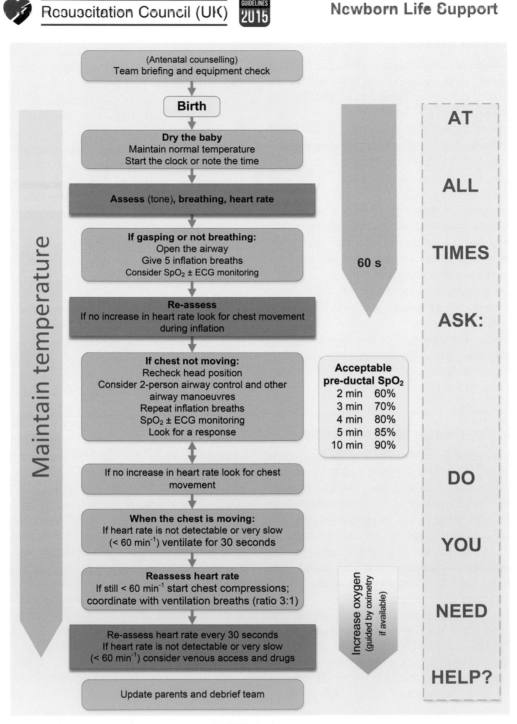

Fig. 38.1 Newborn Life Support Algorithm (2015). (Reproduced with the kind permission of Resuscitation Council UK.)

TABLE 38.1 The Apgar Scoring System

Feature	SCORE		
	0	1	2
Colour	White	Blue	Pink
Tone	None	Poor	Good
Heart rate	<60 bpm	60–100 bpm	>100 bpm
Respiration	None	Gasping	Vigorous
Response to simulation	None	Minimal	Vigorous

From Apgar V. A proposal for a new method of evaluation of the newborn infant. *Curr Res Anesth Analg.* 1953;32(4):260–267.

air. These breaths are designed to inflate lungs that are fluid filled/collapsed. These should be 2- to 3-second sustained breaths using a bag valve mask. If available (and staff are trained), a T-piece resuscitator can provide a set peak inspiratory pressure, usually 25–30 cm H_2O in a term infant, and a positive end expiratory pressure, normally 5 cm H_2O. Use a mask big enough to cover the nose and mouth of the baby with the baby's mouth open (Fig. 38.3).

The best indication of adequate aeration of the lungs is improvement in the heart rate (if this has been low)

or visible chest wall movement. If regular spontaneous breathing has not established after adequate chest inflation, then ventilation breaths should continue at a rate of 30 to 40 ventilations per minute. Ventilation breaths should have a shorter inspiratory phase than inflation breaths. Ventilation of term infants should begin in air; for pre-term infants, a low concentration of oxygen can be used (up to 30%) in the initial stages. Continue to reassess heart rate and chest movement. If there is no increase in heart rate, there are two main explanations. First, and most likely, is inadequate or ineffective aeration of lungs. Second, the baby requires more resuscitation than just aeration of the lungs.

Review points to consider if there has been inadequate aeration of the lungs:
- Is the baby's head in the correct position?
- Is the mask the correct size? Is there a good seal around the mask?
- Do you need to perform a jaw thrust? Do you need to use a two-person technique?
- Is there something obstructing the airway, and can you safely remove it?
- Would an airway adjunct help, such as a Guedel airway?

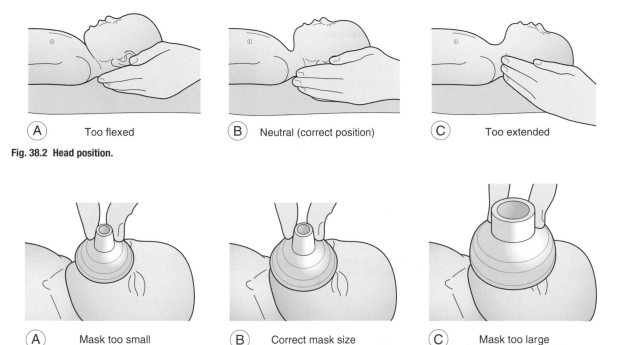

(A) Too flexed (B) Neutral (correct position) (C) Too extended

Fig. 38.2 Head position.

(A) Mask too small (B) Correct mask size (C) Mask too large

Fig. 38.3 Mask positioning.

A Guedel airway should be inserted under direct vision with a laryngoscope, as shown in Fig. 38.4. Using a laryngoscope in this way helps prevent trauma. It helps to keep the relatively large infant tongue out of the way as the airway adjunct is inserted. The correct size of airway adjunct should reach from the middle of the chin to the angle of the jaw.

CIRCULATION

Very few infants will require more than aeration of the lungs. The purpose of cardiac compression is to move a small amount of oxygenated blood to the coronary arteries in order to initiate cardiac recovery. Therefore, there is no point in cardiac compression before the lungs have been inflated.

If the heart rate is not detectable or remains slow (<60 bpm) after five inflation breaths and 30 seconds of effective ventilation, increase the oxygen concentration and commence chest compressions. The most efficient way of doing this in the neonate is to encircle the chest with both hands so that the fingers lie behind the baby and the thumbs are opposed on the sternum just below the inter-nipple line (Fig. 38.5). Compress the chest to one-third of its depth and perform three compressions for each breath. Compressions are ineffective unless interposed breaths are of good quality and inflate the chest. Asynchronous compressions and breaths will not allow adequate ventilation. Even if the baby is intubated, breaths and compressions should remain synchronous with three chest compressions, then one breath. The most common reason for failure of the heart rate to respond, once again, is failure to achieve lung inflation. Once the heart rate is above 60 bpm and rising, cardiac compression can be discontinued.

DRUGS

Drugs are considered when cardiac output does not improve after adequate lung inflation and chest compressions. Airway and breathing must be reassessed as adequate before proceeding to drug therapy. The quickest way to establish reliable vascular access is via an umbilical venous line (if not possible, then an intraosseous needle). Drugs to be considered include:

- Adrenaline (1:10,000) 0.1 mL/kg (epinephrine). If this is ineffective, a dose of 0.3 mL/kg of 1:10,000 can be tried.

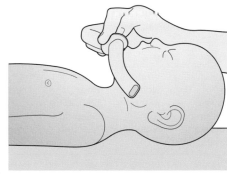

(A) Correct size of Guedel airway

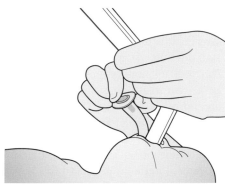

(B) Insertion with a laryngoscope

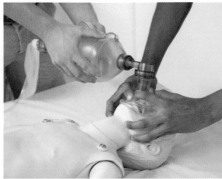

(C) Keeping a seal with the mask

Fig. 38.4 Maintaining the airway. (A) Correct use of Guedel airway. **(B)** Insertion with a laryngoscope. **(C)** Two-person technique.

- Sodium bicarbonate 1 to 2 mmol/kg (2–4 mL/kg of 4.2% bicarbonate solution) given slowly (over >2 minutes).
- 10% dextrose bolus of 2.5 mL/kg

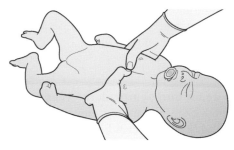

Fig. 38.5 Two-hand technique for cardiac compressions.

Using a wall chart/table of predicted weights and the volume to be administered is safer than trying to do drug calculations in a stressful environment.

Adrenaline (0.5-1mL of 1:10,000) can also be administered via an endotracheal tube. However, absorption via this route is unclear.

Very occasionally, hypovolaemia may be present because of known or suspected blood loss (e.g., in the context of antepartum haemorrhage, placenta praevia or vasa praevia). Volume expansion with 0.9% sodium chloride or O negative blood (if available) may be appropriate.

MONITORING IN NEONATAL RESUSCITATION

Feeling the base of the umbilical cord for pulsation is not always reliable because absent pulsation does not necessarily mean absent cardiac output. Heart rate can be better assessed by feeling apex beat or listening with a stethoscope, though even this is not infallible. Pulse oximetry provides information on pulse and saturations and can guide requirements for additional oxygen. It is important to be aware that there is a normal transition with oxygen saturation from around 60% at birth to >90% at around 10 minutes of age. The saturations probe should be applied to the (dried) right hand/wrist of the baby to give a pre-ductal measurement. If there is reasonable cardiac output, pulse oximetry will also reliably indicate the heart rate.

Electrocardiography (ECG) monitoring can provide a rapid and very accurate examination of the newborn heart rate. In order to be effective, however, there has to be good contact with the skin, that is, a dry baby. It is important to understand that ECG activity does not necessarily mean there is cardiac output.

Temperature control is also an important part of all newborn stabilisation. Hypothermia in newborn infants increases morbidity and mortality. Avoiding hyperthermia, especially in term babies with hypoxic-ischaemic injury, is just as critical. Many resuscitation stations will have skin temperature sensor probes or attachments; these can provide automated regulation of heating to maintain the infant's temperature at 36.5°C to 37.5°C.

PRE-TERM BABIES

The more pre-term a baby is, the less likely it is to establish adequate respirations. Pre-term babies (especially those <32 weeks) are also likely to be deficient in surfactant. The effort required to breathe is greater; yet, the muscles are less developed (see also Chapter 29). Anticipate that babies born before 32 weeks may need help to establish prompt aeration and ventilation. If a pre-term infant is breathing but has signs of respiratory distress or is likely to develop respiratory distress, then commencing continuous positive airway pressure at approximately 5 cm H_2O shortly after birth can provide respiratory support. The paediatric or neonatal team should be called prior to a pre-term birth when possible.

Pre-term babies are more likely to become cold (higher surface-area-to-mass ratio) and more likely to be hypoglycaemic (fewer glycogen stores). The temperature of very pre-term babies can be maintained if they are placed in a plastic bag (without drying), leaving the face exposed, immediately after birth. After delayed cord clamping, the baby should be placed under a radiant heater and the head covered with a hat. The delivery room temperature should be maintained above 26°C.

Discontinuation of Resuscitation

The outcome for a baby born with no detectable heartbeat that remains undetectable after 10 minutes of effective resuscitation is likely to be poor. The decision to discontinue resuscitation should be taken by a senior member of the team – ideally, a consultant.

Debrief and Parental Communication

It is important to keep parents up-to-date and explain what is happening. Time for the baby away from the mother should be minimised when possible. It is important to explain to the parents what has happened, potentially why and what will need to be done (if anything further). A record of events and discussions should be made as soon as possible. Debrief and discussion with team members is just as important. Most infants will do well with minimal need for resuscitation; thus, in the rare/unexpected circumstances in which more intensive efforts are required, it can be stressful. Having a formal debrief can alleviate staff concerns and allow for support. By understanding and reflecting on practice, we may yield positive changes, improving outcomes for the future.

Key Points

- **Prepare for birth, particularly when there is a high chance that resuscitation will be required (e.g., pre-term birth or suspected fetal compromise).**
- **Dry the baby and keep it warm.**
- **Effective airway management and good ventilation are the mainstays of successful neonatal resuscitation.**

Chapter 39

Global Maternal and Neonatal Health

Elizabeth A. Layden

Chapter Outline

Estimates of Global Maternal and Neonatal Mortality

It is estimated that almost 300,000 women worldwide die each year from the complications of pregnancy and childbirth, with 99% of these deaths occurring in low-resource countries. Estimates from 2017 by the World Health Organization (WHO) and other partners show that two-thirds of all maternal deaths occur in sub-Saharan Africa alone and about one-fifth of all maternal deaths occur in Southern Asia. For every woman who dies, around 20 women have serious ill health and lifelong disability as a result of these same complications.

In 2015, the United Nations (UN) adopted 17 Sustainable Development Goals (SDGs), with 169 targets, building on the UN Millennium Development Goals. All UN Member states have agreed to work towards achieving these SDGs by 2030. SDGs 3 and 5 are of particular relevance, although some of the other SDG targets, if achieved, will also positively impact maternal and newborn health.

SDG 3 – 'ensure healthy lives and promote well-being for all ages' – includes specific targets for maternal and neonatal health:

- Reduce the global maternal mortality ratio to less than 70 per 100,000 live births (target 3.1).
- Reduce neonatal mortality to at least as low as 12 per 1000 live births (target 3.2).
- Ensure universal access to sexual and reproductive health care services, including family planning, information and education and integration of reproductive health into national strategies and programmes (target 3.7).

SDG 5 – 'achieve gender equality and empower all women and girls' – also includes several relevant targets, which will impact maternal and newborn outcomes:

- End all forms of discrimination against all women and girls (target 5.1).
- Eliminate all forms of violence against women and girls (target 5.2).
- Eliminate all harmful practices, such as child and forced marriage and female genital mutilation (target 5.3).

- Ensure universal access to sexual and reproductive health and reproductive rights (target 5.6)

Although the latest estimates of maternal deaths published in 2017 suggest a decline in maternal mortality since 1990, there is lack of progress in a number of countries, especially in sub-Saharan Africa and Southeast Asia (Table 39.1).

At least 70% of all maternal deaths globally result from five direct complications that are well understood and can be readily treated: haemorrhage, sepsis, hypertensive disease, complications of obstructed labour and unsafe abortion. This is in contrast to causes of death in countries with low maternal mortality rates, where maternal deaths are more likely to be due to indirect causes (Figs 39.1 and 39.2). In addition to this high number of maternal deaths, an estimated 2.4 million neonatal deaths and 1.9 million stillbirths occur each year. Neonatal deaths account for nearly half of all deaths of children under 5 years of age.

The health and survival of the neonate is closely related to that of the mother. The majority of deaths in the first month of life could also be prevented if interventions were in place to ensure good maternal health (Fig. 39.3). Many birth injuries and birth asphyxia, and most neonatal tetanus, could be prevented with skilled professional care at the time of the birth as well as in the antenatal and postnatal periods. Similarly, many cases of sepsis in the neonate are directly linked to the health of the mother and/or the care she received during childbirth. It is estimated that almost half of all stillbirths in under-resourced countries occur during labour and birth.

Obstetric Causes of Maternal Mortality

The five main causes of direct obstetric maternal mortality are discussed here.

HAEMORRHAGE

Many maternal deaths in resource-poor areas are caused by or associated with haemorrhage. This may be because of antepartum bleeding (e.g., abruption of the placenta), bleeding during birth (e.g., with a ruptured uterus or placenta praevia) or postpartum (e.g., from an atonic uterus or retained placenta).

The risk of dying from haemorrhage is higher if women are already anaemic in pregnancy (Hb <11.0 g/dL). Oxytocics are very effective in preventing postpartum haemorrhage (active management of the third stage), as well as in treating uterine atony, but oxytocics may not be routinely used and/or available. Manual removal of a retained placenta can be carried out by trained midwives and doctors using simple general anaesthesia (e.g., with intramuscular (IM) ketamine). The ability to give intravenous (IV) fluids, safe blood transfusion and anaesthesia is extremely important when pregnancy or birth is complicated by haemorrhage. It is estimated that non-availability of blood for transfusion accounts for about a quarter of deaths associated with haemorrhage.

OBSTRUCTED LABOUR

Most cases of maternal death associated with obstructed labour are attributable to rupture of the uterus

TABLE 39.1   Estimates of Maternal Mortality Ratio, Annual Number of Maternal Deaths, and Lifetime Risk of Maternal Death by WHO Region, 2017

Region	Maternal Mortality Ratio (Deaths per 100,000 Live Births)	Annual Number of Maternal Deaths	Lifetime Risk of Maternal Death
Sub-Saharan Africa	542	196,000	1:37
Northern Africa and Western Asia	84	9,700	1:380
Central and Southern Asia	151	58,000	1:260
Eastern and Southeast Asia	69	21,000	1:790
Latin America and the Caribbean	73	7,700	1:640
Australia and New Zealand	7	26	1:7800
Oceania (excluding Australia and New Zealand)	129	380	1:210
Europe	10	740	1:6500
North America	18	760	1:3100
World	211	295,000	1:190

WHO, World Health Organization.

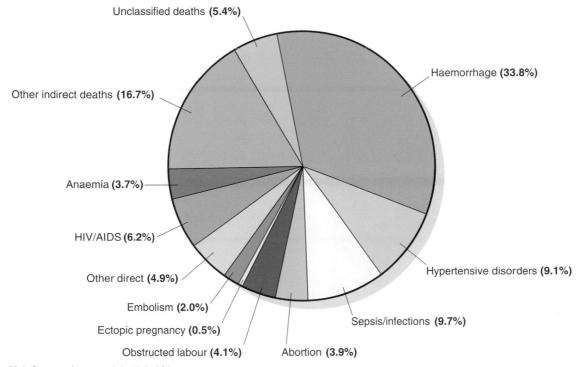

Unclassified deaths **(5.4%)**

Other indirect deaths **(16.7%)**

Haemorrhage **(33.8%)**

Anaemia **(3.7%)**

HIV/AIDS **(6.2%)**

Other direct **(4.9%)**

Embolism **(2.0%)**

Ectopic pregnancy **(0.5%)**

Obstructed labour **(4.1%)**

Abortion **(3.9%)**

Sepsis/infections **(9.7%)**

Hypertensive disorders **(9.1%)**

Fig. 39.1 Causes of maternal death in Africa.

(Figs 39.4A, B). Persistent malposition, for example, transverse lie, is also a cause of rupture of the uterus if unrecognised and allowed to progress (Fig. 39.5). The correct use of a partogram has been shown to be very helpful in making a diagnosis of cephalopelvic disproportion (CPD) or simple failure to progress. The WHO Labour Care Guide (2020) has superseded the basic partogram as an improved tool for labour monitoring (Fig. 39.6), as its adjusted 'alert values' (to prompt a response) reflect the range of acceptable rates of progress in labour, prompting timely diagnosis of failure to progress or CPD but reducing the risk of over-intervention.

In many cases of obstructed labour, women are referred to a health care facility late. The presenting part may be deeply impacted in the pelvis and a vaginal examination may identify oedema and overlapping of the fetal skull bones. The mother will be dehydrated, exhausted, in severe pain from a tonically contracted uterus, or pyrexial as a result of infection and/ or sepsis. If the uterus has ruptured, the fetal heartbeat is usually absent and the fetal parts may be easily palpated abdominally. In addition, the woman may be in shock as a result of bleeding or sepsis. Bleeding during labour should always be a cause for alarm if CPD is suspected.

A woman with CPD in labour may also have a Bandl ring. This is a visible constriction seen in the abdominal contour, which is a warning sign of impending rupture of the uterus. If the presenting part has been impacted in the pelvis for many hours, pressure necrosis of the genital tract as it is compressed between the baby's head and the bony pelvis may lead to obstetric fistulae. Vesicovaginal fistulae are the most common, but rectovaginal and ureterovaginal fistulae also occur. Such fistulae may also occur after difficult obstetric abdominal surgery. Women who suffer from fistulae often have no living child, become outcasts from their society, and may live in poverty. Very many women with fistulae are unable to access suitable care.

In order to try to prevent fistulae, or to encourage small fistulae to close spontaneously, it is important that all women who have survived prolonged

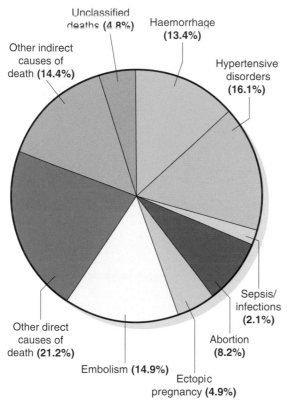

Fig. 39.2 **Causes of maternal death in high-resource countries.**

Unclassified deaths (4.8%)
Haemorrhage (13.4%)
Other indirect causes of death (14.4%)
Hypertensive disorders (16.1%)
Sepsis/infections (2.1%)
Abortion (8.2%)
Ectopic pregnancy (4.9%)
Embolism (14.9%)
Other direct causes of death (21.2%)

or obstructed labour (with or without a caesarean section (CS)) should be treated initially by continuous bladder drainage with an indwelling urinary catheter and, preferably, with antibiotics to minimise the risk of urinary tract infection. Spontaneous closure can occur within 6 to 8 weeks with such conservative management, but most fistulae do not heal spontaneously and require specialised surgical management. Such surgery requires considerable expertise and specialists (obstetrician–gynaecologists and urologists) will need to seek additional training to be able to offer a good surgical repair. Equally important is the provision of good nursing care, physiotherapy and steps towards rehabilitation and reintegration into society for women who have suffered fistulae.

SEPSIS

Sepsis following prolonged membrane rupture or retained products of conception (incomplete miscarriage or unsafe abortion) may lead to overwhelming septic shock, multisystem failure and death. Early recognition and prompt commencement of antibiotic treatment is important. If there are retained products of conception, manual vacuum aspiration (MVA)

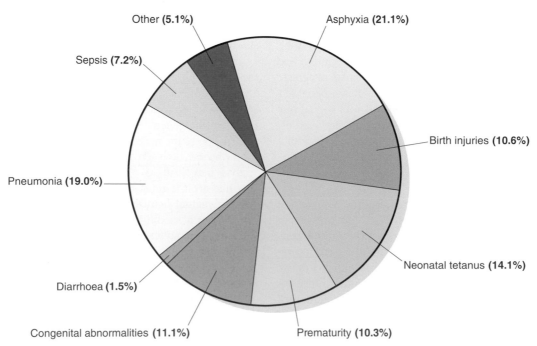

Other (5.1%)
Asphyxia (21.1%)
Sepsis (7.2%)
Birth injuries (10.6%)
Pneumonia (19.0%)
Neonatal tetanus (14.1%)
Diarrhoea (1.5%)
Congenital abnormalities (11.1%)
Prematurity (10.3%)

Fig. 39.3 **Causes of neonatal mortality.**

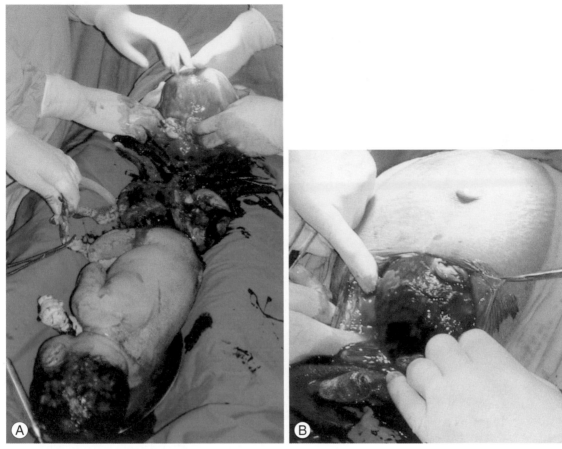

Fig. 39.4 Uterine rupture following obstructed labour with cephalopelvic disproportion.

of retained products of conception can be lifesaving (Fig. 39.7). This has, in many countries, replaced the traditional technique of dilatation and curettage (D&C), which requires general or regional anaesthesia. With good technique, MVA can be performed in early pregnancy under local anaesthesia.

Unrecognised rupture of the membranes during pregnancy risks ascending infection and can lead to chorioamnionitis, premature birth and major systemic sepsis if not recognised and treated during the antenatal period. Prophylactic antibiotics must always be given after prolonged membrane rupture and at the time of a CS.

Untreated sexually transmitted infections (STIs) are common during pregnancy in low-resource settings and may contribute to sepsis. Similarly, underlying impairment of the overall immune response – for example, with human immunodeficiency virus (HIV)

infection – carries an increased risk of opportunistic infections and makes it more difficult to treat sepsis when this occurs.

HYPERTENSIVE DISEASES OF PREGNANCY

Eclampsia, especially if a seizure is prolonged, can lead directly to maternal death. As pre-eclampsia and eclampsia are multi-organ diseases, the exact cause of such a death can often be difficult to ascertain. Cerebral haemorrhage is probably the most common cause of death, but renal or hepatic failure, respiratory failure, coagulopathy or HELLP (*h*aemolysis, *e*levated *l*iver enzymes and *l*ow *p*latelets) syndrome may also contribute.

Recognition of pre-eclampsia by measurement of blood pressure and testing of urine for protein should be available for all women during pregnancy and after birth. Magnesium sulphate reduces the

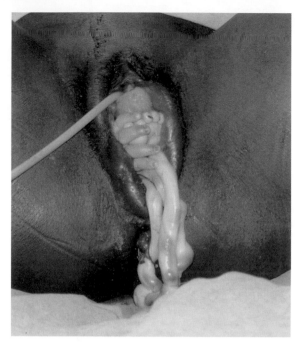

Fig. 39.5 Obstructed labour from a transverse lie, with an arm, leg and cord prolapse.

incidence of seizures in women with severe pre-eclampsia and is the preferred treatment drug for an eclamptic seizure (see Chapter 28). For a woman with severe pre-eclampsia and eclampsia, delivery is needed urgently. This obviously requires the means to expedite birth by induction of labour or by CS. Adequate control of blood pressure with medication is important to prevent cerebral accidents (both haemorrhagic and ischaemic). Close monitoring in a designated high-dependency area of the ward of such sick women is very useful in preventing and treating further complications, which may include pulmonary oedema.

UNSAFE ABORTION

As abortion is illegal in many countries in Africa, Latin America, the Middle East and Asia, attempts at abortion are often carried out by unskilled practitioners outside the existing medical care system, These are known as 'unsafe abortions'. Unsafe abortions may lead directly to maternal death through uterine perforation, sepsis and haemorrhage. Maternal deaths from abortion are more frequently seen with the non-availability of safe abortion services (Fig. 39.8).

The occurrence of unsafe abortion is strongly linked to the non-availability of contraception. Many women do not have access to a full range of contraception. In some instances, they may not be able to use contraception without permission from their husbands and/or family-in-law. Young girls in particular often encounter significant barriers to accessing contraceptives if they are not married or in a recognised and approved relationship (Fig. 39.9).

Medical Conditions Contributing to Maternal Mortality and Morbidity

In addition to the main direct obstetric causes of death, there are often underlying medical conditions during pregnancy which exacerbate the risk of a complication should this occur. In under-resourced countries, these commonly include anaemia, malaria, human immunodeficiency virus/acquired immunodeficiency syndrome (HIV/AIDS) and tuberculosis (TB).

ANAEMIA

It has been estimated that over half the pregnant women in the world have a haemoglobin level indicative of anaemia (Hb <11.0 g/dL). This is usually a chronic anaemia and the mother is frequently asymptomatic at rest. However, she may decompensate easily in labour, is more at risk of postpartum haemorrhage (PPH), and, in the event of any obstetric haemorrhage, she is much more likely to die.

Relatively few studies have comprehensively assessed the aetiological factors responsible for anaemia in pregnancy, but it is likely that anaemia is a result of multiple factors, which will vary between geographical areas and by season. These factors include malaria, micronutrient deficiency (iron, vitamin A), parasitic infestation, recurrent bleeding in pregnancy, chronic infections and infection with HIV.

MALARIA

As well as contributing directly to maternal death in some settings, malaria is most often one of the causes of maternal anaemia and, thus, contributes to maternal deaths indirectly. Malaria should be considered in any pregnant woman presenting with fever in a malaria-prone area. The symptoms and any complications will depend on the intensity of malaria transmission and the

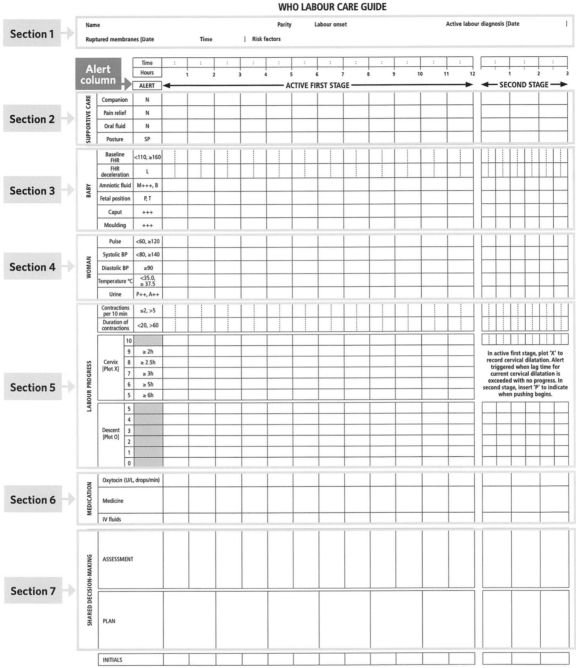

Fig. 39.6 WHO Labour Care Guide. The 'alert' column presents thresholds for abnormal observations that require further action, intervention or referral by the health care provider. (From World Health Organization. *WHO Labour Care Guide: User's Manual.* Geneva: World Health Organization; 2020. https://www.who.int/publications/i/item/9789240017566.)

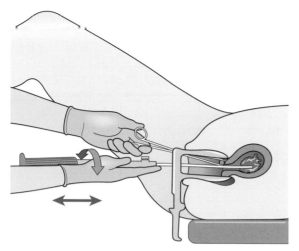

Fig. 39.7 Manual vacuum aspiration.

level of acquired immunity (higher immunity in areas of moderate or high transmission). Pregnant women with severe malaria are prone to hypoglycaemia, pulmonary oedema, anaemia and cerebral malaria. Hypoglycaemia may lead to loss of consciousness.

A thick (blood) film will help detect the parasite and a thin film will identify the species. Of the four types of human malaria, *Plasmodium vivax* and *Plasmodium falciparum* are the most common and *P. falciparum* is the most lethal. Rapid diagnostic tests are increasingly available and widely used in regions of the world where malaria is endemic. If facilities for testing are not available, empirical treatment should be commenced. Treatment depends on the sensitivity profile of the local species. In countries where malaria is common, all pregnant women are recommended routine prophylaxis during pregnancy, and mothers and children should sleep under insecticide-treated bed nets.

HIV/AIDS

Worldwide, about 38 million people are living with HIV infection and about half of all affected adults are female. The largest proportion of maternal deaths associated with HIV infection occur in sub-Saharan Africa and the Caribbean.

Women who are HIV positive have an increased susceptibility to infections. Therefore, they are at higher risk of maternal mortality associated with sepsis. In addition, women may have HIV-associated infections such as TB, cryptococcal pneumonia and meningitis.

Mother-to-child transmission has been by far the most important cause of infection in the estimated 1.8 million HIV-positive children. Pregnant women should be offered screening for HIV early in pregnancy, because appropriate antenatal interventions are needed both to treat the mother and to reduce

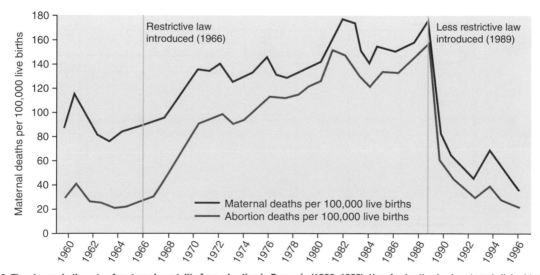

Fig. 39.8 The change in the rate of maternal mortality from abortion in Romania (1960–1996). Unsafe abortion is also strongly linked to the non-availability of contraception.

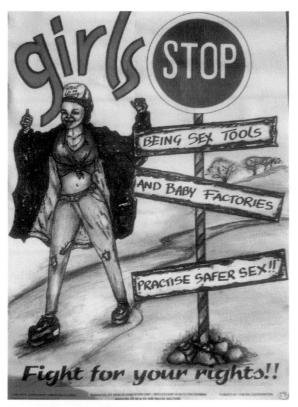

Fig. 39.9 Many women have few fertility choices.

maternal-to-child transmission of HIV infection. This includes antiretroviral therapy (ART) for the mother and to prevent transmission. In addition, consideration should be given to birth by CS and avoidance of breastfeeding when indicated. Choice and type of ART is dependent on viral load and CD4 count. It is also very important to recognise and treat opportunistic infections, including STIs, TB and *Pneumocystis carinii*.

In many countries, being HIV positive carries a significant stigma; thus, many women (and men) do not undergo testing. ART is also still far from widely available in many countries. In addition, HIV health care services are not always integrated within the antenatal or postnatal care services.

TUBERCULOSIS

TB is probably the leading cause of death in women affected by HIV/AIDS. One-quarter of the world population is infected with TB. Sputum smears will be positive for acid fast bacilli (AFB) in the majority of women with pulmonary disease. This is best examined in a specimen of early morning sputum, taken on at least three occasions. A chest X-ray can also be taken (with shielding of the fetus). Treatment involves multiple-drug therapy, usually rifampicin, isoniazid, ethambutol, pyrazinamide and streptomycin (all except streptomycin are considered safe in pregnancy and with breastfeeding). The risk of untreated TB to the pregnant woman and the fetus far outweighs the risk of treatment. Neonatal TB may be congenital or perinatal. A bacillus Calmette-Guérin (BCG) vaccination is recommended for all babies born in areas where there is an increased risk of coming into contact with TB.

Strategies to Improve Global Maternal and Newborn Health

Within the continuum of care for women and their babies, there are two internationally agreed upon key 'care packages' that could reduce maternal and neonatal mortality and morbidity:

- The provision of skilled birth attendance (SBA)
- The availability of emergency obstetric and newborn care (EmONC).

SKILLED BIRTH ATTENDANCE

A skilled birth attendant is an accredited health professional with the midwifery skills necessary to manage normal birth and to diagnose, stabilise and refer obstetric complications. The term 'SBA' encompasses a skilled birth attendant plus the enabling environment, that is, the necessary drugs, equipment, transport and supportive health care system in which the skilled birth attendant works. Maternal mortality is lowest in those countries where the percentage of women who have a skilled birth attendant at delivery is highest (Fig. 39.10).

At least one-third of all women in sub-Saharan Africa give birth without the help of a skilled birth attendant. Many countries are aiming to rapidly increase the number of skilled health care workers. Since 2000, rates of SBA at births in both sub-Saharan Africa and Southern Asia have improved considerably. Training curricula may be revised to be more in line with the competencies needed by a skilled birth attendant or may be adopted to provide fast-track midwifery training. For existing health care professionals, up-skilling

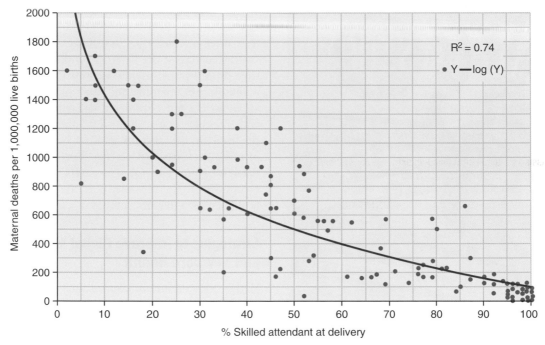

Fig. 39.10 The availability of a skilled birth attendant is strongly associated with a lower maternal death rate.

can enable them to provide a wider range of care. A renewed focus on 'skills and drills' – type competency-based, in-service training is being encouraged in many under-resourced settings (Fig. 39.11). Although a variety of health care provider cadres (midwives, nurses, doctors) are recognised in countries as 'skilled birth attendants', research has shown that they may not be competent to confidently provide skilled care at birth by agreed international standards. As there is often a migration of doctors from the poorer rural parts of many countries to the wealthier cities and a migration of doctors from under-resourced countries to those countries with greater income potential, it often makes sense to focus training on those most likely to remain resident where the need is greatest.

EMERGENCY OBSTETRIC AND NEWBORN CARE (EMONC)

It has been estimated that around 15% of all pregnant women will develop a complication that can become life-threatening if good obstetric care is not available to them. The components of care generally needed in such cases have been bundled into a care package called EmONC. EmONC consists of up to nine

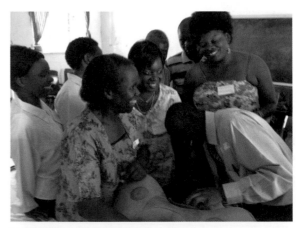

Fig. 39.11 Obstetric skills training in Zambia.

'signal functions' or components (Box 39.1). To reduce maternal mortality, it is important that all women have access to EmONC when an obstetric complication occurs.

EmONC is commonly divided into basic emergency obstetric care (BEmONC) and comprehensive emergency obstetric care (CEmONC). The UN agencies recommend that a minimum of five health care

BOX 39.1 SIGNAL FUNCTIONS OF EMERGENCY OBSTETRIC AND NEWBORN CARE

Basic Emergency Obstetric and Newborn Care (BEmONC)

- IV antibiotics
- IV/IM oxytocics
- IV/IM anticonvulsants
- Manual removal of a retained placenta
- Removal of retained products of conception by manual vacuum aspiration
- Assisted vaginal birth (vacuum extraction or forceps)
- Perform basic neonatal resuscitation (e.g., with bag and mask)

Comprehensive emergency obstetric and newborn care (CEmONC)

All seven BEmONC signal functions, plus:
- Surgery (e.g. caesarean section)
- Blood transfusion

IM, Intramuscular; IV, intravenous.

facilities able to provide EmONC should be available for a population of 500,000, of which at least one health care facility should be able to provide CEmONC and four should be able to provide BEmONC. In many countries, this minimum level of coverage is not yet in place. Designated health care facilities should be able to provide EmONC 24 hours a day and 7 days a week. The distribution of health care facilities must be equitable so that all women in the population have access to this care whether they live in rural or urban areas.

The signal functions or components of EmONC are relatively inexpensive and require basic obstetric knowledge and skills. In practice, in most under-resourced settings, nurse-midwives are able to provide BEmONC and medical doctors CEmONC. There can be many reasons why EmONC signal functions may not be available. Magnesium sulphate, which is relatively inexpensive, is not always available at the health care facility and/or local health care providers may not be familiar with its use. Cheaper broad-spectrum oral antibiotics are generally available, but IV antibiotics and other more expensive antibiotic preparations (which may be needed for drug-resistant strains) may not be available in remote locations. When doctors are not around, nurse-midwives may not be licenced or permitted to give even a starting dose of parenteral antibiotics, an anticonvulsant or to commence an IV infusion. Health care staff in this situation can potentially be supported by systems change, with guidelines supporting wider care provision by nurse-midwives, accompanied by additional training to ensure safety. Virtual health care provision, with remote prescribing, may also enable doctors in urban areas to support health care colleagues in rural areas with fewer doctors, although the significant infrastructure investment required for such technology has limited its use thus far.

MVA can be easily carried out with a simple-operated hand-pump. However, it needs to be purchased, maintained, and sufficient numbers of health care providers trained in its use.

Blood is almost always in short supply. Many hospitals do not have functioning blood banks – often, blood can be given only if a relative or a friend provides it or replaces any blood already available at the health care facility. In some settings, blood can be purchased from a 'private' blood bank. However, since these frequently rely on paid donors, the chance of receiving unscreened blood – with its potential risk of transmission of blood-borne viruses – may be high.

In-depth assessments of availability and coverage of EmONC have shown that in many cases, structures (i.e., health care facility buildings and basic infrastructure) are in place, but these health care facilities cannot offer EmONC. This may be because of a shortage of drugs, equipment or human resources, or of maldistribution of available resources. These challenges often need to be addressed through systems change at a national or international level. The combination of a lack of knowledge and skills is one reason why many beneficial evidence-based practices are still not used by health care workers in many resource-poor settings.

EARLY NEWBORN CARE

Complications of pre-term birth, intrapartum-related complications (asphyxia) and infections are the most frequent sources of neonatal deaths in resource-poor settings (Fig. 39.12). Fourth and fifth are congenital abnormalities and tetanus, respectively. Together, these causes account for over 90% of all newborn deaths globally.

Infections – in particular, sepsis, pneumonia and meningitis – can generally be prevented through good antenatal care, hygienic care during birth, care of the

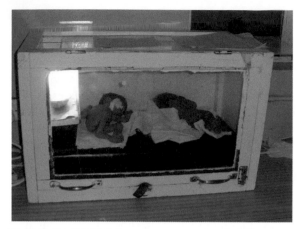

Fig. 39.12 Pre-term birth is a common cause of perinatal loss.

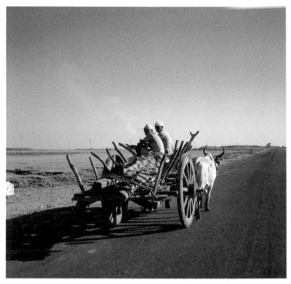

Fig. 39.13 Transporting a mother with obstructed labour to hospital (Bihar, North India).

cord after birth and early exclusive breastfeeding. Recognition and early case management of a baby with infection is needed both at hospital and community level. Postnatal care in the first week of life is crucial to implement this.

Neonatal tetanus is wholly preventable with vaccination of the mother and clean cord care. Complications of pre-term birth can be reduced if a mother is given antenatal corticosteroids when pre-term labour is recognised (see p. 351) and Kangaroo Mother Care (carrying the baby skin-to-skin) is provided to low-birth-weight babies. SBA and EmONC – which includes resuscitation of the newborn – will reduce deaths from asphyxia.

Availability and Quality of Care

Delivering prompt and appropriate health care can be very challenging. In many settings, women and their families do not have access to the health care they need and availability of care may be limited. There are also factors that affect utilisation (or uptake) of health care services, where these are available. Factors affecting utilisation include socioeconomic and cultural factors, accessibility of health care facilities with regard to distance, and cost and the quality of care. Many women will face possible delays in access to care, which include delay in deciding to seek care (phase 1 delay), the speed/ease of identifying and reaching a health care facility (phase 2 delay) and the timeliness and appropriateness of the treatment received (phase 3 delay).

The poor performance of health care services in under-resourced countries is often compounded by broken equipment, poor logistical support and shortages of drugs and equipment. Countries need to ensure a balanced investment not only in human resources but also in infrastructure. Improved management ensuring no stock-outs of drugs, equipment, vaccines, and so on is crucial, as is an established and functional referral pathway from community to health care facility and between health care facilities.

Where services are not free, a lack of money to pay for services can determine when or if at all a woman seeks care. Lack of transportation can delay seeking care (Fig. 39.13) and lack of properly trained staff will increase the risk of poor-quality care that is not timely or appropriate or the risk of failure to recognise that a woman needs care.

While some progress has been made in reducing maternal and child deaths globally, a great deal still needs to be done in regions and countries of the world with the greatest burden of mortality. Increasingly, it is recognised that within countries there are wide disparities between rural and urban populations and between families in the lowest and highest wealth centiles. Recent efforts have seen a renewed focus on ensuring a good-quality evidence base and that respectful woman and baby-friendly care is available for all.

There is need for continued advocacy globally to sustain international aid for resource-poor countries along with ensuring improved governance and accountability.

Epidemics and Pandemics

An epidemic is an increase, often sudden, in the number of cases of a disease above the baseline level expected in a population in a specific area. A pandemic is an epidemic which has spread over several different regions, countries or continents.

Epidemic and pandemic diseases – such as Ebola, Zika, severe acute respiratory syndrome (SARS), Middle East respiratory syndrome (MERS), pandemic influenzas (e.g., H1N1/swine flu) and COVID-19 – often have a disproportionate impact on maternal and neonatal health compared with that of the general population.

DIRECT EFFECTS

Some infections have specific consequences in pregnancy. Pregnancy is a state of relative immunocompromise. Therefore, pregnant women may be both more likely to contract and less physiologically able to mount an immune response to an infection than their non-pregnant counterparts. For instance, pregnant women infected with influenza or malaria are more likely to become severely ill and die as a result than matched non-pregnant women.

The fetus can be affected by maternal infection. Severe maternal illness, regardless of the underlying cause, can increase the risk of miscarriage. However, some infections contracted by the mother also have specific effects on the fetus. For example, rubella and Zika infections usually cause relatively mild systemic illness in adults but have teratogenic effects on the fetus (see Chapter 25).

INDIRECT EFFECTS

A greater impact on maternal and neonatal morbidity and mortality usually comes from the indirect effects of epidemics and pandemics. These significantly impact women's ability to access routine and emergency health care due to hesitation to attend health care facilities out of fear of acquiring infection and/or due to reallocation of health care resources. In an epidemic, health care resources, both human and financial, are often diverted away from 'routine' care towards the new emergency.

In a pandemic, as was seen in the global COVID-19 pandemic in 2020 through 2022, this effect is magnified. National lockdowns and curfews may limit available transportation and reduce women's access to essential health care services. Pandemics also appear to increase the rates of intimate partner violence (IPV), which is associated with worse pregnancy outcomes (see Chapter 23). Many countries worldwide temporarily closed sexual and reproductive health services (including those providing contraception and/or safe abortion), despite the WHO recommendation that these are considered essential services. It is estimated by the UN that in 2020 there may have been as many as 7 million additional unintended pregnancies worldwide as the result of the COVID-19 pandemic, which are likely to have resulted in millions of unsafe abortions and thousands of additional maternal deaths. The causes of the maternal deaths are thought to be complications of unsafe abortion and other obstetric complications exacerbated by lack of access to routine and emergency obstetric care.

Women, including pregnant women, are more likely to be impacted by the effect of epidemics with increased care responsibilities and precarious employment. Women also represent 70% of front-line health and social care workers; thus, they may also be at an increased risk of exposure to infection. Existing gender inequalities usually worsen during disease outbreaks. Advocacy by health care providers for systemic national and international interventions to maintain access to sexual and reproductive health and services for women who experience gender-based violence, as well as gender-sensitive social welfare policies, is important to limit the negative impacts which would otherwise occur.

Key Points

- **Worldwide, approximately 300,000 women die each year from pregnancy- or childbirth-related complications; 99% of these deaths occur in low-resource settings and most are avoidable.**
- **The five main causes of direct obstetric maternal mortality are haemorrhage, sepsis, eclampsia, complications of obstructed labour and unsafe abortion.**

- Globally, there are around 2.4 million neonatal deaths each year and 1.9 million stillbirths.
- Roughly half of all child mortality occurs in the first month of life (neonatal mortality).
- Care packages that are put in place to prevent maternal mortality also reduce neonatal mortality.
- Provision of SBA and availability of EmONC, if added to current care (antenatal care, postnatal care and family planning services), will reduce maternal and neonatal mortality and morbidity.
- Improving maternal health, reducing maternal and neonatal mortality, and improving access to sexual and reproductive health care services are part of the SDGs adopted by the international community in 2015.
- Current rates of reduction in maternal and neonatal mortality must be accelerated in order to achieve the specific SDG targets of reducing the global maternal mortality ratio to <70 per 100,000 live births and neonatal mortality to ≤12 per 1000 live births by 2030.
- Pandemics and epidemics have a disproportionate impact on maternal health and neonatal health, both directly and indirectly.

Self-Assessment

Section Outline

Single Best Answer (SBA) Questions – Part One

Alice Main, Mayank Madhra

Introduction

This is a selection of single best answer (SBA) questions from across this book. This style of questions is increasingly favoured over the traditional multiple choice questions (MCQs) for examinations. The answers and accompanying explanations can be found in Answers to Single Best Answer (SBA) questions – part one.

Questions

Chapter 2

Q1. In which of the following scenarios can a woman be diagnosed as postmenopausal?
  a) When her periods become irregular or lighter
  b) When she develops symptoms such as hot flushes, mood swings and vaginal dryness
  c) When there is more than 3 months between periods
  d) When it has been more than 6 months since her last period
  e) When it has been more than 12 months since her last period

Q2. In obstetric vaginal assessment in labour, which anatomical landmark is used to define the station of the presenting part?
  a) The vaginal opening
  b) The anterior superior iliac spine
  c) The anterior inferior iliac spine
  d) The ischial spine
  e) The pubic symphysis

Q3. A 21-year-old nulliparous women presents to her general practitioner (GP) with 2 days of crampy left iliac fossa (LIF) pain. She is currently on day 14 of her menstrual cycle and has no associated symptoms and no abnormal discharge. Her observations are normal on examination and her abdomen is soft, with some mild LIF tenderness. Urinalysis and human chorionic gonadotropin (hCG) are both negative. On further questioning, she reports she had a similar episode 4 weeks ago. What is the most likely cause of her pain?
  a) Ovarian torsion
  b) Endometriosis
  c) Ectopic pregnancy
  d) Mittelschmerz pain
  e) Pelvic inflammatory disease

Chapter 4

Q1. In the menstrual cycle, a surge of which hormone mid-cycle is the main trigger for ovulation?
  a) Gonadotrophin-releasing hormone
  b) Estrogen
  c) Progesterone
  d) Follicle-stimulating hormone
  e) Luteinizing hormone

Q2. A 14-year-old girl attends her GP with her mother. The mother is concerned that the girl has not yet started her periods like the rest of her friends have. On assessment, she has a normal body weight and normal secondary sexual characteristics. Her mother reports that her own menarche was at age 17 years. What is the recommended management?
  a) Reassurance
  b) 5 days of oral progestogen to induce a withdrawal bleed
  c) A pelvic ultrasound scan to ensure that her anatomy is normal
  d) Referral to gynaecology for further investigation
  e) Advise her to try gaining weight and exercising less

Q3. A 35-year-old woman with a history of polycystic ovarian syndrome presents to her GP due to not becoming pregnant after 1 year of trying to conceive. She is having regular unprotected sex with her male partner and is otherwise fit and well. She has a regular 28-day cycle. You decide to test her progesterone levels to confirm whether she is ovulating. On which day of her menstrual cycle would you arrange for her to have a blood test?
a) Day 1
b) Day 7
c) Day 14
d) Day 21
e) Day 28

Chapter 6

Q1. What is the definition of a missed miscarriage?
a) Passage of some but not all of the pregnancy tissue
b) All pregnancy tissue expelled from the uterus
c) A miscarriage that occurs with no pain or bleeding
d) Pain and bleeding with a closed cervical os
e) Three or more consecutive miscarriages

Q2. A 34-year-old woman attends a recurrent miscarriage clinic following 3 consecutive early miscarriages. She has had no other pregnancies. On further investigation, she is found to have lupus anticoagulant and anti-cardiolipin antibodies, with all other tests returned as normal. What treatment would be recommended to her in her next pregnancy to reduce complications?
a) Progesterone pessaries
b) Low molecular weight heparin (LMWH) and aspirin
c) High-dose folic acid
d) Vitamin D supplementation
e) Wearing compression stockings

Q3. A 28-year-old primigravida attends the early pregnancy assessment centre with vaginal spotting at an estimated 6 weeks' gestation. An ultrasound scan shows a suspected ectopic pregnancy measuring 20 mm in diameter and an empty uterus. She is haemodynamically stable and her hCG shows a fall over the preceding 48 hours from 1200 to 800IU/L. She tells you that she wishes to avoid intervention if possible. What would be your recommended management?
a) Conservative management with hCG monitoring
b) Medical management with methotrexate
c) Medical management with misoprostol
d) Surgical management with salpingectomy
e) Surgical management with salpingotomy

Chapter 8

Q1. A 24-year-old nulliparous woman presents to her GP with chronic pelvic pain and deep dyspareunia and a diagnosis of endometriosis is suspected. What is the gold standard diagnostic investigation that could confirm this diagnosis?
a) Pelvic ultrasound
b) Pelvic MRI
c) Endometrial biopsy
d) Hysteroscopy
e) Diagnostic laparoscopy

Chapter 10

Q1. What is the most common contributing risk factor in pelvic organ prolapse?
a) Pregnancy and childbirth
b) Chronic constipation
c) Chronic cough
d) Obesity
e) High-impact exercise

Q2. A 78-year-old multiparous woman presents with a feeling of a lump in her vagina associated with a dragging sensation. On examination, you find that she has a uterine prolapse with the cervix reaching <1 cm below the plane of the hymen. According to the pelvic organ prolapse quantification system (POP-Q), which stage of prolapse does she have?
a) Stage 0
b) Stage I
c) Stage II
d) Stage III
e) Stage IV

Chapter 12

Q1. A 55-year-old nulliparous, postmenopausal woman presents with a 6-month history of lower abdominal discomfort, bloating and loss of appetite. She

was previously fit and well except for migraines and mild hypertension. She is on no regular medications and is an ex-smoker with a 10-year pack history. On abdominal examination, you find shifting dullness and a fullness in the left lower quadrant. What is the most likely diagnosis?
a) Uterine fibroid
b) Colon cancer
c) Ovarian cancer
d) Coeliac disease
e) Constipation

Q2. A 38-year-old woman undergoes surgery to remove a suspected ovarian tumour. Histologically, the tumour is confined to one ovary, but she is found to have positive peritoneal washings. According to the International Federation of Gynecology and Obstetrics (FIGO) system, what stage of ovarian cancer does she have?
a) Stage Ia
b) Stage Ib
c) Stage Ic
d) Stage IIa
e) Stage IIb

Chapter 14

Q1. The endocervix is lined by which type of epithelium?
a) Simple columnar epithelium
b) Simple squamous epithelium
c) Stratified squamous epithelium
d) Stratified columnar epithelium
e) Simple cuboidal epithelium

Q2. Which two strains of human papillomavirus (HPV) have been identified as the most 'high risk' for cervical cancer?
a) HPV 2 and 4
b) HPV 10 and 12
c) HPV 16 and 18
d) HPV 20 and 21
e) HPV 26 and 28

Chapter 16

Q1. Vulval intraepithelial neoplasia (VIN) is strongly associated with which common sexually transmitted infection?
a) Chlamydia
b) Gonorrhoea

c) Herpes simplex
d) *Treponema pallidum* (syphilis)
e) Human papillomavirus (HPV)

Q2. A 38-year-old woman presents to the gynaecology clinic with a recurrent right-sided Bartholin gland abscess. She has previously undergone several incision-and-drainage procedures on the same side under local anaesthetic, including the use of a balloon catheter on two occasions. Despite this, the abscess has recurred again. What is the next line of treatment you could recommend?
a) Prophylactic antibiotics
b) Incision and drainage under general anaesthetic
c) Marsupialization under general anaesthetic
d) Seton suture insertion
e) Excision of the Bartholin gland

Chapter 18

Q1. A 25-year-old nulliparous woman presents to her GP complaining of a thin green discharge and vulval itchiness for the past 4 days. She is in a long-term relationship and is using combined oral contraception. She is otherwise fit and well with no allergies. On examination, her GP notices an inflamed red cervix with small punctate areas of haemorrhage. What is the most likely diagnosis?
a) Bacterial vaginosis
b) Trichomoniasis
c) Gonorrhoea
d) Vaginal candidiasis
e) Primary syphilis

Q2. A 21-year-old nulliparous woman presents with increased vaginal discharge with a 'fishy' smell. High vaginal swab reveals the presence of clue cells. What treatment would you prescribe her?
a) Metronidazole 400 mg twice a day for 7 days
b) Clotrimazole 1% cream, twice a day for 7 days
c) Doxycycline 100 mg twice a day for 7 days
d) Azithromycin 1 g once only
e) Ceftriaxone 500 mg intramuscular (IM) single dose

Chapter 20

Q1. Which of the following is not a recognised complication of surgical termination of pregnancy?
a) Reduced fertility
b) Haemorrhage

c) Pelvic infection
d) Failure to terminate the pregnancy
e) Retained products of conception

Q2. What is the mechanism of action of the drug mifepristone in termination of pregnancy?
a) Prostaglandin E1 analogue stimulating uterine contractions and cervical ripening.
b) Steroidal anti-progestogen that blocks the action of progesterone in the uterus.
c) Ergot alkaloid stimulating serotonin and alpha-adrenergic receptors in the uterus.
d) Binds to oxytocin receptors, causing uterine contractions.
e) A competitive antagonist of the estrogen receptors in the uterus.

Chapter 23

Q1. Which blood test is not part of routine first-trimester antenatal screening in the United Kingdom?
a) Syphilis
b) Hepatitis B
c) Full blood count
d) Blood group and red cell antibody screening
e) Fasting serum glucose

Q2. A 32-year-old primiparous woman attends antenatal clinic at 36 weeks following diagnosis of polyhydramnios. She is asking how this might impact her pregnancy. Which of the following is a recognised complication of polyhydramnios?
a) Pre-eclampsia
b) Shoulder dystocia
c) Antepartum haemorrhage
d) Cord prolapse
e) Intrauterine growth restriction

Chapter 25

Q1. A 40-year-old primiparous women attends her GP for pre-conception counselling. She and her partner are hoping to start trying for a family but are concerned about the risk of Down syndrome due to her age. What is her background age-related probability of having a baby with Down syndrome?
a) 1 in 1500
b) 1 in 800
c) 1 in 270
d) 1 in 100
e) 1 in 50

Q2. Which of the following conditions cannot be tested for using chorionic villous sampling (CVS)?
a) Fragile X syndrome
b) Down syndrome
c) Phenylketonuria
d) Spina bifida
e) Cystic fibrosis

Chapter 27

Q1. What is the definition of small for gestational age (SGA)?
a) Estimated fetal weight <2 kg at 36 weeks
b) Estimated fetal weight <2.5 kg at 36 weeks
c) Estimated weight is <20th centile for gestational age
d) Estimated weight is <10th centile for gestational age
e) Estimated weight is <5th centile for gestational age

Q2. Which of the following is not a recognised major risk factor for birth of an SGA baby?
a) Maternal depression
b) Recurrent antepartum haemorrhage
c) Pre-eclampsia
d) Smoking >10/day
e) Cocaine use during pregnancy

Chapter 29

Q1. An 18-year-old primiparous women presents at 30 weeks' gestation to obstetric triage with a history of suspected pre-term pre-labour rupture of membranes (PPROM). This is confirmed on sterile speculum. Which is the recommended prophylactic antibiotic in this situation?
a) Clindamycin
b) Co-amoxiclav
c) Gentamicin
d) Nitrofurantoin
e) Erythromycin

Q2. A 35-year-old para 1 attends a pre-term birth clinic at 12 weeks' gestation. She had a previous pre-term birth at 32 weeks and has had 1 previous large loop excision of the transformation zone (LLETZ) procedure to her cervix 4 years ago. The consultant performs a scan to determine her cervical length. In pregnancy, what is the normal length for the cervix?

a) 41 to 45 mm
b) 34 to 40 mm
c) 30 to 35 mm
d) 25 to 30 mm
e) 15 to 25 mm

Q3. A 26-year-old primiparous woman presents at 28 weeks' gestation with a 3-hour history of painful tightenings which are palpable and a 1-cm dilated cervix on speculum examination. She is admitted for monitoring and corticosteroids and is given nifedipine as a tocolytic. What is the mechanism of action of nifedipine in this scenario?
a) Alpha-adrenergic agonist
b) Progesterone agonist
c) Oxytocin receptor blocker
d) Beta-2 receptor agonist
e) Calcium channel blocker

Chapter 31

Q1. A 30-year-old primiparous woman presents in spontaneous labour at 39 weeks' gestation and requests an epidural for analgesia. She is asking you about the risks and side effects. Which of the following is a recognised association with epidural analgesia?
a) Long-term backache
b) Prolongation of the first stage of labour
c) Prolongation of the second stage of labour
d) Increased rate of caesarean section
e) Fetal distress

Q2. You are asked to review the perineum of a 21-year-old woman following spontaneous vaginal birth of her second child, as the midwife suspects that a perineal injury has occurred. On assessment, you identify a tear that involves the vaginal epithelium and the perineal muscles; however, the anal sphincter is completely intact on rectal examination. How would you classify her perineal tear?
a) First-degree tear
b) Second-degree tear
c) Third-degree tear, grade a
d) Third-degree tear, grade b
e) Fourth-degree tear

Chapter 33

Q1. A 28-year-old woman attends her midwife for a routine appointment at 41 weeks' gestation in a low-risk pregnancy. This is her second pregnancy – she previously had an uncomplicated vaginal birth. On examination, her cervix is not favourable and the midwife is unable to perform a membrane sweep. What would you recommend to her?
a) Book an elective caesarean section.
b) Admit to the antenatal ward for observation.
c) Book an induction of labour.
d) Book an artificial rupture of her membranes on the labour ward.
e) Schedule another appointment in 1 week to reassess the favourability of the cervix.

Q2. Which of the following is not a recognised indication for induction of labour?
a) Maternal diabetes
b) Advanced maternal age
c) Prolonged pregnancy (post-dates)
d) Clinically 'large for dates' baby
e) Prolonged pre-labour rupture of membranes

Chapter 35

Q1. You respond to an emergency buzzer on the labour ward for a 37-year-old woman who has suddenly collapsed. She had a vaginal birth of her fifth child 15 minutes ago. On assessment, she is sweaty, peripherally cyanosed, hypotensive and tachycardic. Her bleeding is minimal and there are no signs of infection. What is the suspected diagnosis?
a) Eclamptic seizure
b) Postpartum haemorrhage
c) Amniotic fluid embolus
d) Sepsis
e) Myocardial infarction

Q2. During a labour ward shift, you are called into the room of a 38-year old diabetic woman who is in the second stage of labour at full term. The baby's head had delivered; however, the shoulders have failed to deliver after routine axial traction with the following contraction. After putting out an emergency call, what is the first intervention you should attempt in order to deliver the shoulders?
a) McRoberts position
b) Episiotomy
c) Deliver the posterior arm
d) Fundal pressure
e) Roll the woman onto all fours

Chapter 37

Q1. A 38-year-old woman presents to obstetric triage with reduced fetal movements at 39 weeks' gestation in a previously uncomplicated pregnancy. Unfortunately, there is no fetal heart found and this is confirmed on scan by two senior clinicians. How would this fetal death be legally classified?
   a) Mid-trimester miscarriage
   b) Antepartum stillbirth
   c) Intrapartum stillbirth
   d) Early neonatal death
   e) Late neonatal death

Q2. What is the neonatal survival rate, to discharge home, for a baby born at 24 weeks' gestation?
   a) 30%
   b) 40%
   c) 60%
   d) 80%
   e) 95%

Chapter 39

Q1. What is the most common cause of maternal death in sub-Saharan Africa?
   a) Obstructed labour
   b) Sepsis
   c) Hypertensive disorders
   d) Haemorrhage
   e) Venous thromboembolism

Q2. A 16-year-old primiparous woman presents to Accident and Emergency feeling generally unwell and is found to have a concealed pregnancy of around 36 weeks' gestation. On assessment, her blood pressure is found to be 170/110 and she has significant proteinuria. During your assessment, she becomes unresponsive and appears to be having a generalised seizure. After putting out an emergency call, what is your next line of management?
   a) Administer 10 mg rectal midazolam
   b) Administer IV labetalol infusion
   c) Administer 4 g IV magnesium sulphate
   d) Administer IV phenytoin infusion
   e) Protect her airway and await termination of seizure

Chapter 41

Q1. During ultrasound assessment in late pregnancy, which three measurements are most commonly used to track growth and estimate fetal weight?
   a) Biparietal diameter, thoracic circumference and tibial length
   b) Biparietal diameter, abdominal circumference and femur length
   c) Head circumference, thoracic circumference and tibial length
   d) Head circumference, thoracic circumference and femur length
   e) Head circumference, abdominal circumference and femur length

Q2. A 27-year-old woman is referred from her GP with LIF pain and a history of ovarian cystectomy 4 years ago. What is the recommended first-line imaging technique for suspected ovarian cyst in women?
   a) X-ray pelvis
   b) Pelvic ultrasound
   c) Pelvic CT scan
   d) Pelvic MRI
   e) PET scan

Chapter 44

Q1. A 30-year-old primigravida at 34 weeks' gestation attends obstetric triage complaining of constant severe lower abdominal pain for the last 3 hours, associated with fresh red vaginal bleeding. On assessment, her abdomen is tense and she is tachycardic at 115 bpm. What is the most likely cause of her presentation?
   a) Placental abruption
   b) Placenta praevia
   c) Early labour
   d) Cervical ectropion
   e) Vasa praevia

Q2. A 22-year-old multiparous woman presents to obstetric triage assessment at 35 weeks' gestation with a feeling of 'increased wetness' down below and thinks she may have ruptured her membranes. She is wearing liners only and not soaking through them. She also complains of an associated vaginal itch for the last 2 days. On speculum examination, there is no liquor seen but you notice a plaque-like discharge coating her vaginal walls. What is the most likely diagnosis?
   a) Spontaneous rupture of membranes
   b) Bacterial vaginosis
   c) Vaginal candidiasis
   d) Physiological discharge
   e) Urinary incontinence

Single Best Answer (SBA) Questions – Part Two

Olivia Foster, Mayank Madhra

Introduction

This is a selection of single best answer (SBA) questions from across this book. This style of questions is increasingly favoured over the traditional multiple choice questions (MCQs) for examinations. The answers and accompanying explanations can be found in Answers to Single Best Answer (SBA) questions – part two.

Questions

Chapter 1

Q1. A 48-year-old woman reports symptoms of uterine prolapse and urinary incontinence which have developed over time following the births of her three children. On examination, she is noted to have laxity of her pelvic floor muscles. Which of the levator ani muscles inserts into the perineal body?
   a) Ischiococcygeus
   b) Iliococcygeus
   c) Puborectalis
   d) Obturator internus
   e) External anal sphincter

Q2. A 35-year-old woman wishes to have a laparoscopic sterilization. When performing this procedure, which portion of the fallopian tube should be occluded?
   a) The ampulla
   b) The isthmus
   c) The mesosalpinx
   d) The infundibulum
   e) The mesovarium

Chapter 3

Q1. A 7-year-old girl has developed secondary sexual characteristics and is being investigated for precocious puberty. Which of the following statements is true of precocious puberty?
   a) Investigations and follow-up can be managed by the child's own general practitioner (GP).
   b) All children require treatment, as symptoms can progress quickly.
   c) A multicystic appearance to the ovaries on ultrasound suggests constitutional puberty.
   d) Café-au-lait skin pigmentation can be a sign of a common cause of precocious puberty.
   e) Long-bone radiological skeletal survey is the first-line investigation.

Q2. A 12-year-old girl and her mother are concerned as she has not shown any signs of puberty. Which of the following statements is most correct for delayed puberty?
   a) Delayed puberty is defined as the absence of physical manifestations of puberty by 14 years of age.
   b) Short stature is not a typical sign of constitutional delay.
   c) X-ray for bone age is a first-line investigation.
   d) Induction of puberty may not be indicated when constitutional delay is the cause.
   e) Anorexia is not a known cause of hypogonadotropic hypogonadism.

Chapter 5

Q1. A 35-year-old woman is being investigated for primary subfertility. Which of the following statements is not an appropriate first-line investigation?
a) Day 21 progesterone
b) Measure Body Mass Index
c) Hysteroscopy
d) Hysterosalpingography
e) Measure Anti-Mullerian Hormone

Q2. A couple are being investigated for possible male factor infertility. Which of the following statements is the single best answer?
a) A testicular biopsy is purely for diagnostic purposes.
b) Donor insemination (DI) at the time of ovulation has a chance of live birth of 6% per cycle.
c) Multivitamins have been associated with an improvement in sperm parameters.
d) Varicocele correction surgery is associated with an improvement in fertility.
e) If a vasectomy is reversed 12 years after the original procedure, pregnancy rates are around 10%.

Chapter 7

Q1. A 37-year-old para 2 woman presents with heavy menstrual bleeding. An ultrasound scan is performed which shows the presence of a single fibroid (leiomyoma) measuring 2 cm which does not distort the endometrial cavity. What is the most appropriate treatment option?
a) Myomectomy
b) Total abdominal hysterectomy
c) Uterine artery embolization
d) Levonorgestrel-releasing intrauterine system (LNG-IUS)
e) Gonadotropin releasing hormone (GnRH) analogue

Q2. Taking tranexamic acid during menstruation reduces blood loss by around 50%; therefore, it is a drug used often in the management of heavy menstrual bleeding. What is the mode of action of this drug?
a) Suppresses the effects of progesterone withdrawal on the endometrium.
b) Inhibits cyclo-oxygenase, which is required for the synthesis of prostaglandins.
c) Inhibits the binding of adenosine diphosphate to its platelet receptor.

d) Inhibits plasminogen activator.
e) Suppresses ovulation.

Q3. A 22-year-old para 0 + 0 woman presents with a 9-month history of increasing pain during menstruation. The pain typically occurs 3 to 4 days before menstruation and lasts throughout. She also reports deep dyspareunia, and wishes to continue using condoms with her new partner. What is the most appropriate initial management?
a) A trial of the progesterone-only pill
b) A trial of the LNG-IUS
c) An ultrasound of the pelvis
d) High vaginal swab, including tests for chlamydia and gonorrhoea
e) Diagnostic laparoscopy

Chapter 9

Q1. A 36-year-old woman with a history of depression managed with medication presents with a history of increasingly distressing hot flushes with associated nausea and palpitations. These are not any worse or better during her periods, which are regular. She reports that her mother went through menopause at 50 years old. What is the most likely diagnosis?
a) Thyroid dysfunction
b) Premature ovarian insufficiency (POI)
c) Pre-menstrual syndrome (PMS)
d) Phaeochromocytoma
e) Side effect of tricyclic antidepressants

Q2. A 48-year-old woman wishes to commence hormone replacement therapy (HRT). She has been amenorrhoeic for 18 months and is suffering from severe vasomotor symptoms. She is a long-term smoker, with a BMI of 30, and has a history of previous breast cancer. Which of the following would be an absolute contraindication to her commencing systemic HRT?
a) Presence of antiphospholipid antibodies
b) Uterine fibroids
c) Obesity
d) History of endometrial hyperplasia
e) History of breast cancer

Q3. A 52-year-old woman attends her GP wishing to commence HRT. Her last menstrual period was 9 months ago and she reports increasingly distressing vasomotor symptoms. She has no significant medical history. What treatment is most likely to effectively manage her symptoms?

a) Continuous estrogen-only HRT
b) Cyclical combined HRT
c) LNG-IUS
d) Clonidine
e) Evening primrose oil

Chapter 11

Q1. A 65-year-old woman reports a history of involuntary loss of urine on sneezing and coughing. What is the first investigation you will perform?

a) Cystoscopy
b) Post-void ultrasound measurement
c) Urodynamic studies
d) Urinalysis
e) Pelvic ultrasound

Q2. A 66-year-old woman with a background of incontinence, poorly controlled hypertension and early-onset Alzheimer disease is reporting worsening incontinence when coughing or sneezing since starting a new medication. Which of the following medications is most likely responsible?

a) Ramipril
b) Amlodipine
c) Memantine
d) Mirabegron
e) Doxazosin

Chapter 13

Q1. A 62-year-old woman presents with postmenopausal bleeding. What percentage of women with postmenopausal bleeding will have an underlying malignancy?

a) 10%
b) 2%
c) 2.5%
d) 7.5%
e) 5%

Q2. A 54-year-old woman presents to her GP with postmenopausal bleeding. The pelvic examination is normal. What is the most appropriate initial investigation for this woman?

a) Endometrial biopsy
b) Hysteroscopy
c) Full blood count and coagulopathy screen
d) Ultrasound scan
e) Colposcopy

Q3. Following an endometrial biopsy, a 65-year-old woman is found to have endometrial changes in keeping with endometrial adenocarcinoma. Which of the following risk factors is most commonly associated with a higher risk of developing endometrial carcinoma?

a) Polycystic ovary disease
b) Personal history of breast or colon cancer
c) Late menopause
d) Early menarche
e) Obesity

Q4. A woman with endometrial adenocarcinoma on an endometrial biopsy has cross-sectional imaging in the form of an MRI. This shows the endometrial cavity to be distended by the tumour with para-aortic and pelvic node involvement. It appears that there is no invasion of the bladder or bowel mucosa. What International Federation of Gynecology and Obstetrics (FIGO) stage is the described endometrial carcinoma?

a) FIGO II
b) FIGO IIIC1
c) FIGO IVA
d) FIGO IIIC2
e) FIGO IVB

Chapter 15

Q1. An 18-year-old woman in her first pregnancy is 10^{+3} weeks pregnant based on her LMP. She is referred to gynaecology triage with vaginal bleeding and ongoing hyperemesis despite regular oral antiemetics prescribed by her GP. An ultrasound confirms the appearance of a complete hydatidiform molar pregnancy. Which of the following statements is the single best answer?

a) Medical evacuation may be appropriate for a partial mole.
b) An oxytocin infusion should be commenced preoperatively.
c) In a complete molar pregnancy, there is fetal and placental tissue present.
d) Follow-up after evacuation should be organised by the local Early Pregnancy Unit.
e) Following evacuation of a complete molar pregnancy, there is an approximately 25% chance of persistent disease and the development of malignancy.

Q2. A woman with a complete molar pregnancy undergoes a surgical evacuation of the uterus and is followed up. Her hCG levels are as follows:
- Day 1 hCG = 5500 IU/L;
- Day 7 hCG = 3450 IU/L;
- Day 14 hCG = 4897 IU/L;
- Day 21 hCG = 8678 IU/L

What is the most appropriate next step?
a) Repeat uterine evacuation.
b) Repeat hCG in 48 hours.
c) Commence chemotherapy.
d) CT scan.
e) Consent for hysterectomy.

Chapter 19

Q1. A 55-year-old man is seen by his GP with a history of erectile dysfunction. He has a BMI of 35, has been married for over 20 years, and has no significant medical history. Following a full sexual history, what is the most appropriate initial management?
a) Referral to urology
b) Clinical examination of genitalia
c) Serum testosterone, glucose and lipids
d) Commence sildenafil 50 mg as required
e) Check blood pressure

Chapter 21

Q1. A 29-year-old woman wishes to commence the combined-oral-contraceptive pill. Which of the following is a contraindication (UKMEC category 4) to prescribing this contraceptive?
a) Age 35 years and smoker of <15 cigarettes per day
b) Family history of breast cancer
c) Family history of thromboembolic disease in first-degree relatives <45 years old
d) Women undergoing hepatocellular adenoma surveillance
e) Migraine without aura
Q2. A 23-year-old woman wishes to switch from the desogestrel progesterone-only pill (POP) and has come to discuss this with you. In regard to all other POPs, which of the following statements best describes the mode of action?
a) Prevents endometrial proliferation
b) Inhibits ovulation
c) Decreases tubal motility

d) Thickens cervical mucous
e) Toxic to corpus luteum

Chapter 24

Q1. A 24-year-old female attends her GP following a positive pregnancy test at home and estimates herself to be 5 weeks pregnant as per her last menstrual period. She wishes to continue with the pregnancy. However, as she has a diagnosis of epilepsy, she is concerned about her medication. Which of the following medications is recommended for epilepsy in pregnancy?
a) Phenobarbitone
b) Phenytoin
c) Lamotrigine
d) Carbamazepine
e) Sodium valproate
Q2. A 32-year-old primagravid woman is currently at 26 weeks' gestation. She has a BMI of 32 and is, therefore, offered an oral glucose tolerance test. Her results are as follows:
- Fasting blood glucose level = 5.3 mmol/L
- 2-hour blood glucose level = 10.3 mmol/L

What is the most appropriate next step in the management of this patient in addition to starting blood glucose monitoring?
a) Commence metformin 500 mg twice daily.
b) Commence metformin 1 g twice daily.
c) Lifestyle advice with follow-up in 2 weeks.
d) Commence insulin.
e) Commence gliclazide 40 mg once daily.

Chapter 26

Q1. A 31-year-old woman has a vaginal birth of a healthy baby but shortly after loses an estimated 1250 mL of blood. Which of the following is not a risk factor for primary postpartum haemorrhage (PPH)?
a) Polyhydramnios
b) Pre-eclampsia
c) Prolonged labour
d) Epidural analgesia
e) Macrosomia
Q2. A 28-year-old primigravid woman attended the obstetric assessment area. She reports a small amount of postcoital vaginal bleeding which has now stopped. She is 32 weeks' gestation. There is

no uterine activity or abdominal pain. An ultrasound shows the baby to be active and cephalic, with a normal liquor volume and the placenta in a posterior position, with the leading edge 18 mm from the cervix. What plan of care would be the most appropriate?

a) Speculum and digital vaginal examination
b) Antenatal corticosteroids
c) Admission to hospital for observation
d) Caesarean section
e) Intravenous magnesium sulphate

Chapter 28

Q1. A 27-year-old woman at 32^{+2} weeks' gestation is referred by her community midwife with a blood pressure of 162/110 mmHg and a urine dipstick with protein +++. On examination, she is noted to have marked oedema of her ankles but otherwise feels well. Which of the following best describes the initial management?

a) Caesarean section, following a course of corticosteroids
b) Oral labetalol
c) IV magnesium sulphate
d) IV furosemide
e) Oral methyldopa

Q2. A 22-year-old woman at 34 weeks' gestation is admitted with a frontal headache and seeing 'flashing lights'. On assessment, she is found to be hypertensive, with proteinuria. Which of the following is not regarded as a predisposing factor for developing gestational hypertension/pre-eclampsia?

a) Obesity
b) Extremes of maternal age
c) Family history of pre-eclampsia with mother and sister affected
d) Parity
e) Twin pregnancy

Chapter 30

Q1. A 32-year-old woman is 36^{+5} weeks pregnant with monochorionic diamniotic twins. Which of the following best describes the formation of this particular set of twins?

a) Embryo division occurred at or before the eight-cell stage.
b) Embryo division occurred at the blastocyst stage.
c) Two ova are fertilized and implanted separately into the decidua.
d) Embryo division occurred between 8 and 14 days.
e) Embryo division occurred after 14 days.

Q2. A 29-year-old patient is pregnant with monochorionic twins. She has had a routine scan at 22 weeks' gestation, following which she is told that there are concerns regarding twin-to-twin transfusion syndrome (TTTS). Which of the following statements is true regarding this condition?

a) TTTS accounts for around 5% of perinatal mortality in twins.
b) If the bladder is seen in both twins, then it is Stage II.
c) Without treatment, TTTS is associated with a 50% intrauterine death rate.
d) Evidence suggests that serial amniodrainage is the most effective intervention.
e) Laser ablation is associated with a lower rate of neurological morbidity.

Chapter 32

Q1. A 29-year-old multiparous woman with one previous caesarean section and one vaginal birth previously has progressed well through the first stage of labour. She is now fully dilated, with occipito-anterior position and new meconium staining of the liquor and you are asked to review her cardiotocography (CTG). The baseline rate is 115 beats per minute, variability has been less than 5 beats for 1 hour, and variable deceleration has been present for the last 20 minutes. What would your next steps be?

a) Prepare for caesarean section.
b) Obtain a fetal blood sample.
c) Encourage active pushing and prepare for assisted vaginal birth.
d) Have the woman change position and obtain fluids.
e) Stop active pushing and prepare for assisted vaginal birth.

Chapter 34

Q1. A 32-year-old female at 36 weeks' gestation in her second pregnancy is reviewed by her community midwife. On abdominal palpation, the midwife suspects that the baby is in breech position. She refers the patient for discussion regarding mode of birth in which she is offered external cephalic version (ECV). What is the success rate for this procedure for this woman?

a) 8%
b) 40%
c) 50%
d) 60%
e) 80%

Q2. A 28-year-old primiparous patient presents to the labour ward at 39+6 weeks' gestation in spontaneous labour. She has progressed well through the first stage of labour, is now fully dilated, and has been actively pushing for 2 hours. Which of the following is not associated with a prolonged second stage of labour?

a) Epidural anaesthesia
b) Pudendal nerve dysfunction
c) Fetal macrosomia
d) Persistent occipitoposterior position
e) Spinal kyphosis or scoliosis

Chapter 36

Q1. A 26-year-old nulliparous patient has progressed through the first stage of labour and has been fully dilated and pushing for 2 hours. On examination, the station is +2 but the CTG shows deep variable decelerations. She gives consent for ventouse to assist with the birth of baby. Which of the following is more strongly associated with vacuum extraction than with forceps?

a) Lower Apgar score at 5 minutes
b) Maternal perineal trauma
c) Neonatal phototherapy
d) Neonatal cephalohaematoma
e) Need to revert to caesarean section

Q2. A 37-year-old nulliparous patient has progressed well in labour. She is now fully dilated and has been pushing with no significant descent. The fetal position is thought to be occipito-posterior. Which of the following instruments is best suited for rotating the fetal head from occipito-posterior to occipito-anterior?

a) Piper forceps
b) Simpson forceps

c) Kielland forceps
d) Non-toothed forceps
e) Wrigley forceps

Chapter 40

Q1. The first pharyngeal arch is important in the development of what?

a) The larynx
b) The face
c) The upper limbs
d) The eye
e) The ductus arteriosus

Q2. What does the hindbrain (the rhombencephalon) give rise to?

a) The optic nerve
b) The cerebellum
c) The spinal cord
d) The thalamus
e) The hypothalamus

Chapter 42

Q1. A 30-year-old female is 26 weeks pregnant and attends for review with her community midwife. Her antenatal check is normal but she does report a faster breathing rate than normal over the past few weeks. She is reassured by the midwife that this is normal in pregnancy due to an increase in ventilation. Which of the following physiological changes is also normal in pregnancy?

a) Plasma volume increases
b) Red blood cell volume decreases
c) Stroke volume decreases
d) Cardiac output increases
e) All of the above

Q2. A 32-year-old nulliparous woman is admitted at 8 weeks' gestation with nausea and vomiting. A scan confirms an intrauterine pregnancy and she is reassured this is common in early pregnancy. Which of the following is also true of the gastrointestinal system during pregnancy?

a) Increase in gut motility
b) Diarrhoea
c) Increased gastric emptying
d) Increased gastro-oesophageal reflux
e) Reduced formation of gallstones

Objective Structured Clinical Examination (OSCE) Practice Cases

Sophie Mackay, Mayank Madhra

Chapter Outline

Introduction

Objective Structured Clinical Examinations (OSCEs) are commonly used as part of medical school assessments. They allow assessment of clinical performance and important skills which are difficult to assess in written examinations. These include key domains such as clinical skills, communication skills, judgement, leadership and professionalism.

In many countries over the past decade, OSCEs have moved away from a rigid 'checklist'-based scoring system to assessment by global competency scoring, usually assessing different domains at each station. The practice cases given here do include a checklist as part of the answer scheme because they are designed to allow readers to practice OSCE stations with peers, with one taking the part of the candidate and the other the examiner and/or model patient.

Gynaecology Cases

STATION 1

Information for Candidate

Part 1

Ms AB, 32 years old, and Mr TB, 34 years old, have attended the clinic with a 3-year history of not being able to conceive. Please take a concise history.

Part 2

What initial investigations would you request?

Part 3

Please interpret these results. What is the diagnosis? What treatment options may be available?

    See Chapter 5.

Further Information for Model Patient

Part 1

    AB. You have never been pregnant before (para 0+0). You have a history of regular periods, 5 days in 28, which are not heavy or particularly painful. You do not experience bleeding between your periods. Your last smear was 1 year ago and was normal. You have previously used the combined oral contraceptive pill but stopped this 3 years ago. You and your partner have been actively trying for a pregnancy for 3 years. You do not have any history of abnormal discharge and, as far as you know, have never been diagnosed with a pelvic infection. Your past medical history includes asthma only. Your drug history includes use of a salbutamol inhaler only. You are a non-smoker and drink 4 units alcohol per week and take regular exercise. You are a primary school teacher.

    TB. You have no children from previous relationships. Your past medical history includes type 1 diabetes. You have no history of testicular trauma, surgery nor infection. You smoke 20 cigarettes a day and drink 8 units of alcohol per week. You work in the construction industry.

Part 3

Please provide the following investigation results:

Investigations:

Rubella IgG antibodies: Negative
Day 21 Progesterone: (normal   35 ng/mL
   >10 ng/mL)
Day 3 LH, FSH, Estradiol levels   All normal

Semen Analysis

	Normal Value	Result
Volume (mL)	>1.5	2
Vitality (%)	>58	65
Count (million/mL)	15	0.5
Morphologically normal (%)	4	5
Motility (progressive) (%)	>32	40
Motility (total) (%)	>40	50

Answer

Part 1

A history should include:

- A pregnancy history from Ms AB and whether Mr TB has any children from other relationships
- Menstrual history, including pattern and amount and last menstrual history. A history of oligomenorrhoea or amenorrhoea will point towards an anovulatory cause.
- Use of contraception
- Length of time trying to conceive
- Pelvic pain and dyspareunia, which may point towards endometriosis
- Abnormal vaginal discharge or a previous history of pelvic infection
- Past medical history
- Drug history
- Smoking status
- Lifestyle factors, including occupation
- Psycho-sexual problems

Part 2

Initial investigations should include:

- LH, FSH, estradiol, Anti-Mullerian Hormone
- Rubella serology
- D21 serum progesterone (test of ovulation)
- Hysterosalpingogram (HSG; test of tubal patency)
- Semen analysis.

Other options: Pelvic ultrasound, laparoscopy, hysteroscopy, prolactin, thyroid function tests, testosterone, sex hormone binding globulin, sperm function, mixed agglutination; anti-sperm antibodies may be relevant based on initial investigation results and specific history.

Part 3

Male factor infertility/oligospermia.

In vitro fertilization (IVF) with intracytoplasmic sperm injection. In this scenario, an HSG is not required, as the requirement for IVF means the fallopian tubes are 'bypassed'. An ultrasound is required to look for hydrosalpinx, because the presence of hydrosalpinges reduces the success of each IVF cycle.

See Chapter 5.

STATION 2

Information for Candidate

Ms CB has presented with bleeding at 10 weeks of pregnancy. An ultrasound demonstrates: (1) an intrauterine gestation sac, (2) a fetal pole, (3) crown-rump length of 9 mm and (4) the absence of fetal heart activity. She has been told that, sadly, she has experienced a miscarriage. Please speak to her regarding her options at this point.

See Chapters 6.

Further Information for Model Patient

Possible questions for you to ask:

- Why has this happened? Is this really unusual?
- What are the risks of management? Will there be any impact on my future fertility?
- Will I be able to get pregnant in the future? When can I try for another pregnancy?
- Are there any investigations I should have? Is there any treatment available?

Answer

It is important to be understanding and sympathetic. It is a good idea to start by recognising that this is a distressing situation.

The incidence of miscarriage is about 20%, increasing significantly with age.

A woman may ask why this has happened. It is helpful to be reassuring that the woman's actions have not caused a miscarriage. In at least 50% of cases, no reason can be found. Some 50% of cases appear to be caused by chromosomal abnormalities within the fertilized egg. Rarer causes include autoimmune conditions, such as anti-phospholipid syndrome or poorly controlled diabetes. It is unclear whether structural abnormalities of the uterus play a part. Smoking cessation advice should always be given.

Options for management include:

- Expectant management (a 'wait-and-see' approach)
- Medical management of miscarriage, with synthetic prostaglandins (misoprostol)
- Surgical management of miscarriage, usually under general anaesthetic whereby a suction curette is used to aspirate the contents of the uterus. Cervical preparation with misoprostol is usually used beforehand.

Risks include:

- Retained products of conception
- Infection–women should be specifically told to report whether they have any symptoms, such as fever, heavy bleeding, pain, offensive discharge
- Haemorrhage and, in rare cases, blood transfusion
- In the case of surgical management, trauma to the genital tract, including perforation of the uterus and cervical trauma. In the case of perforation, further surgery, such as laparoscopy or laparotomy, may be required to diagnose and treat any complication, such as bowel or bladder injury.

In terms of impact on future fertility, there is no clear evidence that either method impacts on future fertility. Asherman syndrome is a rare condition which has been described after uterine evacuation whereby adhesions and scarring of the endometrium cause secondary amenorrhoea.

If asked when it is okay to become pregnant again, it is appropriate to say that it is usually when a woman feels emotionally and physically ready.

Investigations for rarer causes of miscarriage are usually performed only in cases of recurrent miscarriage, which is defined as 3 or more miscarriges. Only a small percentage have an identifiable and treatable cause. However, even in these cases, the chance of a successful future pregnancy is 60% to 75%. Counselling and reassurance are currently the mainstays of treatment, although this is an area of ongoing research. Unproven treatments should be avoided.

See Chapters 6.

STATION 3

Information for Candidate

Ms EF has arrived in the emergency department with a 1-day history of vaginal spotting and severe abdominal pain. She had an episode of fainting while in the waiting room. You are the on-call emergency department doctor. Please discuss with the examiner how you will assess her.

See Chapters 6 and 44.

Further Information for Examiner

Encourage a systematic approach. Provide information when specifically asked. The woman is lying still on a hospital trolley. She looks pale. She is conscious but not answering questions clearly and keeps saying she feels really unwell. No one is available to provide a collateral history.

A. Airway is patent.

B. Respiratory rate (RR) is 12, oxygen saturation 98%, chest is clear on auscultation.

C. Heart rate (HR) is 120 beats per minute, regular. Heart sounds pure. Cool peripheries, peripheral capillary refill 4 seconds, central capillary refill less than 2 seconds. Blood pressure (BP) 110/65 mmHg. Ask what actions would you take at this point. Expect intravenous (IV) access; bloods, including full blood count (FBC) and blood group; and fluid replacement with crystalloid.

D. Blood glucose 6.3, Glasgow Coma Scale (GCS) 15.

E. Abdomen tender and peritonitic. Pregnancy test is positive. Left shoulder pain.

Ask about differential diagnoses.

Ask initial management.

Ask whom they would like to contact for assistance. Ask them to make the phone call.

Ask about further management.

Answer

In an emergency situation, it is helpful to take a structured ABCDE approach.

An ectopic pregnancy should always be considered in collapse of a woman of childbearing age.

A. Airway

B. RR, oxygen saturations, auscultate chest

C. HR, BP and capillary refill. Actions: gain IV access (large bore, 2 cannulas), take bloods tests including FBC, renal function, and blood group. Start IV fluid circulating volume resuscitation with crystalloid fluid.

D. Blood sugar and GCS.

E. Expose, palpate abdomen, looking for evidence of bleeding (external and concealed), shoulder pain.

A urinary catheter should be inserted to obtain urine for a urinalysis, perform a urinary pregnancy test and guide fluid replacement.

A speculum should be inserted to look for vaginal bleeding or an open cervical os, which may suggest miscarriage.

Young healthy women typically compensate well in the early stages of ongoing bleeding. By the time their vital signs are abnormal, they are very unwell. Therefore, a normal BP in this case is not reassuring. This woman is showing signs of haemorrhagic shock, including tachycardia, dizziness and cool peripheries. A peritonitic abdomen and positive pregnancy test point towards an ectopic pregnancy test being the most likely cause. It is important to recognise the seriousness of the situation and escalate appropriately. An appropriate person to contact on this occasion would be the on-call gynaecology registrar or consultant.

Good communication is key and could take an SBAR approach. For example:

Situation—I'm phoning with regard to a 23-year-old woman who I suspect has an ectopic pregnancy. She has signs of severe hypovolaemia and has collapsed once already.

Background—She has a short history of abdominal pain, vaginal bleeding and dizziness.

Assessment—On examination, she is tachycardic with cool peripheries. Her abdomen is peritonitic. Her pregnancy test is positive.

Recommendation—I have gained IV access and taken bloods, including blood group, and started IV fluids. I would like you to come and review her with a view to urgent surgery.

A pelvic ultrasound would be useful in determining the diagnosis but should not delay management,

which, in this case, will be transfer to theatre for surgery. A FAST (Focused Assessment with Sonography for Trauma) scan in the Emergency Department may be useful to look for the presence of free fluid in the abdomen, which in this context, is intraperitoneal blood.

See Chapters 6 and 44.

STATION 4

Information for Candidate

Part 1

Ms GH is a 49-year-old solicitor who has been referred to gynaecology triage by her general practitioner (GP) with heavy vaginal bleeding. Please take an appropriate history.

Part 2

What investigations would be appropriate at this point?

Part 3

What is your differential diagnosis?

See Chapter 7.

Further Information for Model Patient

You have a 6-week history of constant bleeding. Your GP started a course of tranexamic acid and norethisterone 2 weeks ago, which helped while you took it, but as soon as you stopped this, the heavy bleeding came back.

Prior to this, your periods were regular, bleeding for 5 days in 28. They have been heavier over the last year and have become significantly more painful. You have had time off work because off this, which is very unusual for you. You are para 2+0 having had 2 vaginal births in the past. You have not had any postcoital bleeding and do not have any pain with sexual intercourse. Your smears have always been normal in the past, although it is 10 years since you had one. You do not use contraception, as your husband has had a vasectomy. You have had no new sexual partners.

You have been feeling very run down recently. Your past medical history includes hypothyroidism, for which you take thyroxine. You are allergic to penicillin. Your mother had a hysterectomy in her 50s, although you are not sure what this was for.

Answer

Part 1

A gynaecology history should include:

- Menstrual history, including whether periods are regular or irregular, length, heaviness and any associated pain. Irregular periods may suggest an anovulatory disorder. Painful periods raise the possibility of endometriosis or adenomyosis. Heaviness can be subjective—it is useful to ask about impact on quality of life, as what may be acceptable for one woman could be unbearable for another.
- Intermenstrual bleeding, which may point towards structural abnormality
- Postcoital bleeding, which might suggest cervical pathology, or infection.
- Cervical screening history—in particular, abnormal tests or missed tests
- Sexual history—a new partner may increase the risk of sexually transmitted infection
- Dyspareunia—deep dyspareunia may suggest endometriosis, or infection.
- Pelvic pain, whether cyclical or non-cyclical
- Pregnancy history, future fertility wishes, date of last period and considering the possibility of the woman being pregnant and unaware of it
- Contraception, including iatrogenic causes. For instance, sudden cessation of a progestogen is likely to cause a withdrawal bleed.
- Any easy bruising/frequent nose bleeds etc – which might point towards a coagulation disorder. Any fatigue or light-headedness, which may suggest anaemia.
- Past medical history
- Current medication, allergies
- Relevant family history
- Investigations performed to date
- Symptoms related to menopause.

Part 2

Given her age (>45 years) and recent change in bleeding pattern, it is necessary to investigate further, including endometrial sampling. In a younger woman, when history and examination do not suggest pathology, a trial of treatment is an appropriate first-line step. However, investigations should be initiated in the event of treatment failure.

Investigations should include:
- FBC and haematinics (ferritin, iron stores) to look for anaemia
- Examination and pelvic swabs, including endo-cervical swab
- An ultrasound to look for structural abnormalities, such as a submucosal fibroid or polyp
- An endometrial biopsy to look for endometrial hyperplasia or cancer
- A hysteroscopy, depending on initial investigations, for structural abnormalities in the uterus.

Part 3

A differential for possible causes of heavy menstrual bleeding includes:
- Endometrial and cervical polyps
- Adenomyosis
- Fibroids, particularly submucus and intramural
- Malignancy, including cervical and endometrial
- Coagulopathy
- Iatrogenic related to contraception or exogenous hormones
- Ovulatory dysfunction, or approaching menopause.
- Endometrial origin (when other causes excluded).

This is often the conclusion of an OSCE question. Sometimes, the questions are designed to test how systematic your approach is and how wide your differential diagnoses are rather than to specifically test whether you reached the correct diagnosis.

See Chapters 2 and 7.

STATION 5

Information for Candidate

IH is a 28-year-old para 1 who has been experiencing heavy periods. She has had a normal examination, recently had negative vaginal swabs, a normal pelvic ultrasound and has a normal cervical smear history. She would like to discuss treatment options. She feels that her periods are ruining her life.

Please discuss this with her.

See Chapter 7.

Further Information for Model Patient

If asked, you are not currently trying for another pregnancy but are not sure if your family is complete.

You would specifically like more information on intrauterine contraception, including side effects and risks.

Answer

Medical options for managing heavy periods include:

- The levonorgestrel-releasing intrauterine system (LNG-IUS)—also offers contraception for up to 5 years and 95% reduction in blood loss at 12 months, with many women experiencing amenorrhoea. Side effects include irregular bleeding, particularly in the first 3 to 6 months, and expulsion rate is about 5%. There is a small risk of perforating the uterus on insertion. There is an increased risk of pelvic infection. If pregnancy does occur, there is an increased risk of ectopic pregnancy. However, overall lower numbers of pregnancies also means fewer ectopic pregnancies.
- Tranexamic acid and mefenamic acid—tranexamic acid is an antifibrinolytic. It can reduce blood loss by about 50%. Side effects include gastric upset and tinnitus. It is not suitable in individuals at high risk of venous thromboembolism (VTE). Mefenamic acid is a non-steroidal anti-inflammatory drug. It reduces blood loss by 25% and acts as a painkiller. Side effects include headache, dizziness and gastric upset. This is the best option for women trying to conceive, as other medical options also act as contraceptives.
- Oral contraception—can be taken in a cyclical fashion to cause a withdrawal bleed, or 'back to back'. There is an approximate 50% reduction in blood loss. Not always appropriate for those at high risk for venous thrombosis aged over 35 years and experiencing persistent migraine with aura. The progesterone-only pill may be suitable for some women who cannot take the combined contraception pill.
- Cyclical norethisterone—may be used to regulate an irregular cycle, although it does not appear to reduce blood loss.
- Injected long-acting progestogens—depot-injectable progestogen frequently results in amenorrhoea when taken for an extended period. Side effects include irregular bleeding initially, bloating, breast tenderness, headaches, increased appetite and skin changes. It can sometimes take 12 to

18 months for periods and fertility to resume once the injections are stopped.
- GnRH analogues which cause amenorrhoea by pituitary downregulation would not be an appropriate first-line treatment in a 28-year-old.
- Both endometrial ablation and hysterectomy are inappropriate in this case, as IH wishes to preserve her future fertility.

See Chapter 7 and 21.

STATION 6

Information for Candidate

Part 1

JK is a 21-year-old woman who presents to the emergency department with severe abdominal pain. Her initial systemic observations are normal and a urinary pregnant test is negative. Please take an appropriate history.

Part 2

What would you look for on examination?

Part 3

Please suggest a differential diagnosis. What initial investigations would you send?

See Chapters 8 and 44.

Further Information for Examiner/Model Patient

Part 1

JK has had severe 9/10 pain in her left lower abdomen for the last 6 hours. It is constant and sharp. This was a sudden, almost instant onset and associated with vomiting initially. She has taken co-codamol with no improvement. The pain is particularly bad when she moves or tries to go the toilet. It does not radiate anywhere. There is no change in bowel habit. There are no urinary symptoms.

Her last menstrual period was 3 weeks ago; her periods are usually light and regular. She reports no intermenstrual or postcoital bleeding. She has a new sexual partner whom she has been dating for 3 months. They are using condoms. She reports no new vaginal discharge. She had surgical termination of pregnancy 2 years ago but no other pregnancies. Her past medical history includes a previous laparoscopic appendicectomy. She takes no regular medications and is allergic to latex.

Part 2

Vital signs are normal. On general inspection, JK looks very uncomfortable and is struggling to mobilise with the pain. She has tenderness and guarding in the left iliac fossa. A speculum demonstrates a normal vulva, vagina and cervix. There is cervical excitation and a mass is felt in the left adnexa.

Answer

Part 1

When asking about acute pelvic pain, it is necessary to ask about site, onset, characteristics, radiation, severity, exacerbating and relieving factors, relationship to menstrual cycle and analgesia requirement. A sudden onset of severe pain may point towards an ovarian cyst accident (ovarian torsion, ovarian cyst rupture or haemorrhage into a cyst).

Associated gastrointestinal symptoms should be sought. Vomiting and nausea may be a feature of ovarian torsion; gastrointestinal upset can be a symptom of a ruptured ectopic pregnancy. These symptoms may also point towards a non-gynaecological cause, such as appendicitis or diverticulitis. Associated urinary symptoms such as dysuria or frequency may point towards a UTI, while haematuria or loin to groin pain may suggest renal colic.

A detailed menstrual history is important, including frequency and character, any intermenstrual bleeding, or postcoital bleeding.

A sexual history should be taken. Ask about changes in vaginal discharge. It is necessary to ask about deep and superficial dyspareunia. In addition, ask for specifics regarding contraception and smear history.

Part 2

Examination should include general inspection—is the woman able to move and talk without significant discomfort?

An abdominal examination would include inspection of the abdomen for distension and masses, palpation for tenderness, rebound tenderness, guarding and auscultation for bowel sounds.

A speculum and bimanual examination should be carried out, looking specifically for cervical excitation and adnexal masses.

Part 3

A differential diagnosis might include:
- Ovarian torsion
- Ovarian cyst accident
- Pelvic inflammatory disease.

Appropriate investigations would include:
- Urinalysis, urinary pregnancy test
- Bloods, including FBC and C-reactive protein (CRP) to assess markers of infection
- High vaginal and endocervical swabs
- Pelvic ultrasound to look for evidence of ovarian cysts and tubo-ovarian abscess. An ovary with a large cyst is more likely to tort, and sometimes colour Doppler can be performed to give information on the likelihood of torsion.

In cases of severe, unresolved pain, a diagnostic laparoscopy may be appropriate. If torsion is suspected, expediting surgical management will relieve symptoms and give the best chance of salvaging healthy ovarian tissue in the case of torsion.

See Chapters 8 and 44.

STATION 7

Information for Candidate

LM, a 25-year-old, returns to your clinic for a follow-up appointment. She has recently had a diagnostic laparoscopy due to chronic pelvic pain. This has demonstrated superficial endometriosis on the left pelvic side wall and in the pouch of Douglas, which has been excised. She has been told she has endometriosis but does not know what it is. Please discuss the operation findings with her.

See Chapter 8.

Further Information for Model Patient

Questions you ask could include:
- What is endometriosis?
- What causes it?
- Can it be cured?
- I have heard that you cannot get pregnant if you have endometriosis. Is this true?
- How can endometriosis be treated? Will I have to have more surgery?

Answer

A question like this tests your communication skills. It is important to explore what the woman already understands and what she is concerned about. An explanation should be clear and should avoid using medical jargon when possible. It may be helpful to look at patient information leaflets or websites to get an idea for how to explain medical ideas simply.

Endometriosis is the presence of endometrial-like tissue outside of the uterus. This is usually in the pelvis, such as the uterosacral ligaments or pelvic peritoneum but more rarely can affect more distant sites. These tissues respond to hormones in the same way that endometrium does, causing inflammation and pain. The incidence is reported to be between 4% and 43%. It is unclear what causes it—theories include retrograde menstruation and metaplasia. It is difficult to know why it affects some women and not others, although there may be genetic or immunological factors. Typically, it causes pain just before or during a period, although some women also experience chronic pain unrelated to their cycle. Other symptoms include pain during sex, pain during ovulation, pain on defecation, cyclical or menstrual symptoms and subfertility. There is a poor correlation between the extent of disease found at laparoscopy or on imaging and the severity of the symptoms. There is an association with subfertility, but it is not the case that all women with endometriosis will have problems conceiving.

Management options can be split into analgesia, ovulation suppression or surgery. Ovulation suppression may be with combined or progesterone-only contraceptives, or with LNG-IUS. GnRH analogues are second line and usually limited to 4 to 6 months, with add-back hormone replacement. Surgery can include treatment of superficial disease, a pelvic clearance or treatment of deep infiltrating disease in a specialist centre.

There is an association with subfertility. Treatment of minimal to mild disease does appear to improve fertility, but the role in moderate to severe endometriosis is less clear. Removal of large endometriotic cysts may improve fertility. Assisted reproductive techniques may be required more often than in the non-endometriosis population.

See Chapter 8.

STATION 8

Information for Candidate

Part 1

Mrs ML is a 65-year-old woman who has been experiencing urinary incontinence. Please take an appropriate history.

Part 2

Please suggest possible management options.
   See Chapter 11.

Further Information for Model Patient

You have been experiencing incontinence for several years. You find that you need to go to the toilet up to 10 times daily, including many times overnight and sometimes will not make it to the toilet in time. You have not noticed any leakage of urine when coughing or sneezing.

You are a para 4, having had 4 vaginal births. Your favourite drink is tea and you do not tend to drink anything else. When out for the day, you will not drink anything at all to avoid needing the toilet. You are a smoker and do not drink alcohol. You have not been aware of a prolapse.

This is having a huge impact on your confidence and quality of life.

Answer

Part 1

History:

- Frequency, urgency, nocturia (all of these point towards an overactive bladder)
- Urinary incontinence—is it exertional (i.e., stress incontinence) or constant or related to urgency?
- Voiding symptoms, such as hesitancy or straining, poor or intermittent urinary stream; post-micturition symptoms include a feeling of incomplete emptying
- Red flag symptoms include haematuria, persistent pain, recurrent bladder infection
- Any suggestion of organ prolapse
- Impact on quality of life, or sex life
- Bowel dysfunction
- Past medical history and drugs
- Risk factors, including previous pregnancies
- Lifestyle factors, including caffeine usage, alcohol use, smoking status, carbonated drinks

Part 2

The history in this case of frequency, urgency and nocturia, with episodes of incontinence not related to coughing or sneezing, point towards a diagnosis of overactive bladder, rather than urinary stress incontinence or mixed incontinence.

Possible treatments include lifestyle advice, such as normalising fluid intake, reducing alcohol, caffeine, and carbonated drinks, smoking cessation, and weight loss if appropriate. Bladder retraining involves gradually increasing the time between voids to achieve a normal micturition pattern. Anticholinergic medication—such as oxybutynin, solifenacin and tolterodine—may be helpful (use with caution in the elderly.)

More specialist treatments include Botox injections to the bladder muscle.

See Chapter 11.

STATION 9

Information for Candidate

Part 1

Mrs QR is a 70-year-old retired clerical worker who has been referred by her GP with a history of vaginal bleeding. Please take an appropriate history.

Part 2

Please see the result of the pelvic ultrasound. What further investigation(s) should she have? What would your differential diagnosis be?

See Chapter 13.

Further Information for Model Patient

Part 1

You have had 3 episodes of bleeding over the last 4 months. On each occasion, the bleeding has been fresh red and there has been enough to soak your underwear. You have not had any associated pain, but have had a continuous brown vaginal discharge for the past 4 months.

You went through menopause 15 years ago and have never been pregnant. Your past medical history includes type 2 diabetes, hypertension and osteoarthritis. You are waiting for a hip operation, but your orthopaedic surgeon told you that you should try to lose some weight first.

Part 2

Investigations:
Transvaginal pelvic ultrasound demonstrates a 5-cm-long uterus with an endometrial thickness of 8 mm. No adnexal pathology is seen.

Answer

Part 1

History:
- Bleeding history includes amount and timing
- Presence of vaginal discharge
- Pain
- Pregnancy history—nulliparity is a risk factor for endometrial hyperplasia
- Time of menopause—late menopause is a risk factor for endometrial cancer
- Cervical smear history
- Past medical history, including obesity, tamoxifen use, polycystic ovarian syndrome or other ovarian tumour, breast cancer, colorectal cancer and smoking status.

Part 2

An endometrial thickness of 8 mm is abnormal after menopause, particularly in the presence of postmenopausal bleeding. An endometrial biopsy needs to be obtained to look for evidence of endometrial hyperplasia or cancer. This can be done in the clinic during speculum examination. A hysteroscopy is considered the gold standard investigation.

Differential diagnoses would include endometrial hyperplasia, endometrial cancer, cervical cancer, endometrial polyp, cervical polyp and atrophic vaginitis.

See Chapter 13.

STATION 10

Information for Candidate

Part 1

Ms ST is a 31-year-old primary school teacher who has recently had the result of a smear test: 'High grade (moderate) dyskaryosis'.

Please explain this result to her.

Part 2

Ms ST has been advised that she should attend for colposcopy. Please explain this procedure.

See Chapter 14.

Further Information for Model Patient

You are worried about the results of your smear test. All your smears in the past have been normal, and you are anxious about the need for further investigations.

Possible questions to ask:
- Does this mean I have cancer?
- Will I get an anaesthetic? Will it be painful?

Answer

A question like this is designed to test your communication skills. It is important to explore what the woman already understands and what she is concerned about. Explanations should be clear and should avoid using medical jargon when possible. It may be helpful to look at patient information leaflets or websites to get an idea of how to explain medical ideas simply.

Part 1

Abnormal cells found on the surface of the cervix can be described as dyskaryosis. If these cells are left untreated, they can develop into cancer.

It does not mean that you have cancer, but you may require further investigation or treatment.

Part 2

Colposcopy is a procedure whereby the cervix is examined in more detail using a type of microscope called a colposcope. During the procedure, the woman is positioned with her legs in lithotomy position and a speculum is used to visualize the cervix. Substances such as acetic acid or iodine may be applied to the cervix to help visualize abnormal cells. If high-grade changes are suspected, a biopsy may be taken or the area may be excised in a 'see and treat' approach (large loop excision for transformational zone (LLETZ)). To take a biopsy, the cervix is infiltrated with local anaesthetic and an instrument with cautery is used to excise the areas of concern. If the findings during colposcopy are reassuring, no treatment may be required. There is typically some short-lasting pain associated with a cervical biopsy or LLETZ.

See Chapter 14.

STATION 11

Information for Candidate

Please demonstrate how you would perform a speculum examination and take vaginal swabs.

See Chapter 2.

Further Information for Examiner

Prompts.
- What should you ensure before starting?
- What position should the woman be in?
- What are you are looking for on inspection?

Answer

- Ensure a private room. Have a chaperone present, and document the chaperone's name and role in the clinical notes.
- Explain the procedure and confirm that consent is given.
- Allow privacy for the woman to undress.
- The woman should lie on her back with heels together and knees apart.
- Inspection—features to comment on include hair distribution, vulval skin conditions, scars, visible prolapse.
- To perform a speculum examination, lubricate with gel and hold so that the blades are vertical and the speculum is closed. Part the labia and gently insert, rotating until the blades are horizontal. Insert fully and gently open to visualize the cervix.
- Inspect the vagina for atrophic vaginitis or discharge and the cervix for lumps, cysts, warts, tumours and the threads of an intrauterine device.
- A high vaginal swab should be taken from the vaginal fornices. An endocervical swab should also be taken for chlamydia and gonorrhoea. You should familiarise yourself with what these different swabs look like in your hospital.
- To remove the speculum, open further and remove beyond the cervix before rotating back around, closing and removing.
- Allow privacy to dress.
- Explain the findings to the woman, answer any questions and explain how the results of any investigations will be reported to her.

See Chapter 2.

STATION 12

Information for Candidate

Ms RS attends the emergency department after 3 days of increasing abdominal pain and vaginal bleeding.

She had a medical termination of pregnancy 6 days ago. On arrival her temperature is 39.7°C, pulse is 112 beats per minute, RR is 25 breaths per minute, oxygen saturation is 98% on air, BP is 105/62 mmHg.

Please perform an initial assessment.

See Chapters 20, 35 and 44.

Further Information for Examiner

Please provide information when asked.

A. Patent airway
B. Chest sounds clear on auscultation, RR elevated.
C. HR 112 beats per minute, regular bounding pulse, capillary refill <2 seconds, warm peripheries. Ask what actions you would take.
D. Alert, blood glucose 5.6, temperature 39.7°C.
E. Abdomen soft, tender suprapubically. Positive pregnancy test. Urinalysis—1+ leucocytes. There is moderate and offensive vaginal bleeding.

Ask what the likely diagnosis is. Ask about initial management.

Answer

Pyrexia, tachypnea and tachycardia raise the possibility of sepsis. In an emergency situation, it is usually helpful to use a structured ABCDE approach.

A. Airway patent
B. RR, oxygen saturation, chest auscultation
C. HR, pulse rate, oxygen saturation. Gain IV access and take bloods
D. Blood glucose, temperature
E. Expose the woman, palpate her abdomen, obtain urinalysis, pregnancy test

Perform speculum to assess bleeding and take vaginal swabs.

The woman is tender suprapubically, with moderate offensive vaginal discharge. In the context of a recent termination of pregnancy, a likely diagnosis is endometritis or retained pregnancy tissue, which are recognised complications.

Appropriate initial management includes IV access, blood tests (including full blood count FBC, serum lactate, renal function, blood cultures), fluids and broad-spectrum antibiotics according to local protocols.

A pelvic ultrasound to look for retained products of conception will be useful.

See Chapters 20, 35 and 44.

Obstetric Cases

STATION 1

Information for Candidate

Part 1

Ms AB is a 34-year-old woman who is currently 32 weeks pregnant. She has been referred to obstetric triage by her GP, with a history of vomiting for treatment of hyperemesis.

Please take an appropriate history.

Part 2

What investigations would you like to perform? What is your differential diagnosis at this point?

Part 3

Please review the following investigation results. What is your differential diagnosis?

See Chapter 24.

Further Information for Model Patient

Part 1

You are 32 weeks into your first pregnancy. You are rhesus positive. You had hyperemesis in the first trimester but have had no problems with vomiting since 15 weeks. You have had a booking scan and anomaly scan, which were both normal.

You have been vomiting and feeling generally unwell and tired for the past 3 days. You have abdominal pain, which is constant and in the upper part of your abdomen; you have never had pain like this before. You are passing urine more frequently but have no pain with urination. You feel constantly thirsty.

You have not had any vaginal bleeding or vaginal discharge. The baby's movements have been reduced in the last 24 hours. You have not had any headaches or visual disturbance, but have noticed some mild swelling of your hands and feet.

Further Information for Examiner

Part 2

On examination, the woman looks jaundiced. She has a gravid abdomen, with a symphysis fundal height (SFH) appropriate for dates. On palpation, the fetus has a longitudinal lie and is cephalic. The woman's abdomen is soft, with right upper quadrant (RUQ) tenderness but no guarding. Bowel sounds are present.

Her heart and respiratory rates, temperature and oxygen saturations are within normal limits. BP is 149/92 mmHg.

Ask: What investigations would you like to perform?

Part 3

Provide the following information:

Investigations

Hb: 105	(normal: 95–150)
Platelets: 110	(normal: 146–429)
Urea: 5	(normal: 1.1–3.0)
Creatinine: 80	(normal: 35–80)
ALT: 1053	(normal: 2–25)
Bilirubin: 50	(normal: 1.7–18.8)
Amylase: 58	(normal: <100)
ALP: 300	(normal: 38–229)
Glucose: 1.9	

Abdominal Ultrasound:
No gallstones. Common bile duct not dilated.
Urine: 1+ protein, 2+ ketone.
CTG: Normal and reassuring pattern.

If suitable differential not provided, prompt: Is there anything that is particularly concerning about these results?

Answer

Part 1

Obstetric history taking

- Vomiting in pregnancy does not always mean hyperemesis; a careful history should still be taken to exclude other pathology (suggest as urine infection). New-onset vomiting starting in the third trimester is very unlikely to be hyperemesis and these women need careful review. Ask about associated diarrhoea, urinary symptoms, abdominal pain, infective contacts. If abdominal pain is present, ask about site, onset, severity, exacerbating and relieving factors, analgesia, and so on.
- In all pregnant women, gestation, parity, pregnancy history, rhesus status, scans to date (typically, booking and anomaly scan and any additional scans, including growth scans) should be noted.
- Enquire about past obstetric history, medical history, family history, current medications, and allergies.

- Always ask specifically about fetal movements (after 20 weeks), the presence of vaginal bleeding, and any symptoms that may suggest rupture of membranes.
- Ask specifically about headache, visual disturbance, limb swelling, and epigastric pain, which may suggest pre-eclampsia toxaemia (PET).

Part 2

Non-obstetric causes of upper abdominal pain in pregnancy include gastritis/gastric ulcers, cholecystitis, and pancreatitis. It is also worth remembering that the presentation of some pathology, such as appendicitis, may be atypical due to displacement of the appendix by the gravid uterus, and can present with RUQ pain. Rare obstetric causes of upper abdominal pain include PET, HELLP (*h*aemolysis, *e*levated *l*iver enzymes and *l*ow *p*latelets) syndrome, and acute fatty liver disease. While not suggested by the history here, placental abruption and pre-term labour should always be considered in a pregnant woman presenting with abdominal pain. Investigations should include blood tests: FBC, urea and electrolytes (U+E), liver function test (LFT), urate, glucose, lactate, amylase, and coagulation screen.

Urinalysis should be performed to look for proteinuria, ketones (which can be a marker of poor food and fluid intake), and evidence of infection. An abdominal ultrasound scan could be performed to look for gallstones and dilatation of the biliary tree. After 26 weeks, a cardiotocography (CTG) should be performed to assess fetal well-being

Part 3

Acute fatty liver of pregnancy is a rare but serious complication of pregnancy with high rates of maternal and fetal mortality. It typically presents with vomiting in the third trimester with abdominal pain, malaise, jaundice, thirst, polyuria, and polydypsia. Deranged liver function test results, a high urate level, and hypoglycaemia are features. There may also be hypertension and proteinuria. The woman may be very unwell.

The key thing to recognise here is that these results are very abnormal and should raise significant concern. There should be urgent escalation to a senior obstetrician.

See Chapter 24.

STATION 2

Information for Candidate

Part 1

Ms BC is a 26-year-old para 0+0 woman who is currently 32 weeks pregnant. She is attending the antenatal clinic for review, as she has a body mass index (BMI) of 42 kg/m². During the consultation, she mentions that she has noticed some chest discomfort the last few days.

Please take an appropriate history.

Part 2

What is your differential? What investigations would you like to arrange? What would you like to do next?

See Chapter 24.

Further Information for Model Patient

You have had pain in the centre of your chest for the last 4 days. This started quite suddenly, and is 4/10 in severity. There is no radiation. Taking a breath in makes it worse. You have not noticed any tenderness. You have been feeling a bit short of breath for several weeks, but this has been worse over the last 4 days. You have not had a cough or haemoptysis. You have noticed some swelling and tenderness in your right calf. You are not short of breath on lying flat.

You are a smoker (of 10 cigarettes per day). Your mother has previously had a deep vein thrombosis (DVT) with no obvious cause. You have been much less mobile than usual recently due to symphysis pubis dysfunction. You have no history of travel, surgery nor dehydration.

Answer

Part 1

- Shortness of breath (SOB) is a common presentation in pregnancy and is often physiological. Serious possible underlying causes such as cardiac disease or VTE need to be investigated.
- While cardiac disease is uncommon, it accounts for a fifth of maternal deaths. Ask about orthopnoea, paroxysmal nocturnal dyspnoea, oedema, syncope and palpations.
- Acute-onset SOB is more suspicious of VTE than a gradual-onset history.
- Enquire about the nature of chest pain. Pleuritic chest pain suggests a pulmonary embolism

(PE). Severe central chest pain radiating to the back may suggest aortic dissection. Pain which radiates with associated autonomic symptoms may point towards ischaemic heart disease. Pain which is reproducible on palpation of the chest wall is more likely to be musculoskeletal.

- Symptoms of a DVT should be enquired for.
- Risk factors for thromboembolism should be identified: age >35 years, obesity, parity >3, gross varicose veins, current infection, pre-eclampsia, immobility, recent caesarean or other surgery, personal or family history of venous thrombosis, smoker, multiple pregnancy, IVF
- Respiratory symptoms such as cough, wheeze and haemoptysis may point towards another diagnosis.
- In all pregnant women, gestation, parity, pregnancy history, rhesus status, scans to date (typically, booking and anomaly scan and any additional scans, including growth scans) should be noted.
- Enquire about past obstetric history, medical history, family history, current medications and allergies.
- Always ask specifically about fetal movements (after 20 weeks), the presence of vaginal bleeding, and any symptoms that may suggest rupture of membranes.

Part 2

- In this case, PE needs to be investigated. There is a history of sudden-onset pleuritic chest pain with associated breathless. There are risk factors for VTE, including family history, raised BMI and smoking history.
- Appropriate investigations include an ECG and chest X-ray (CXR) to look for alternative causes for chest pain and breathlessness. Women should be advised that CXR is safe in pregnancy and that the risk to the baby is negligible. Lead aprons are sometimes given to pregnant women having a CXR to provide additional protection to the baby.
- The CXR may reveal an alternative cause for her symptoms, such as pneumonia or pneumothorax.
- Bloods, including FBC (anaemia can cause SOB), liver and renal function, troponin. Do not

perform D-dimer. It is typically raised in pregnancy, and lacks negative predictive value in the pregnant population.

- Diagnosis of PE requires either a lung perfusion scan or a computed tomography pulmonary arteriogram (CTPA). A CTPA carries a greater lifetime risk of breast cancer when performed in pregnancy; therefore, a perfusion scan may be recommended first. A lung perfusion scan works less well if the CXR is abnormal.
- There is a small association with an increase in childhood malignancy (1 in 250,000) with this investigation that women should be informed of.
- If a PE is suspected, women should be admitted and treated with treatment dose low-molecular-weight heparin (LMWH) until investigations have been carried out. Twice-daily dosing of LMWH is required in pregnancy.

See Chapter 24.

STATION 3

Information for Candidate

Part 1

Ms DE is a 28-year-old para 0+0 woman who is currently 34 weeks pregnant. She has been referred to obstetric triage with a headache.

Please take an appropriate history.

Part 2

What further assessment would you like to make?

Part 3

What would you recommend in this case, considering these results?

See Chapter 28.

Further Information for Model Patient

Part 1

You are a 28-year-old para 0+0 and are currently 34 weeks pregnant. Your pregnancy has been uncomplicated so far. You had a normal booking and anomaly scan. You have had an intermittent frontal headache for 4 days, which is worse today. You have also noticed some 'floaters' in front of your vision. Your hands and feet have been more puffy the last week. Your baby is moving well. Your past medical history includes asthma, for which you occasionally use a salbutamol

inhaler. Your mother had pre-eclampsia when she was pregnant with you. You have no allergies.

Further Information for Examiner

Part 2

Ask specifically which blood tests, if they are mentioned.

Part 3

Provide the following information:

The woman's BP readings are 165/95, 160/93 and 159/91 mmHg.

Urinalysis, 3+ protein

On examination, there is oedema to the knees and elbows. Reflexes are brisk and there is 1 beat of clonus. Abdomen is soft and non-tender, with an symphysis-fundal height of measuring 31 cm. CTG is normal.

Investigations:

Hb: 105	(normal >105)
Platelets: 130	(normal >150)
Urea: 4.5	(normal <3.9)
Creatinine: 60	
Urate: 0.48	(normal <0.34)
ALT: 35	(normal <50)
Clotting Screen:	Normal

Answer

Part 1

- Headaches are common in pregnancy and may be migraines or tension-type headaches. As with assessing headache in non-pregnant women, 'red flag' symptoms should be sought which might prompt further investigation, such as imaging or lumbar puncture: sudden onset, severe, loss of consciousness, history of headache, trauma, vomiting, symptoms of meningism (photophobia, rash, neck stiffness, fever).
- Headache, visual disturbance, oedema and epigastric pain may all be symptoms of PET and should be asked about.
- Pregnancy is a pro-thrombotic state; therefore, cerebral sinus thrombosis is more common. Ask about postural association, effect of valsalva manoeuvres, visual disturbance and vomiting. Ask about other thrombosis risk factors.
- A headache after an epidural or spinal anaesthetic may be the result of dural puncture. This

manifests as a headache that is worse when sitting or standing.

- Pregnancy history—Parity, gestation, any issues so far, scans. Pre-clampsia is more common if present in a previous pregnancy, if is the first pregnancy, or if there has been a significant pregnancy interval (>10 years).
- Past medical history—Obesity, pre-existing hypertensive or renal disease, diabetes, connective tissue diseases, inherited thrombophilias, smoking, all increase the risk of PET.
- Personal family history—a family history of PET is a risk factor.

Part 2

- BP and urinalysis are essential first-line tests in any pregnant woman.
- If an initial BP is high, a 'BP profile' is usually commenced, which looks at 3 to 5 readings 10 to 15 minutes apart.
- Proteinuria should be quantified using an albumin: creatinine ratio (ACR) or protein:creatinine ratio (PCR) or 24-hour collection.
- Appropriate IV access and blood tests include FBC, U+Es, LFTs, urate, blood group and save. Always bear in mind pregnancy-specific ranges.
- A neurological examination should be performed. If available, fundoscopy could be performed to assess for papilloedema, which would be an indication of raised intracranial pressure, and to consider further imaging.
- When assessing a woman with suspected PET, look for peripheral oedema, assess reflexes and look for clonus. Significant clonus and brisk reflexes can be a sign of severe pre-eclampsia.
- Palpate the abdomen, assess growth. In this case as the baby is measuring small for dates, a growth scan should be arranged.
- While not indicated here, if an intracranial bleed is suspected, a CT head may be indicated. A CT or MRI venogram is required to exclude cerebral sinus thrombosis.

Part 3

The combination of severe hypertension, significant proteinuria and raised urea/creatinine make the diagnosis of PET likely.

BP must be urgently controlled (less than 150/100 mmHg) to avoid cerebral vascular accidents. First-line treatment would usually be oral labetalol 100 to 200 mg (contraindicated in asthma) or nifedipine 10 to 20 mg with IV treatment labetalol or hydralazine sometimes required in refractory cases.

The woman should be admitted to hospital and should be discussed with senior obstetrician.

In severe PET, an accurate fluid balance is important. Magnesium sulphate IV may be considered to reduce the risk of eclampsia. The timing of birth will depend on the maternal condition, fetal condition and gestational age. If antenatal corticosteroids are indicated, the safety of delaying birth until after these have been taken, is taken into account.

See Chapter 28.

STATION 4

Information for Candidate

Part 1

Ms EF has presented to triage with vaginal bleeding at 26 weeks' gestation with a singleton pregnancy. The bleeding stopped prior to arriving in triage. She has had her observations checked, which are normal, and the fetal heart rate has been auscultated and is normal.

Please take an appropriate history.

Part 2

How would you examine this woman? How would you manage the care of this woman?

See Chapter 26.

Further Information for Model Patient

Ms FE is a para 1, having had an emergency caesarean for failure to progress in the first stage of labour in her last pregnancy. She noticed fresh red blood on her underwear and in the toilet about 2 hours ago. She is not sure how much but thinks it might have been a couple of spoonfuls. She has had a mild cramping pain since, but no further fresh red bleeding. She is happy, with baby's movements. She has had no watery discharge. The bleed did not happen after intercourse. This is the first bleed she has had in pregnancy.

Her booking scan was normal. However, she was told at her anomaly scan that her placenta was low and at the front and she has another ultrasound arranged for 32 weeks 'to see if it has moved'. She is up-to-date with her cervical smears and they have always been normal. She is a non smoker.

On assessment, her abdomen and uterus are soft and non-tender. There is no evidence of ongoing bleeding.

Answer

Part 1

When assessing vaginal bleeding in pregnancy, it is important to know:

- Rhesus status? A rhesus-negative woman may require anti-D.
- Where is the placenta? A low placenta on ultrasound may represent a placenta praevia; these women are a higher risk of significant bleeding. A low, anterior placenta in the context of a previous caesarean section raises the question of potential placenta accreta (the invasion of the placenta into the uterine scar of the previous caesarean section).

Ask about onset of bleeding, amount of bleeding and colour. Brown PV loss suggest old bleeding and less of a concern than fresh red loss. Spotting or bleeding <5 mL is usually of less concern whereas ongoing bleeding >50 mL may be an obstetric emergency.

Was the bleed following intercourse? A postcoital bleed may suggest a cervical ectropion or polyp or, more rarely, cervical cancer. Ask about smear history—missed smears or previously abnormal smears increase the likelihood of cervical cancer, especially in women who smoke.

Are there any symptoms or signs of labour? Is the woman sore or contracting? Is there a history of watery loss that may suggest rupture of membranes? Ask about symptoms of thrush or infection, such as itchiness or offensive discharge.

Could this be a placental abruption? Abruption typically presents with a history of bleeding (although it may be concealed) and pain. On assessment, there is a hard, 'woody' uterus and usually fetal distress or fetal death. Smoking, hypertension and pre-eclampsia are risk factors.

Part 2

An abdominal examination should be performed. Palpate to assess for softness or tenderness. A hard, tender uterus is highly suggestive of an abruption, which is an obstetric emergency. Pads should be checked for further bleeding, as ongoing bleeding is a concern.

Given the history of a low-lying placenta, it is inappropriate to perform a speculum examination on this woman (in some cases, it may be performed but this should be discussed with a senior obstetrician first.) A digital vaginal examination is definitely contra-indicated, as there is a risk of provoking significant bleeding.

Admission for observation is warranted, as this has been a significant antepartum haemorrhage (APH). Ensure wide bore IV access and send bloods, including an FBC and blood group. Let your senior know about the admission, discuss with the senior whether antenatal corticosteroids are needed, and discuss the situation with neonatologists/paediatricians in case pre-term birth becomes necessary.

STATION 5

Information for Candidate

Ms GF is a 36-year-old woman, para 0+0, who is currently 8 weeks pregnant. She is concerned about the chance of her baby having Down syndrome and would like additional information on what tests will be done. In your unit, Down syndrome (T21) screening is done using combined screening.

Please counsel her with regard to Down syndrome screening.

See Chapter 25.

Further Information for Model Patient

Questions to ask:

- How common is Down syndrome?
- Will this test tell me if my baby has Down syndrome?
- Do I have to have an amniocentesis or chorionic villous sampling? Are there any risks associated with either procedure?

Answer

It is important to remain neutral when proving counselling, as your expressions and language may imply judgement and influence someone's decision—for instance, saying that there is a 95% of a baby being unaffected may be understood differently compared with saying that there is a 5% risk of an abnormality.

The chance of Down syndrome increases with age. The chance of having a baby with Down syndrome is 1 in 1500 for women in their 20s, but this rises to 1 in 270 over the age of 35 years and 1 in 50 over the age of 45 years.

It is a personal decision whether to screen for Down syndrome. Women will be counselled by their midwives early in pregnancy as to whether they want a screening test.

A screening test only identifies babies with a higher chance of having the condition; it is not diagnostic and would need to be followed up with a diagnostic test if required.

In the first trimester (up to 14 weeks), T21 screening involves measuring the thickness of the nuchal fluid behind the fetal head (NT) at the booking scan and combining this measurement with information from a blood test (free human chorionic gonadotrophin (hCG) and pregnancy-associated plasma protein A (PAPP-A)). This generates a score, with 'high risk' being defined as a risk of greater than 1 in 150. Different cutoffs can be used; however, this cutoff has a 90% sensitivity for detecting Down syndrome, that is, 1 in 10 babies with Down syndrome will not be identified by screening. The woman then has the option of undergoing a diagnostic test.

Amniocentesis can be performed after 15 weeks. It involves passage of a needle through the abdomen into the amniotic sac under ultrasound guidance and extracting a small amount of amniotic fluid. The miscarriage risk from the procedure is 1%. Chorionic villus sampling (CVS) can be performed after 10 weeks and involves passing a needle under ultrasound guidance to take a sample of placental tissue. The risk of miscarriage from CVS is around 1%.

Non-invasive prenatal screening test (NIPT) is a newer test, but not always widely available. It is a blood test which looks to identify cell-free fetal DNA from maternal blood, which can then be screened for genetic abnormalities. It is more sensitive and specific than conventional screening tests. At present in the United Kingdom, women who have a high risk NIPT result are usually offered a confirmatory diagnostic test, that is, CVS or amniocentesis.

See Chapter 25.

STATION 6
Information for Candidate

Ms GH had a straightforward vaginal birth of a baby girl yesterday. As part of her discharge check, you have been asked to discuss contraception with her.

Please counsel her with regard to postnatal contraception.

See Chapter 21.

Further Information for Model Patient

You are 31-year-old, now para 2. You would like a long-acting form of contraception and intend to breastfeed. You have previously had issues with heavy periods and have no other past medical history of note.

Questions to ask:
- Is it safe to breastfeed?
- What are the side effects?
- How long does the contraception last?
- Does it always work?

Answer

Currently, the World Health Organization recommends a 24-month pregnancy interval. A pregnancy interval of less than 12 months is associated with an increased risk of pre-term birth, low birth weight, stillbirth and neonatal death. Therefore, discussing contraception is an essential component of postnatal care.

The combined oral contraception pill carries an increased risk of VTE and should not be used within 6 weeks postnatally if breastfeeding or within 3 weeks postnatally if not breastfeeding (UKMEC 4 Category)—unacceptable risk).

Nexplanon (etonogestrel) is a low-dose progestogen-only implant which works by preventing ovulation. It is safe to start immediately postnatally (off-licence use) and can be safely used with breastfeeding. A minor surgical procedure is necessary to put it in the upper arm, which can be associated with bruising. There is a small risk of infection and a very small risk of vascular injury. It lasts for up to 3 years and is highly effective, <1 in 1000 pregnancy rate. The most common side effect is irregular bleeding; about 1 in 3 women with Nexplanon change to another contraceptive method due to this.

The progestogen-only pill works by thickening cervical mucus and preventing ovulation. It can be started immediately. The pill must be taken every day at about the same time. It has a medium efficacy (9 pregnancies per 100 women in 1 year). Side effects include irregular bleeding and skin changes. Fifty percent of women will experience amenorrhoea after 1 year.

Depo-Provera (medroxyprogesterone acetate) is a progestogen-only injection which works by preventing ovulation. It can be started immediately postnatally (off-licence use). It has a medium efficacy (6 pregnancies per 100 women in 1 year). It involves an injection every 13 weeks. Fifty percent of women will experience amenorrhoea. Side effects include irregular bleeding, weight gain and skin changes. There can be a delay of up to 1 year after cessation before periods and fertility returns. Long-term use can cause loss of bone density, which is regained upon stopping.

The copper coil and LNG-IUS can be inserted within 48 hours of birth or after 4 weeks postnatally. Contraindications involve risk factors for infection (prolonged rupture of membranes or sepsis.) They are highly effective (99%) and can last for up to 5 years. Some brands of LNG-IUS last 3 years; some types of copper coil last 10 years. There is an increased risk of expulsion when placed postnatally—1 in 7 risk of expulsion compared with 1 in 20 usually. Typically, women should have a 6-week examination to check that the threads are present. There is a risk of infection (1/100) and uterine perforation (1/200). The LNG-IUS coil contains progestogen. It usually makes periods lighter (90% reduction in bleeding at 1 year) but can cause erratic bleeding, particularly in the first 3 to 6 months. The copper coil contains no hormones and works by inhibiting fertilization. It can make periods heavier, longer and more painful; thus, it may be best avoided in women who have had problems with their periods prior to pregnancy.

See Chapter 21.

STATION 7

Information for Candidate

You are working on the postnatal ward as a junior doctor. An emergency buzzer has been pulled and you find that Mrs JK, a 29-year-old para 1 woman who gave birth vaginally to a baby boy 4 hours ago, has collapsed. There is blood on the bed. Please make an appropriate assessment.

See Chapters 26 and 35.

Further Information for Examiner

 A. Airway is patent, oxygen saturations are 90% on room air.

 B. Chest is clear, respiratory rate 20, trachea central.

 C. HR 130 beats per minute, BP 95/65 mmHg, capillary refill 2 seconds, cool peripheries.

 D. Temperature 37°C, Glasgow Coma Scale 15.

 E. There is a significant amount of blood on the bed and on the floor.

When the candidate starts examining the abdomen provide this additional information:

The senior doctor has now arrived. The senior doctor examines the woman and finds that the fundus is above the umbilicus and the uterus is boggy. Multiple clots are expelled from the cervix on vaginal examination. Blood loss is estimated to be at 1.5 L and is ongoing. Preparations are made to transfer the woman to theatre.

Ask:

1. What are the possible causes of a primary postpartum haemorrhage?
2. How can uterine atony be reversed?

Answer

Ensure that help is on the way by making an emergency call if needed. Check environment for hazards.

 A. Maintain airway patency, give oxygen if appropriate via face mask, check oxygen saturations.

 B. Assess RR and auscultate chest

 C. Monitor HR and BP. This woman's BP is 95/60 mmHg and her heart rate is 130/min. IV access should be gained. Two wide-bore peripheral cannulas should be inserted and bloods sent, including FBC, coagulation, urea and electrolytes and liver function tests. Crossmatch is appropriate at this stage if not already done. There is evidence of haemorrhagic shock; therefore, IV fluid resuscitation with a crystalloid fluid should be given.

 D. Assess GCS and temperature.

 E. Expose the woman.

This is a major obstetric haemorrhage— a primary postpartum haemorrhage. The 4 causes are atony (most common), trauma, coagulopathy and retained placental tissue. There are often multiple causes. If the uterus is atonic, bimanual compression is often effective as initial management.

Pharmacological uterotonics include:

- IV/IM oxytocin bolus, which can be followed by an infusion
- IV/IM ergometrine (avoid in hypertensive disorders)
- IM carboprost (avoid in women with asthma)
- PR misoprostol

IV fluids, blood and blood products should be given. Tranexamic acid can also be given to assist with haemostasis.

Surgical interventions include inserting an intra-uterine balloon to apply pressure to the placenta bed, a 'brace' suture across the uterus, such as a B-Lynch (requires laparotomy), and, as a last resort, hysterectomy. Uterine artery embolization is an interventional radiological procedure.

See Chapters 26 and 35.

STATION 8

Information for Candidate

You are working on the postnatal wards as a junior doctor. You are asked to review Ms LM, who is a 29-year-old, now para 2, who had a caesarean birth of a baby girl 6 hours ago. You are told that she suddenly looks very unwell.

See Chapter 35.

Further Information for Examiner

A. Airway is patent, oxygen saturations 89% on room air.

B. RR is 35 breaths per minute, chest sounds clear.

C. BP is 93/60 mmHg. HR is 130/min. Peripheries feel cool to elbows and have mottled appearance.

D. Temperature 40°C, GCS 15, BMI 4.1.

E. Abdomen is soft, uterus is tender, contracted to 2 cm below the umbilicus.

There are no rashes. The lochia is offensive.

Ask what the diagnosis and initial management is.

After 1.5 L IV fluids, the woman's observations are as follows: BP 85/60, RR 40, temperature 40°C, saturations 95% (on 15 litres/min oxygen). The lactate on an arterial blood gas was 5.

Whom would you want to contact?

Answer

A. Maintain airway patency, give 15 L oxygen via face mask, check oxygen saturations.

B. Assess RR and auscultate chest

C. Monitor HR and BP. IV access should be gained and blood test taken. IV fluid resuscitation with crystalloid fluid should be given.

D. Assess GCS and temperature

E. Assess abdomen and fundus. If the woman is catheterized, assess urine output. Look for signs of bleeding.

This woman is pyrexic, tachycardic, with a high RR, an oxygen requirement and a low BP. This indicates severe sepsis. Within 12 hours of birth, chorioamnionitis is a likely cause, although other causes such as pneumonia or renal tract infection should be considered. Mastitis is another cause of sepsis postnatally.

She is very sick and needs prompt resuscitation and escalation of care. IV access should be gained and IV fluid challenge should be given (i.e., 1 L crystalloid fluid stat.)

FBC/U+E/LFTs/CRP/lactate, coagulation screen and glucose should be sent. An arterial blood gas would be indicated in this situation to assess acid-base status and lactate.

A bacteriological survey would include urine cultures, a high vaginal swab, throat swabs, placental swabs and blood cultures. A CXR can be considered. She should be catheterized and urine output monitored and broad-spectrum antibiotics should be given within 1 hour ('sepsis 6 bundle').

This woman will need urgent care from a senior obstetrician and critical care doctor.

See Chapter 35.

STATION 9

Information for Candidate

Ms NM is currently 24 weeks pregnant and has been referred by her midwife to the antenatal clinic due to concerns about significant varicose veins. As part of the consultation, your consultant has asked you to perform a thromboembolism risk assessment.

Part 1

What are risk factors for thromboembolism would you look for in the history?

Part 2

You decide that Ms NM meets the criteria for thromboprophylaxis from 28 weeks' gestation. Please council Ms NM appropriately.

See Chapters 23 and 24.

Further Information for Model Patient

This woman has 3 risk factors: varicose veins, maternal age (she is 36 years old) and smoking history.

Questions for the woman to ask:

- How do I take it?
- Are there any risks to the baby?
- What are the risks if I choose not to take it?
- Will this affect how I give birth to my baby?

Answer

Part 1

Thromboprophylaxis with LMWH may be recommended with the following major risk factors:

- Major pelvic surgery
- Personal history of VTE
- Heritable and acquired thrombophilia
- Caesarean section

Thromboprophylaxis with LMWH may be recommended postnatally when 2 risk factors are present, from 28 weeks with 3 of the following minor risk factors, or from the second trimester if 4 of these risk factors are present:

- Age (>35 years)
- Obesity (BMI >30)
- Parity (> Para 3)
- Gross varicose veins
- Current infection
- Pre-eclampsia
- Immobility, for example, severe pelvic girdle pain, long-distance travel
- Major current illness
- Family history
- Smoking
- Multiple pregnancy
- Hyperemesis, dehydration
- IVF
- Postpartum haemorrhage
- Operative vaginal birth
- Pre-term birth
- Prolonged labour

Part 2

Ultimately, it is the woman's choice whether she wishes to take LMWH. It is being recommended to reduce the increased risk to her of a PE, which would carry the risks of a serious cardiac event or death. The risks of thromboembolism should be discussed and women should be aware of the signs and symptoms of PE and DVT.

LMWH is a subcutaneous injection given once or twice daily, usually in the thigh or abdomen. Women should be shown how to perform the injection and dispose of the needles safely. It is safe to use in pregnancy and does not cross the placenta. Spinal anaesthetic is not usually given within 12 hours of LMWH; therefore, women should be advised to stop injections if they have any bleeding or show any signs of labour.

See Chapters 23 and 24.

STATION 10

Information for Candidate

Ms LP is attending the antenatal clinic at 36 weeks of pregnancy for a routine check.

Please perform an abdominal palpation.
See Chapter 2.

Answer

Ensure privacy and gain consent. Consider position—examine with the woman in a semi-recumbent position (this usually involves moving the back of the bed down) but try to minimise the amount of time that a pregnant woman spends lying flat on her back.

Inspect the abdomen, noting distension, any asymmetry, fetal movements, any striae gravidarum, the presence of a linea nigra or any scars.

Measure the symphysis-fundal SFH (measure between the symphysis pubis and the fundus). After 20 weeks, this is usually equivalent to the number of weeks' gestation ± 2 cm, that is, 32 cm at 32 weeks.

Gently palpate to feels for fetal 'poles', that is, head and bottom. This will allow you to identify the lie of the fetus (longitudinal, transverse or oblique) and the presentation (cephalic, breech or legs or limbs). Work out which side the fetal back is on. Assess how far down in the pelvis the presenting part is—how many fifths palpable is it and is it engaged? An assessment of liquor volume can be made depending on how tense the abdomen feels and how easily palpable the fetal parts are.

Assess the fetal heart by placing a Doppler transducer over the anterior shoulder of the fetus. Remember to wipe away any ultrasound gel on the woman's abdomen.

Allow the woman privacy to get dressed. Record the measurements in her notes and plot the SFH measurements on the chart.

See Chapter 2.

STATION 11

Information for Candidate

Part 1

You are a junior doctor working in the obstetric assessment area. Ms RS is a 24-year-old para 1 who is currently 33 weeks pregnant. She has presented to obstetric triage with a 12-hour history of lower abdominal pain and tightening.

Please take an appropriate history.

Part 2

On examination, the woman is distressed by the pain. There are palpable tightenings, 2 to 3 every 10 min. Her abdomen is soft between contractions. The fetus palpates as cephalic. The CTG looks normal.

You have asked your registrar to supervise you performing a speculum examination. Please demonstrate on the model how you would perform a speculum examination.

See Chapter 2 and 29.

Further Information for Model Patient

Part 1

Ms RS has had lower abdominal pain for 12 hours now. This is intermittent, initially happening once every 20 minutes, but she is now aware of it every few minutes. The pain lasts about 30 seconds when it is there and is severe—she is unable to talk when she has the pain. Yesterday, she was aware that she was leaking fluid for most of the day, enough to soak her underwear and clothes. The fluid was clear and odourless. She has not had any vaginal bleeding. She is happy with fetal movements. She reports no urinary or bowel symptoms, no nausea or vomiting.

She is para 1 having a spontaneous vaginal birth at 33 weeks in her last pregnancy. In this pregnancy, she has been attending the pre-term birth clinic and has had growth scans and cervical length scans, which have been normal. She is usually fit and well outside of pregnancy. She is taking no medications and has no allergies.

Part 2

A speculum examinations demonstrates a liquor pooling in the vagina. The cervix looks closed.

Ask: What is the recommended treatment?

Answer

Part 1

- Abdominal pain—site, onset, character, relieving and exacerbating factors, severity
- Any vaginal discharge, including history of bleeding or history suggestive of spontaneous rupture of membranes (SRM). Pre-term pre-labour rupture of membranes and bleeding in the first and second trimester increase the risk of pre-term labour.
- Fetal movements
- Urinary symptoms, bowel symptoms, nausea and vomiting. Urinary tract infections are associated with pre-term birth.
- Pregnancy history, including parity, history of complications in this and previous pregnancies. Previous pre-term birth is a risk factor for another pre-term birth.
- Scan history—fetal growth restriction, polyhydramnios, congenital abnormalities and placenta praevia are associcated with pre-term birth.
- Medical history – Congenital uterine structural anomalies are associated with pre-term birth.

The history is suggestive of pre-term pre-labour SRM and pre-term labour. This woman is high risk, having had a previous pre-term birth. Examination to look for liquor to confirm this and assess the cervix is appropriate.

Part 2

It is very important to use an aseptic technique when performing a speculum examination when SRM is suspected. Sterile gloves should be used, and the vulva may be washed with an antiseptic solution.

Ensure privacy and explain the procedure. Obtain consent and have a chaperone present. To perform the examination, the woman should be in recumbent position—minimise the amount of time a pregnant woman spends lying supine. Lubricate the blades of the speculum with gel and insert with blades in a horizontal position, rotating around to vertical as the speculum is advanced. When the speculum is fully inserted, gently open the speculum.

Membrane rupture is diagnosed when liquor is seen pooling in the vagina. Liquor may be seen coming through the cervix, particularly when the woman is asked to cough. It is important to take a high vaginal swab, in particular to look for group B streptococcus. The cervix should be inspected to assess whether it is open. A digital examination should be avoided where possible unless labour is suspected, as this may introduce infection.

Fetal fibronectin is a swab test that is sometimes performed when pre-term labour is suspected. A speculum examination is done without lubricating gel and a swab is taken from the posterior fornix. A negative result gives a less than 5% chance of labouring in the next week. There is no need to perform this in cases of confirmed rupture of membranes, as these women are already high risk of pre-term labour (and it will be positive).

A diagnosis of pre-term pre-labour rupture of membranes can be made. A diagnosis of pre-term labour cannot be made, as cervical change has not be demonstrated, but this is suspected. She has a high chance of pre-term birth.

An ultrasound should be performed to check presentation. The woman should be admitted, likely to a labour ward initially. Antibiotics are given following pre-term pre-labour rupture of the membranes, as they have been shown to benefit the baby—typically, 10 days of oral erythromycin. Corticosteroids should be considered after discussion with a senior obstetrician, as pre-term birth is more likely. These are usually given as two IM injections 24 hours apart (dexamethasone or betamethasone). Magnesium sulphate may also be considered for neuroprotection if pre-term birth appears likely although generally reserved for the more pre-term gestations.

See Chapters 2 and 29.

STATION 12

Information for Candidate

Part 1

You are a junior doctor working in an obstetric antenatal clinic. Ms TN has been advised by her community midwife that she should attend for an oral glucose tolerance test, as she has a family history of diabetes. She is unsure what this test is or why she is having it.

Please explain the test to Ms TN.

Part 2

Investigations:
  Results:
  Fasting glucose level 7.1 (abnormal >5.6)
  2-hour glucose level 9.3 (abnormal >7.8)

Please explain this result to Ms TN and how this might affect her care in pregnancy.

See Chapter 24.

Further Information for Model Patient

Part 1

You are 31 years old and this is your first pregnancy; you are currently 28 weeks pregnant. Your BMI is 34 and you have no past medical history of note. Your mother has type 2 diabetes.

Part 2

Questions to ask:
- Does this mean that I now have diabetes?
- What treatment will I need? Will I have to inject insulin?
- How will this affect my baby?
- Does this mean I will need to have an induction?
- Will I get diabetes again in the future?

See Chapter 24.

Answer

Part 1

Gestational diabetes is a type of diabetes that develops during pregnancy.

In the United Kingdom, women are currently offered testing for gestational diabetes between 24 and 28 weeks if they have risk factors—family history, high BMI, previous large baby, or if they belong to an ethnic group with higher rates of diabetes. This is usually done by offering a 2-hour 75-g glucose tolerance test.

To perform this test, women fast from midnight the night before. They have 2 blood tests to measure blood glucose—one fasting and one 2 hours after consuming a carbohydrate drink. If these values are higher than the recommended cut-offs, a diagnosis of gestational diabetes is made.

Part 2

Treatment aims to keep blood sugar levels controlled while avoiding hypoglycaemia. Women will be encouraged to check their blood sugars frequently and keep a record of these results. The first step is treatment with dietary modification. Women are usually seen in dedicated clinics where they can get multidisciplinary advice from midwives, obstetricians, endocrinologists and dieticians. If targets are not achieved, metformin and, subsequently, insulin are the next steps.

Women with gestational diabetes have an increased risk of fetal macrosomia. This can increase the likelihood of labour and birth complications, including induction of labour, caesarean and shoulder dystocia. For this reason, growth and liquor volume scans are usually performed from 28 weeks. There is also an increased risk of polyhydramnios, prematurity, pre-eclampsia, stillbirth, neonatal hypoglycaemia and jaundice. Good blood sugar control reduces these risks. The timing of birth is individualised to the woman. Induction of labour is not necessarily required in women with gestational diabetes.

Women with gestational diabetes in one pregnancy have a 75% chance of having gestational diabetes in subsequent pregnancies. Monitoring and treatment is usually started early in these pregnancies. They also have an increased risk of developing type 2 diabetes in the future.

See Chapter 24.

Answers to Single Best Answer (SBA) questions – part one

Alice Main, Mayank Madhra

Answers

Chapter 2

Q1. Answer: e – When it has been more than 12 months since her last period
Explanation: Menopause can only be diagnosed retrospectively, which is 12 months after the last menstrual period. Symptoms of hot flushes, mood swings and vaginal dryness are common when a woman is 'perimenopausal'. However, these are suggestive of low levels of estrogen and not specifically for being postmenopausal.

Q2. Answer: d – The ischial spine
The ischial spines are a pair of bony prominences of the pelvis that can be palpated through the posterior vaginal wall during examination. The station of the presenting part is measured in centimetre in relation to the level of the spine from 0 to −5 above or from 0 to +5 below the spine. It is used as a marker of progression in labour.

Q3. Answer: d – Mittelschmerz pain
Mittelschmerz is mid-cycle pain caused by the process of ovulation. Commonly, it is a cramping or dull one-sided pain which can continue for 1 to 2 days. This woman is mid-cycle and has no other concerning signs or symptoms; it is the most likely cause ovarian torsion tends to be sudden onset and associated with vomiting. Endometriosis typically causes painful periods and women tend to present with a longer history of pain. Ectopic pregnancy is excluded with a negative pregnancy test. Pelvic inflammatory disease is also possible but is usually associated with vaginal discharge.

Chapter 4

Q1. Answer: e – Luteinizing hormone

Ovulation is triggered by the mid-cycle surge in luteinizing hormone. It causes rupture of the mature follicle with release of the oocyte.

Q2. Answer: a – Reassurance
Primary amenorrhoea is only diagnosed once aged 16 years or older. The reassuring points in this case are that she has normal secondary sexual characteristics and a normal body weight. Further investigation is only warranted after the age of 16 years and, even then, with normal secondary sexual characteristics, it is most likely to be a physiological delay.

Q3. Answer: d – Day 21
If ovulation has occurred, progesterone levels peak 7 days before menstruation, on day 21 of a 28-day cycle. Therefore, this is the best day to measure progesterone levels. This is a commonly used test during fertility investigations. Progesterone is produced by the corpus luteum, which strongly implies that ovulation has taken place.

Chapter 6

Q1. Answer: c – A miscarriage occurs with no pain or bleeding
Answer *a* describes an incomplete miscarriage. Answer *b* is a complete miscarriage. Answer *d* is a threatened miscarriage. Answer *e* is recurrent miscarriage.

Q2. Answer: b – Low molecular weight heparin (LMWH) and aspirin
This woman has antibodies that confirm antiphospholipid syndrome. Untreated, she will have a miscarriage rate of 70% to 80%. Low-dose aspirin and heparin help reduce the risk of miscarriage and obstetric complications related to placental

dysfunction. Because of variation between laboratories when testing for anti-phospholipid antibodies, a positive result should be repeated in the same laboratory after an interval of 12 weeks.

Q3. Answer: a – Conservative management with hCG monitoring

The woman meets the criteria for conservative management as she is stable, pain free with a falling hCG of <1500 IU/L, and the ectopic pregnancy is <35 mm in diameter. All of the options should be discussed with her but she has stated that she would like to avoid intervention if possible. Therefore, conservative management seems to be an appropriate option for her.

Chapter 8

Q1. Answer: e – Diagnostic laparoscopy

Although pelvic ultrasound and MRI may detect large endometriotic lesions, diagnostic laparoscopy remains the gold standard test and can often provide a tissue diagnosis. Endometrial biopsies and hysteroscopy are used to detect abnormalities in the endometrial lining of the uterus.

Chapter 10

Q1. Answer: a – Pregnancy and childbirth

All of these answers are potential contributors in the development of pelvic organ prolapse. However, the most common and most likely cause is pregnancy and childbirth, with one-third of women who have had children developing symptomatic prolapse.

Q2. Answer: c – Stage II

Stage II is when the most distal portion of the prolapse is 1 cm or less proximal or distal to the plane of the hymen. Stage 0 is no prolapse, Stage I is more than 1 cm above the plane of the hymen, Stage III is more than 1 cm below but protrudes no further than 2 cm less than the total vaginal length, and Stage IV is essentially complete eversion of the total length of the lower genital tract (also known as a procidentia).

Chapter 12

Q1. Answer: c – Ovarian cancer

Symptoms are often insidious in ovarian cancer but common symptoms are abdominal discomfort, bloating, early satiety, loss of appetite and urinary frequency. Her age, nulliparity and smoking history are all risk factors. No change in bowel habit

is mentioned; therefore, colon cancer, coeliac disease and constipation are all unlikely. Uterine fibroids tend to present in the reproductive years.

Q2. Answer: c – Stage Ic

The fact that the cancer is confined to the ovaries makes it Stage I and the finding of positive peritoneal washings makes it Ic. There is no mention of extension to other organs or peritoneal spread; therefore, it does not fit into the Stage II or III classification.

Chapter 14

Q1. Answer: a – Simple columnar epithelium

The endocervix is lined by simple columnar epithelium and the ectocervix is lined by squamous epithelium. They meet at the transformation zone which is vulnerable to cytological abnormalities.

Q2. Answer: c – HPV 16 and 18

A strong association has been observed between HPV serotypes 16 and 18 (and others) and preinvasive disease and invasive cervical cancer. Other strains may be linked but do not appear to be as 'high risk' as 16 and 18.

Chapter 16

Q1. Answer: e – Human papillomavirus (HPV)

In a similar manner to cervical intraepithelial neoplasia (CIN) and cervical cancer, HPV can predispose to vulval intraepithelial neoplasia and vulval cancer. The other infections listed do not have a strong association with VIN.

Q2. Answer: c – Marsupialization under general anaesthetic

Given the recurrent nature of this woman's abscess, it would be recommended to offer her marsupialization of the abscess under general anaesthetic. This involves suturing the edges of the abscess to the surrounding skin to prevent the incision from closing over the abscess cavity and the abscess reforming. Antibiotics tend to have minimal effect in this scenario. Further incision and drainage is unlikely to prevent recurrence. Seton sutures are used in perianal fistulas and not Bartholin gland abscesses.

Chapter 18

Q1. Answer: b – Trichomoniasis

A thin or 'frothy' green discharge paired with an inflamed (strawberry) cervix and vaginal itchiness is typical of *Trichomonas vaginalis*. Bacterial vaginosis tends to produce a thin white 'fishy' discharge, which is usually not itchy. Gonorrhoea is asymptomatic in the majority of cases, or causes a mucopurulent discharge. Candidiasis causes a thick 'cottage cheese'–like discharge and itch. Primary syphilis presents with a painless chancre on the genital region.

Q2. Answer: a – Metronidazole 400 mg twice a day for 7 days
The presence of clue cells on a swab paired with a fishy discharge suggests a diagnosis of bacterial vaginosis (BV), the treatment of which is metronidazole. Clotrimazole is used to treat vaginal candidiasis. Doxycycline is used to treat chlamydia or suspected pelvic inflammatory disease (PID). Azithromycin and ceftriaxone are often used together to treat gonorrhoea.

Chapter 20

Q1. Answer: a – Reduced fertility
There is no established positive association between previous termination of pregnancy and future subfertility, ectopic pregnancy or placenta praevia. There may be a slight increase in risk of subsequent miscarriage and pre-term birth with mid-trimester termination of pregnancy, although the evidence is unclear. The other answers are all recognised complications; women should be counselled for them prior to undergoing surgical termination of pregnancy.

Q2. Answer: b – Steroidal anti-progestogen that blocks the action of progesterone in the uterus
Answer *a* is the action of misoprostol. Answer *c* describes ergometrine. Answer *d* is the mechanism of oxytocin. Answer *e* is the mechanism of clomifene and tamoxifen.

Chapter 23

Q1. Answer: e – Fasting serum glucose
If a woman has risk factors for gestational diabetes mellitus (GDM), an oral glucose tolerance test is indicated at 24 to 28 weeks or sooner if there is a personal history of GDM. All of the other blood tests are part of the routine tests offered in the first trimester.

Q2. Answer: d – Cord prolapse
Women with polyhydramnios should be counselled for the risk of cord prolapse, especially if planning artificial rupture of membranes. The other risks listed are not recognised associations.

Chapter 25

Q1. Answer: d – 1 in 100
The risk of chromosomal abnormality increases with maternal age. At age 40, the risk is 1 in 100. Answer *a* is the risk at age 20, *b* is the risk at age 30, *c* is the risk at age 35 and *e* is the risk at age 45.

Q2. Answer: d – Spina bifida
CVS is usually performed between 11 and 13+6 weeks and can detect chromosomal conditions such as Down syndrome and genetic disorders such as cystic fibrosis, fragile X syndrome and phenylketonuria. Spina bifida is a neural tube defect, a structural abnormality and is usually diagnosed by ultrasound.

Chapter 27

Q1. Answer: d – Estimated weight is <10th centile for gestational age
The definition is based on centiles for head circumference and abdominal circumference; the cutoff for diagnosing small for gestational age (SGA) is <10th centile.

Q2. Answer: a – Maternal depression
There is no clear link between maternal depression and having an SGA baby. All of the other answers are recognised major risk factors for SGA and should prompt further monitoring in pregnancy.

Chapter 29

Q1. Answer: e – Erythromycin
The Royal College of Obstetrics and Gynaecologists recommends that a 10-day course of oral erythromycin be administered following the diagnosis of pre-term pre-labour rupture of membranes (PPROM) as it reduces the risk of chorioamnionitis and neonatal infection. Clindamycin and gentamicin have been proven to not be as effective. Co-amoxiclav should not be prescribed, as its use is associated with an increased risk of necrotising enterocolitis for the neonate. Nitrofurantoin can cause fetal haemolysis when used in the third trimester; thus, it is best to avoid it.

Q2. Answer: b – 34 to 40 mm
Cervical length is assessed using transvaginal ultrasound and the normal length is 34 to 40 mm with no funnelling at the internal os. If cervical shortening (<25 mm) is found, interventions such as a cervical suture can be considered.

Q3. Answer: e – Calcium channel blocker
Nifedipine acts to inhibit the inward calcium flow across cell membranes, thus, reducing uterine contractility. Atosiban is an oxytocin antagonist. Terbutaline is a beta-2 receptor agonist. Progesterone agonists and alpha-adrenergic agonists are not used for tocolysis.

Chapter 31

Q1. Answer: c – Prolongation of the second stage of labour
There is an association between epidural analgesia and prolonged second stage of labour with an increased rate of assisted vaginal birth. There is no proven association between epidural and the other answers.

Q2. Answer: b – Second-degree tear
First-degree tears involve the vaginal epithelium and vulval skin only. Second-degree tears involve perineal muscles but not the anal sphincter. Third-degree tears involve the anal sphincter complex and are graded a, b or c depending on the extent of the involvement. Fourth-degree tears involve the anal sphincter and anal/rectal mucosa.

Chapter 33

Q1. Answer: c – Book an induction of labour.
The risk of stillbirth increases after week 41 of pregnancy and, once she is 42+ weeks, the perinatal mortality doubles compared with term. For this reason, induction of labour should be planned between 41 and 42 weeks. As her cervix is unfavourable, artificial rupture of membranes would not be possible. Thus, she will likely need an induction agent prior to this. There is currently no indication for a caesarean section.

Q2. Answer: d – Clinically 'large for dates' baby
In the absence of any other indications, induction of labour should not be carried out simply because a health care professional suspects that a baby is large for gestational age. Women who are aged 40 years or above are routinely offered induction at term due to increased risks of stillbirth. Women with pre-existing or gestational diabetes are routinely offered induction at or before term. Post-dates induction is recommended between 41 and 42 weeks to reduce the risk of stillbirth. Women who have not gone into spontaneous labour 24 hours after rupturing their membranes are recommended to consider induction of labour to reduce the risk of infection.

Chapter 35

Q1. Answer: c – Amniotic fluid embolus
Amniotic fluid embolism (AFE) most commonly presents in labour or immediately after birth. Risk factors include multiparity (as in this case), multiple pregnancy, polyhydramnios, abdominal trauma and precipitate labour. Cyanosis and respiratory distress are the most common early presenting signs of AFE. These are shortly followed by cardiovascular collapse ± coma. There is no mention of blood pressure problems or seizure activity in this case; thus, eclampsia is unlikely. Bleeding is minimal; thus, it is unlikely to be the cause of her collapse. AFE often leads to a profound coagulopathy.

Q2. Answer: a – McRoberts position
The McRoberts position involves flexion and abduction of the maternal hips with positioning of the maternal thighs onto the abdomen and is the recommended first-line manoeuvre once shoulder dystocia is recognised. This should be followed by suprapubic pressure. Fundal pressure should never be used. Episiotomy is not always necessary but should be considered if not already performed. The next steps include internal manoeuvres such as internal rotation or delivery of the posterior arm. If this is unsuccessful, change the woman's position to all fours.

Chapter 37

Q1. Answer: b – Antepartum stillbirth
In the United Kingdom, the death of a baby between 24 weeks and birth (with no signs of life) is known as a stillbirth. In this case, the woman was not in labour; thus, it would be classified as an antenatal stillbirth as opposed to intrapartum if she was in labour. It would be classified as a miscarriage had it occurred before 24 weeks. Early neonatal death is a death within the first 7 days of life and late neonatal death is from 7 to 28 days.

Q2. Answer: b – 40%
In the United Kingdom, the survival rate to discharge for a baby born at 24 weeks' gestation is 60%. It is 30% at 22 weeks, 40% at 23 weeks, 80% at 26 weeks and 95% at 31 weeks.

Chapter 39

Q1. Answer: d – Haemorrhage

Maternal haemorrhage is responsible for around a third of maternal deaths in Africa. This is compared with around 13% in high-income countries. Oxytocin is very effective in preventing postpartum haemorrhage but may not be routinely used or available globally.

Q2. Answer: c – Administer 4g IV magnesium sulphate

Magnesium sulphate is the most effective agent for the treatment of eclampsia – it can be given intramuscularly or intravenously. If her blood pressure remains elevated, she will then need additional anti-hypertensive medication, such as IV labetalol. Following this, you would need to make an immediate plan for birth.

Chapter 41

Q1. Answer: e – Head circumference, abdominal circumference and femur length

These are the three parameters measured in later pregnancy to monitor growth and estimate fetal weight. It is recognised that these measurements have a margin of error; thus, clinical decisions should not be made based on small changes on the growth charts.

Q2. Answer: b – Pelvic ultrasound

Pelvic ultrasound is the first-line imaging technique used in gynaecology. Both the transabdominal and transvaginal routes allow an excellent assessment of the uterus and the adnexae. Pelvic X-ray has little use other than assessing tubal patency in hysterosalpingography. CT scanning is often used in suspected malignancy for staging purposes. MRI may be used following ultrasound to further characterise ovarian masses, fibroids or severe endometriosis. PET scans are reserved for assessing malignancy.

Chapter 44

Q1. Answer: a – Placental abruption

Pain and bleeding in late pregnancy is placental abruption until proven otherwise. This is an obstetric emergency; she should be transferred to the labour ward or theatre immediately. Bleeding from placenta praevia, vasa praevia or cervical ectropion tends to be painless. Early labour would cause contraction-like pain and should not be constant.

Q2. Answer: c – Vaginal candidiasis

Vaginal candidiasis, or 'thrush', is common in pregnancy and causes a vaginal itch associated with a plaque-like white discharge on examination. It is common for women to feel an increased 'wetness' due to the discharge it causes. There is no liquor on examination; thus, it is unlikely she has ruptured her membranes. Physiological discharge is more like milk than plaque-like and bacterial vaginosis commonly causes a fishy, thin discharge. It is also not uncommon for pregnant woman to mistake urine leakage as their waters break; thus, it is important to check the urine for signs of infection.

Answers to Single Best Answer (SBA) questions – part two

Alice Main, Mayank Madhra

Answers

Chapter 1

Q1. Answer: c – Puborectalis
Laterally, the muscle sheets of the iliococcygeus and ischiococcygeus are oblique/transverse. The medial fibres of the puborectalis are inserted into the upper part of the perineal body and the succeeding fibres turn medially behind the anorectal flexure, and are inserted into the anococcygeal raphe and the tip of the coccyx.

Q2. Answer: b – The isthmus
Female sterilization involves occluding the entire lumen of both tubes, which is best performed in the narrow isthmic portion, using clips, sutures, rings or diathermy.

Chapter 3

Q1. Answer: c – A multicystic appearance to the ovaries on ultrasound suggests constitutional puberty.
Children with precocious puberty should be under the care of a paediatric endocrinologist, although not all children will need treatment. Café-au-lait skin pigmentation suggests McCune–Albright syndrome, which is very rare. A radiological skeletal survey of the long bones is indicated if this syndrome is suspected; otherwise, an X-ray of the hand to determine bone age is more appropriate. A multicystic appearance to the ovaries on ultrasound is seen in normal puberty, and so may be seen with constitutional or cerebral precocious puberty.

Q2. Answer: c – X-ray for bone age is a first-line investigation.
X-ray for bone age is a first-line investigation for both delayed and precocious puberty. Delayed puberty in girls is defined as the absence of physical manifestations

of puberty by the age of 13 years. Short stature is commonly seen with constitutional delay. Reassurance may suffice for management of constitutional delay. Anorexia is a recognised cause of hypogonadotrophic hypogonadism.

Chapter 5

Q1. Answer: c – Hysteroscopy
Hysteroscopy should only be performed selectively to assess for structural intrauterine abnormalities. Hysterosalpingography assesses for tubal patency, and AMH and luteal phase progesterone (which is taken on day 21 for women with a 28-day cycle) are all first-line investigations, as is BMI.

Q2. Answer: c – Multivitamins have been associated with an improvement in sperm parameters.
Multivitamins are recommended for all men whose partners are trying to conceive.

Testicular biopsy can confirm non-obstructive azoospermia (in men with a raised FSH and azoospermia); this is not purely diagnostic, as islands of spermatogenesis can be identified on occasion. Sperm can be extracted at the time of testicular biopsy and used for intracytoplasmic sperm injection (ICSI).

The chance of live birth is 14% per cycle for unstimulated donor insemination (DI) and 15% for stimulated DI.

Surgery is no longer recommended for varicocele in otherwise asymptomatic men, as there is no evidence that this improves sperm count. Pregnancy rates are around 30% following re-anastomotic surgery more than 10 years after the original vasectomy.

Chapter 7

Q1. Answer: d – Levonorgestrel-releasing intrauterine system (LNG-IUS)
The IUS can be considered when fibroids measure less than 3 cm and cause no distortion of the uterine

cavity. Fibroids of this size are unlikely to be causing pressure-related symptoms to surrounding organs, nor do they significantly contribute to heavy menstrual bleeding as the cavity is undisturbed. Myomectomy and hysterectomy carry a risk of surgical complications (and myomectomy would be technically challenging with such a small fibroid). Uterine artery embolisation (UAE) and Gonadotropin releasing hormone (GnRH) analogues have more side effects than the LNG-IUS.

Q2. Answer: d – Inhibits plasminogen activator.
Antifibrinolytics, such as tranexamic acid, work by inhibiting plasminogen activator, thereby reducing the fibrinolytic activity in the endometrium. This stabilises clot formation in the spiral arterioles and reduces menstrual blood loss.

Q3. Answer: d – High vaginal swab, including tests for chlamydia and gonorrhoea
This woman describes secondary dysmenorrhoea, which requires investigation. This refers to dysmenorrhoea developing over many years after menarche and is the result of an underlying pathology. Pain usually starts 3 to 4 days before the onset of the period. Possible causes include endometriosis, adenomyosis, pelvic inflammatory disease and fibroids. Swabs are helpful in excluding active pelvic infections, which are generally more prevalent in younger, sexually active populations. If pelvic masses such as fibroids are suspected on examination, a pelvic ultrasound may be useful. A trial of the progesterone-only pill or LNG-IUS would be reasonable after excluding sexually transmitted infections. If this is unsuccessful, or symptoms persist, diagnostic laparoscopy could be considered. However, since this carries risks of operative complications, it would not be the first investigation indicated.

Chapter 9

Q1. Answer: e – Side effect of tricyclic antidepressants
Vasomotor symptoms may be caused by calcium channel antagonists and antidepressant drugs, especially the tricyclic class of medication. Premature ovarian insufficiency (POI) is less likely given that she has a regular menstrual cycle. Hyperthyroidism can cause palpitations, but is unlikely to cause hot flushes. Phaeochromocytoma can cause episodes of palpitations and nausea, but these are usually associated with sweating rather than hot flushes. Premenstrual syndrome does not usually cause vasomotor symptoms.

Q2. Answer: e – History of breast cancer
Use of estrogen-containing hormone replacement therapy (HRT) is widely considered to be contraindicated following breast carcinoma (including intraductal carcinoma) and following endometrial carcinoma. Uterine fibroids do not preclude the use of HRT. Women with a history of endometrial hyperplasia who wish to use HRT can use an LNG-IUS for continuous progesterone cover while taking systemic estrogen or consider continuous combined HRT. Obesity and anti-phospholipid antibodies are relative risk factors for venous thromboembolism (VTE) and not absolute contraindications to the use of HRT.

Q3. Answer: b – Cyclical combined HRT
The commonest indication for starting HRT is for the relief of vasomotor symptoms. This woman has a uterus; therefore, the HRT must have estrogen and progesterone, that is, combined. The progesterone is important as unopposed estrogen therapy would increase her risk of developing endometrial hyperplasia and endometrial malignancy. The LNG-IUS can be used with systemic estrogen for endometrial protection; however, when used alone, it will not affect her vasomotor symptoms. Clonidine is no more effective than placebo at managing vasomotor symptoms. There is no conclusive evidence that evening primrose oil is effective.

Chapter 11

Q1. Answer: d – Urinalysis
Every woman presenting with lower urinary tract symptoms should have a urinalysis performed. The presence of leucocytes and nitrites can suggest a lower urinary tract infection (UTI), which may be causing or worsening the woman's symptoms. If the woman is symptomatic of a UTI, treatment with an empirical antibiotic is started and a mid-stream specimen of urine is sent. Recurrent UTI and/or presence of haematuria should prompt cystoscopy and ultrasound of the upper renal tracts. The presence of glycosuria may suggest diabetes, which can predispose to recurrent UTIs and urinary frequency due to higher volumes of urine being passed.

Q2. Answer: e – Doxazocin
Doxazosin is an alpha-1 receptor antagonist, which may worsen symptoms of stress incontinence by relaxing the bladder outlet and urethra.

Chapter 13

Q1. Answer: e – 5%

Q2. Answer: d – Ultrasound scan
Ultrasound is the first-line diagnostic tool for identifying structural abnormalities. Transvaginal ultrasound, the first-line investigation in postmenopausal bleeding, can be used to measure the endometrial thickness in postmenopausal women. If the thickness is equal to or more than 4 mm, further investigation with endometrial biopsy is warranted. The chance of underlying endometrial cancer in women with postmenopausal bleeding who have an endometrial thickness under 4 mm is under 1%.

Q3. Answer: e – Obesity
It is thought that a third of cases of endometrial malignancy are related to obesity. The majority of endometrial cancers are associated with conditions in which there are higher levels of estrogen production. Obesity results in the aromatisation in body fat of peripheral androgen to estrogen (specifically, estriol), thereby stimulating the growth of the endometrium, which can lead to hyperplasia and cancer in the long term.

Q4. Answer: d – FIGO IIIC2
Stage for stage, endometrial cancer has a prognosis similar to that of cancer of the cervix. The details of this case are categorised as FIGO IIIC2.

Chapter 15

Q1. Answer: a – Medical evacuation may be appropriate for a partial mole.
Partial molar pregnancies contain 69 chromosomes, 23 from the mother, and the other 46 derived from the father. In contrast to partial molar pregnancies, in complete molar pregnancies, there are 46 chromosomes all derived from the father, and no fetal tissue present. Following an ultrasound scan suggestive of a molar pregnancy, uterine evacuation is required. In a complete molar pregnancy such as that described here, the evacuation should be performed by suction procedure. It is recommended that oxytocin be avoided until after the uterine evacuation is completed to minimise risk of distant spread of molar cells in venous blood by uterine contractions. Medical evacuation may be appropriate for a partial mole, particularly if larger fetal parts are present. Following

the evacuation of a complete molar pregnancy, there is an approximately 10% to 15% chance of persistent disease and development of malignancy. In the United Kingdom, follow-up and monitoring of hCG after a diagnosis of molar pregnancy is arranged by registering the woman with one of three centres in London, Sheffield or Dundee.

Q2. Answer: c – Commence chemotherapy
Approximately 10% to 15% of complete molar pregnancies are persistent and will require chemotherapy after surgical evacuation. An indication for treatment after a molar pregnancy is persistent of serum hCG. After a successful medical or surgical procedure, a large and sustained drop in the hCG level would be expected. The majority of women receive treatment with single-agent chemotherapy, which has a high cure rate and is generally well tolerated.

Chapter 19

Q1. Answer: e – Check blood pressure
Erectile dysfunction is often the first sign of cardiovascular disease. Therefore, all men presenting with this symptom must have their cardiovascular risk status assessed.

Chapter 21

Q1. Answer: d – Women undergoing hepatocellular adenoma surveillance
UKMEC category 4 refers to a condition which represents an unacceptable health risk if the contraceptive method is used. These include current and/or history of ischaemic heart disease, hypertension, liver disease (severe cirrhosis, active viral hepatitis, tumours) or migraine with aura at any age or for women within 6 weeks postpartum and breast feeding. Women smoking >15 cigarettes per day are also considered as UKMEC category 4 for combined oral contraceptives.

Q2. Answer: d – Thickens cervical muocus
All progesterone-only pills (POPs) thicken cervical muocus, thus preventing sperm penetration into the upper reproductive tract. Some POPs also inhibit ovulation. POPs containing norethisterone or levonorgestrel inhibit ovulation in up to 60% of cycles. The desogestrel POP inhibits ovulation in up to 97% of cycles.

Chapter 24

Q1. Answer: c – Lamotrigine

There is an increased incidence of fetal anomalies in association with older antiepileptic drugs, such as phenytoin and carbamazepine. Single-drug regimens are less teratogenic. Sodium valproate carries the highest risk of teratogenesis (10%). Risk of congenital malformations appears lower with lamotrigine and levetiracetam.

Q2. Answer: c – Lifestyle advice with follow-up in 2 weeks

Monitoring blood glucose is essential to guide further treatments for mother and baby. Treatment should aim to keep fasting glucose <5.5 mmol/L and postprandial level <7.8 mmol/L. The pattern and levels of blood glucose on home monitoring will determine and assess the response to lifestyle changes and whether oral medication is needed in the first instance. Insulin is sometimes started in preference to metformin when the fasting blood glucose is over 7 mmol/L.

Chapter 26

Q1. Answer: d – Epidural analgesia

All of the other factors are known risk factors for post-partum haemorrhage (PPH).

Q2. Answer: c – Admission to hospital for observation

This woman has a low-lying placenta and has experienced an antepartum haemorrhage. The bleeding has stopped, and the lack of abdominal pain is less suggestive of an abruption or pre-term labour. Some might advise a speculum to exclude a local cause of postcoital bleeding on the basis that a transvaginal scan is sometimes recommended for placenta praevia. Performing a digital vaginal examination in this case can lead to catastrophic and sudden bleeding. Magnesium sulphate for fetal neuroprotection and antenatal corticosteroids can be considered if there is felt to be a high change of birth in the near future. Her history does not suggest this, and the use of magnesium sulphate is more common under 30 weeks' gestation. An immediate caesarean section would expose the baby to the risks of prematurity and the mother to surgery, when there is a good chance that later in the pregnancy the placenta may not be low lying and a vaginal birth could be pursued with little additional risk.

Chapter 28

Q1. Answer: b – Oral labetalol

The woman has pre-eclampsia. Labetalol or nifedipine are used as first-line antihypertensive treatment. Expediting birth should be offered to women before 34 weeks only if there is a poor response to maximal antihypertensive treatment or if the woman's condition worsens, (e.g., abnormal blood results, deteriorating symptoms), or if there are significant concerns for fetal well-being.

IV magnesium sulphate can be used when a woman has severe pre-eclampsia to prevent progression to eclampsia. It is not solely used to lower blood pressure. Methyldopa can be used, particularly in women with pre-pregnancy hypertension, but is not first-line treatment due to the increased risk of postnatal depression.

Furosemide should not be used to treat hypertension in pregnancy because the mother is usually relatively intravascularly depleted despite high blood pressure.

Q2. Answer: d – Parity

Increasing parity does not increase the risk of pre-eclampsia. First pregnancy is a moderate risk factor. Obesity, multiple pregnancy and extremes of maternal age are all recognised risk factors. A family history in a first-degree relative increases the risk of pre-eclampsia four to eight times, illustrating a strong genetic influence.

Chapter 30

Q1. Answer: b – Embryo division occurred at the blastocyst stage.

Monochorionic diamniotic is the most common form of monozygotic twins. Embryo division at the blastocyst stage (8–14 days post-fertilization) occurs after the chorion has started to differentiate; therefore, the babies share an outer chorion (placenta and outer chorionic membrane).

Q2. Answer: e – Laser ablation is associated with a lower rate of neurological morbidity.

Twin-to-twin transfusion syndrome (TTTS) accounts for around 15% of perinatal mortality in twins. Without treatment, TTTS is associated with a >80% intrauterine death rate. Evidence suggests that laser ablation is the most effective intervention and is also associated with a lower rate of significant neurological morbidity.

Chapter 32

Q1. Answer: c – Encourage active pushing and prepare for assisted vaginal birth.

The overall situation would be classified as high risk because of the previous caesarean section and meconium-stained liquor. Being in the second stage means that the option of assisted vaginal birth for expediting birth is available. The cardiotocography (CTG) would be classified as non-reassuring. This woman has had a vaginal birth previously, therefore, there is a high chance the baby would be born this way again. Should a delay be encountered, starting preparation for an assisted birth is prudent. Active pushing would help avoid additional morbidity from forceps or vacuum extraction if the baby was born before additional procedures were required. Position change and fluids as well as fetal blood samples would be helpful only in a limited number of scenarios, for example, when an assisted vaginal birth was unacceptable to the woman. A caesarean section would probably be considered in this scenario if a vaginal birth proved impossible and the CTG concerns continued.

Chapter 34

Q1. Answer: d – 60%

The success rate of external cephalic version (ECV) can mean the proportion of babies who are turned to cephalic presentation at the end of the ECV or the proportion of babies who are cephalic when labour starts. For ECV in general, the success of the procedure is 50%. For multiparous women, the success is around 60%. For primiparous women, it is 40%. The chance of a baby spontaneously changing presentation to cephalic is around 8%, and the chance of a baby changing back to breech presentation after a successful ECV is also around 8%.

Q2. Answer: b – Pudendal nerve dysfunction

Fetal macrosomia and persistent occipitoposterior position are associated with a prolonged second stage of labour because they increase the chance of delays due to the size of the presenting part of the baby passing through the pelvis. Narrowing of the maternal skeleton can also make it less favourable for the baby to pass through the pelvis. Epidural analgesia is thought to reduce the effectiveness of maternal effort in the second stage. However, a deliberate delay (passive second stage) for 1 to 2 hours reduces the need for operative vaginal birth.

Chapter 36

Q1. Answer: d – Neonatal cephalohaematoma

Vacuum extraction is less likely to be associated with significant maternal perineal trauma, and has similar rates of caesareans, low Apgar scores and need for neonatal phototherapy.

Q2. Answer: c – Kielland forceps

Kielland forceps are the only ones of those listed which are designed to rotate. Simpson and Wrigley forceps are for mid-cavity non-rotational and outlet forceps, respectively. Piper forceps have longer shanks and are used when forceps are required for the aftercoming head during a vaginal breech birth. Vacuum devices or manual rotation can be used to rotate the position of the baby before birth in the scenario. Non-toothed forceps are a different device to hold tissues and surgical needles.

Chapter 40

Q1. Answer: b – The face

The first pharyngeal arch develops into the maxilla and mandible and the muscles of mastication, amongst others. The sixth arch on the left side develops into the ductus arteriosus and most of the structures of the larynx. The eye and upper limbs develop from other structures.

Q2. Answer: b – The cerebellum

The hindbrain develops into the medulla, pons and cerebellum as well at cranial nerves V to XII. The thalamus and hypothalamus are derived from the midbrain. The spinal cord develops from the neural tube, and the eye from a combination of mesoderm and ectodermal tissues.

Chapter 42

Q1. Answer: a – Plasma volume increases

Ventilation rates are known to increase in pregnancy due to increased demand for oxygen and increased basal metabolic rate. The plasma volume increases, which results in an increased heart rate, stroke volume and cardiac output. The plasma volume increases by up to 50% and the red blood cell volume increases by about 20% to 30%.

Q2. Answer: d – Increased gastro-oesophageal reflux
The effect of pregnancy on smooth muscle is of relaxation. This is partly driven by progesterone. As a
result, there is delayed gastric emptying, reduced gut
motility and increased gastric reflux. The relaxation of
muscle at the lower oesophageal sphincter can result
in reflux. This can add to symptoms of nausea and
lower the threshold for vomiting. Other effects on the
chemo-receptor trigger zone further lower the triggers
for nausea and vomiting. These changes are particularly significant during induction of general anaesthesia during pregnancy, as stomach acid is much more
likely to aspirate into the lungs unless specific precautions are taken to prevent it. Constipation is more
common, particularly with the alteration of position
and compression of the large bowel at later gestations.
Reduction in the contractility of the gallbladder results
in a higher chance of gallstone formation.

INDEX

Page numbers followed by 'f' indicate figures, 't' indicate tables, 'b' indicate boxes, and 'e' indicate online content.